Microsurgery of Retinal Detachment

Second Edition

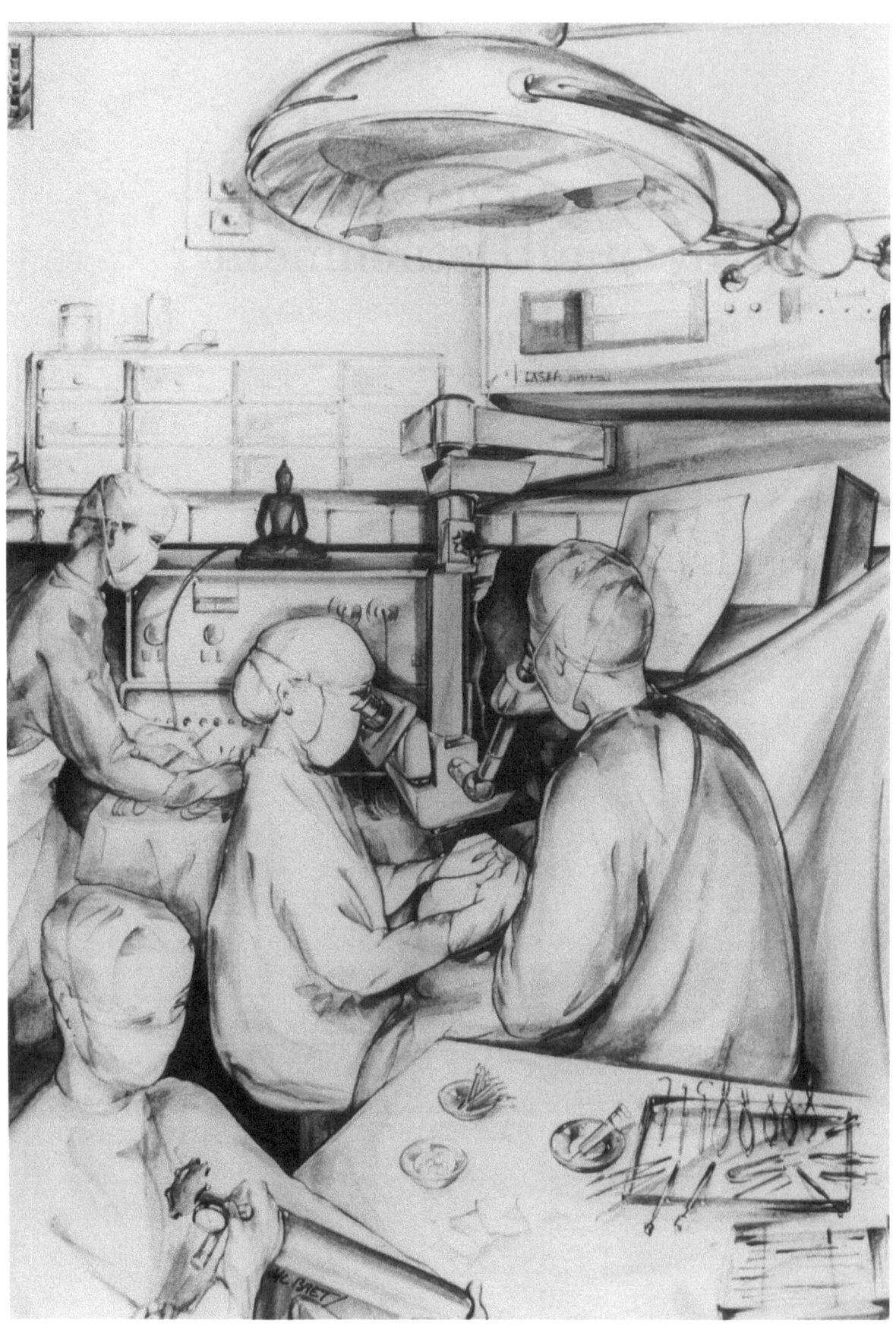

Microsurgery of Retinal Detachment

Second Edition

Mireille Bonnet, M.D.

Professor and Chairman
Department of Ophthalmology
Croix-Rousse Hospital
University of Lyon
Lyon, France

Illustrated by Hélène Bret

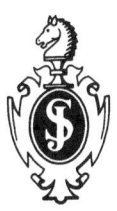 Springer-Verlag Berlin Heidelberg GmbH

Copyright © 1989, Springer-Verlag Berlin Heidelberg
Originally published by Field and Wood, Medical Publishers, Inc. in 1989
Softcover reprint of the hardcover 2nd edition 1989

ISBN 978-3-662-08733-6   ISBN 978-3-662-08731-2 (eBook)
DOI 10.1007/978-3-662-08731-2

Library of Congress Catalog Card Number: 89-080877

To my colleagues, residents, fellows, and visitors, of the Croix-Rousse Hospital Eye Clinic

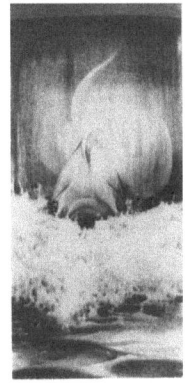

"He who wishes to catch the exceptional fish must not be afraid of turbulent water."
                    —Ingen Zengi (1592–1673)

Contents

IV

Types of Retinal Detachment: Clinical Characteristics and Surgical Management

155

Index

Foreword

Microsurgery of Retinal Detachment is an important contribution to the practice of vitreoretinal surgery. In this comprehensive volume, Dr. Bonnet shares her extensive experience in the management of conditions ranging from retinal tears and primary retinal detachment to giant retinal breaks and vitreoretinal surgery.

The field of microsurgery has continued to evolve over the last twenty years, both for the anterior segment surgeon and, since 1970, for the vitreoretinal surgeon. Although there have been extensive descriptions of vitrectomy techniques, little has been written about microsurgical techniques for scleral buckling operations This subject is well covered in the present edition, which consequently will be a valuable resource to the majority of retinal surgeons who do not as a rule employ microsurgery in the repair of retinal detachments.

Dr. Bonnet has succeeded admirably in producing a well-organized and appropriately illustrated text while maintaining a writing style that allows easy assimilation. In so doing, she provides a great service to those of us who have not routinely employed microsurgical techniques in the management of retinal detachment.

William Tasman, M.D.

Acknowledgments

This book would not have been accomplished without the warm assistance of the staff members of the Croix-Rousse Hospital Eye Clinic, and the encouragement of my friends and colleagues. In particular, I am deeply endebted to the staff of the operating unit, especially Andrée Soubeyrat for her tireless assistance, to my friend and secretary, Many Hoffmann, for typing the manuscript, to Mr. Estero for the photographs, to Christian Blanchet for his support for correction of the manuscript by "la traduction médicale," to the Merck Sharp & Dohme–Chibret documentation center of Clermont-Ferrand for providing references, and to my labradors, Jean and Crunch, for keeping quiet beneath my desk for so many hours, and harbouring no resentment when they miss the enjoyment of a stroll in a balmy forest or a swim in a cool pond.

Introduction

The microsurgical approach to retinal detachment management was born in the early 1970s. Microsurgical techniques were initially restricted to selected surgical steps, such as cryotreatment,[1] visualization of tiny retinal breaks,[2] subretinal fluid release,[3,4] and vitreous surgery.[5–9] Initially, the operating microscope was routinely used in the management of all retinal detachments and during the performance of all surgical steps by a only small number of retina surgeons.[10,11] At present, microsurgical techniques are routinely used in retinal detachment management by an increasing number of retina surgeons.

The gradual change that has occurred in retinal detachment surgery over the last 15 years is related to three main reasons: (1) evolution of ideas, (2) improvement of the instrumentation, and (3) development of vitreous surgery.

Eye surgeons were pioneers in the development of microsurgery. However, microsurgical techniques were initially developed for the anterior segment of the eye only.[12–15] In addition, a long period of time elapsed before microsurgery was widely accepted and routinely performed by all anterior segment surgeons.

An even longer period of time elapsed before microsurgical techniques were developed for retinal detachment management. During this time period, eye surgeons who performed both anterior segment and posterior segment surgery were confronted with a paradoxical situation: They experienced the advantages of the operating microscope when they performed relatively easy operations on the anterior segment of the eye. In contrast they had to withdraw the operating microscope when they dealt with the most important and the most fragile part of the eye, the retina. As a surgeon of both the anterior segment and the posterior segment of the eye, this author felt deeply frustrated by such a paradoxical situation; and thus pioneered the development of routine microsurgical management of retinal detachment.

Since its introduction by Schepens,[16] binocular indirect ophthalmoscopy was considered the only valid method for intraoperative examination of the retina. However, increased experience of slit lamp examination of the fundus using the three-mirror contact lens during preoperative examination and during argon laser photocoagulation treatment showed that the latter technique could also be used intraoperatively, provided proper instrumentation be developed.

Routine use of the operating microscope for retinal detachment surgery required the development of specific instrumentation, mainly an operating microscope that permits proper visualization of both the internal and external parts of the posterior segment. Until 1976 the operating microscopes available in ophthalmology could be used only for external surgery of the posterior segment of the eye. They could not be used for fundus examination, and therefore, were not suitable for retinal detachment microsurgery. Intraoperative biomicroscopy of the fundus with a three-mirror contact lens requires that a slit lamp be attached to the microscope. As a mandatory requirement the angle between the slit beam and the observation axis of the microscope must range between 5° and 10°. The operating microscopes designed specifically for anterior segment surgery were equipped with a slit lamp, the minimum angle of which was generally about 40°. Therefore, they were not suitable for retinal detachment surgery. Some surgeons, conscious of the advantages of biomicroscopy of the fundus during surgery, attached a prism to their microscope in order to reduce the angle of the slit lamp. However, the operating microscopes equipped with a slit lamp and a reducing prism allowing intraoperative biomicroscopy of the fundus remained prototypes. At Klöti's[6] and Machemer's[5] requests, Carl Zeiss developed a mobile slit lamp that could be moved within ± 30°. This slit lamp can be attached to the Zeiss OPMI I and OPMI 6 microscopes. The equipment has two main advantages: (1) Intraoperative biomicroscopy of the fundus can be performed when the slit lamp is positioned at approximately 5°; and (2) the same equipment can be used for anterior segment microsurgery, since the slit lamp can easily be moved to a 30° angle. The mobile slit lamp designed by Carl Zeiss was initially developed for vitreous surgery through the pars plana rather than retinal detachment surgery. The equipment, however, revealed more helpful in routine microsurgical management of retinal detachment than in vitreous surgery. Indeed the mobile slit lamp developed by Carl Zeiss made routine examination of the fundus with the three-mirror contact lens and the operating microscope feasible. Therefore, the equipment made it possible to develop routine microsurgery for retinal detachment management. In contrast, in the management of retinal detachments that require vitreous surgery, the slit lamp is only an adjunct to other illumination sources.

Vitreous surgery through the pars plana, initially developed by Machemer[5] in the United States and Klöti in Europe[6] brought the most significant advancement in the microsurgical approach to retinal detachment management. Vitreous surgery has made desperate and hopeless retinal detachments amenable to surgical management. It has brought a new and valuable alternative to conventional methods in the management of selected retinal detachments, such as retinal detachments with macular holes, which were difficult to manage with scleral buckling. Vitreous surgery has also contributed to the acceptance of routine microsurgery in retinal detachment repair, merely because it has removed the barrier between anterior segment surgeons and retinal detachment surgeons. Vitreous surgery has led retina surgeons to experience the advantages of the operating microscope. Consequently, an increasing number of retina surgeons extend the use of the operating microscope to the management of all retinal detachments and the performance of all surgical steps.

ADVANTAGES OF MICROSURGERY AS COMPARED TO CONVENTIONAL SURGERY IN RETINAL DETACHMENT MANAGEMENT

Improved visual control is the major advantage of microsurgery as compared to conventional surgery, therefore use of the operating microscope should not be restricted to only a few difficult and severe cases or certain surgical steps. To the contrary, the operating microscope is advantageously used in all retinal detachments and every surgical step.

During the surgical stages that do not require simultaneous observation of the fundus, the advantages of the operating microscope are the accuracy and the safety provided by improved visual control. Use of the operating microscope makes certain surgical steps, such as subretinal fluid release, paracentesis of the anterior chamber, scleral dissection, and placement of scleral sutures, easier and less hazardous to perform as compared to conventional surgery. Dissection and suture of periocular tissues can be performed with accuracy and minimal trauma, hence postoperative complications related to these surgical steps can be avoided. Even more importantly, improved visual control makes it possible to decrease the incidence of serious intraoperative complications that may lead to surgical failure or poor visual results.

The advantages of using the operating microscope during surgical stages that require simultaneous observation of the fundus should also be stressed. Improved visualization of vitreoretinal anatomy and fundus details, as well as the ability to observe the inner part and the outer part of the eye with the same optical equipment are two major advantages of the operating microscope as compared to conventional surgery combined with indirect ophthalmoscopy. In most rhegmatogenous retinal detachments, the postoperative outcome depends only on identification and proper treatment of all retinal breaks. Identification of retinal breaks and control of treatment depend mainly on proper visualization of the fundus preoperatively and intraoperatively. Therefore, the methods used for preoperative and intraoperative fundus examination are of primary importance in retinal detachment management. Binocular indirect ophthalmoscopy, introduced by Charles Schepens, has brought about dramatic improvement in fundus examination. It is not, however, the only valuable method for fundus examination. Preoperative and intraoperative biomicroscopy of the fundus shares most advantages of binocular indirect ophthalmoscopy. In addition to the advantages shared by indirect ophthalmoscopy, biomicroscopy has four specific advantages: (1) observation of the vitreoretinal anatomy is made in an optical cross section of the tissues; (2) observation of fundus details can be performed under high magnification; (3) intraoperative observation of the fundus is done with no need for the surgeon to change instruments; and (4) in most cases, clear visualization of the fundus does not require that the lights in the operating room be turned off. However, biomicroscopy of the fundus has one disadvantage in comparison with indirect ophthalmoscopy: the range of observation of the ocular fundus is much more limited. This is a disadvantage in preoperative evaluation of the topography of the retinal detachment rather than in intraoperative control of the fundus. In fact, in most rhegmatogenous retinal detachments, the retinal breaks are the only fundus lesions to be dealt with intraoperatively. Owing to their limited size, most retinal breaks are entirely visible in the small field of observation provided by slit lamp examination. In addition, the surgeon, who has acquired sufficient expertise in intraoperative biomicroscopy of the fundus, can easily and rapidly explore the entire fundus by the combined use of the three mirrors of the Goldmann contact lens and the X/Y coupling system of the microscope. Examination of the entire fundus is done with no need for the surgeon to change position. Intraoperative indirect ophthalmoscopy using coaxial illumination of the microscope and a 40-diopter-lens can also be performed as an adjunct to biomicroscopy in selected cases. In the future, improvement of the operating microscopes may make direct observation of the fundus possible without any contact lens.

OBJECTIVES AND RESULTS OF MICROSURGERY IN RETINAL DETACHMENT MANAGEMENT

With regard to the objectives and the results of microsurgery, retinal detachments should be categorized into two separate groups: (1) easy retinal detachments and (2) difficult retinal detachments.

Easy retinal detachments account for the majority of cases. They include most rhegmatogenous retinal detachments that are not associated with actual or potential proliferative vitreoretinopathy. Retinal detachments associated with disinsertion at the ora serrata and round atrophic holes in lattice degeneration belong to this group. Most retinal detachments associated with a single horseshoe tear (or group of tears) that involves less than two clock hours of the peripheral retina, and does not show a curled posterior edge, also belong to this group. In such retinal detachments an anatomical success rate close to 100% is achieved by experienced surgeons using either conventional surgery or microsurgical techniques. However, the anatomical success rate achieved by surgeons who have less expertise are not as satisfactory. In easy retinal detachments most failures to permanently reattach the retina with a single operation are related to unrecognized retinal break(s), mispositioning of the scleral buckle(s), or intraoperative complications. Following failed primary surgery, a number of easy detachments become difficult cases. In such cases, reoperation(s) will provide a lower anatomical success rate as compared to that achieved by proper primary surgery. In addition, the visual results are rather disappointing in a significant number of patients. In spite of a reattached retina, central vision does not improve or

even becomes worse postoperatively. Poor visual results following retinal detachment repair are mainly related to macular changes. Certain macular changes, such as cystoid macular degeneration and pigment epithelium atrophy, are directly related to the duration of preoperative macular detachment. Certain macular puckers are related to specific preoperative clinical characteristics of the retinal detachment. Certain macular changes in eyes operated on for retinal detachment are related to associated fundus diseases, such as senile macular degeneration and myopia. However, other postoperative macular changes, such as macular hemorrhages, heavy pigment deposits in the subretinal space, cystoid macular edema, and certain macular puckers, are related to the surgical trauma for retinal detachment repair rather than the primary retinal disease.

The objectives of microsurgery in easy retinal detachments are threefold: (1) to increase the number of eye surgeons capable of adequately managing such retinal detachments, (2) to decrease the incidence of failures related to inadequate primary surgery, and (3) to improve visual results. In France, microsurgery has fulfilled these objectives. The number of eye surgeons trained in microsurgery who are capable of repairing easy retinal detachments with excellent results has gradually increased over the last 15 years. Most easy retinal detachments are repaired with a single operation. Easy detachments that require more than one operation for permanent retinal reattachment account for less than 5% of cases.[17] The incidence of failures of a primary operation related to unrecognized retinal break(s), mispositioning of the scleral buckle(s), and intraoperative complications has become virtually nil. Most failures of primary operations are related to the inability of young surgeons to determine the best surgical approach according to the clinical characteristics of the retinal breaks, rather than improper surgical technique.[17]

Owing to the wide variety of macular changes that may interfere with postoperative visual recovery, objective evaluation of the visual results after retinal detachment repair is difficult. Case selection rather than surgical technique may account for the differences of visual results in various series. Comparing the final visual acuity to the visual acuity a few days before the occurrence of retinal detachment is a clinical method that partially eliminates the bias of methods traditionally used for evaluating the postoperative visual results. Unfortunately, the visual acuity preexisting to the occurrence of retinal detachment is not known by the retina surgeon in the vast majority of patients referred. Therefore, such analysis can be conducted only in a smaller series. In a series of patients with aphakic retinal detachment the macula was preoperatively detached in 62.5% of eyes. In spite of that, 69% of those patients recovered a final visual acuity equal to their visual acuity before the occurrence of retinal detachment.[18]

The incidence of postoperative macular changes that are likely related to surgical trauma is rather low in eyes repaired by microsurgery.[19] In particular, the incidence of pigment deposits in the subretinal space and macular hemorrhage is virtually nil in eyes primarily managed by microsurgery. Similarly, postoperative cystoid macular edema disclosed by routine fluorescein angiography is less frequent after microsurgical repair as compared to conventional surgery. The overall incidence of angiographic cystoid macular edema is 14.6% after microsurgery[20] versus 30%[21] to 43%[22] after conventional surgery. In aphakic eyes, which are more prone to develop postoperative cystoid macular edema, the incidence of postoperative macular edema disclosed by fluorescein angiography is lower after microsurgical repair (30%)[20] as compared to conventional surgery (64%).[22]

Difficult retinal detachments account for the vast majority of cases referred to retina centers. They are rather uncommon, however, as compared to easy retinal detachments. They include a variety of rhegmatogenous and/or traction detachments that can be categorized into two distinct groups: (1) retinal detachments difficult to manage by conventional scleral buckling and (2) retinal detachments that were desperate and nearly hopeless before the development of vitreous microsurgery.

Retinal detachments difficult to manage by conventional scleral buckling include retinal detachments associated with multiple and large horseshoe tears, macular holes in highly myopic eyes, retinal breaks situated posteriorly to the equatorial region, and initial stages of proliferative vitreoretinopathy. Development of microsurgery has made it possible to manage such difficult cases by techniques that are more appropriate and less traumatic as compared to conventional surgery. Retinal detachments that were nearly hopeless before the development of vitreous microsurgery include most traction detachments, in particular detachments complicating proliferative diabetic retinopathy, penetrating injuries of the eye, and late stages of retinopathy of prematurity. They also include most retinal detachments associated with giant retinal tears and all retinal detachments associated with severe proliferative vitreoretinopathy. Development of microsurgery has made such desperate and hopeless detachments amenable to surgical management with reasonable chances of success. The anatomical success rate presently achieved with difficult and desperate retinal detachments clearly shows that microsurgery has brought dramatic improvement in the management of such cases. Actually, at present, most mechanical problems encountered in the management of difficult retinal detachments can be overcome by microsurgi-

cal techniques. However, a significant number of eyes with severe retinal detachments still fail to permanently reattach. In most cases recurrent detachment of the retina is related to the development of severe proliferative vitreoretinopathy postoperatively. In the future, decreased incidence of failures to permanently reattach the retina in such eyes will likely be achieved by pharmacological means used as adjuncts to surgery, rather than improved microsurgical techniques.

DEFINITION AND CHARACTERISTICS OF MICROSURGERY FOR RETINAL DETACHMENT MANAGEMENT

Basically, microsurgery for retinal detachment management merely consists of applying the basic rules of microsurgery to this specific field, so as to carry out well controlled surgery with minimal operative trauma.

In practice, microsurgery for retinal detachment management implies that three main conditions be fulfilled: (1) special training, (2) special instrumentation, and (3) choice of the surgical procedure that can provide the highest success rate with the least surgical trauma.

Training is obviously required for any surgeon who plans to perform microsurgery, whatever the field of application. This basic rule applies to microsurgical management of retinal detachment. The retina surgeon should become familiar with use of the operating microscope and should practice using the operating microscope so that no more brain effort is necessary than to drive a car. There is general agreement among microsurgeons that performing several microsurgical operations every week is a mandatory requirement to acquire and maintain skill. The retina surgeon who wishes to perform proper microsurgical operations should use the operating microscope routinely. Retina surgeons who restrict the use of the microscope to selected surgical procedures and/or selected surgical steps, often complain that the operating microscope is rather troublesome and makes the operation longer to perform. In contrast, retina surgeons who routinely use the operating microscope for all surgical procedures and all surgical steps acquire the necessary skill to perform microsurgery as rapidly as conventional surgery.

To become an experienced microsurgeon in vitreoretinal work, the eye surgeon has to learn and master many more techniques than the anterior segment surgeon, mainly because the operating microscopes that are presently available do not allow for a direct view of the fundus. Special lenses and illumination devices are required for observation of the vitreous gel and retina during surgery. The retina microsurgeon should, therefore master all techniques for observation of the fundus and vitreous gel, particularly slit lamp biomicroscopy of the retina and vitreous gel. The retina microsurgeon should master the techniques for maneuvering instruments under direct, as well as indirect observation of the surgical field through the microscope. It should be stressed, however, that mastering these techniques does not require more training than indirect ophthalmoscopy.

Vitreoretinal microsurgery has benefited from the development of ergonomics for microsurgery, as has any microsurgery.[23–24] In many circumstances the vitreoretinal microsurgeon has to work within the limits of human technical ability: to discriminate fine details only by vision, never by touch, and to control subtle movements, and handle fragile tissues without trauma. Thanks to improved instrumentation, this ability is no longer limited to a few gifted surgeons. With training any retina surgeon can acquire the ability to perform microsurgery.

Vitreoretinal microsurgeons, who deal with the most difficult retinal detachments, often have to work on the same eye for several hours at length to ensure error-free surgery during the entire surgical procedure. The surgeon must keep his mental and physical abilities at their best for several hours at a time. This implies that certain physical activities should be avoided before performing surgery,[23–24] and it may also require that life style be modified in accordance with the mandatory requirements of microsurgery.

Mastering all techniques for surgery and fundus examination using the operating microscope is a mandatory requirement for all microsurgeons of the posterior segment of the eye. Surgical skill, however, is not, by far, the only requirement. Thorough knowledge of vitreoretinal diseases is an even more important requirement. Knowledge of vitreoretinal diseases rather than surgical skill makes the difference between young vitreoretinal microsurgeons and experienced surgeons. Deep knowledge of vitreoretinal diseases requires more work and takes more time than mastering microsurgical techniques.

One of the main goals of microsurgery in retinal detachment management is to achieve permanent retinal reattachment with the least surgical trauma in a single operation, so as to improve the visual results. However, choice of the most appropriate surgical approach to achieve this goal, in any given case, may not be easy for less experienced surgeons.

Difficulty, commonly encountered by residents in establishing an accurate prognosis, and in choosing the most appropriate surgical approach has led the author to extend the contents of the present book

to a thorough description of her understanding of retinal detachment. That is the reason why the new version of the book has not been restricted to mere description of the basic surgical techniques of retinal detachment microsurgery.

Retinal detachment is a clinical syndrome rather than a disease. Retinal detachments that require surgical management are related to several distinct causes. Surgical management is aimed at the cause(s) of accumulation of subretinal fluid rather than the subretinal fluid itself. Subretinal fluid will be absorbed spontaneously when the cause for its accumulation is properly treated. Retinal detachment requiring surgical management may be related to retinal break(s) or traction on the retina. The clinical significance of retinal breaks varies depending on their pathogenesis. Retinal breaks associated with major vitreous changes and clinical evidence of vitreous traction, such as horseshoe tears, should be differentiated from retinal breaks that are not associated with significant vitreous changes, such as atrophic holes and nontraumatic oral dialyses. When retinal breaks are properly sealed surgically, the prognosis for permanent retinal reattachment is excellent in the latter group, whereas it may be guarded in the former group. Similarly the clinical significance of traction on the retina varies, depending on the vitreoretinal changes. Traction may be either dynamic and occur only during vitreous gel movements induced by eye rotation, or static with permanent pull on the retina.[25]

Since the causes for accumulation of subretinal fluid show significant clinical variations, the surgical approach to retinal detachment management should be determined according to the fundus changes that resulted in the development of retinal detachment. There is not a single surgical procedure that could be applied to any retinal detachment, regardless of the cause, and still provide a high anatomical and visual success rate. On the contrary, the retina surgeon must master several basic surgical approaches to retinal detachment management. In any given case, choice of the most appropriate surgical approach will depend on the clinical significance of the findings disclosed by fundus examination.

REFERENCES

1. Hilsdorf C: Cryocoagulation rétinienne sélective et de dosage exact. Bull Mem Soc Fr Ophtalmol 84:120–124, 1971
2. Urrets-Zavalia A: Retinal surgery under the microscope. Dev Ophthalmol 2:195–201, 1981
3. Gärtner J: Release of subretinal fluid with the aid of the microscope. Report of 100 cases. Mod Probl Ophthalmol 15:127–133, 1975
4. Draeger J: The microscope as a tool in the management of the sclera. Dev Ophthalmol 2:202–207, 1981

5. Machemer R, Parel JM, Buettner H: A new concept for vitreous surgery (1) Instrumentation. Am J Ophthalmol 73:1–7, 1972

6. Klöti R: Vitrectomie. Bull Mem Soc Fr Ophtalmol 86:251–253, 1973

7. Tolentino F, Banko A, Schepens A, et al: Vitreous surgery: New Instrumentation for vitrectomy Arch Ophthalmol 93:667–672, 1975

8. O'Malley C, Heintz RM: Vitrectomy with an alternative instrument system Ann Ophthalmol 7:585, 1975

9. Michels RG: Vitreous surgery. St. Louis, C.V. Mosby Company, 1981

10. Bonnet M: Les avantages de la chirurgie sous microscope du décollement de la rétine Bull Soc Ophtalmol Fr 75:1111–1112, 1975

11. Bonnet M, Bonamour G: Les avantages de la microchirurgie du décollement de la rétine Mod Probl Ophthalmol 18:373–375, 1977

12. Barraquer J, Ruttlan J, Troutman R: Surgery of the anterior segment of the eye New York, McGraw-Hill, 1964

13. Barraquer JI: Compilation of reprints, Vol 1: refractive keratoplasty Bogota, Colombia, 1970, Instituto Barraquer de America

14. Harms H, Mackensen G: Ocular surgery under the microscope Chicago, Year Book Medical Publishers, Inc. 1967

15. Troutman R: Microsurgery of the anterior segment of the eye St. Louis, CV Mosby Company, 1977

16. Schepens CL: Un nouvel ophtalmoscope binoculaire pour l'examen du décollement de la rétine Bull Soc Belge Ophtalmol 82:9–13, 1945

17. Bonnet M: Microsurgery for retinal detachment repair In New microsurgical concepts J Draeger and R Winter, eds. Dev Ophthalmol 14:5–9, 1987

18. Bonnet M, Nagao M: Microsurgery of aphakic retinal detachment Ophthalmologica 186:177–182, 1983

19. Bonnet M, Lenail B: Prophylaxie des complications maculaires du décollement de la rétine par microchirurgie J Fr Ophtalmol 3:83–88, 1980

20. Bonnet M, Bievelez B, Noel A, et al: Fluorescein angiography after retinal detachment microsurgery Graefe's Arch Clin Exp Ophthalmol 221:35–40, 1983

21. Meredith TA, Reeser FH, Topping TM, Aaberg TM: Cystoid macular edema after retinal detachment surgery Ophthalmology 87:1090–1095, 1980

22. Lobes LA, Grand MG: Incidence of cystoid macular edema following scleral buckling procedure Arch Ophthalmol 98:1230–1232, 1980

23. Patkin M: Ergonomics and microsurgery Excerpta Medica International Congress N° 465 Microsurgery. Proceedings of the 5th international congress of the International Microsurgical Society, 305–308

24. Patkin M: Ergonomics and the operating microscope Adv Ophthalmol 37:53–63, 1978

25. Scott JD: Static and dynamic vitreous traction Trans Ophthalmol Soc UK 91:175–188, 1971

I
Preoperative Examination

1
Examination of the Anterior Segment

Slit lamp examination of the anterior segment of both eyes is performed before and after dilation of the pupils.

Measurement of the intraocular pressure and gonioscopy are performed in all cases.

The main goal of anterior segment examination is to disclose changes of clinical significance with regard to retinal detachment management.

Examination of the anterior segment can also provide useful information about the etiology of the retinal detachment in selected cases, such as retinal detachments after blunt trauma and retinal detachments in eyes with congenital abnormalities.

Anterior segment changes of clinical significance with regard to surgical management of retinal detachment may involve the cornea, the lens, the iris, and the intraocular pressure.

CORNEA

Corneal opacities may interfere with visualization of the fundus. Dense opacities that prevent identification of the retinal breaks are uncommon, however.

Endothelial degeneration, such as advanced cornea guttata, may result in corneal decompensation after selected surgical procedures for retinal detachment management. Whenever possible, vitrectomy should be avoided in aphakic eyes with significant endothelial cell loss. Repeated paracentesis of the anterior chamber are avoided in phakic eyes with cornea guttata.

Special care should be taken to avoid increased intraocular pressure intraoperatively and postoperatively, in eyes with recent corneal wounds after penetrating injury and anterior segment surgery.

In aphakic eyes after penetrating trauma and cataract surgery great care is taken to recognize vitreous strands adhering to the corneal scars. In such eyes, relief of anterior posterior vitreous traction by vitrec-tomy is often required to achieve permanent retinal reattachment.

LENS

Lens opacities may interfere with visualization of the fundus. However, identification of the retinal break(s) using the three-mirror contact lens and the slit lamp with bright illumination is possible in most eyes with cortical opacities and/or dense nuclear sclerosis. In eyes with lens opacities, krypton laser photocoagulation is used rather than argon laser photocoagulation to seal retinal breaks in attached retina. Rarely, lens opacities are so dense that lens removal is required as a preliminary step to retinal detachment surgery. Choice of the technique for lens removal depends mainly on the patient's age.

Anterior chamber paracentesis to decrease intraocular pressure intraoperatively is contraindicated in most eyes with ectopia lentis and/or lens subluxation.

In pseudophakic eyes, mainly eyes with iris-supported lens and an anterior chamber lens, special intraoperative measures must be taken to avoid endothelial damage from the lens (see p. 258)

IRIS

Poor pupillary dilation may lead to difficulty in accurate examination of the fundus periphery. Failure to obtain wide pupillary dilation may result from a number of causes that are either related or unrelated to retinal detachment. In eyes with a pupil diameter under 3 mm, deep scleral depression may be required to accurately examine the retina peripheral to the equator. Intraoperatively, various means to decrease intraocular pressure (see p. 63) can make such deep scleral depression easier and less hazardous.

In aphakic eyes that require vitrectomy for retinal detachment management, a small pupil can be enlarged at the beginning of the operation so as to obtain a satisfactory view of the vitreous cavity and the retina (see p. 146).

Posterior iris synechiae may be related to previous or active intraocular inflammation. Active intraocular inflammation, with iris edema and flare of the anterior chamber, may be related to either retinal detachment or associated intraocular changes. Intraocular inflammation is common in rhegmatogenous retinal detachment of long standing duration, recent onset detachment associated choroidal detachment, retinal detachment complicated by severe proliferative vitreoretinopathy, retinal detachment secondary to an underlying inflammatory disease, and a number of pseudophakic eyes. Anti-inflammatory medications, such as corticosteroids, are indicated preoperatively in selected cases.

Ischemia of the anterior segment should be suspected in eyes that underwent previous surgery for retinal detachment and that exhibit iris atrophy with posterior synechiae. In such eyes, great care should be taken so as to avoid further ischemia of the anterior segment induced by further scleral buckling procedures.

INTRAOCULAR PRESSURE

In most rhegmatogenous retinal detachments the intraocular pressure is decreased in the eye with retinal detachment as compared to the other eye. A severe decrease in intraocular pressure may be associated with choroidal detachment.

Primary or secondary glaucoma may be associated with retinal detachment. Owing to common decrease in intraocular pressure in eyes with retinal detachment, diagnosis of glaucoma is based on the patient's history, the intraocular pressure of the other eye, and examination of the optic disc, rather than the intraocular pressure of the affected eye. Selected surgical procedures for retinal reattachment, such as gas injection, are avoided in eyes with glaucoma.

2
Examination of the Posterior Segment

Proper management of retinal detachment mandatorily requires that thorough fundus examination be performed preoperatively. The goal of preoperative fundus examination is to recognize any finding of clinical significance with regard to correct choice of the surgical procedure. Any finding of clinical significance is recorded on a fundus chart in all cases. Charts of cross-sections of the vitreous cavity are made when the retinal detachment is associated with significant vitreous changes. Fundus findings are recorded on the preoperative chart in relation to anatomical fundus landmarks, mainly the long ciliary arteries and nerves, the short ciliary nerves, the vortex veins, and the ora serrata.

Time spent by the surgeon in preoperative fundus examination is of great value, because it will result in correct choice of the surgical procedure and will save time during the operation, when the surgeon has become familiar with the fundus changes to be dealt with intraoperatively, mainly retinal breaks. Finally, the preoperative examination is an opportunity for the surgeon to inform the patient about fundus disease and treatment. The latter point is of great importance in difficult cases and when intravitreal gas injection is planned.

METHODS OF EXAMINATION

Examination of the posterior segment is performed with full mydriasis of the pupil. Two methods are used for preoperative fundus examination: (1) binocular indirect ophthalmoscopy and (2) slit lamp biomicroscopy using the three-mirror contact lens. Both techniques are combined with scleral depression for examination of the retina peripheral to the equator.

Indirect ophthalmoscopy is of value in providing a wide field of observation. In contrast, the range of observation obtained by slit lamp examination using the three-mirror contact lens is minimal. However, slit lamp examination has two major advantages for detailed evaluation of the fundus: (1) the scale of magnification is high and (2) the fundus is observed in an optical cross section.

Binocular indirect ophthalmoscopy is useful for rapid evaluation of retinal detachment anatomy. Slit lamp examination using the three-mirror contact lens is mandatory to accurately evaluate vitreoretinal details of clinical significance with regard to surgical management and prognosis.

Quality of the contact lens and the slit lamp is of great importance to obtain a clear view of vitreoretinal details in any part of the fundus. The slit lamp must fulfill specific requirements for biomicroscopic examination of the fundus. Slit lamps that were designed mainly for examination of the anterior segment may not be adequate for fundus examination. The author routinely uses either the Haag-Streit slit lamp 900 or the Carl Zeiss slit lamp 30 SL. The Haag-Streit slit lamp 900 with a stereopsis angle changer is of great value in providing perfect stereopsis in any part of the fundus. In difficult cases slit lamp examination of the fundus is performed using the Zeiss OPMI 6 microscope preoperatively. Prolonged examination with scleral depression is necessary in difficult cases, and is easier to perform with the patient lying comfortably.

As with any method for fundus examination, slit lamp examination will be helpful in the accurate evaluation of fundus disease provided two main requirements are fulfilled; (1) the surgeon should master the technique and (2) he or she, should be familiar with the normal variations of fundus anatomy, in particular the peripheral region. Both requirements can be achieved through clinical training and by reading books that are basic references for any retina surgeon.[1–6]

FUNDUS FINDINGS OF CLINICAL SIGNIFICANCE

Fundus examination is conducted methodically. The detachment, the retinal break(s), the vitreous cavity, the vitreoretinal relationship, and associated lesions of clinical significance are routinely evaluated and recorded on preoperative chart(s).

Retinal Detachment

Retinal detachment features of clinical significance include: (1) detachment shape, (2) location and extent of subretinal fluid, (3) detachment height, (4) presence and clinical characteristics of retinal folds, (5) detachment of the pars plana epithelium (6) signs of detachments with gradual progression, (7) macular changes, and (8) shifting subretinal fluid.

DETACHMENT SHAPE

The shape of the detachment is correlated with the cause of subretinal fluid accumulation. The de-

tachment may be either rhegmatogenous or tractional.

The anterior surface of rhegmatogenous retinal detachment is convex. The anterior surface of purely tractional detachment is concave. Tractional retinal detachment commonly shows a tent-like configuration.

When tractional retinal detachment is associated with a dome-shaped configuration, careful search is indicated to disclose a rhegmatogenous component.

LOCATION AND EXTENT OF SUBRETINAL FLUID

In rhegmatogenous retinal detachment subretinal fluid accumulation and spread are correlated with the retinal break(s) location.[2,7] The location and extent of subretinal fluid thereby, provide guidelines to forecast the site of the retinal break(s). These guidelines are helpful in retinal detachments associated with small retinal breaks that may be difficult to disclose.

When a small break is located in an upper quadrant, subretinal fluid tends to sink into the lower quadrants. At the time of diagnosis the retina may be highly detached in the lower quadrants, whereas the detachment may be very shallow in the upper

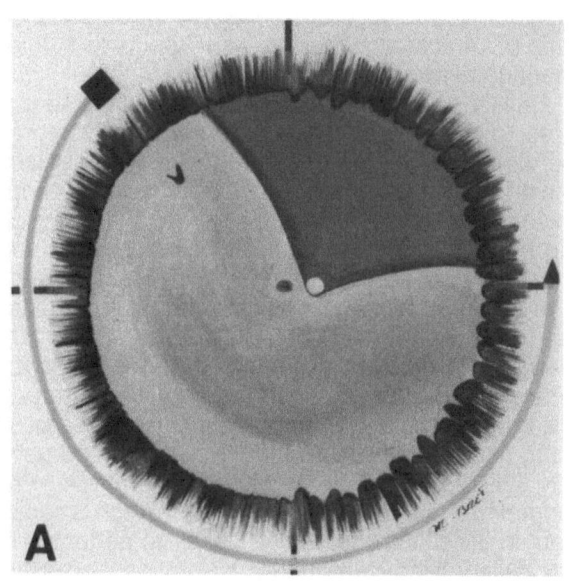
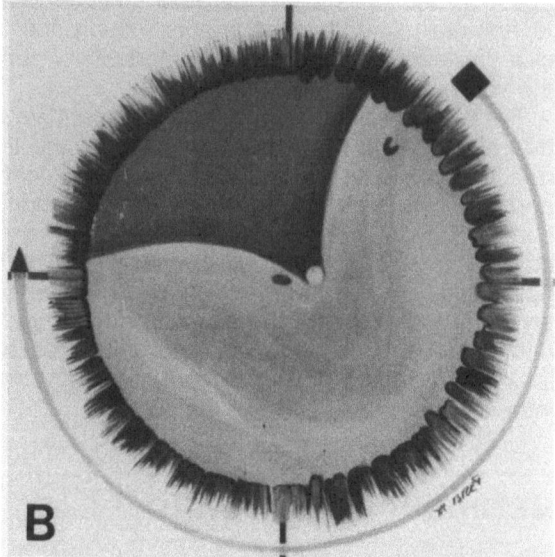

Figure 1. Relationship of subretinal fluid accumulation and retinal break side (A) Subretinal fluid spread from a retinal break in the superior temporal quadrant (B) Subretinal fluid spread from a retinal break in the superior nasal quadrant (C) Subretinal fluid spread from a retinal break in an inferior quadrant. Superior border of the detachment is higher on the side of the break (D) Subretinal fluid spread from a retinal break at 6 o'clock. Superior border of the detachment is at the same level in both inferior quadrants (E) Subretinal fluid spread from a retinal break near 12 o'clock. Lower border of the detachment is on the side of the break (F) Subretinal fluid spread from a retinal break at 12 o'clock. Lower border of the detachment is approximately at the same level on both sides.

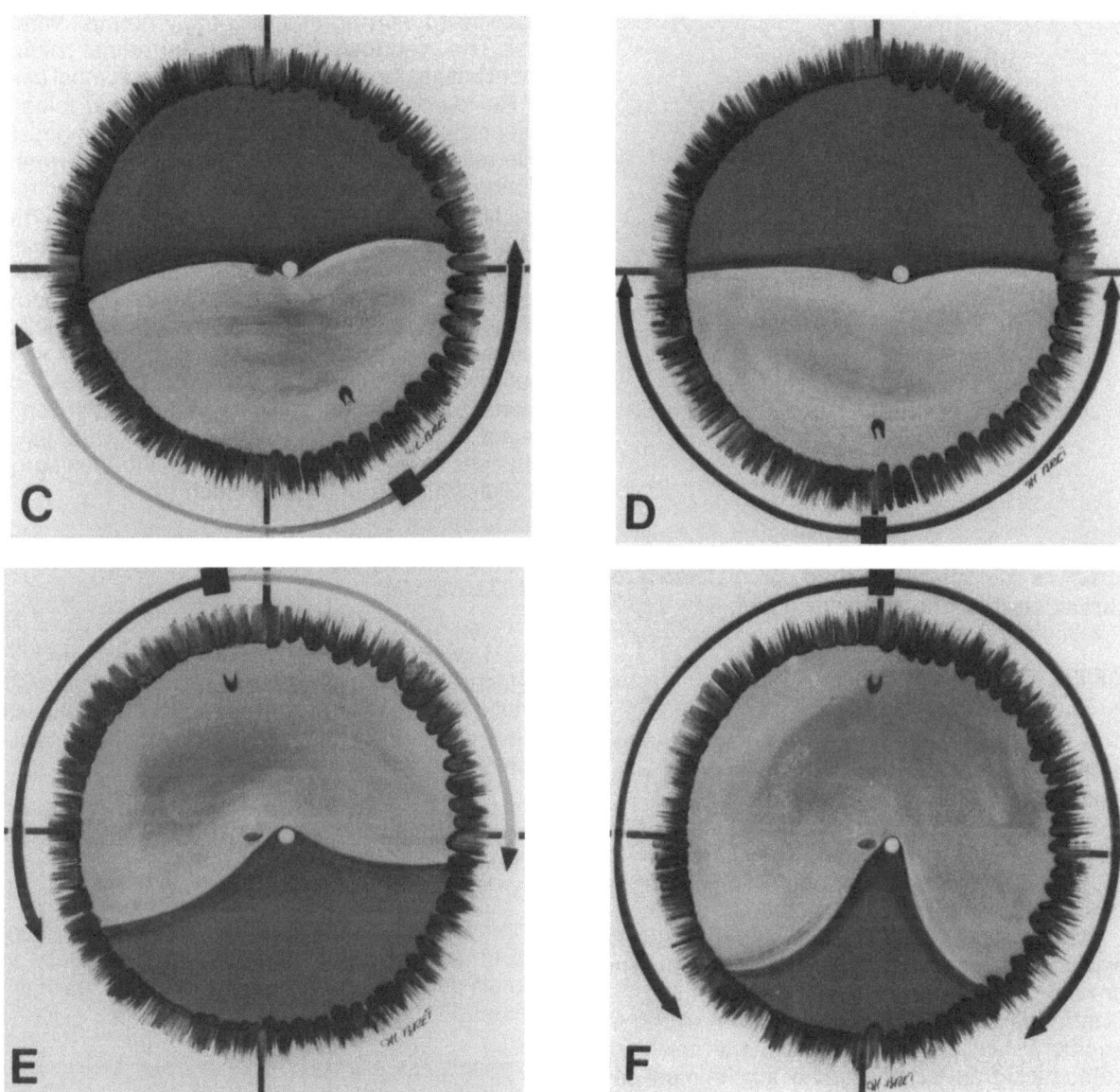

Figure 1. (Continued)

quadrant where the break is located. As a rule, these small breaks are present in the upper quadrant contiguous to the lower quadrant where the retina is the most highly and extensively detached. The upper limit of the inferior detachment is on the side of the break (Figs. 1A and B). Small breaks located in the lower quadrants result in inferior detachments, which are relatively shallow. When an inferior detachment is bullous, the break is located in a superior quadrant. When a small break is located in a lower quadrant, the superior limit of the detachment is higher on the side where the break is located (Fig. 1C). When the break is at or near 6 o'clock, the superior limit of the detachment is at the same level in both inferior quadrants (Fig. 1D). Total detach-

ments or superior detachments that cross the 12 o'clock meridian, arise from breaks at or near 12 o'clock (Fig. 1E and F). When the break is located on the posterior pole, or in close vicinity of the posterior pole, the maximal height of detachment is on the posterior pole or midperiphery. The retina anterior to the equator shows a shallow detachment or no detachemnt (Fig. 2). When a retinal break is found and the extent of subretinal fluid is not as expected from the break location, further fundus examination should be performed so as to disclose the other break(s).

In purely tractional retinal detachment, subretinal fluid accumulation and spread are correlated with the site(s) of static vitreoretinal traction.

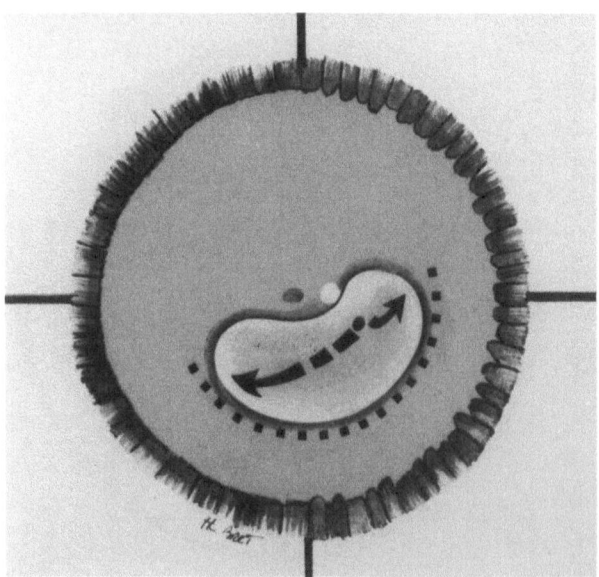

Figure 2. Subretinal fluid spread from a retinal break close to the posterior pole.

DETACHMENT HEIGHT

In rhegmatogenous retinal detachment the height of the detached retina is mainly correlated with the status of the vitreous gel.

Bullous retinal detachments indicate lack of retinal support by the vitreous gel. They are associated with significant vitreous gel liquefaction and posterior vitreous detachment.

Most shallow retinal detachments are associated with normal, or nearly normal vitreous gel and limited or no posterior vitreous detachment.

Intraoperative difficulty encountered in the management of bullous retinal detachments can be overcome by current surgical techniques in most cases. However, the prognosis for permanent retinal reattachment may be more guarded in bullous detachments as compared to shallow detachments. The prognosis is correlated to vitreous changes associated with the retinal detachment rather than the amount of subretinal fluid itself.

In tractional retinal detachment, the height of the detached retina is correlated with the degree of static vitreoretinal traction. The maximal height of the detachment is at the site(s) of vitreoretinal traction.

RETINAL FOLDS

Retinal folds are correlated with the presence and degree of vitreous gel and epiretinal changes associated with the detachment.

Most rhegmatogenous retinal detachments that exhibit a smooth surface without retinal folds are associated wtih normal, or nearly normal, vitreous gel. The prognosis for permanent retinal reattachment after scleral buckling is excellent in most cases.

Retinal detachments that show retinal folds are associated with significant vitreous gel changes. Mobile retinal folds that exhibit undulating movements during fundus examination are indicative of vitreous gel liquefaction and posterior vitreous detachment. Deep retinal folds may hide retinal breaks. Radial folds may involve the posterior edge of a horseshoe tear (Fig. 3) and can predispose to the development of the fishmouth phenomenon after scleral buckling. Intravitreal gas injection as an adjunct to scleral buckling is indicated in a number of such eyes. Fixed retinal folds are indicative of static traction on the retina. Traction may be related to vitreous gel changes or epiretinal membranes. Vitreous surgery is indicated in a number of such eyes.

DETACHMENT OF THE PARS PLANA EPITHELIUM

A few retinal detachments are associated with detachment of the pars plana epithelium. This finding is usually indicative of significant traction of the vitreous base. Specific surgical management is required in most cases.

DETACHMENTS OF GRADUAL PROGRESSION AND LONG DURATION

In eyes without significant vitreous changes, retinal detachment may progress very gradually and remain unrecognized for an extended period of time.

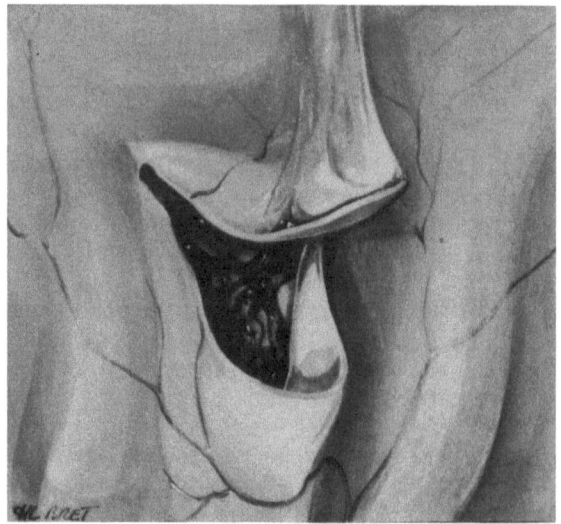

Figure 3. Radial retinal fold at the posterior edge of a horseshoe tear.

Such detachments show specific signs that enable the physician to determine their approximate duration. Signs of long-standing detachment include: (1) cystic degeneration of the detached retina, (2) demarcation lines, and (3) subretinal proliferation.

Cystic appearance, increased thickness, and increased transparency of the detached retina characterize cystic degeneration of the retina secondary to longstanding detachment. Microcystic degeneration of the detached retina may be associated with large intraretinal cysts (Fig. 4). Large intraretinal cysts usually take at least a year to develop.[8] They require no specific treatment and flatten spontaneously after the retinal break has been sealed.

Demarcation lines show the appearance of hyperpigmented arch-shaped lines at the level of the pigment epithelium (Fig. 5). They develop at the junction of the attached and detached retina and are commonly multiple and concentric. Multiple demarcation lines indicate gradual a increase in the extent of retinal detachment. It takes at least 3 months for a demarcation line to develop.[9] Therefore, the number of demarcation lines provides an indication in evaluating detachment duration.

Longstanding retinal detachments are commonly associated with clinical evidence of subretinal proliferation. White lines or thick, white cords, are present in the subretinal space (Fig. 6). The central part of the white lines usually shows an arch-shaped configuration similar to that of pigmented demarca-

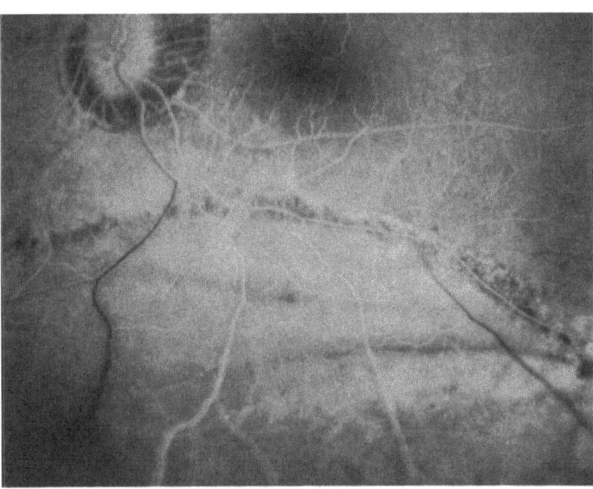

Figure 5. Fluorescein angiography of multiple demarcation lines in a longstanding retinal detachment. The retinal detachment was associated with two atrophic holes in lattice degeneration at 6 o'clock.

tion lines. The peripheral parts show an interlacing network of white lines. Multiple concentric retroretinal white lines are common. In contrast to epiretinal proliferation, subretinal proliferation is not an obstacle to retinal reattachment, even when thick subreti-

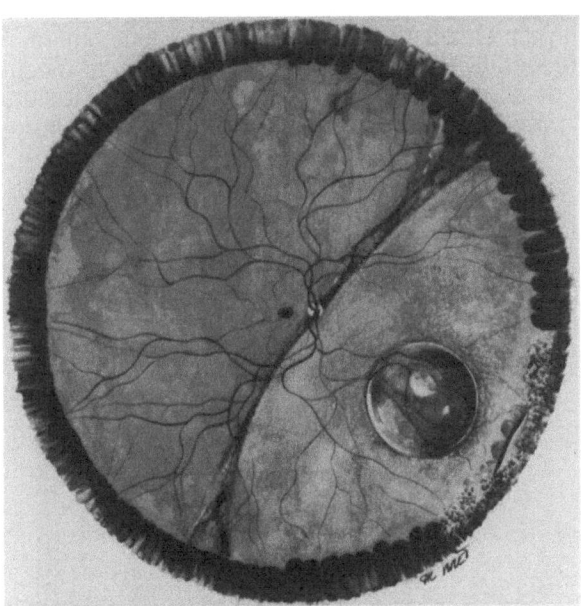

Figure 4. Longstanding retinal detachment after blunt trauma. The detachment is associated with a small dialysis at the anterior border of the vitreous base, increased transparency of the detached retina, and large intraretinal cyst.

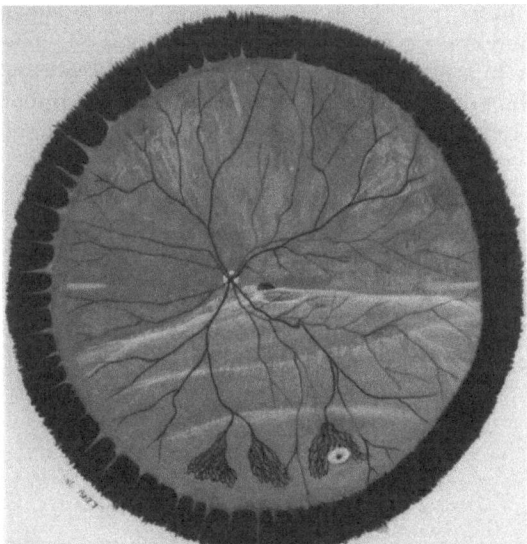

Figure 6. Longstanding retinal detachment with subretinal proliferation. The detachment is related to a small atrophic hole at 5 o'clock. Newvessels in the equatorial region are secondary to the long-duration retinal detachment (Courtesy of BONNET M. and URRETS-ZAVALIA J, J Fr Ophtalmol 9:615–624, 1986.

nal cords are present. It requires no specific treatment.

The prognosis of retinal detachments with clinical evidence of gradual progression and long duration is excellent in most cases. The excellent prognosis is likely related to the absence of significant vitreous changes.

MACULAR CHANGES

Preoperative macular changes are of great value in predicting final visual acuity after retinal detachment repair.

Preoperative macular changes may be related to either the detachment or associated retinal diseases. In most cases macular changes unrelated to the detachment cannot be recognized preoperatively when the macula is detached. However, examination of the other eye may provide useful information in patients with bilateral macular diseases, such as senile macular degeneration.

In eyes with an attached macula, surgical management should be performed as soon as possible to avoid extension of the detachment to the macula. However, an attached macula preoperatively does not guarantee optimal central visual acuity after retinal detachment repair. In spite of an attached macula, visual acuity may be decreased preoperatively owing to macular lesions unrelated to the detachment, such as degenerative changes in highly myopic eyes, cystoid macular edema in aphakic and pseudophakic eyes, and senile macular degeneration. In addition, macular changes related to the detachment or surgical management may develop postoperatively and can result in decreased central

visual acuity after retinal detachment repair. The main macular changes that may develop postoperatively include cystoid macular edema and macular pucker. An attached macula preoperatively does not preclude the development of such postoperative complications. Postoperative cystoid macular edema is more likely to occur in aphakic and pseudophakic eyes,[10–12] and in patients 60 years of age or older.[13] Postoperative macular pucker is more likely to develop in eyes with horseshoe tears that show a curled posterior edge,[14,15] retinal detachments with fixed retinal folds preoperatively,[14] giant tears and retinal detachments with horseshoe tear(s), and incomplete posterior vitreous detachment.[15] In such eyes a premacular membrane may be visible preoperatively (Fig. 7) and can increase postoperatively.

In eyes with a macula detached preoperatively, cystoid macular edema and macular pucker may also develop postoperatively. Predisposing factors are similar to those in eyes with an attached macula. In addition, two main parameters will interfere with postoperative visual recovery: The duration and the height of macular detachment.

Optimal visual recovery can be expected in eyes with macular detachment of less than a week's duration. In eyes with macular detachment for over a week's duration, the likelihood of poor visual recovery is correlated with three main parameters: (1) duration of macular detachment, (2) preoperative macular changes, and (3) height of the detachment. The final visual acuity shows a progressive decline with increased duration of macular detachment.[16] Preoperative macular changes secondary to macular detachment of long duration are predicting factors of poor visual recovery after retinal detachment re-

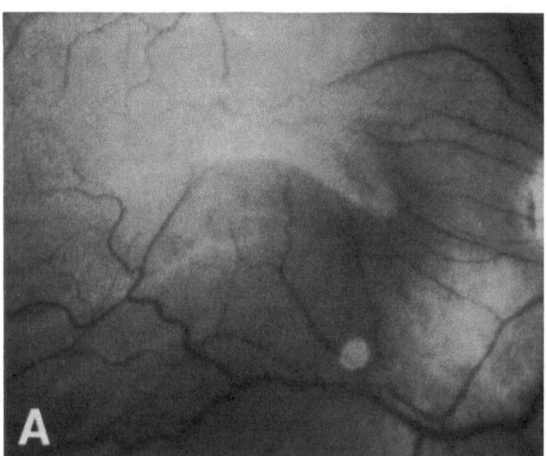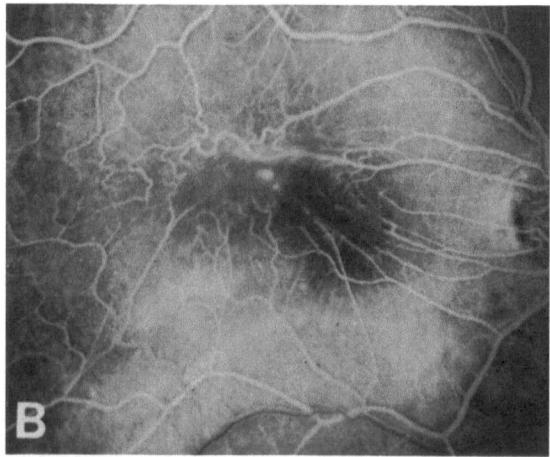

Figure 7. Premacular membrane present preoperatively in an eye with retinal detachment of the superior temporal quadrant associated with two horseshoe tears with a curled posterior edge. (A) Preoperative fundus photograph (B) Preoperative fluorescein angiography.

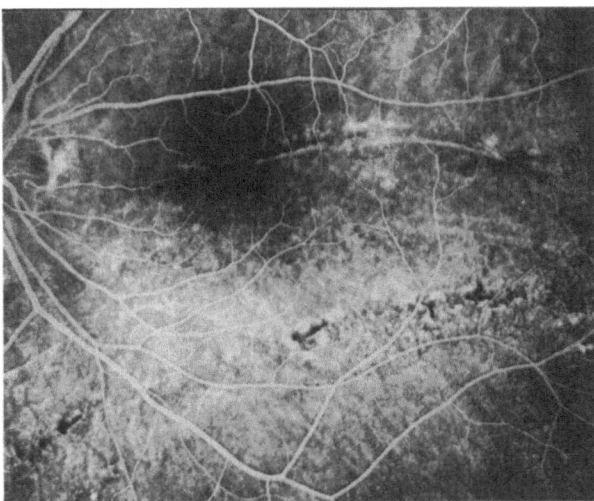

Figure 8. Fluorescein angiography after surgical repair of a longstanding retinal detachment. Pigment epithelium atrophy and demarcation lines involving the macula.

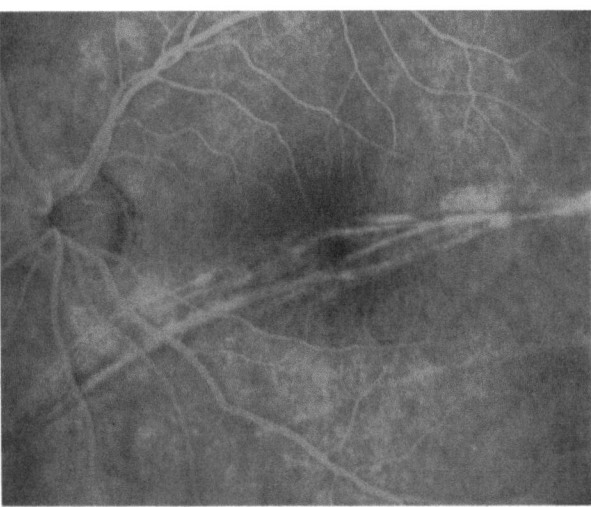

Figure 9. Fluorescein angiography after surgical repair of a longstanding retinal detachment. White cords of subretinal proliferation in the macular area.

pair. Macular changes secondary to macular detachment of long duration include cystoid macular degeneration, demarcation lines on the posterior pole (Fig. 8), and subretinal proliferation involving the macula (Fig. 9). Height of macular detachment is also an important factor in predicting postoperative visual acuity.[16] Eyes with a highly detached macula of over a week's duration are likely to recover poor visual acuity postoperatively.

SHIFTING SUBRETINAL FLUID

The term shifting subretinal fluid designates the phenomenon characterized by immediate change in the configuration of the detachment following eye movements or change of the patient's head position. Rapid change in detachment configuration is caused by movement of the subretinal fluid in the subretinal space to the most dependent part of the eye. Shifting subretinal fluid is a clinical sign that is common in nonrhegmatogenous retinal detachment and most uncommon in rhegmatogenous detachment. It may be observed in long standing rhegmatogenous detachments associated with tiny tears or holes, especially in aphakic eyes.

Retinal Breaks

In rhegmatogenous retinal detachment, retinal breaks are the most important fundus change to

be carefully evaluated preoperatively since sealing of all retinal breaks is a mandatory requirement to achieve permanent retinal reattachment. In easy retinal detachments, surgical management is restricted to proper sealing of the retinal break(s). In difficult detachments, surgical adjuncts to retinal break sealing are commonly required, although sealing every retinal break is mandatory in all cases. Therefore, any retinal break in a detached or attached retina must be disclosed by preoperative examination. In addition, the clinical characteristics of retinal breaks are factors of great value in choosing the correct surgical procedure and in predicting the prognosis for permanent retinal reattachment.

With regard to surgical management and prognosis, retinal breaks can be categorized into two main groups: (1) retinal breaks unrelated to significant vitreous changes, and (2) traction retinal breaks.

RETINAL BREAKS UNRELATED TO SIGNIFICANT VITREOUS TRACTION

Retinal breaks that are clinically unrelated to significant vitreous changes are the least common. They include round atrophic holes in lattice degeneration and nontraumatic oral dialyses. Management of retinal detachments associated with such breaks is easy in most cases. Permanent retinal reattachment can be achieved in all cases provided the retinal breaks are properly sealed. Risk of postoperative proliferative vitreoretinopathy and recurrent detachment is virtually nil.

TRACTION RETINAL BREAKS

Traction retinal breaks are the most frequent. They are usually associated with significant vitreous changes. They include two distinct groups: (1) retinal breaks whose formation is related to dynamic vitreous traction and (2) retinal breaks whose formation is related to static traction. In both groups degenerative changes of the retina may predispose to retinal break formation.

Retinal breaks whose formation is related to dynamic and transient vitreous traction develop at the time of acute posterior vitreous detachment. They are the most common and include: (1) horseshoe tears, (2) giant tears that are an extreme form of horseshoe tears, (3) postequatorial paravascular tears in myopic eyes, and (4) most retinal breaks after blunt trauma, in particular dialysis. With regard to surgical management, such retinal breaks can be categorized into three distinct groups:

1. Breaks that remain under dynamic vitreous traction
   Dynamic and discontinuous, vitreous traction on the tear flap is related to vitreous gel movements induced by eye movements.
2. Breaks that are no more under traction
   The tear flap has parted from the retina (operculated tear).
3. Breaks under subsequent static traction
   Static traction on the break develops following tear formation. Traction is permanent. It gradually increases in a number of eyes. It is independent from eye movements. It is related to either contraction of the vitreous base (tears at the posterior border of the vitreous base) or development of preretinal membranes.

The amount of surgery necessary to achieve permanent sealing of the break(s) and retinal reattachment varies according to the break group. For example permanent sealing of a break that is no longer under traction, such as an operculated tear, can be achieved merely through choroidal irritation and intravitreal gas injection. Permanent sealing of an equatorial tear that remains under dynamic vitreous traction usually requires scleral buckling. However, a temporary scleral buckle may be sufficient to permanently close the tear and reattach the retina. In contrast, permanent sealing of a retinal tear under static vitreous traction will require either permanent scleral buckling and/or vitreous surgery.

Retinal breaks whose formation is related to static traction are uncommon. They result from a permanent and increasing traction on the retina. Static traction may result from either fibrovascular prolifera-

tion into the vitreous cavity or preretinal membranes. Two examples of retinal breaks caused by static traction are (1) dialyses associated with traction detachment after penetrating trauma and (2) posterior paravascular tears that occur in retinal detachments complicated by severe proliferative vitreoretinopathy. In most cases such breaks gradually increase in size as static traction increases. Permanent sealing of such breaks requires rather heavy surgery, which must include both high scleral buckles and vitreous surgery.

Vitreous Body

The status of the vitreous body and the vitreoretinal relationship are of particular importance with regard to the choice of surgical procedure and prognosis. They are carefully evaluated by slit lamp examination using the three-mirror contact lens. Vitreous gel findings of clinical significance that may be associated with retinal detachment include (1) normal vitreous gel without posterior vitreous detachment, (2) vitreous gel liquefaction and posterior vitreous detachment, (3) vitreoretinal traction, and (4) vitreous hemorrhage.

NORMAL VITREOUS GEL

Normal viscous vitreous gel closely applied to the inner layers of the retina is uncommon in eyes with retinal detachment. However, certain rhegmatogenous retinal detachments, such as detachments associated with nontraumatic oral dialyses and round atrophic holes in lattice, develop in eyes with normal or nearly normal vitreous gel, which remains continuous with the internal limiting lamina. Scleral buckling is the procedure of choice in the management of such detachments. Intravitreal surgery is contraindicated in most cases. Prognosis for permanent retinal reattachment is excellent in most cases.

VITREOUS GEL LIQUEFACTION AND POSTERIOR VITREOUS DETACHMENT

Most retinal detachments that require surgical management are associated with vitreous gel syneresis and posterior vitreous detachment. The degree of vitreous gel liquefaction, the extent of posterior vitreous detachment, and the mobility of the detached posterior vitreous face are carefully evaluated preoperatively.

In most cases the degree of vitreous gel liquefaction and the severity of the retinal detachment are positively correlated. The more extensive the vitreous gel syneresis, the more severe the retinal detachment.

In eyes with rhegmatogenous retinal detachment, posterior vitreous detachment may be either total with collapse of the vitreous gel in the lower part of the vitreous cavity, or incomplete with the vitreous gel still attached to the posterior pole and the inferior half of the retina. Incomplete posterior vitreous detachment with vitreous gel still attached to the posterior pole may predispose to the development of macular pucker postoperatively. The extent of posterior vitreous detachment and the degree of vitreous gel liquefaction are positively correlated in a number of eyes. There are, however, numerous exceptions to this rule. In eyes with severe vitreous gel syneresis, very large vitreous lacunae may mimic total posterior vitreous detachment. Actually, a thin layer of cortical vitreous gel remains adherent to the retina. Severe proliferative vitreoretinopathy is more likely to develop in such eyes.

In eyes with traction retinal detachment, posterior vitreous detachment is incomplete. The anatomy of the retinal detachment is determined by the site(s) of the vitreoretinal attachment(s) and the severity of vitreoretinal traction.

The detached posterior vitreous face is mobile in eyes with rhegmatogenous retinal detachments that are not complicated by proliferative vitreoretinopathy. In contrast the detached posterior vitreous face is immobile in eyes with traction retinal detachments and rhegmatogenous retinal detachments complicated by severe proliferative vitreoretinopathy. Vitreous surgery is indicated in such eyes.

VITREORETINAL TRACTION

The presence and type of vitreoretinal traction should be carefully evaluated, since they are the determining parameters in the choice of the surgical procedure.

Vitreoretinal traction may be either dynamic or static.[17]

Dynamic vitreous traction occurs during movements of the vitreous gel induced by eye movements. Most retinal detachments with horseshoe tears of the equatorial region are associated with dynamic vitreous traction. Traction is related to vitreous fibrils, that remain adherent to the tear flap. Scleral buckling is required to seal the retinal break(s) in most eyes with significant dynamic traction on the tear flap. However, permanent relief of traction is unnecessary to achieve permanent retinal reattachment in most cases.

Static vitreous traction is continuous. In a number of eyes, the traction forces that pull on the retina increase as the vitreous changes worsen. Vitreous base changes, vitreoretinal attachments in eyes with incomplete posterior vitreous detachment, condensed vitreous strands, and cellular membranes are the most common causes of static traction on the retina. Permanent relief of traction is required to achieve permanent retinal reattachment in such eyes. This can be achieved by permanent scleral buckling and/or vitreous surgery.

VITREOUS HEMORRHAGE

Vitreous hemorrhages that do not prevent fundus examination are not taken into account in the choice of the surgical procedure for retinal detachment management.

In eyes with dense vitreous hemorrhage preventing fundus examination, diagnosis of retinal detachment is made by A- and B-scan ultrasonography. vitrectomy is indicated as the first step of the operation for retinal detachment management.

Associated Findings

Choroidal detachment and sequelae of previous surgery for retinal detachment management are the main associated findings of clinical significance that may be present.

CHOROIDAL DETACHMENT

Choroidal detachment may be associated with rhegmatogenous retinal detachment (see p. 165), retinal detachment after penetrating injury, and retinal detachments following inflammatory eye diseases. It is a clinical finding of poor prognosis. Specific management is commonly required in such eyes (see p. 166).

SEQUELAE OF PREVIOUS SURGERY

Accurate evaluation of fundus changes is often more difficult in eyes that have previously undergone retinal detachment surgery and failed to reattach. Sequelae of previous surgery of clinical significance with regard to reoperation include: (1) chorioretinal scars, (2) scleral buckles, and (3) clinical evidence of previous complications such as choroidal and/or vitreous hemorrhage, vitreous and/or retinal incarceration in a drainage site or a pars plana incision, and iatrogenic retinal breaks after vitrectomy.

Choice of the surgical approach is based on identification of the cause(s) for the failure of previous surgery. Failed surgery may be related to four main causes: (1) improper management of the primary retinal break(s) or an unrecognized primary break, (2) development of subsequent retinal breaks, (3) development of proliferative vitreoretinopathy, and (4) iatrogenic lesions, such as iatrogenic retinal breaks and vitreous gel or retinal incarceration in a pars plana incision.

Prognosis for retinal reattachment is good in eyes that failed to reattach after improper management of retinal break(s) and eyes with retinal break(s) that were not recognized and left untreated. When there is no clinical evidence of proliferative vitreoretinopathy, such eyes are managed by revision of the scleral buckle(s) and cryotreatment. Intravitreal gas injection as an adjunct to scleral buckling is required in selected cases. Identification of the retinal break(s) may be difficult in eyes with atrophic scars following extensive and heavy cryotreatment. Great difficulty may be encountered intraoperatively owing to scar tissue or scleral erosion beneath previous buckles. In eyes that underwent previous vitrectomy, sealing of inferior retinal breaks may be very difficult to achieve owing to lack of retinal support by the vitreous gel.

Prognosis for retinal reattachment is good in most eyes with recurrent detachment related to the development of subsequent retinal breaks. Such breaks, however, usually indicate the presence of a continuing disease with increasing vitreous traction. The subsequent tears are commonly situated at the posterior edge of the vitreous base. Circumferential scleral buckling of the vitreous base is often required to achieve permanent retinal reattachment in such eyes.

In failures related to the development of proliferative vitreoretinopathy, surgical management and prognosis depend on the degree and extent of the proliferative process (see p. 231).

In failed eyes with iatrogenic changes, the surgical approach varies depending on the iatrogenic changes and associated lesions. Significant retinal incarcerations in a drainage site or a pars plana incision are managed by scleral shortening in most cases. Retinotomies are considered only in eyes that fail to reattach after scleral shortening. Eyes with large iatrogenic retinal breaks are often inoperable.

FUNDUS EXAMINATION OF THE OTHER EYE

The posterior segment of the other eye is examined with full mydriasis. In patients with rhegmatogenous retinal detachment, the main objective of fundus examination of the other eye is to recognize asymptomatic retinal breaks and degenerative

changes that may predispose to subsequent retinal detachment. Thorough examination of the peripheral retina and the vitreous gel will enable the physician to determine whether prophylactic treatment is required.

Prophylactic treatment is usually performed on asymptomatic retinal breaks, regardless of the status of the vitreous gel.

In eyes with vitreoretinal degeneration of the equatorial region, such as lattice degeneration and snailtrack degeneration, the indications for prophylactic treatment are based on the status of the vitreous gel.

Prophylactic treatment is restricted to eyes that exhibit no posterior vitreous detachment. Prophylactic treatment is unnecessary in eyes that exhibit clinical evidence of posterior vitreous detachment with vitreous gel collapse.

REFERENCES

1. Urrets-Zavalia A: Le décollement de la rétine. Paris, Masson, 1968
2. Schepens CL: Retinal detachment and allied diseases. Philadelphia, W.B. Saunders Co, 1983
3. Piñero Carrion A: Tratamiento del despredimiento de la retina Publicaciones de la Universidad de Sevilla, Spain, 1974
4. Mackenzie Freeman H, Hirose T, Schepens CL: Vitreous surgery and advances in fundus diagnosis and treatment. New York, Appleton Century Crofts, 1977
5. Busacca A, Goldmann H, Schiff-Wertheimer S: Biomicroscopie du corps vitré et du fond d'oeil. Paris, Masson, 1957
6. Eisner G: Biomicroscopy of the peripheral fundus. New York, Springer-Verlag, 1973
7. Lincoff H, Gieser R: Finding the retinal hole. Arch Ophthalmol, 85:565–569, 1971
8. Hagler WS, North AW: Intraretinal macrocysts and retinal detachment. Trans Amer Acad Ophthalmol Otolaryngol 71:442–454, 1967
9. Benson WE, Nantawan P, Morse PH: Characteristics and prognosis of retinal detachments with demarcation lines. Am J Ophthalmol 84:641–644, 1977
10. Lobes LA, Grand MG: Incidence of cystoid macular edema following scleral buckling procedure. Arch Ophthalmol 98:1230–1232, 1980
11. Meredith TA, Reeser FH, Topping TM, Aaberg TM: Cystoid macular edema after retinal detachment surgery. Ophthalmology 87:1090–1095, 1980
12. Bonnet M, Bievelez B, Noel A, et al: Fluorescein angiography after retinal detachment microsurgery. Graefe's Arch Clin Exp Ophthalmol 221:35–40, 1983
13. Bonnet M, Fernandez-Pastor D: Rupture de la barriére hémato-rétinienne après, microchirurgie du décollement de la rétine. Ophtalmologie 1:29–31, 1988
14. Lobes LA, Burton TC: The incidence of macular pucker after retinal detachment surgery. Am J Ophthalmol 85:72–77, 1978
15. Bonnet M: Proliferative vitreoretinopathy after retinal detachment surgery: Grade B, a determining risk factor. Graefe's Arch Clin Exp Ophthalmol 226:201–205, 1988
16. Tani P, Robertson DM, Langworthy A: Prognosis for central vision and anatomic reattachment in rhegmatogenous retinal detachment with macula detached Am J Ophthalmol 92:611–620, 1981
17. Scott JD: Static and dynamic vitreous traction Trans Ophthalmol Soc UK 91:175–188, 1971

3
Systemic Examination

Systemic examination is carried out by an internist and the anesthesiologist. The main objectives of systemic examination are threefold: (1) to recognize contraindications to general anesthesia, or occasionally to local anesthesia, (2) to evaluate associated systemic diseases that may require specific management before and after the operation for retinal detachment management, and (3) to avoid systemic complications postoperatively.

Contraindications to retinal detachment surgery related to associated systemic diseases are uncommon. However, medical preparation for a few days prior to surgery is necessary in a number of patients with systemic diseases, such as diabetes mellitus, increased blood pressure, and heart and vascular diseases. Careful systemic examination is also important to recognize contraindications to certain medications, such as antiinflammatory agents and diamox, which are used as an adjunct to surgery in selected retinal detachments. Systemic complications after retinal detachment surgery are uncommon since the patient is allowed to move around normally on the first postoperative day in most cases. Medical preparation of the patient is of great importance to avoid complications that may occur after any surgical trauma and general anesthesia, particularly in elderly patients.

II
Instrumentation

4

The Surgical Microscope: Technical Equipment

The surgical microscope must fulfill specific requirements for external surgery, trans-scleral surgery with simultaneous observation of the fundus, and vitreous surgery.

SURGERY WITHOUT SIMULTANEOUS OBSERVATION OF THE FUNDUS

The technical characteristics of the surgical microscope used for external microsurgery are the same as for microsurgery of the anterior segment of the eye. The use of the surgical microscope during the surgical steps that do not require simultaneous observation of the fundus has the same purpose as in surgery of the anterior segment. High magnification and uniform illumination without a shadow on the operating area allow for well controlled surgery. Thus surgical microscopes designed for surgery of the anterior segment can be used for the stages of retinal detachment microsurgery that are carried out without simultaneous observation of the fundus. However, surgical microscopes designed for anterior segment microsurgery cannot be used without special fittings for the stages of retinal detachment surgery, which must be carried out with simultaneous observation of the fundus.

SURGERY WITH SIMULTANEOUS OBSERVATION OF THE FUNDUS

For trans-scleral surgery with simultaneous biomicroscopic examination of the fundus, the surgical microscope must be equipped with a slit illuminator. In addition to this, some special equipment is very useful, since it makes biomicroscopy of the vitreous cavity easier during surgery.

Illumination

COAXIAL ILLUMINATION

Coaxial illumination is used for indirect ophthalmomicroscopy.[1] This technique has two major advantages: (1) the wide field of observation and (2) the variable magnification. It also has its own limits and disadvantages, however (see p. 50). Therefore, its use is restricted to fundus examination without simultaneous surgery, fundus photographs, and films. Observation of the fundus through a contact lens is possible with coaxial illumination. Nevertheless, illumination of the fundus is diffused, and observation of the retina is difficult because of the reflection of the light on the surface of the contact lens. Thus, surgical microscopes equipped solely with coaxial illumination are not suitable for retinal detachment microsurgery.

SLIT ILLUMINATOR

At present a slit lamp is the only means for suitable observation of the fundus with a surgical microscope during the steps of external surgery that require simultaneous control of the fundus. The slit illuminator allows for an optical cross section of the vitreous body and the retina.

The angle between the microscope axes and the slit lamp must be approximately 5° in order to make biomicroscopic examination of the retina possible.

25

The surgical microscopes equipped with a slit lamp designed for anterior segment surgery cannot be used for retinal detachment surgery without modification, since the angle of the slit lamp usually varies between 30° and 40°.

Such a wide angle can be reduced by means of a prism. The prism is not provided by the manufacturers unless there is a special request. The reducing prism of the Zeiss firm, which can be placed on Zeiss microscopes OPMI 2, OPMI 3, and OPMI 5, does not reduce the angle of the slit lamp beam below 11°.

The surgical biomicroscope designed by Zeiss in the 1960s was equipped with a slit lamp whose angle could vary from 50° to 5°. Unfortunately, the position of the slit lamp was not suitable for biomicroscopic examination of the retina. To date the mobile surgical slit lamp manufactured by Zeiss is the most suitable equipment for biomicroscopic examination of the fundus during surgery (Fig. 10). It can be adjusted on the Zeiss microscopes OPMI 1 and OPMI 6 (Figs. 11 and 12). The slit illuminator can be moved either by motor or manually about 30° to either side of the central position without the slit image being dis-

placed from the center of the object field. The optimum position of the slit lamp for biomicroscopy of the fundus during surgery is situated at the edge of either of the eyepieces. In effect, this position corresponds exactly to an angle of 5°. Of course, the position of the slit illuminator should not be modified during fundus observation. The only advantage of the motorized slit illuminator is to permit the surgeon to use the same microscope and slit illuminator both for fundus surgery, with a narrow angle, and anterior segment surgery, with a wide angle.

The Zeiss mobile surgical slit lamp was originally designed for vitreous surgery at Machemer's[2] and Klöti's[3] request. However, this source of illumination has been withdrawn by most vitreous surgeons owing to the fact that endoillumination by a fiberoptic probe provides better visualization of the vitreous gel.[4] The author still routinely uses the slit lamp illuminator in vitreous surgery. In most cases it is used in conjunction with endoillumination. The slit beam, which should be narrow, is used to provide improved stereopsis. In particular it provides a clearly visible landmark to locate the posterior lens capsule when working in the anterior vitreous cavity. The

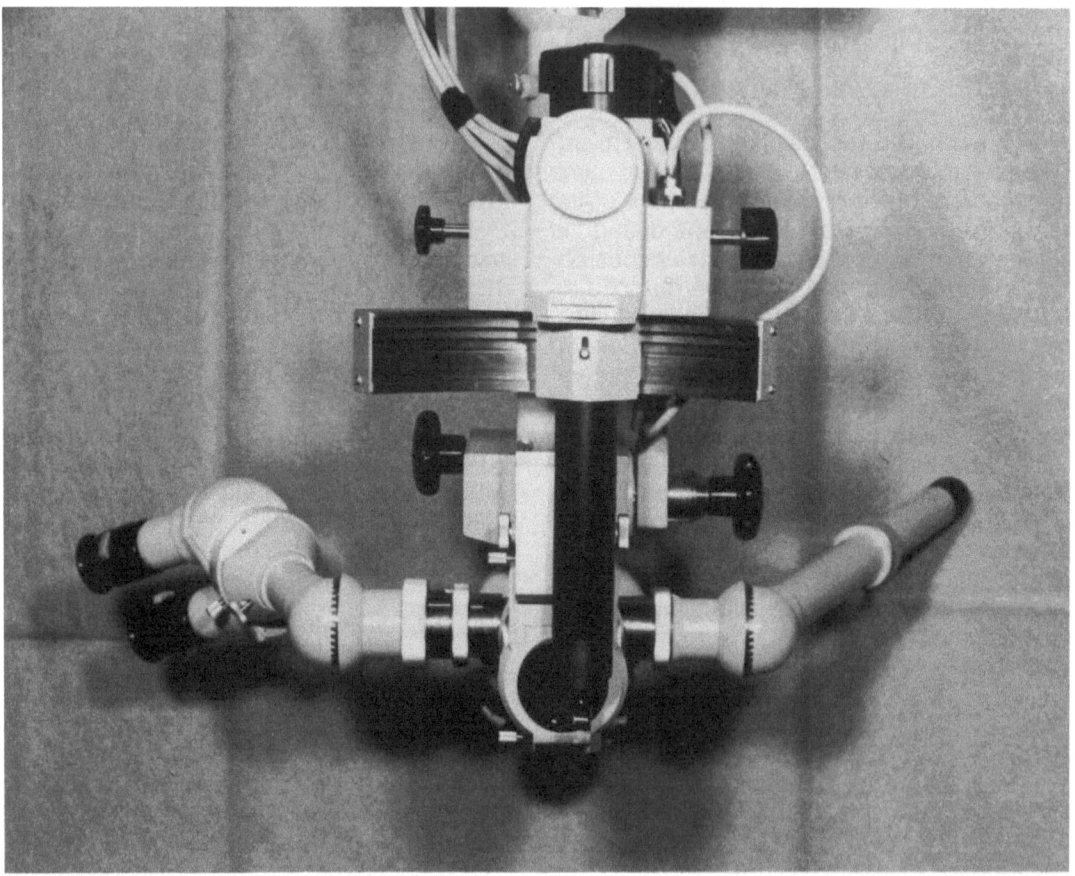

Figure 10. The mobile surgical slit lamp manufactured by Zeiss. The slit illuminator can be moved 30° to either side of the central position.

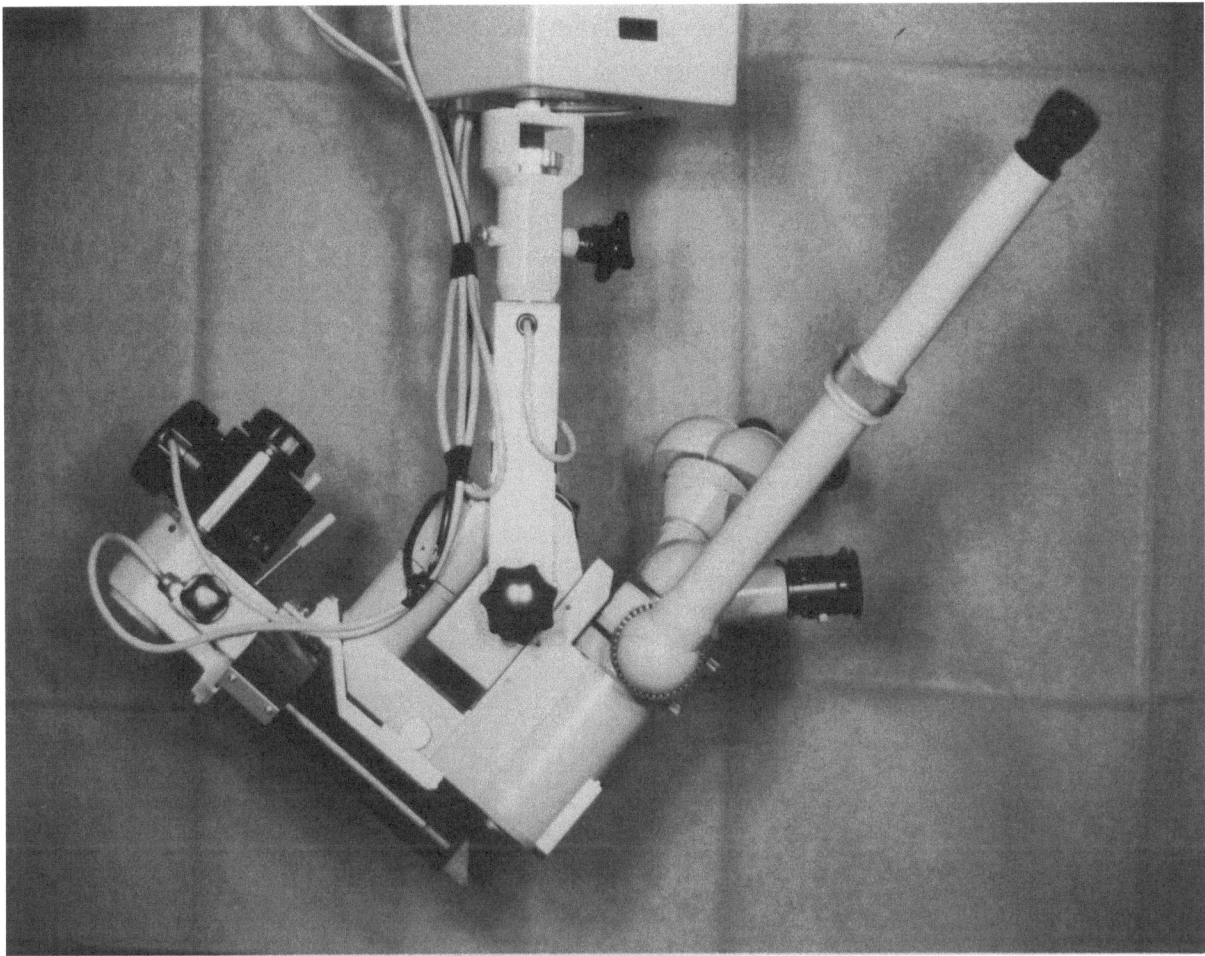

Figure 11. Lateral view of the Zeiss OPMI 6 microscope equipped with the mobile slit lamp.

slit illuminator is also occasionally used as the only illumination source during selected steps of endosurgery which require simultaneous use of the three-mirror contact lens.

Special Fittings

The most useful special fittings of the surgical microscope for retinal detachment surgery are the electric zoom system, a control for increasing power of the slit lamp filament, the X/Y coupling system, the foot switch control, and binocular microscope eyepieces for the assistant.

VARIABLE MAGNIFICATION

Variable magnification is very useful at every surgical stage. A continuously adjustable motorized zoom system is preferable to the Galilean changer, be-cause it allows for regular variation of magnification without down time and without altering focus. Electric foot control of the zoom system, which leaves both of the surgeon's hands free, is mandatory for vitreous surgery. In addition, it allows for more rapid external surgery with simultaneous observation of the fundus. Indeed, localization of retinal breaks and control of choroidal indentation are usually easier and more rapidly performed under low magnification, while cryo-application and moulding the choroidal indentation in front of the retinal tear itself are more accurately carried out under high magnification.

The range of magnification provided by the zoom system varies within wide limits depending on the focal length of the objective and the eyepieces (Table 1). The author uses a Zeiss OPMI 6 microscope equipped with an objective with a focal length F or 175 mm and a pair of 12.5 x eyepieces. With this latter equipment the range of magnification varies from 4.5 to 22.3. This range, when used to the maximum of its possibilities, would appear to be sufficient.

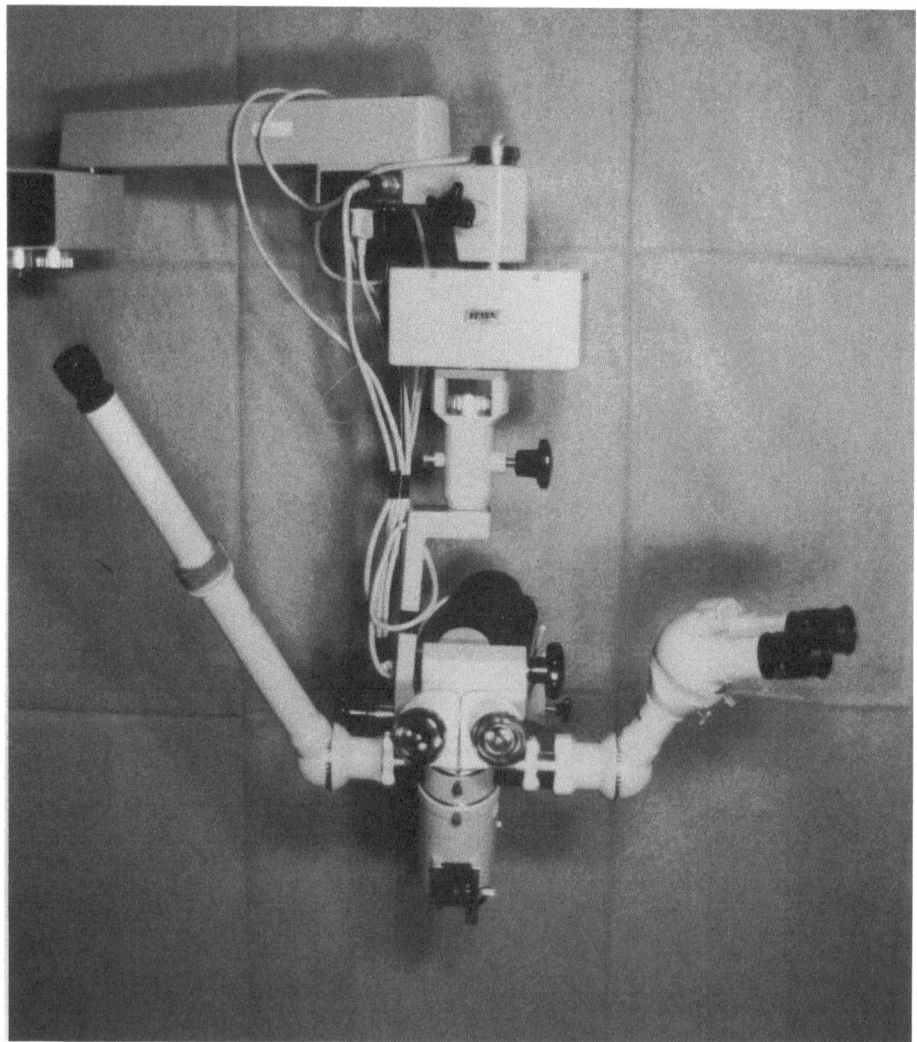

Figure 12. Frontal view of the Zeiss OPMI 6 microscope.

POWER OF THE SLIT LAMP

The illumination of the fundus and the vitreous cavity provided by a 6-V, 25 W filament lamp is sufficient in most cases. However, more powerful illumination is sometimes necessary, especially for vitreous surgery, for the localization of a very small retinal tear, and/or for cryoapplication when the media are not quite clear and when operating under very high magnification. This illumination can be obtained by increasing the power of the filament lamp. A slit illuminator fitted with fiber optics is the most suitable.

X/Y COUPLING SYSTEM

The X/Y coupling system for motorized two-dimensional movement in a horizontal plane of the micro-scope head is most useful in any stage of retinal detachment microsurgery. It allows for easy and rapid centering of the microscope head. It is especially useful during endosurgery and during external surgery with simultaneous observation of the fundus. The X/Y coupling system used in conjunction with the three-mirror contact lens permits easy and rapid examination of the entire peripheral fundus, as well as the posterior pole, without the necessity of rotating the eye or changing the surgeon's position.

ELECTRIC FOOT SWITCH CONTROL

All motorized functions of the surgical microscope should be activated by a remote control equipment operated by the surgeon. The author uses the single multifunction foot pedal of the Zeiss OPMI 6 micro-scope. This electric foot switch control is convenient

Table 1
Range of Magnification Provided by Zoom System

Zoom System Factor	Eyepieces							
	10 ×		12.5 ×		16 ×		20 ×	
	β	φ	β	φ	β	φ	β	φ
0.5	3.6	55.6	4.5	44.4	5.7	35.1	7.1	28.2
1.0	7.1	28.2	8.9	22.5	11.4	17.5	14.3	14
1.5	10.7	18.7	13.4	14.9	17.1	11.7	21.4	9.3
2.0	14.3	14	17.9	11.2	22.9	8.7	28.6	7
2.5	17.9	11.2	22.3	9	28.6	7	35.7	5.6

Table 1. Microscope magnifications and field-of-view diameters of the surgical slit lamp with 1:5 zoom system (OPMI 6), fitted with main objective $f = 175$ mm, inclined binocular tube $fr = 125$ mm, and four different magnifying eyepieces.

for surgeons with small sized feet. Its use requires training, however. Use of the multifunction foot pedal of the microscope can be difficult when the surgeon has to simultaneously use additional foot pedals for the remote control of other instruments. Certain motorized functions of the microscope can be controlled by other devices, such as voice controlled devices.

BINOCULAR EYEPIECES FOR THE ASSISTANT

The surgical microscope should be equipped with binocular eyepieces for the assistant. Unfortunately, the assistant eyepieces of the Zeiss OPMI 6 microscope have a major disadvantage as compared to the equipment used in anterior segment microsurgery. The beam-splitter provides only one of the two images observed by the surgeon through each of his eyepieces, therefore, the assistant has no true stereoscopic view of the surgical field.

The Zeiss OPMI 6 microscope has made development of retinal detachment microsurgery possible. However, improvements of the surgical microscopes used in this specific field of microsurgery are still required. The necessity of using a contact lens to obtain a clear view of the vitreous body and retina is the major disadvantage of the available microscopes, as compared to the conditions of observation obtained in anterior segment surgery. There is a need for a surgical microscope that would permit the vitreoretinal surgeon to work within the posterior segment of the eye under the same optical conditions as those obtained for external work and anterior segment surgery. A binocular indirect ophthalmoscope-microscope for noncontact wide-angle vitreous surgery has been developed;[5] however, this device still needs improvements. The ideal ophthalmoscope-microscope that can be easily used for both external surgery and endosurgery should fulfill five main requirements; (1) it should provide a clear view of the entire vitreous cavity and retina with no need to use a contact lens; (2) it should provide a wide field of observation with uniform illumination for both endosurgery and external surgery; (3) a special device should erect the inverted image of the fundus provided by the ophthalmoscope;[6] (4) moving from external view to internal view of the surgical field, and vice versa, should be easy and rapid; and (5) the ophthalmoscope-microscope should not be cumbersome.

5

Contact Lenses

As long as the ideal ophthalmoscope-microscope remains to be designed, the vitreoretinal microsurgeon will need a series of contact lenses for observing the vitreous body and the retina during surgery. There is not a single contact lens that fulfills all requirements for vitreoretinal microsurgery; and therefore, the vitreoretinal microsurgeon should have a series of different contact lenses available at all times. Each of them will be used by the surgeon according to the specific technique that is to be carried out.

The set of contact lenses should include at least two three-mirror contact lenses of different sizes, a plano concave contact lens, and a biconcave lens. A plano concave lens with a 30° or 45° prism may also be useful under certain circumstances.

CONTACT LENSES FOR EXTERNAL SURGERY WITH SIMULTANEOUS OBSERVATION OF THE FUNDUS

A Goldmann three-mirror contact lens is used for observation of the fundus during localization of the retinal break(s), cryotreatment, laser photocoagulation treatment, and control of the choroidal indentation after scleral buckling.

Any Goldmann three-mirror contact lens can be used, but during surgery the contact lens is sometimes cumbersome. It may thus hinder the passage of the marker and the cryoprobe between the eye and the orbit wall. To date, the most suitable three-mirror contact lens for biomicroscopy during surgery is the Goldmann three-mirror contact lens number 630, reference number 180041 D, manufactured by Haag-Streit (St. Gallen, Switzerland). Its characteristics are shown in Figure 13. At present this three-mirror contact lens remains unsurpassed for this specific utilization. The mirrors are large enough to allow for satisfactory observation of any part of the

fundus and vitreous gel. Its small size makes the simultaneous maneuvering of the cryoprobe and the marker along the sclera quite easy.

However this three-mirror contact lens is still too large for practical use when surgical instruments are placed or maneuvered anteriorly to the ora serrata. Such is the case in particular during scleral depression of the pars plana and during pars plana vitrectomy. In such circumstances the author uses the smallest three-mirror contact lens reference number 138614A.AZ, which was designed by Haag Streit for use in young children. The 10 mm diameter of its corneal side does not interfere with simultaneous scleral depression of the pars plana. The contact lens can also be used at any time of vitreoretinal microsurgery through the pars plana.

A contact lens with a single peripheral mirror was designed by Urrets-Zavalia[7-8] for retinal detachment microsurgery. The flattened surface opposite the mirror allows for easy passage of the instruments along the sclera; however, its single 70° mirror does not allow for easy observation of the entire fundus during surgery.

Some contact lenses designed for endosurgery, such as the plano-concave lens and the biconcave lens, are also occasionally used in surgical procedures that do not include a vitrectomy.

CONTACT LENSES FOR ENDOSURGERY

Planoconcave Contact Lens

The lens that is most commonly used during endosurgery through the pars plana is a plano concave contact lens. The emmetropic eye has a refractive power of + 58.6 diopters. Most of the refractive power takes place in the anterior cornea where light passes from air, whose refractive index is 1,000, to the cornea, whose refractive index is 1,376. A

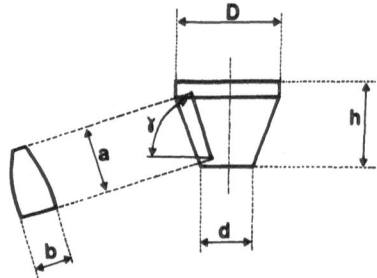

3 - MIRROR CONTACT LENS h. 630	D	d	h	ɣ	a	b
	30	18	19	59°	13	13
				66°	13,4	13
				73°	13	13

Figure 13. The Goldmann three-mirror contact lens number 630, manufactured by Haag-Streit (Reference number 180041 D).

contact lens with a flat anterior surface reduces the refractive power of the anterior surface of the cornea from 48.8 diopters to 14.5 diopters. Consequently, the fundus is easily seen. A direct image of the fundus is the main advantage of the plano concave lens. However, none of the various means for keeping the lens well-centered on the cornea during the surgical procedure is entirely satisfactory. The various systems for suturing the lens posteriorly to the limbus have the main disadvantage of preventing the surgeon from using the three-mirror contact lens during certain steps of the procedure. Plano concave lenses kept on the cornea merely by suction forces are the most easily maintained in place and the most rapidly removed for temporary use of the three-mirror contact lens. Unfortunately, the optical qualities of these lenses are rather poor. In the author's own experience, the most convenient plano concave lenses for use during vitreoretinal work through the pars plana remain those that are kept centered on the cornea by the assistant. All of them have the main advantage of application upon and removal from the cornea very rapidly. Most models available have good optical qualities. Unfortunately, keeping the lens well-centered on the cornea during a lengthy and difficult vitreoretinal procedure can be satisfactory performed only by a good-willed and well-trained assistant. This apparently simple task may be difficult when the surgeon works under very high magnification. Under such circumstances it is difficult for the assistant to keep visual control on both the surgical field in the fundus and the position of the contact lens on the cornea because under very high magnification the external surgical field beyond the cornea is no longer in the field of observation provided by the microscope.

Prismatic Contact Lens

Plano concave contact lenses provide a clear view of the posterior pole. When the surgeon has to work in the equatorial region, however, rotation of the eye and tilting of the contact lens result in a distorted image of the fundus. Improved visualization of the peripheral fundus is obtained by using prismatic contact lenses.[9–10]

Biconcave Contact Lens

When the vitreous cavity of a phakic eye is filled with gas, the posterior surface of the crystalline lens becomes strongly refractive. The total refractive power of an emmetropic eye increases from 59 diopters to 102 diopters.[11] Thus the fundus cannot be seen through a plano concave lens. Biconcave contact lenses can reduce the refractive power of the eye to that of an emmetropic eye with a plano concave lens.[11] Various biconcave corneal contact lenses have been developed.[11–14] They allow for examination, argon laser photocoagulation, and cryotreatment of the posterior pole in the gas-filled phakic eye. The biconcave lens is routinely used for control of the central retinal artery on the optic disc after gas injection into the phakic eye.

Panfunduscope

The T-model of the Rodenstock Panfunduscope, originally designed for fundus observation during laser treatment, can also be used during vitreoretinal microsurgery.[15] The wide field of observation is the main advantage of the lens.

Although useful under certain circumstances, the panfunduscope cannot be used at the exclusion of other corneal lenses during vitreoretinal microsurgery. The main disadvantages of the lens are as follows: (1) the lens is rather cumbersome; (2) the field depth provided is poor; (3) the far periphery of the fundus cannot be seen; (4) the optical qualities of the lens are poor under very high magnification; (5) the lens gives an indirect image of the fundus.

A stereoscopic diagonal inverter adapted to the surgical microscope[6] makes it possible to overcome the latter disadvantage. The device permits the image of the fundus to be vertically inverted and laterally reversed. The main advantage of this equipment used in combination with the panfunduscope, which has been cut to allow easy access of the instruments through the pars plana, is to provide a stereoscopic and wide field of observation, even through a small pupil.

6

Instruments

Modifications have been made to instruments used in conventional retinal detachment surgery. A series of instruments conventionally used only for anterior segment microsurgery have been included with little or no modification in the set of instruments routinely used for retinal detachment repair. In addition, a series of instruments have been especially developed for retinal detachment microsurgery.

INSTRUMENTS FOR EXTERNAL SURGERY WITHOUT SIMULTANEOUS OBSERVATION OF THE FUNDUS

As in anterior segment surgery, use of the surgical microscope has led to miniaturization of the instruments. Indeed, use of the microscope points out the need for modifying some instruments in order to change the harmful and sometimes inaccurate macromanipulations of conventional surgery into less traumatic and more precise micromanipulations. Most instruments that were used for tissue dissection in conventional retinal detachment surgery are not used in retinal detachment microsurgery. Under the microscope magnification, those instruments appeared to be inappropriate for gentle and accurate dissection of the conjunctiva, Tenon's capsule, and sclera. The instruments presently used for tissue dissection and suturing are either instruments originally developed for anterior segment microsurgery or instruments of conventional retinal detachment surgery that have been modified according to the requirements of microsurgery (Fig. 14).

Instruments Initially Developed for Anterior Segment Microsurgery

A series of instruments that were originally developed for anterior segment microsurgery, such as the Bonn forceps, the Kuhnt-Bregeat straight needle, the needle holders, the corneal scissors, and the Castroviejo scissors are routinely used in retinal detachment microsurgery. Some of these instruments have been slightly modified so as to make their strength, length, and curvature more suitable for scleral surgery.

BONN FORCEPS

Bonn forceps are used for holding the conjunctiva and Tenon's capsule, holding the scleral flap during dissection and suturing of a lamellar scleral pocket, parting of the edges of the sclerotomy for subretinal fluid drainage, and holding the edges of pars plana sclerotomies during suturing. The claws and shaft of Bonn forceps used for scleral work have been made slightly stronger than those of Bonn forceps used for corneal work.

DIATHERMY FORCEPS

Diathermy forceps are used for precise hemostasis of conjunctival and episcleral vessels without unnecessary coagulation of adjacent tissues.

KUHNT-BREGEAT STRAIGHT NEEDLE

The Kuhnt-Bregeat straight needle for cataract discision is perfectly suitable for puncture of the choroid. Its slender tip makes such a tiny hole in the choroid that drainage can be accurately controlled. It is also used as the instrument of choice to perform anterior chamber paracentesis in phakic eyes.

SCISSORS

Castroviejo scissors and corneal scissors are used for dissection of periocular tissues.

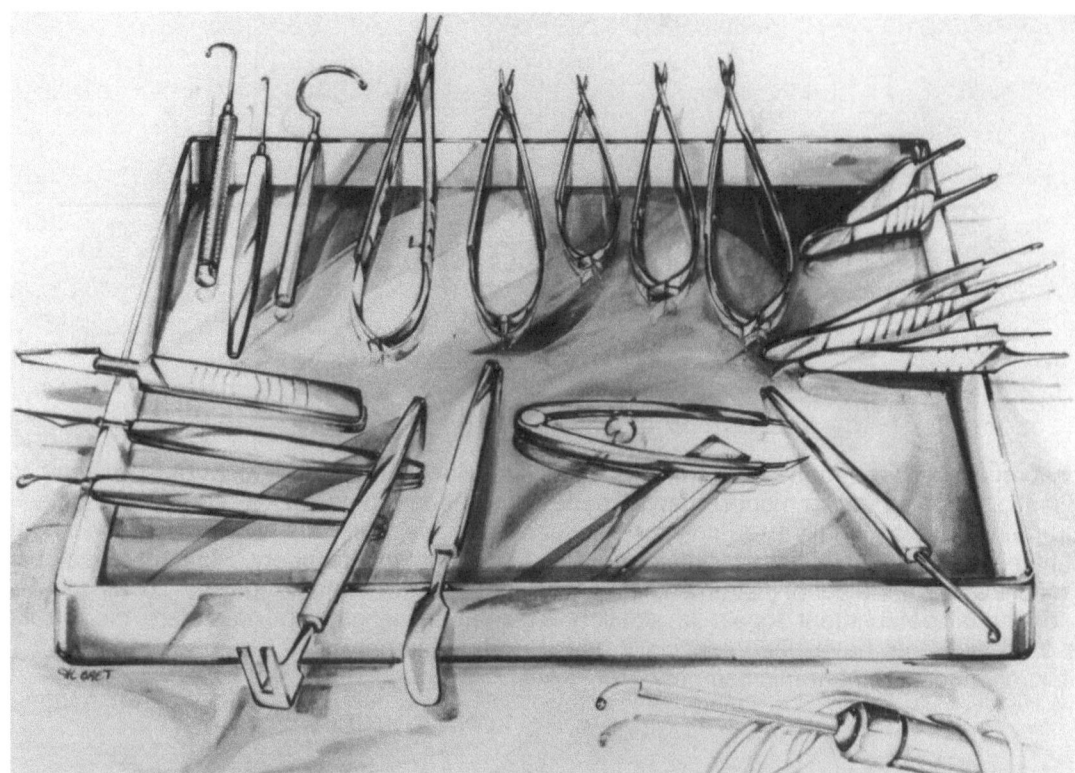

Figure 14. Basic set of instruments used in external surgery with and without simultaneous observation of the fundus. Clockwise from top left: Muscle hook, vortex vein hook, hook for scleral buckling of the posterior pole, needle-holder for thick needles, needle-holder for thin needles, Vannas blunt scissors, corneal scissors, Castroviejo scissors, Paufique forceps, Castroviejo forceps, Bonn forceps, scleral marker, compass, Bonn speculum, Gobin speculum, microdissector, discision straight needle, and razor-knife. A cryoprobe is in front of the instrument tray.

INSTRUMENTS OF DENUDATION OF VORTEX VEIN

When the retinal tear is located in a very posterior position behind a vortex vein ampulla, denudation of the intrascleral portion of the vein makes it possible to carry out a very posterior intrascleral implant without destroying the vortex vein.[16] Dissection of the scleral fibers around the vortex vein is performed with a Strampelli corneal microdissector and Vannas blunt scissors. A small blunt hook similar to the Thyrel iris hook is used for lifting the intrascleral part of the vortex vein, which has been exposed, in order to allow for the placing of fascia lata behind and beneath the vein.

Modified Instruments of Conventional Retinal Detachment Surgery

Instruments originally designed for conventional retinal detachment surgery, such as the muscle hook and needle holders, have been modified so as to be easily maneuvered under the surgical microscope. Shortening of the instrument handle is a common modification. Instrument handles are shortened to eliminate any risk of inadvertent contact with the microscope. The common rule is to keep the instrument handle just long enough to extend from the tip of semiflexed fingers to the thumb cleft.[17–18] The handle thickness of most conventional instruments, and in particular the needle holders, was decreased so as to increase precision of instrument grip. Three types of needle holders are used depending on the thickness and shape of the needles used. A needle holder with thin jaws and a short shaft is used for sutures 0–7 or thinner. A stronger needle holder with a longer shaft is used for needles mounted on thicker sutures. Needle holders with concave-convex jaws are helpful for holding round-bodied needles.

The shaft of instruments used in the close vicinity of the posterior pole, in particular forceps and scissors, is also modified. As a general rule shaft thick-

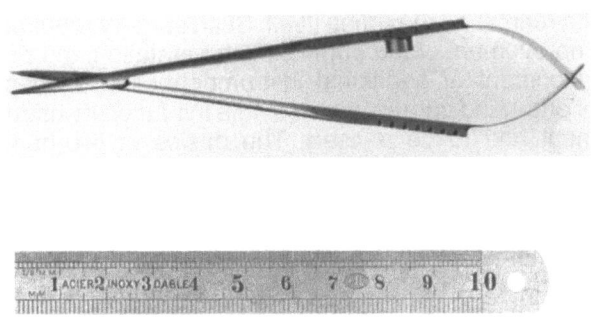

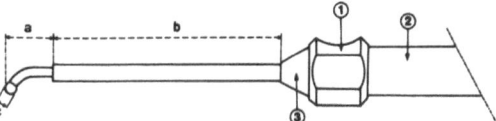

Figure 17. Diagram of the cryoprobe for retinal detachment surgery under microscope. 1: reference point on the handle where the surgeon places index finger; 2: protective capsule; 3: conical connection; a: 10 mm; b: 50 mm; and c: 2.5 mm [Optikon (Rome)].

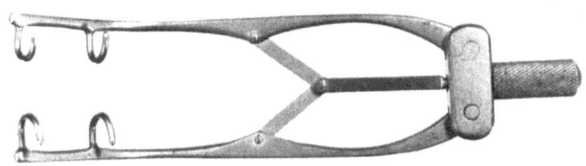

Figure 15. Microscissors for tissue dissection in the retroequatorial region [Moria (Paris)].

ness is decreased and shaft length increased to facilitate instrument maneuvering in the retroequatorial region[19] (Fig. 15).

Use of the most appropriate instrument for each surgical step is most important so as to produce the least damage to ocular tissues and keep the qualities of the most fragile instruments.

INSTRUMENTS FOR EXTERNAL SURGERY WITH SIMULTANEOUS OBSERVATION OF THE FUNDUS

Most of the instruments used when the three-mirror contact lens is held on the cornea have been modified so as to make maneuvering of the instruments along the sclera easier.[20]

Eyelid Speculum

On the usual eyelid speculum the stems holding the posterior face of the eyelids hinder the shifting

of the marker, the scleral depressor, and the cryoprobe between the upper and the lower quadrants of the sclera and the orbit wall. Therefore, the Castroviejo eyelid speculum has been modified. Each stem has been replaced by two blunt hooks that less impede the passage of the instruments along the sclera (Fig. 16).

Scleral Marker

The Meyer-Schwickerath marker is perfectly suitable for locating the retinal tear under biomicroscopic control of the fundus, since its handle is thin and suitably long.

Cryoprobe

The cryoprobes available in conventional retinal detachment surgery are too thick and too short to be easily shifted between the orbit wall and the eyeball covered by the contact lens.

To date the most suitable cryoprobe for retinal detachment surgery under biomicroscopic control of the fundus is shown in figures 17 and 18. This

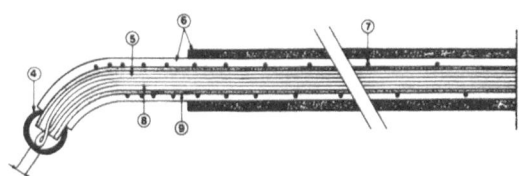

Figure 18. Cutaway cross section of the cryoprobe for retinal detachment microsurgery. 4: the active tip of silver; 5: the thermocouple; 6: the isolation sheath; 7: resistance for keeping the outer part of the cryoprobe at room temperature; 8: thermocouple; stainless-steel tube [Optikon (Rome)].

Figure 16. Castroviejo eyelid speculum modified for retinal detachment surgery under microscope. The stems holding the posterior faces of the eyelids have been replaced by two blunt hooks [Moria (Paris)].

cryoprobe is thin and long enough to reach the most posterior retinal breaks without rotating the eye or inducing passage of air between the contact lens and the cornea. An insulating sheath covers the whole length except for the active tip (Figs. 17 and 18), and prevents freezing of the conjunctiva and Tenon's capsule. The small size of the active tip allows for great accuracy in cryoapplication. This cryoprobe is manufactured by the Optikon Company (Rome).

Movable Scleral Depressor Attached to the Contact Lens

A movable scleral depressor attached to the contact lens is sometimes necessary when the retinal break is treated by argon laser photocoagulation before the positioning of the buckle.

The various movable scleral depressors attached to the contact lens, which are available for preoperative examination, are not suitable for surgical use because the funnel is too cumbersome.

The author uses a model designed by the Ophtalux cie. It has the following characteristics: it is adaptable on the three-mirror contact lens number 630, manufactured by Haag Streit; the space taken up by the attachment to the contact lens is reduced to a minimum (height: 18.8 mm, minimum diameter: 18.2 mm, maximum diameter: 35 mm); and the stem of the depressor is malleable steel.

INSTRUMENTS FOR VITREORETINAL ENDOMICROSURGERY

Since the introduction of closed vitrectomy by Machemer[2] and Klöti[3] in the early 1970s, instrumentation and techniques for vitreoretinal endomicrosurgery have been significantly improved by a number of surgeons and technicians[4,21–35]

The primary instrument for vitreous gel removal still maintains the basic characteristics that make such surgery feasible. Satisfactory removal of the vitreous gel can only be achieved with an instrument that simultaneously aspirates and cuts the vitreous components. The basic characteristics of the instrumentation were originally developed by Parel and Machemer.[2] However, with the development of closed vitrectomy, it soon appeared that, under many circumstances removal of the vitreous gel was only part of more complicated surgical procedures. To achieve retinal reattachment the surgeon had to deal directly with membranes in close relationship with

the retina and the retina itself. Such surgery required improvement of the original instrumentation and development of additional instruments. The concept of one-hand surgery with a single full-function instrument had to be revised. The basics of two-hand endosurgery with two or three entry sites through the pars plana were primarily developed by O'Malley.[24] Simultaneous miniaturization of the instruments, improvements of the vitreous machines, and development of additional instruments have made it possible to perform sophisticated vitreoretinal microsurgery. There is no doubt that the instrumentation currently used will still be improved in the future.

Automation, miniaturization, distant control rather than manual command, and specialization are the main requirements of instruments used in vitreoretinal endomicrosurgery.

Vitreous Probe

Removal of the vitreous gel is satisfactorily achieved with an instrument that permits the surgeon to simultaneously aspirate and cut the vitreous components.[2]

ASPIRATION SYSTEMS

Aspiration of the vitreous components into the vitreous probe was initially achieved manually. It was performed by the assistant with a syringe connected to the aspiration tube of the vitreous probe. Manual aspiration had several disadvantages. It required a skillful and well-trained assistant. Control of the suction pressure had to rely on adequate manual manipulation of the syringe by the assistant, according to his or her own observation of vitreous motions at the port of the vitreous probe. The onset of aspiration was quite abrupt. Monitoring the suction force according to vitreous movements into the port was uneasy and rather approximate. These disadvantages could result in hazardous surgery when the instrument port was in the close vicinity of a detached retina.

Better control of suction pressure was achieved with a mechanical syringe drive,[30] which eliminated the hazards of manual manipulation. The peristaltic pump system[34] was another step towards the improvement of suction control during vitrectomy. At present linear suction systems[26–35] provide the best control of suction forces to be used during vitrectomy. The maximum suction pressure to be safely used during the procedure is preset on the vitreous console before starting the operation. During vitrectomy, the suction force, under the preset maximum level, is controlled by the surgeon with a foot-pedal. The more the surgeon presses the foot pedal, the more suction is obtained up to the preset maximum. At any time a sound signal of increasing intensity informs the surgeon of the suction pressure which is being used. The suction force is monitored by the surgeon through visual observation of vitreous movements at the port of the vitreous probe and in any part of the vitreous cavity that is in the observation field. A basic rule of vitrectomy is to use the minimal suction force sufficient to remove vitreous gel. The linear suction system makes it easy to apply this basic rule. Elimination of abrupt onset of suction is another major advantage of linear suction systems.

CUTTING DEVICES

Vitreous cutters can be divided into two groups, the linear and the oscillating type cutters. Both systems have proven to be efficient. The original oscillating systems had the main disadvantage of winding vitreous gel around the rotating blade when the blade was not sharp enough. This led to excessive vitreore-

tinal traction and could result in severe retinal complications. The introduction of alternating rotating movements of the blades has removed this major disadvantage. Whatever system, sharpness of the cutting device is imperative. Although obvious, this requirement is apparently not recognized by the many vitreous systems presently available on the market. Sharpness of the cutter device should last long enough to make it possible to use the same instrument at maximum efficiency for successive numerous surgical procedures. Resharpening of the instruments should also be possible. In the author's experience, the vitreous stripper designed by Ortli at the request of Klöti[35] perfectly fulfills the requisite qualities for adequate cutting of the vitreous components and prolonged utilization of the same instrument before resharpening becomes necessary (Fig. 19). The outer cutting tube of the guillotine like system can be placed into three different positions. Hence if it appears during the surgical procedure that cutting is no longer satisfactory, the surgeon can place the trephination tube into the next position and a new perfectly cutting segment is immediately at the surgeon's disposal.

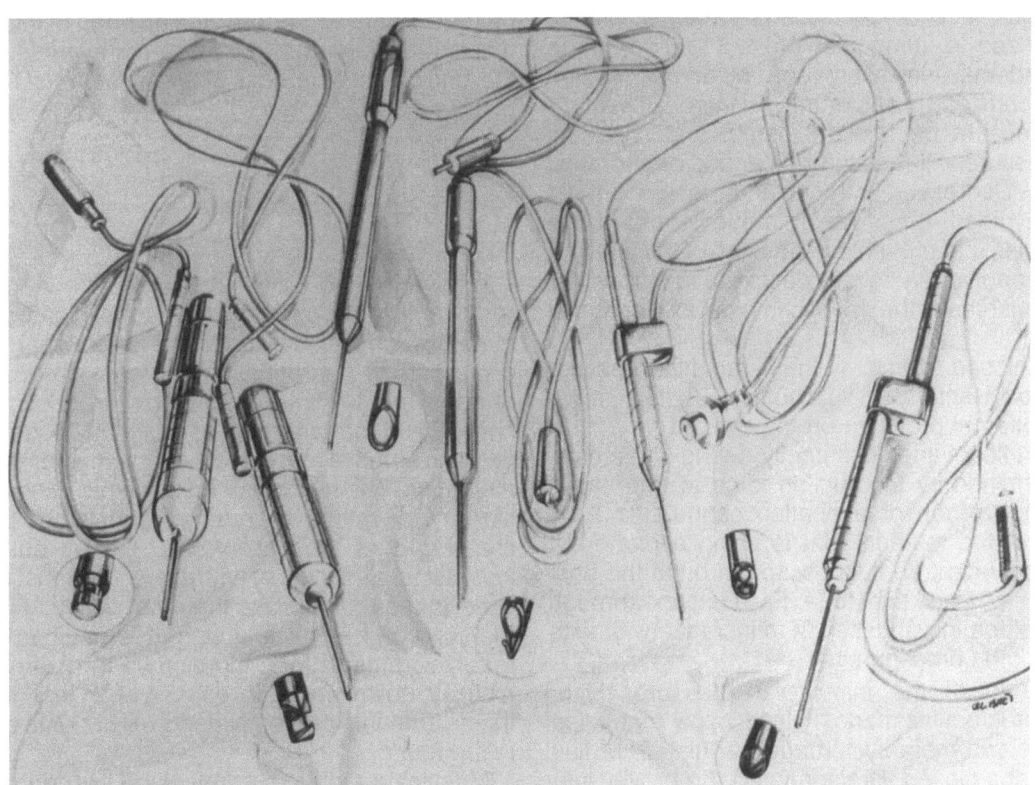

Figure 19. Basic set of instruments used in vitreous surgery for retinal detachment management. From left to right: vitreous stripper, automatic microscissors, fiberoptic probe, hooked fiberoptic probe, combined fiberoptic and suction probe, and bipolar endodiathermy [Örtli (St. Gallen, Switzerland)].

Infusion Systems

Fluid infusion into the vitreous cavity is necessary during closed vitrectomy in order to compensate fluid outflow and maintain the intraocular pressure. On the initial full function probe, the infusion system was part of the working instrument.[2,3] At present an infusion sleeve can still be adjusted to any of the working instruments, however, this infusion system is rarely used. Under most circumstances, an infusion cannula separate from the working instrument is more advantageous.[34] A separate infusion cannula offers three main advantages: (1) it decreases the diameter of the working instrument; (2) it increases the distance between the infusion and suction ports and decreases the turbulence within the vitreous cavity; and (3) it makes it easy to perform simultaneous fluid-gas exchange.

Intraocular Pressure Control

The intraocular pressure should be kept close to physiological level during closed vitrectomy. Significant increase in intraocular pressure will result in corneal edema, which prevents clear observation of the vitreous cavity and retina. An increase in intraocular pressure beyond the retinal and choroidal blood pressure will result in retinal and/or choroidal ischemia. Decreased intraocular pressure should also be avoided. It can result in miosis and striate corneal folds that prevent observation of the vitreous cavity. In addition, a severe decrease in intraocular pressure increases the risk of choroidal and/or retinal bleeding.

During closed vitrectomy the intraocular pressure depends on 3 factors: (1) fluid outflow, (2) fluid inflow, and (3) external pressure on the eye.

Fluid outflow varies constantly during vitrectomy. It is determined by the suction force at the port of the vitreous probe or aspiration cannula and the viscosity of the material that is being aspirated. It is also dependent on fluid escape through the pars plana incisions and pilot tube. Fluid escape through the pars plana incisions tends to increase with time during lengthy procedures.

Monitoring of the intraocular pressure during closed vitrectomy is made by fluid inflow regulation. There are two main systems for regulation of fluid inflow during closed vitrectomy: (1) the gravity infusion system and (2) the electronic feedback system.

In the gravity infusion system, fluid infusion is determined by the bottle height and the diameter and length of the tubing system from the bottle to the cannula introduced through the pars plana. Fluid infusion can be increased by increasing the bottle height and vice versa. Simplicity and low cost are the two main advantages of the gravity infusion system. Lack of accuracy and time required for modification of the bottle height by the nurse during the surgical procedure are the two main disadvantages.

In the electronic feedback system, fluid infusion is determined by intraocular pressure. Intraocular pressure is measured several thousand times per second. The information is transmitted at any time to a computer that controls a peristaltic pump. The intraocular pressure to be maintained during the surgical procedure is preset before starting surgery. Decreased intraocular pressure will automatically and instantly result in fluid infusion increase and restoration of the preset intraocular pressure level. Similarly, increased intraocular pressure will automatically and instantly result in a decrease or a stop of intraocular inflow. The preset intraocular pressure level can be modified at any time during vitrectomy, merely by rotating a button of the vitrectomy console. Accuracy of intraocular pressure control, and the easiness and rapidity of any modification of the pressure level during the surgical procedure are the two main advantages of the electronic system. The system permits the surgeon to concentrate attention on the surgical procedure with no need to think about the intraocular pressure level being monitored by the computer. The cost of the system is the main disadvantage.

Additional Instruments

In complicated retinal detachments, vitreous gel removal is only part of more sophisticated procedures, which include additional maneuvers such as dissection of periretinal membranes, repositioning of an inverted retina, removal of intraocular foreign bodies, and management of bleeding vessels. Each of these surgical maneuvers requires specific instrumentation. The number of instruments used in endosurgery for retinal detachment repair has been increasing over the past years. This is due to the increasing audacity of vitreous surgeons and the specific requirements of the most difficult situations the surgeon has to deal with. It is obvious that the list of instruments for endomicrosurgery remains potentially unlimited. It is conceivable that some of the instruments presently used will become obsolete in the future.

Most instruments currently used in endomicrosurgery for retinal detachment repair have the same basic characteristics: (1) miniaturization of the working tip, (2) standardization of the shaft diameter, (3) specialization for specific function, (4) automation with remote control, and (5) lightweight for limiting hand fatigue (Fig. 19).

VITREOUS SCISSORS

Vitreous scissors are used for cutting dense vitreous strands that cannot be aspirated and cut with the aspirating vitreous probe. They are also used for segmentation of the condensed posterior vitreous face and segmentation of preretinal membranes. At present automatic microscissors with remote command are used in most circumstances. The membrane peeler-cutter, designed by Grieshaber at Machemer's request was the first instrument based on this concept.[33] Since then other manufacturers have designed vitreous scissors with similar characteristics. The author uses Klöti's microscissors manufactured by Ortli. They are 20 gauge for compatibility with the incision size and used with the same console and foot pedal as the vitrectomy system. The cutting rate is controlled with the foot pedal. It can also be used for single cutting strokes. The blades are right angled so as to facilitate segmentation of epiretinal membranes. Only the upperblade is moving. The bottom blade is nonmoving so as to decrease retinal trauma. The characteristics of the automatic microscissors have enhanced the safety and versatility of preretinal membrane surgery.[33] In spite of miniaturization, however, the nonmoving blade is still too large in selected circumstances. The ideal automatic microscissors should have an interchangeable working tip with several types of blades. In addition to automatic microscissors, a variety of other vitreous scissors such as Sourdille's reverse scissors[36] manufactured by Grieshaber may be useful in selected circumstances. Each surgeon has his or her own preference and personal instruments.

VITREOUS FORCEPS

The retinal microsurgeon should have at his or her disposal a set of different vitreous forceps for removal of intraocular foreign bodies. The shape and size of each forceps should be adapted to the size and shape of any intraocular foreign body to be removed.

Except for intraocular foreign body removal, the indications for use of intravitreal forceps are infrequent in endosurgery for retinal detachment repair. Microforceps with remote or hand control can be used to hold preretinal membranes during bimanual delamination and segmentation. However, membrane holding with an aspirating cannula connected to linear aspiration system is less traumatic than any forceps. The aspiration cannula allows the surgeon to lift preretinal membranes with minimal traction on the underlying retina. Hand fatigue is limited to a minimum. The fiberoptic attached to the cannula allows bimanual endosurgery without additional endoillumination.

MEMBRANE DELAMINATORS

A large variety of membrane delaminators have been designed (see p. 245).

INSTRUMENTS DESIGNED FOR ANTERIOR SEGMENT MICROSURGERY

A variety of instruments that have been designed for anterior segment microsurgery can be used for endomicrosurgery through the pars plana. Such is the case for the Kuhnt-Bregeat straight needle and a variety of blunt spatulas. The Kuhnt-Bregeat straight needle used for needling of secondary cataracts in anterior segment surgery is useful for making a hole in a condensed posterior vitreous face, which cannot be aspirated and opened by the vitreous probe. Spatulas are used for delamination of preretinal membranes and freeing synechiae between the iris and the anterior vitreous surface.

BIPOLAR ENDODIATHERMY

A bipolar coaxial microprobe for endodiathermy is used for coagulation of bleeding vessels. The current flows only at the probe tip. The very small size of the instrument active tip allows pinpoint coagulations of small bleeding vessels. The probe is connected to the vitreous console and the current is monitored with a foot pedal. The instrument provides the minimum level necessary for coagulation. The probe can be used safely on the retina surface and close to the optic nerve head. It is also used for direct coagulation of the retina, in particular when the surgeon wants to make a landmark on the margin of a retinal tear to facilitate further localization of the tear through a gas bubble. The coagulation should be light and the instrument withdrawn from the retina very gently. Coagulation at too high a level would result in the sticking of the instrument to the retina and rapid withdrawal of the instrument may create a new retinal tear.

INTRAOCULAR MAGNET

An intraocular magnet is useful for removal of magnetic foreign bodies. The instrument should be powerful and the magnetic force must be focused at the tip of the magnet so that the magnetic foreign body is pulled towards the magnet tip.

In conclusion, at present, the ideal equipment for

endomicrosurgery should embody the following features: (1) linear aspiration controlled by the surgeon, (2) electronic feedback system for automated control of the intraocular pressure, (3) a single foot pedal for control of the linear aspiration and all automated instruments, such as the vitreous cutter, scissors, forceps, bipolar endodiathermy, endolaser, and cryoprobe; (4) a single console for connection of all instruments cables; and (5) clear labelling of all cables for easy, rapid, and error-free assistance of the operating room staff during the surgical procedure.

A large variety of instruments for use through the pars plana should be at the surgeon's disposal. All instruments should have the same shaft diameter to minimize as much fluid escape through the incisions as possible. At present, 20 gauge is the standard size, however, it is conceivable that the standard size could be decreased in the future with improved miniaturization of the instruments. The smaller the pars plana incisions, the less likelihood of postoperative complications related to tissue incarceration in the wound.

Illumination for Endomicrosurgery

Adequate illumination of the surgical field during endomicrosurgery can be obtained with either the operating microscope or fiberoptic probes. Each illumination system has its own advantages and disadvantages, and each of the illumination can be considered more advantageous under selected circumstances than the others. Therefore, one illumination device should never be used at the exclusion of the others.

EXOILLUMINATION WITH THE OPERATING MICROSCOPE

Coaxial Illumination. Coaxial illumination of the operating microscope is rarely used for endomicrosurgery with the microscopes presently available for retinal detachment microsurgery. When used in conjunction with a contact lens, the reflexes of coaxial light on the anterior surface of the corneal lens prevent adequate visualization of the vitreous gel and retina. Coaxial illumination is only used when working in the anterior part of the vitreous gel in aphakic eyes. In this specific circumstance no contact lens is used. The anterior vitreous surface and its relationship with the iris and corneal wound are better seen with coaxial illumination than any of the other illumination devices.

Coaxial illumination can also be used to look at the posterior part of the fundus in phakic eyes after intravitreal gas injection. No corneal lens is used. The microscope should be focused 4 cm above the cornea. An inverted image of the fundus is obtained. The increased working distance from the patient is a disadvantage.

Slit Lamp Illumination. Slit lamp illumination is used as the only mode of illumination during three steps of endomicrosurgery: (1) at the beginning of the procedure to verify (along with the three-mirror contact lens) the position of the infusion cannula inserted through the pars plana, (2) at the end of endosurgery for examination of the peripheral fundus before placing the sutures on the incisions of the pars plana, and (3) for observation of the fundus after gas injection in aphakic eyes.

During vitrectomy, slit lamp illumination is used in combination with endo illumination. In this circumstance the slit beam is used to improve stereopsis rather than for illumination of the vitreous cavity. The slit beam provides an optical cross section of the surgical field and gives landmarks for localization of the posterior surface of the lens and the retina.

ENDOILLUMINATION WITH FIBEROPTICS

At present, endoillumination with fiberoptics is the most effective modality for illumination of the endosurgical field. The fiberoptic illumination system can be attached or separate from the working instrument.

Fiberoptic Illumination System Attached to the Working Instruments. Initially the fiberoptic illumination system was attached to the full function vitreous probe.[2–3] At present such attachment is rarely used. An increase in instrument diameter is the main disadvantage. In addition, the fiberoptics attached to the vitreous probe illuminates only the cutter tip and surrounding vitreous.

The fiberoptic endoillumination can be combined with any of the working instruments. In addition to the suction cannula, the retinal hook and delaminator are the most commonly used. The shaft diameter of these instruments combined with the fiberoptics is 20 gauge. The combination of fiberoptic illumination with working instruments makes true bimanual endomicrosurgery feasible.

Fiberoptic Separate from the Working Instruments. Fiberoptic endoilluminators separate from the working instruments provide the best illumination of the surgical field. The illumination system can be either mobile or sutured to the pars plana. Mobile illuminating probes are the most commonly used. The probe is held by one of the surgeon's hands. It can be oriented in any direction and allows for illumination of any part of the fundus. It allows for retro illumination, which provides the best visualization of clear vitreous gel.

The fiberoptic endoilluminator separate from the working instruments can also be combined with the infusion cannula in the pars plana region.[36] This attachment enables the surgeon to use two working instruments simultaneously. The fiberoptic provides a 55 degree field of observation. The light can be moved into several directions by the assistant.

Powerful light sources for fundus illumination are useful during certain steps of endomicrosurgery and for making photographs and films. However the vitreous surgeon should keep in mind the retinal hazards of light toxicity (see p. 66).

LASER INSTRUMENTATION FOR INTRAOPERATIVE USE

Argon laser photocoagulation is the only laser treatment currently used during surgery for retinal detachment repair. Argon laser photocoagulation treatment during surgery can be performed either through the pupil or through the pars plana.

Instrumentation for Argon Laser Photocoagulation through the Pupil

The attachment of the argon laser to the surgical microscope[37] consists of four components: (1) fiberoptics that can be connected to either side of the microscope, (2) an optical system that makes the laser beam parallel and allows for focusing it on the retina, (3) a micromanipulator that allows for moving the laser beam within a field of 8 × 10 mm and (4) a protecting filter for the surgeon (Fig. 20). The protecting filter is automatically set into action when the surgeon presses the laser foot command. The position of the protecting filter is controlled by a computer. The laser beam can be delivered only when the protecting filter is in the proper position.

The equipment enables argon laser photocoagulation to be performed during surgery under the same optical conditions as with an argon laser connected to a slit lamp for photocoagulation in a seated patient. The slit lamp of the microscope is used for observing the fundus during laser treatment. The laser fiberoptics is connected to the surgical microscope only when the surgeon has to perform photocoagulation treatment. Connecting and disconnecting the fiberoptics to or from the microscope is most rapid.

The equipment can be used in any surgical procedure for retinal detachment management.

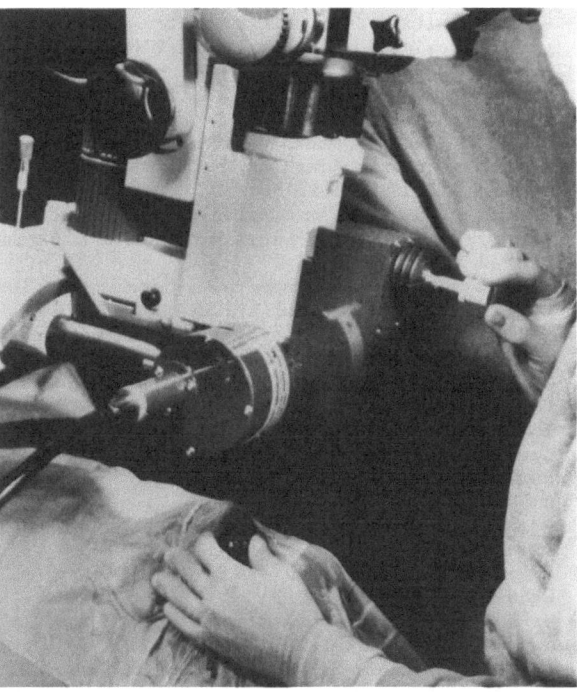

Figure 20. Instrumentation for intraoperative argon laser photocoagulation. Attachment of the biophysic medical argon laser to the Zeiss OPMI 6 microscope.

Instrumentation for Endolaser Photocoagulation

The instrumentation for endolaser photocoagulation via the pars plana is made up of the same laser source, surgeon's protecting filter, and foot command as for photocoagulation through the pupil. The only additional item of equipment necessary is the fiberoptic and laser probe for endophotocoagulation. The probe is 0.89 mm in diameter. The laser beam and endoillumination are conducted by the same probe.

In the future other types of lasers will likely be available for intraoperative use. In particular, continuous wave CO_2 wetfield laser,[38–40] Yag laser,[41–42] and endoexcimer laser systems may be routinely used in the future to cut vitreous strands. A contact laser scalpel using a Yag laser and sapphire rod tip for trans-scleral burns may also be available.[43]

REFERENCES

1. Dominguez A: Oftalmoscopia cinematografica de imagen invertida. Arch Soc Espan Ophthalmol 41:701–702, 1981
2. Machemer R, Parel JM, Buettner H: A new concept for vitreous surgery. 1—Instrumentation. Am J Ophthalmol 73, 1:1–7, 1972

3. Klöti R: Vitrecktomie: ein neves instrument Für die hintere vitrecktomie. Graefe's Arch Klin Exp Ophthalmol 187:161–170, 1973

4. Parel JM, Machemer R, Aumayr W: A nex concept for vitreous surgery. 4—Improvements in instrumentation and illumination. Am J Ophthalmol 77:6–12, 1974

5. Spitznas M: A binocular indirect ophthalmomicroscope (BIOM) for non contact wide-angle vitreous surgery. Graefe's Arch Klin Exp Ophthalmol 225:13–15, 1987

6. Spitznas M, Reiner J: A stereoscopic diagonal inverter (SDI) for wide-angle vitreous surgery. Graefe's Arch Klin Exp Ophthalmol 225:9–12, 1987

7. Urrets-Zavalia A: Retinal surgery under the microscope. Dev Ophthalmol Karger, Basel, 1981, Vol 2, 195–201

8. Urrets-Zavalia A: New concepts and techniques for retinal detachment under microscope control, in Boyd Highlights of ophthalmology, Silver University Vol. 1 pp. 264–277 Tennessee, Kingsport Press, 1982

9. Tolentino FI, Freeman HM: A new lens for closed pars plana vitrectomy. Arch Ophthalmol 97:2197–2198, 1979

10. Stenkula S: A new type of contact lens for vitrectomy. Am J Ophthalmol 87:575–576, 1977

11. Landers MB, Stefansson E, Wolbarsht ML: The optic of vitreous surgery. Am J Ophthalmol 91:611–614, 1981

12. Sebestyen JG: Biconcave contact lens for vitreous surgery. Am J Ophthalmol 87:719–720, 1977

13. Sebestyen JG: An improved contact lens for trans pars plana vitreous surgery. Am J Ophthalmol 93:122–123, 1982

14. Stefansson E, Mc Cuen BW, Mc Pherson SD: Biconcave contact lens for examination and laser treatment of the fundus in normal and gas-filled phakic eyes. Am J Ophthalmol 98:806–807, 1984

15. Malbran ES: Methods for improved observation of vitreoretinal cavity, in Boyd Highlights of Ophthalmology—Atlas and textbook of microsurgery and laser surgery. 30th Anniversary, Vol 1, 64–70, Tennessee, Kingsport Press, 1985

16. Bonnet M: Les avantages de la chirurgie sous microscope du décollement de la rétine Bull Soc Ophthalmol Fr 1975, 75:1111–1112

17. Patkin M: Ergonomics and microsurgery Excerpta Medica International Congress N° 465 Microsurgery Proceedings at the 5th International Congress of the International microsurgical society, Bonn, October 4–7, 1978, pp 305–308

18. Patkin M: Selection and care of microsurgical instruments Adv ophthalmol (Karger, Basel) 37:23–33, 1978

19. Bonnet M, Nagao M: Poche sclerale sur le pôle postérieur dans le traitement des décollements de la rétine par trou maculaire J Fr Ophthalmol 5, 8–9, 505–513, 1982

20. Bonnet M: Biomicroscopy of the ocular fundus during retinal detachment surgery Ocular therapy surgery 1–2, 50–54, 1982

21. O'Malley C, Heintz RM: Vitrectomy with an alternative instrument system. Ann Ophthalmol 7:585–594, 1975

22. Freeman HM, Schepens CL, Tolentino FI: The current status of vitreous membrane surgery. Mod Probl Ophthalmol 15:261–271, 1975

23. Douvas NG: Microsurgical roto-extractor instrument for vitrectomy. Mod Probl Ophthalmol Vol 15:253–260, 1975

24. O'Malley C, Heintz RM: Advances in Vitreous Surgery. Springfield Il, Charles C. Thomas Publishers, 1976

25. O'Malley C, Tripp RM, Heintz RM: Recent modifications in closed eye intraocular surgery, in Mc Pherson A (ed): New and Controversial Aspects of Vitreoretinal Surgery. St. Louis, C.V. Mosby Company, 1977, 190–194

26. Federman JL: The "site" instrument (suction infusion tissue extractor), in Mc Pherson A (ed): New and Controversial Aspects in Vitreoretinal Surgery. St. Louis, C.V. Mosby Company, 1977, 184–189

27. Karlin D: Ultrasonic and laser techniques in vitreoretinal surgery in Mc Pherson A (ed): New and Controversial Aspects in Vitreoretinal Surgery, St. Louis, C.V. Mosby Company, 1977, 274–280

28. Klöti R: What is the present status of pars plana vitreous surgery in Zurich? Mod Probl Ophthalmol 18:187–194, 1977

29. L'Esperance FA: Vitreolysis. Mod Probl Ophthalmol 18:224–235, 1977

30. Charles S: Ancillary techniques for pars plana vitrectomy, in Mc Pherson A (ed): New and Controversial Aspects of Vitreoretinal Surgery, St. Louis, C.V. Mosby Company, 1977, 195–198

31. Spitznas M: New developments in instrumentation for vitreous surgery. Mod Probl Ophthalmol 18:201–204, 1977

32. Machemer R: Present status of pars plana vitreous surgery in Miami. Mod Probl Ophthalmol 18:180–182, 1977

33. Parel JM, Machemer R, Blankenship G, Hickingbotham D, Nose I, Denham D, Aumay R: The membrane peeler-cutter. Poster 33 Annual meeting, American Academy Ophthalmology, 1980

34. Charles S: Vitreous microsurgery. Baltimore, Williams and Wilkins, 1981

35. Klöti R: From vitreous loss to vitrectomy Ophthalmologica 187/2:108–113, 1983

36. Sourdille Ph: Instrumentation review. 5th Vail vitreoretinal seminar, March 9–14, 1986

37. Bonnet M: Adaptation du laser á l'argon sur le microscope opératoire. J Fr Ophthalmol 13, 2:127–128, 1980

38. Miller JB, Smith MS, Pi F, Stockert M: Transvitreal carbon dioxide laser photocautery and vitrectomy. Ophthalmology 85:1195–1200, 1978

39. Karlin DB, Patel CK, Wood OR, Llovera I: CO_2 laser in vitreoretinal surgery 1—quantitative investigation of the effects of CO_2 laser radiation on ocular tissue. Ophthalmology 86:290–298, 1979

40. Miller JB, Smith MR, Boyer DS: Miniaturized intraocular carbon dioxide laser photosurgical system for multi-incision vitrectomy. Ophthalmology 88:440–442, 1981

41. Frankhauser F, Kwasniewska S, Van Der Zypen E: Vitreolysis with the q-switched laser Arch Ophthalmol 103:1166–1171, 1985

42. Williams G: Development of an endoexcimer laser system. 5th Vail vitreoretinal seminar, March 9–14, 1986

42. Fumitaka A, Federman J: Contact laser scalpel in the management of severe diabetic retinopathy and for retinal photocoagulation. 5th Vail vitreoretinal seminar, March 9–14, 1986

III

Surgical Technique

7

Fundus Examination During Surgery

Two methods are used for fundus examination during retinal detachment microsurgery: (1) biomicroscopy using the slit illuminator and a contact lens and (2) indirect ophthalmoscopy using the microscope and a 40 diopter lens. In addition to this, endoillumination and special devices are used during vitrectomy (see p. 40).

BIOMICROSCOPY OF THE FUNDUS AND THE VITREOUS CAVITY

In microsurgical management of retinal detachment, intraoperative observation of the ocular fundus and vitreous cavity is mainly done using the microscope slit illuminator in conjunction with the Goldmann three-mirror contact lens.[1-8] Use of other techniques for fundus examination are restricted to selected circumstances (see p. 40). Biomicroscopic examination of the fundus can be carried out at any stage of the surgical procedure, whatever the surgical technique used for retinal detachment repair. Biomicroscopy is also routinely used for simultaneous visualization of the fundus during certain surgical steps such as, in particular, localization of the retinal breaks, cryotreatment, and fluid-gas exchange.

In order to overcome the particular difficulties of biomicroscopic observation of the ocular fundus during surgery, certain simple general rules must be followed.

The particular difficulties of biomicroscopy of the fundus during surgery are due to the following: the patient is in a supine position, the conjunctiva is incised, and precise manipulation should be performed while observing the fundus through the microscope.

The difficulties are easily overcome if the following precautions are taken: correct position, efficient protection of the cornea, and precise hemostasis.

Correct Position

The microscope and its slit illuminator, the contact lens, the surgeon and the patient's eye should all be in the correct position.

POSITION OF THE SURGICAL MICROSCOPE

For easy examination of the entire fundus with the slit illuminator in conjunction with the three-mirror contact lens, the observation axis of the microscope must be parallel to the optical axis of the patient's eye. In most cases the patient's eye is immobilized in the straight ahead position, therefore, the microscope observation axis should be strictly perpendicular to the center of the cornea.

In simple retinal detachments with a single retinal break or contiguous breaks located in the same quadrant, intraoperative observation of the fundus is often restricted to the retinal break(s) area and the optic disc. In such cases it may be advantageous to slightly tilt the microscope. The microscope observation axis is slightly tilted towards the surgeon when the surgeon is seated in front of the retinal quadrant where the break(s) is/are located. It is tilted in the opposite direction when the surgeon is seated opposite the retinal break quadrant.

POSITION OF THE SLIT ILLUMINATOR

Biomicroscopic examination of the fundus mandatorily requires that the slit illuminator be positioned at a 5° to 8° angle. With such a narrow angle, the slit beam will pass very close to the center of the pupil. Thus it will reach the retina even when the pupil is not widely dilated. In addition slit illumination of the retina coincides with the observation axis (Fig. 21).

The slit illuminator should not be placed at a central position between both eyepieces of the microscope. In fact, if the slit lamp were to be placed at a central position, the angle of the beam would be zero; therefore, observation of the fundus in an optical cross section would no longer be possible since the views of the various planes would be placed exactly on top of each other. When the beam angle is zero, biomicroscopic examination is not used, but rather binocular observation under focused illumination (Fig. 22).

The slit illuminator should not be positioned at an angle superior to 10°. With such a wide angle, the slit beam passing through the contact lens will coincide with the periphery of the pupil or even the iris. Thus the slit illumination cannot reach the fundus

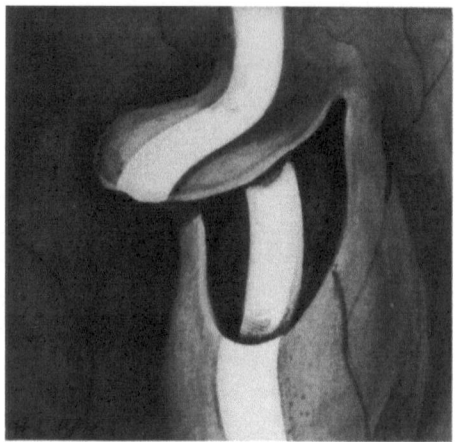

Figure 22. View of a retinal tear obtained by placing the slit illuminator at a central position between both eye pieces of the microscope. The retinal tear is observed under focused slit illumination rather than in an optical cross-section.

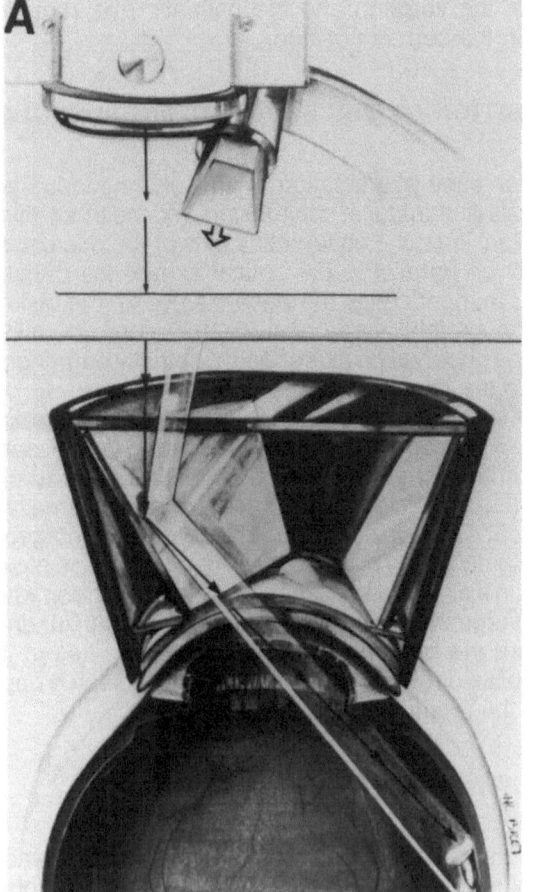

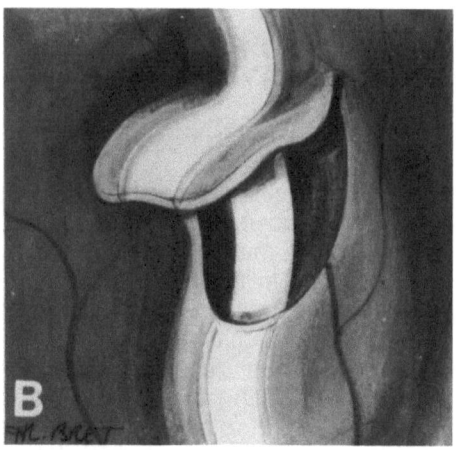

Figure 21. Correct position of the slit illuminator for biomicroscopic examination of the fundus using the three-mirror contact lens. (A) The slit illuminator is approximately at a 5° angle; slit illumination of the fundus coincides with the observation axis. (B) Optical cross-section of retinal tear obtained by placing the slit illuminator at 5°.

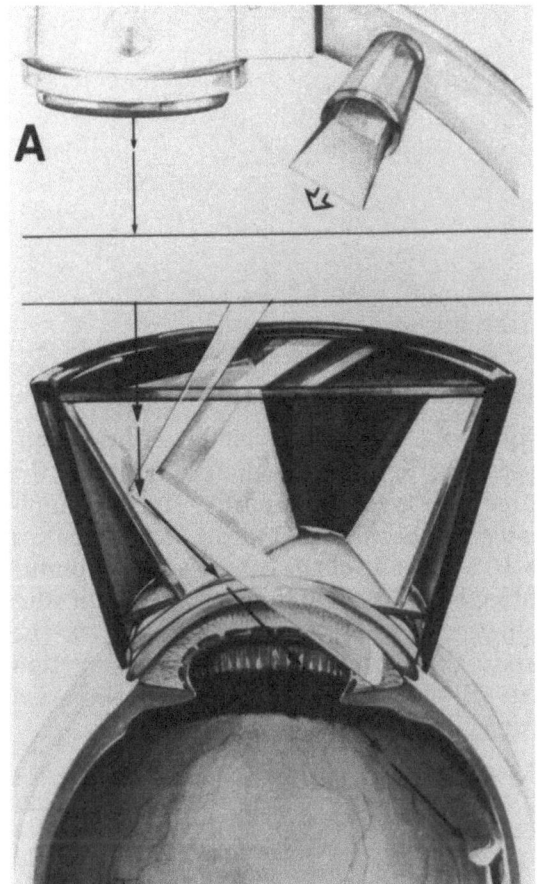

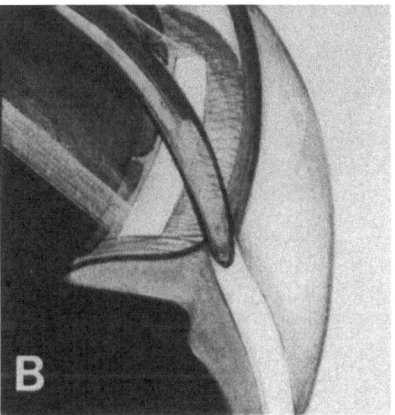

Figure 23. Error to avoid in fundus examination using the slit illuminator and the three-mirror contact lens. (A) The slit illuminator has been positioned at an angle superior to 10°. Slit illumination cannot reach the fundus through a small pupil. (B) Slit illumination of the iris rather than the fundus is obtained.

(Fig. 23). When the pupil has been widely dilated, the slit beam can pass through the pupil, but slit illumination of the retina does not coincide with the axis of observation: slit illumination of the retina is much too far from the area of the fundus, which is in the observation axis (Fig. 24).

Of course, the slit illuminator should not be moved on its arc during fundus observation. Observation of all parts of the fundus is obtained by the use of the X/Y coupling system combined with the use of the central and the peripheral mirrors of the contact lens.

Coaxial illumination of the microscope, which would cause undesirable reflection of the surface of the contact lens, is switched off during biomicroscopic examination of the fundus. However, it is more advantageous when maneuvering instruments and as a guarantee for asepsis to leave the lights on in the operating room.

POSITION OF THE CONTACT LENS

During surgery the three-mirror contact lens is used in the same way as during routine examination with the slit lamp focused on the seated patient. The cavity of the contact lens is three-quarters filled with a sterile 2% methylcellulose solution. To avoid flooding the surgical field with methylcellulose solution, it is advisable not to completely fill the cavity of the contact lens. Passage of air and/or blood between the contact lens and the cornea is the major difficulty that beginners encounter in biomicroscopy of the fundus during surgery. Simple rules make it possible to overcome this difficulty. Before placing the contact lens on the cornea, hemostasis must be as complete as possible; when the corneal epithelium has been cleaned with balanced solution, blood and serum must be removed from the fornix with surgical sponges. The contact lens must be centered

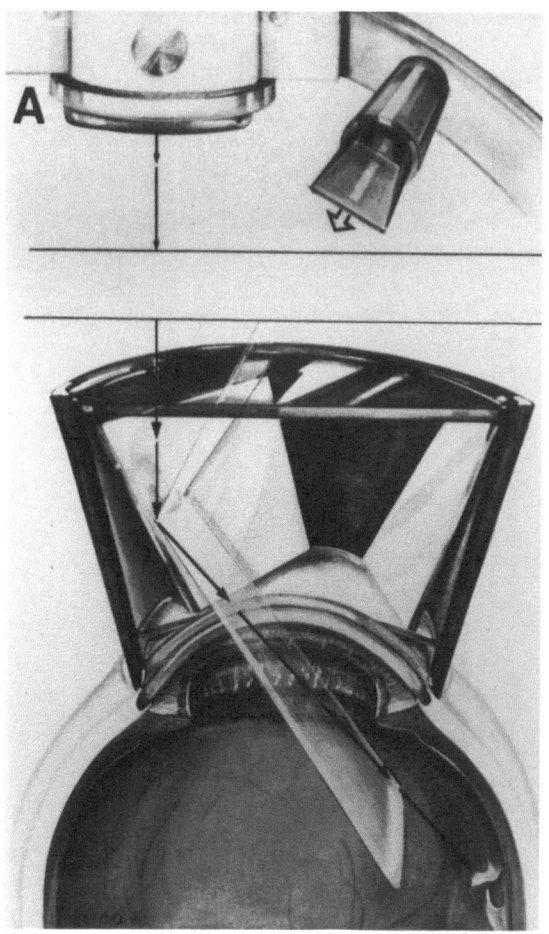

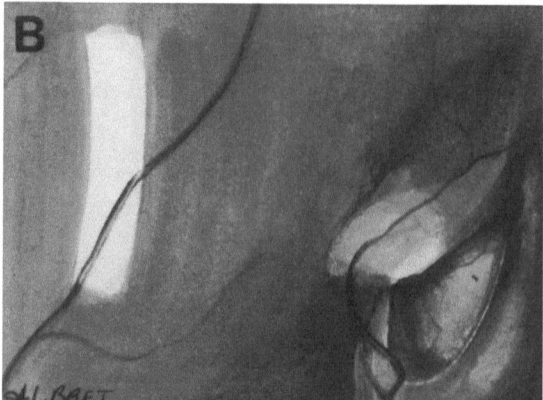

Figure 24. Error to avoid in fundus examination using the slit illuminator and the three-mirror contact lens. (A) The slit illuminator has been placed at an angle superior to 10°. The slit beam can reach the fundus through a widely dilated pupil, but slit illumination of the retina is distant from the area of the fundus which is in the observation axis (B) the retinal tear in the observation axis is in the shadow.

accurately on the cornea, and it should be held in place with only light pressure (Fig. 25). Simultaneous manipulation of the instruments along the sclera should be carried out according to precise rules (see below).

The central mirror is used when treating retinal tears close to the posterior pole and for checking the retinal circulation on the optic disc. The 66° mirror is used for looking at lesions located near the ora serrata. The 73° mirror is used for observations of the equator and the adjacent regions.

Cleaning the contact lens during surgery requires great care since the contact lens must be free of any stain, blood in particular. Caution should be taken so as not to damage the surface of the lens, caused especially by scratches through repeated, hard rubbing. It is, therefore, advisable not to clean the contact lens with a surgical compress, but to gently wipe it with a piece of soft material.

POSITION OF THE SURGEON

The surgeon should be seated, whenever possible, in front of the retinal quadrant where the retinal

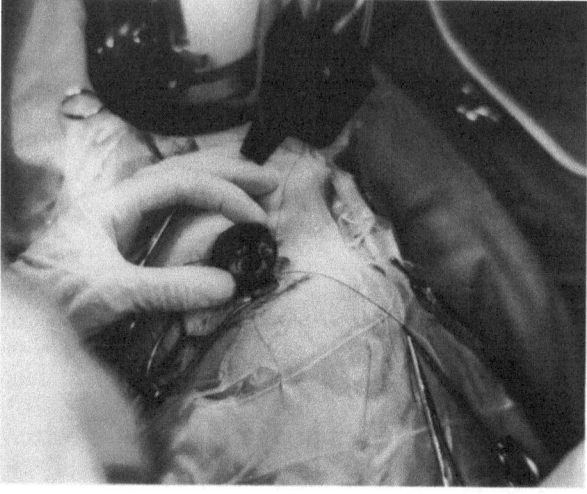

Figure 25. Handling of the three-mirror contact lens during surgery. The contact lens has been accurately centered on the cornea. It is held in place with very light pressure.

break is located. In fact, this position allows for dual control—external control of the sclera and internal control of the retina. This dual control makes the cryoapplication and especially the locating of the break easier. Indeed, the beam of the slit lamp, which is projected on the retinal break, can be seen through the sclera. Being able to see it through the sclera permits the immediate placing of the marker into the desired position (see p. 861).

The position of the surgeon in front of the retinal quadrant where the break is located is convenient and comfortable when operating on the temporal quadrants and the upper nasal quadrant. In contrast, this position is not convenient and is very uncomfortable for the lower nasal quadrant and for retinal breaks located at the 6 o'clock position. The surgeon must then sit at the head of the operating table, but in this position simultaneous scleral control is no longer possible during biomicroscopy of the fundus.

When several retinal tears located in two or three different quadrants have to be treated, it is possible to keep dual control, external and internal, without changing position as follows: If a myotomy of one rectus muscle has been performed, it is easy to induce a cyclophoria by pulling on the stitches placed in the muscle insertion and consequently aligning each quadrant in turn with the surgeon.

POSITION OF THE EYE

As a general rule the patient's eye should be placed in the straight ahead position. In addition to this, the eye must be immobilized in this position. Immobilization of the eye is important because the shifting of the marker and the cryoprobe along the sclera tends to rotate the eye. Rotation of the eye changes the conditions of observation of the fundus and it frequently causes passage of air and blood between the contact lens and the cornea. Immobilization of the eye is obtained by attaching the bridle sutures to the surgical drapes with hemostatic forceps (Fig. 26).

Protection of the Cornea

As in any retinal detachment surgery, effective protection of the corneal epithelium is necessary to ensure that observation of the fundus is possible, right up to the end of the operation. When the contact lens is placed on the cornea, the precorneal film of 2% methylcellulose solution ensures effective protection of the epithelium.

During the surgical stages that do not require simultaneous observation of the fundus, protection

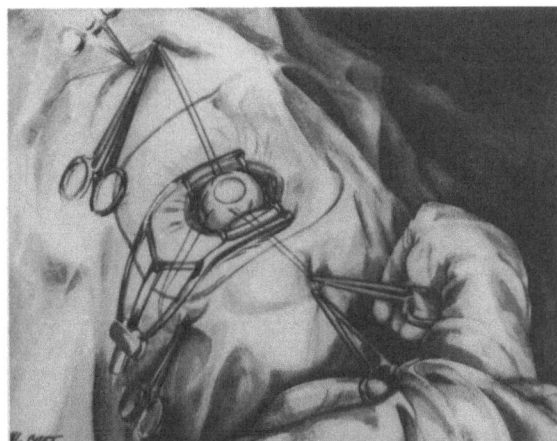

Figure 26. Immobilization of the eye in the straight ahead position for biomicroscopic observation of the fundus during simultaneous shifting of instruments along the sclera. Two opposite bridle sutures are attached to the surgical drapes using hemostatic forceps.

of the corneal epithelium is ensured with a pellucid membrane (see p. 52) (Fig. 27).

Hemostasis

Precise and complete hemostasis is a mandatory requirement to avoid passage of blood under the contact lens. Microsurgery allows accurate and com-

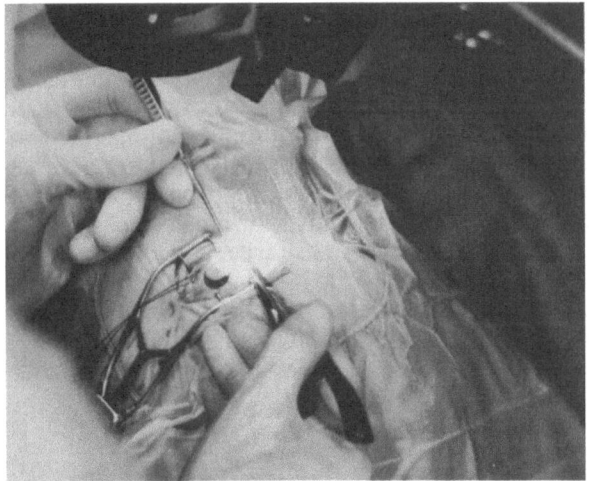

Figure 27. During surgical stages that do not require simultaneous observation of the fundus, a piece of egg pellucid membrane ensures protection of the corneal epithelium and prevents light damage to the retina.

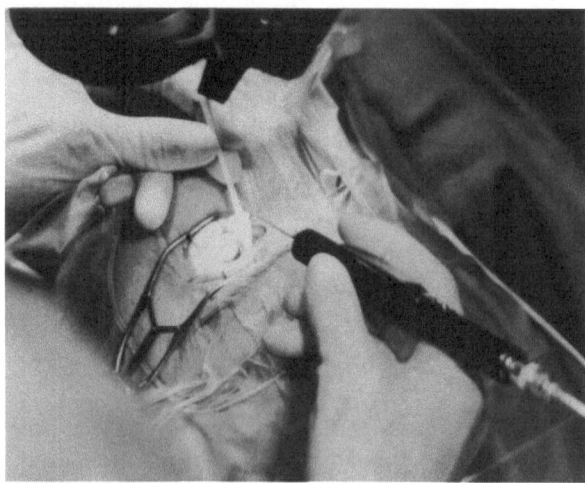

Figure 28. Accurate hemostasis under microscope.

plete hemostasis without excessive tissue destruction (see p. 61) (Fig. 28).

INDIRECT OPHTHALMOSCOPY WITH THE SURGICAL MICROSCOPE

Indirect ophthalmoscopy with the surgical microscope is also used in selected circumstances. The method was originally developed by Dominguez.[9] Its major advantage as compared to slit lamp biomicroscopy is to provide a large field of observation as in any technique for binocular indirect ophthalmoscopy. Its major advantage as compared to conventional indirect ophthalmoscopy is the high magnification provided by the surgical microscope. However, as in any technique for indirect ophthalmoscopy, indirect ophthalmoscopy with the surgical microscope does not provide an optical cross section of the fundus and vitreous cavity, and this is a disadvantage as compared to biomicroscopy. In addition, the amount of light entering the eye is significantly higher as compared to slit lamp examination.

In spite of these disadvantages, indirect ophthalmoscopy with the surgical microscope may be helpful for the retina surgeon, who was primarily trained using indirect ophthalmoscopy, but who would like to experience the advantages of microsurgery in retinal detachment repair. Use of the surgical microscope for performing binocular indirect ophthalmoscopy, has the advantage of eliminating the need to change instrumentation to look at the fundus during surgery.

At present the author restricts the use of intraoperative indirect ophthalmoscopy with the surgical microscope to the following indications: (1) fundus examination in babies with very narrow eyelid slits that do not permit the use of a three-mirror contact lens, in particular premature babies and (2) performing films and photographs.

Indirect ophthalmoscopy with the surgical microscope is performed using the coaxial illumination and a 40 diopter lens. The surgical microscope is raised by approximately 4 cm. The increased working distance is a disadvantage when accurate surgical maneuvers, such as cryotreatment, should be performed during fundus examination.

REFERENCES

1. Bonnet M: Les avantages de la chirurgie sous microscope dans le traitement du décollement de la rétine Bull Soc Ophthalmol Fr 75:1111–1112, 1975
2. Bonnet M: L'utilisation du verre á trois miroirs dans le traitement du décollement de la rétine J Fr Ophtalmol 2:209–216, 1979
3. Bonnet M: New concepts and techniques for retinal detachment surgery In Boyd B. Highlights of Ophthalmology 1980 Monthly letter vol 8, 407:1–5
4. Bonnet M: Microsurgery of retinal detachment In Boyd Highlights of ophthalmology, Silver anniversary edition 1981, 1:239–261
5. Urrets-Zavalia A: Retinal surgery under the microscope Dev Ophthalmol 2:195–201 (Karger, Basel, 1981)
6. Bonnet M: Biomicroscopy of the ocular fundus during retinal detachment surgery Ocular Therapy and Surgery 1:50–54, 1982
7. Bonnet M: Biomicroscopie peropératoire du fond d'oeil dans la chirurgie du décollement de la rétine Ann Instituto Barraquer 16:503–533, 1982–1983.
8. Bonnet M: Microsurgery for retinal detachment repair Dev Ophthalmol 14:5–10 (Karger-Basel 1987)
9. Dominguez A: Oftalmoscopia cinematografica de imagen invertida Arch Soc Esp Oftal 41:701–702, 1981

8

Surgical Steps Common to All Surgical Procedures

Surgical steps common to all procedures for retinal detachment management include proper dilation of the pupil, keeping a clear cornea through the entire operation, incision and suture of the conjuncitva and Tenon's capsule, isolation, disinsertion and repositioning of the extraocular muscles, proper hemostasis, monitoring of the intraocular pressure, protection against light damage to the retina, and subretinal fluid release.

None of these surgical steps belongs to the basic surgical procedure for retinal reattachment. All of them are performed with the only goal of making the basic surgical procedures for retinal reattachment feasible or easier to perform. Hence these surgical steps may be considered as negligible. However, proper performance of these steps is most important since it will make surgical management of the retinal detachment easy and rapid to perform, as well as most accurate. Proper completion of these surgical steps is a basic requirement to avoid certain intraoperative complications and ensure an uneventful postoperative course.

In contrast, poor performance of the surgical steps that are not basically required to achieve permanent retinal reattachment may be the main cause of intraoperative complications as well as postoperative patient discomfort and/or postoperative complications. Poor intraoperative pupillary dilation, clouding of the cornea, bleeding and inadequate exposure of the sclera will result in poor visualization of the surgical field and the ocular fundus. Poor visualization during surgery is a major cause of intraoperative difficulties: waste of time, lack of accuracy or serious intraoperative complications, which may result in failure to permanently reattach the retina and/or achieve satisfactory visual results. Poor monitoring of the intraocular pressure is a major cause of intraoperative difficulties and hazards. Improper dissection and suture of the conjunctiva and Tenon's capsule will result in postoperative eye discomfort, difficulties in

postoperative examination of the fundus, and abnormal scars. Conversely, careless isolation, disinsertion, or repositioning of the extraocular muscles may result in permanent muscle imbalance and diplopia.

All these difficulties and complications can be avoided by careful performance of the "minor" surgical steps.

PUPILLARY DILATION

Inducing and maintaining a wide pupillary dilation throughout the operation is of primary importance in retinal detachment surgery. This is achieved in most cases by a combination of sympathomimetic and anticholinergic agents. Preoperative instillations of 1% atropine and 10% phenylephrine eye drops are combined with a subconjunctival injection of 0.2–0.3ml of 0.5% atropine and 0.5% phenylephrine at the beginning of the operation. Phenylephrine is contraindicated in a few patients with vascular disease. Oxybuprocaine has been shown to have a significant inhibitory effect on surgically induced miosis,[1] 0.4% oxybuprocaine eye drops are instilled ten and five minutes preoperatively.

Miosis during retinal detachment surgery is considered as a complication because it prevents adequate visualization of the fundus. Miosis induced by surgery is due to a number of factors, including decreased intraocular pressure, trigeminal nerve stimulation, prostaglandin release, and release of substance P from sensory nerves ending within the eye.[2] Intraoperative miosis is more likely to occur when lensectomy through the pars plana is associated with vitreoretinal surgery and when decreased intraocular pressure occurs during certain surgical steps, in particular subretinal fluid release and fluid gas exchange, as well as removal of high buckles in eyes previously operated on. Iris trauma during lensectomy through the pars plana can be avoided by proper technique in most cases (see p. 145). Topical prostaglandin inhibitors administered preoperatively may be helpful to help maintain a wide pupil in eyes requiring a lensectomy.[3] Severe decrease in intraocular pressure induced by subretinal fluid release can also be avoided in most cases (see p. 68).

Intraoperative miosis that prevents proper completion of the operation is treated by medications to redilate the pupil. However, repeated instillations are often ineffective. A1:10000 epinephrine solution can be injected into the anterior chamber. Higher epinephrine concentrations should not be used because they are toxic to the corneal endothelium.[4]

KEEPING A CLEAR CORNEA

In retinal detachment management, perfect visualization of the fundus is a mandatory requirement for proper surgery, therefore, keeping a clear cornea during the entire surgical procedure is of primary importance. This can easily be achieved in most cases, including complicated retinal detachments that require lengthy procedures, provided precise rules are followed during the entire procedure.

At any stage of the surgical procedure, one or several mistake(s) may lead to a cloudy cornea and prevent the performance of well-controlled surgery. Avoiding such mistakes should be a major concern of the retina surgeon.

A cloudy cornea during surgery may result from epithelial damage, Descemet's membrane folds, and/or endothelial damage.

Epithelial Damage

Epithelial damage is the most frequent cause of corneal clouding during retinal detachment surgery. The most common causes of epithelial damage are (1) inadvertent trauma, (2) dessication, (3) blood deposit on the epithelial surface, (4) epithelial desquamation induced by topical drugs, and (5) increased intraocular pressure.

INADVERTENT TRAUMA

Inadvertent trauma to the epithelium surface may occur at any stage of the surgical procedure. Epithe-

lial erosion by an instrument, or a bridle suture used to rotate the eye, are the most frequent errors of beginners. Such errors are easy to avoid.

EPITHELIAL DESSICATION

Epithelial dessication results in desquamation of the superficial epithelial layers and may lead to a cloudy cornea. Epithelial dessication may develop just before surgery and during surgery.

Undetected lagophthalmia during the initial steps of general anesthesia is the most common cause of epithelial dessication occurring before any surgical maneuver. This can easily be avoided by keeping the eyelids closed with an adhesive strip from the time of anesthesia induction until preparation of the surgical field.

Dessication during surgery more rapidly develops when surgery is performed using the surgical microscope. It is prevented by placing a piece of egg pellucid membrane on the cornea during the surgical steps that do not require simultaneous observation of the fundus. The pieces of egg pellucid membrane are prepared in advance (Fig. 29) and stored in alcohol. They are washed in a balanced salt solution for approximately ten minutes before use. The membrane is coated with 2% methylcellulose solution before placing it onto the cornea and should be kept moist with a balanced salt solution. Use of an egg pellucid membrance has three advantages: (1) it keeps the corneal epithelium moistened; (2) it protects the corneal epithelium from the mechanical trauma due to direct moistening; and (3) it provides protection against light damage to the retina.

BLOOD DEPOSIT

Blood deposit on the corneal surface may predispose to epithelial damage. Blood clots stick to the corneal epithelium. Their removal with a balanced salt solution may result in mechanical damage to the superficial epithelial layers.

Blood deposit on the cornea can be avoided through proper hemostasis (see p. 62). When blood seeps onto the corneal surface, it is immediately washed using a balanced salt solution, so as to prevent the formation of blood clots that would adhere to the epithelium.

DRUG INDUCED EPITHELIAL DESQUAMATION

Touching the cornea with solutions used for sterile preparation of the operative field should be avoided.

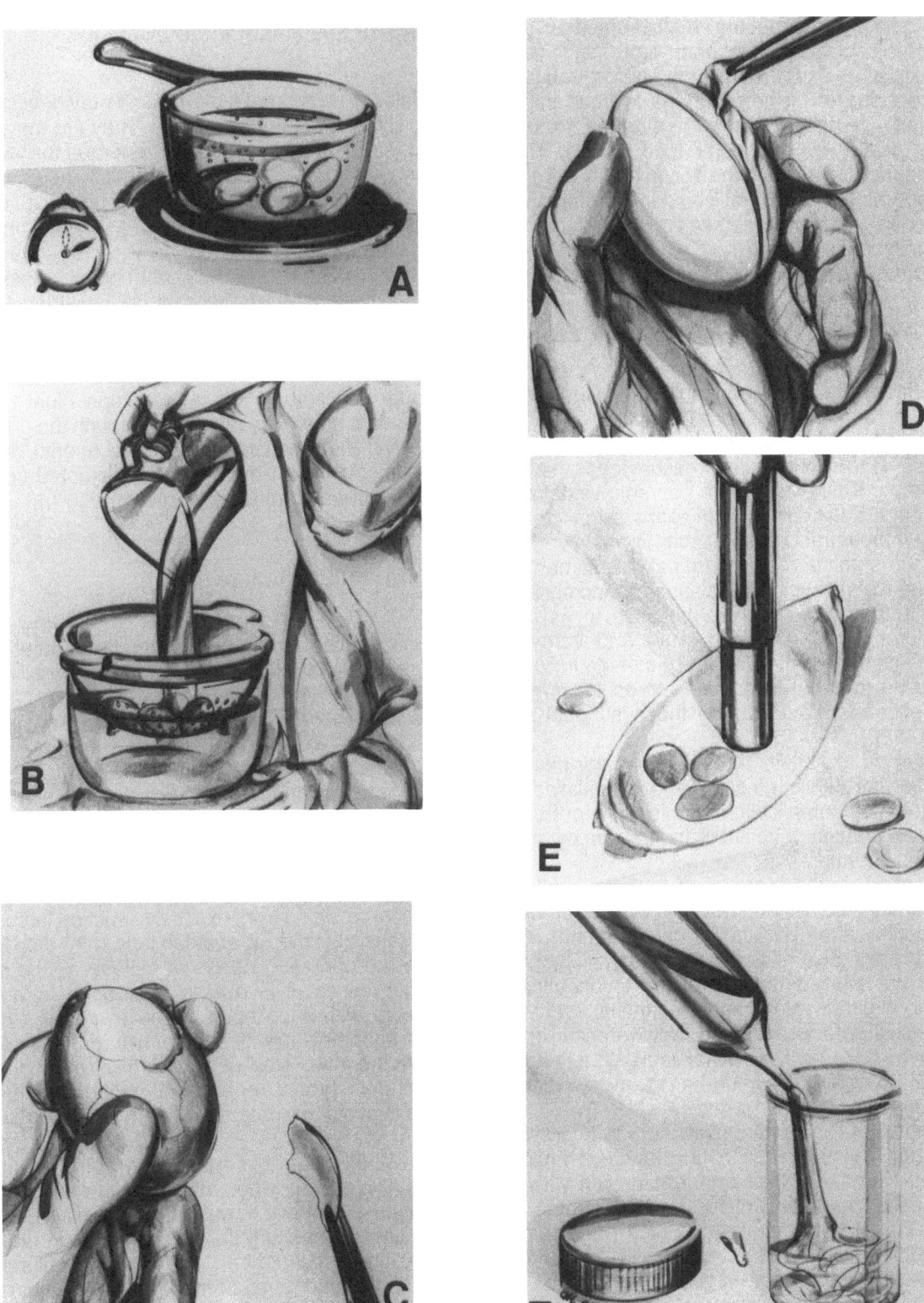

Figure 29. Preparation of egg pellucid membrane pieces for corneal protection. (A) Eggs are boiled for ten minutes (B) Further manipulations are made using sterile gloves and instruments. Boiled eggs are cooled with sterile water (C) The egg shell is removed (D) A cruciform incision of the pellucid membrane is made to isolate four main parts (E) Pieces are removed from the main parts using a 11 mm trephine (F) Pieces are stored in alcohol.

Sloughing of the corneal epithelium may result from the use of topical phenylephrine.[5] Topical phenylephrine should be avoided before retinal detachment surgery. Phenylephrine is used subconjunctivally in association with atropine to obtain proper dilation of the pupil (see p. 51). During subconjunctival injection the solution may seep onto the cornea. The assistant should, therefore, wash the cornea with a balanced salt solution during subconjunctival injection.

INCREASED INTRAOCULAR PRESSURE

An intraoperative increase in intraocular pressure is the most common cause of epithelial damage during retinal detachment surgery. A rapid and significant increase in intraocular pressure leads to epithelial edema. Epithelial edema prevents visualization of the fundus. In addition, epithelial erosions develop rapidly if the intraocular pressure is not lowered.

Certain surgical steps of retinal detachment surgery are well known to predispose to increased intraocular pressure. Such is the case in particular for scleral buckling (see p. 106) and intravitreal gas injection (see p. 127). Specific measures make it possible to avoid increased intraocular pressure and epithelial edema during these surgical steps (see p. 62).

Pulling on the bridle sutures is a major cause of increased intraocular pressure and epithelial edema. This potential complication should be kept in mind whenever rotating or immobilizing the eye by means of the bridle sutures.

Increased intraocular pressure and epithelial edema may also develop during scleral depression, in particular when performing cryotreatment of the retinal breaks. Scleral depression with the cryoprobe should be relieved between each cryoapplication so as to avoid development of epithelial edema.

Epithelial defects are more likely to occur in diabetic eyes because the epithelium is loosely adherent to Bowman's membrane in many diabetic patients.[6]

Removal of the corneal epithelium to improve intraoperative visualization of the fundus should be avoided. Removal of the corneal epithelium will result in increased hydration of the corneal stroma and folds in Descemet's membrane. Folds in Descemet's membrane become more severe with time and will interfere with intraoperative visualization of the fundus. When an epithelial defect occurs during the operation, the corneal surface is coated with sodium hyaluronate and the utmost care is taken to keep the intraocular pressure as near to normal as possible during the entire surgical procedure.

Folds in Descemet's Membrane

Folds in Descemet's membrane may develop during retinal detachment surgery. They are more likely to occur in aphakic eyes after repeated surgery and in lengthy procedures. These folds increase with time and make fundus visualization difficult or impossible. Large epithelial defects, a large volume of irrigating solution used during vitrectomy, and prolonged hypotonia are the most common causes of folds in Descemet's membrane. When striate keratopathy occurs, coating the inner surface of the cornea with sodium hyluronate may be helpful to improve fundus visualization.[7] Sodium hyaluronate is injected through the limbus with a 30-gauge blunt needle. Great care should be taken not to touch the endothelium and the lens capsule with the needle. A small amount of sodium hyaluronate is injected so as to avoid increased intraocular pressure.

Endothelial Damage

Endothelial damage during retinal detachment surgery is an infrequent cause of intraoperative and/or postoperative corneal edema. However, this severe complication may occur in aphakic and pseudophakic eyes under specific circumstances.

Severe endothelial damage by the intraocular lens may occur during retinal detachment surgery in pseudophakic eyes. This complication is more likely to occur in eyes with an anterior chamber lens. Corneal touch by the intraocular lens may occur during vitrectomy. This is due to a shallowing of the anterior chamber resulting from excessive suction force. Corneal touch by the intraocular lens may also occur when the operation does not include a vitrectomy. In such cases, it is due to decreased intraocular pressure with a collapse of the eye wall. Coating of the endothelium with sodium hyluronate is carried out as the initial step of any surgical procedure for retinal detachment repair in all pseudophakic eyes so as to avoid this potential and most severe complication.

Endothelial damage may occur during vitrectomy in aphakic eyes or when difficulties are encountered during lens removal through the pars plana. Excessive suction force, turbulence of the irrigating solution in the anterior chamber, use of large volumes of irrigating solution, use of inadequate irrigation solutions, and toxic effects of pharmacologic agents are the most common causes of endothelial damage during vitrectomy in aphakic eyes and lens removal through the pars plana.[6] Improved irrigating solutions have been shown to be helpful in maintaining the endothelial structures during vitrectomy,[8-13] and should be used by preference in patients with low cell densities or morphologic abnormalities of the endothelium, in particular, aphakic and diabetic patients. Epinephrine has a toxic effect on the endothelium.[4] For that reason it is not added to the irrigating solution to improve pupillary dilation during vitrectomy. Phenylephrine solution also has a toxic effect on the endothelium when applied topically in eyes with epithelial defects because the drug penetrates the anterior chamber in a higher concentration.[5]

INCISION AND SUTURE OF THE CONJUNCTIVA AND TENON'S CAPSULE

Incision of the Conjunctiva and Tenon's Capsule

The operating microscope makes it easier to obtain satisfactory exposure of the sclera without unnecessary cutting of tissues that would result in intraoperative bleeding and postoperative cicatricial adhesions.

Juxtalimbal incision, associated with two radial incisions, is performed by preference whenever possible. It has three advantages over the limbal incision developed by Hudelo and Massin: (1) hemostasis of the cut edge of the narrow limbus based flap is easy to perform; (2) the limbal vascular arcades are undamaged; and (3) tight suturing of the anterior conjunctival incision can be performed at the end of the procedure.

Juxtalimbal incision also has five advantages over conjunctival incision in the fornix: (1) there is less bleeding; (2) hemostasis is easy to obtain without excessive tissue coagulation; (3) when vitrectomy is required, exposure of the pars plana region is excellent; (4) there is less postoperative scar; and (5) the conjunctiva and Tenon's capsule can be reflected in one piece.

The juxtalimbal incision is made at 2mm from the limbus (Fig. 30). It is made parallel to the limbus. It is limited to the quadrant(s) of sclera to be exposed. It is made using corneal scissors. A radial incision is made at each end. Both relieving incisions are extended towards the fornix. The relieving incisions are made using Castroviejo scissors. The scissors are superficially shifted under the conjunctiva so that the anterior extensions of Tenon's capsule and the episcleral vessels are not unnecessarily damaged. When all four quadrants have to be exposed, a 360° incision parallel to the limbus is performed. It is asso-

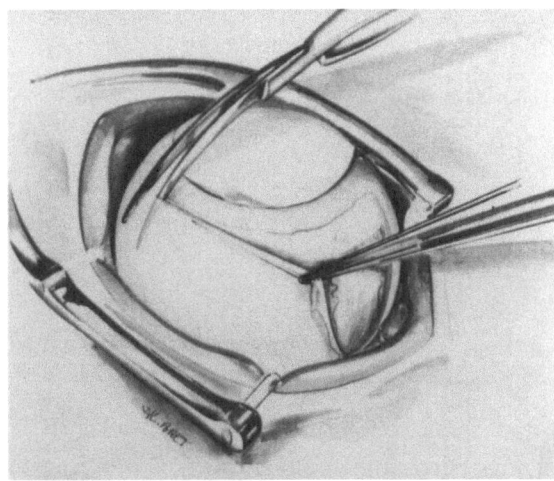

Figure 30. Juxta limbal incision of the conjunctiva in a retinal detachment associated with a single retinal break situated at the 11 o'clock meridian of the left eye. The incision is parallel to the limbus. It is made approximately 2 mm from the limbus. The relieving incisions are made at the inferior border of the medial rectus muscle and the lateral border of the superior rectus muscle so that placement of the bridle sutures in the muscles insertions can be performed under visual control.

ciated with two relieving incisions at the 6 and 12 o'clock meridians, or at the 3 and 9 o'clock meridians.

Tenon's capsule is opened 5 to 6mm posterior to the limbus using Castroviejo scissors and Severin's blunt scissors (Figs. 31 and 32). The scissors are conducted close to the sclera so as to free Tenon's capsule without damaging the anterior extensions of the muscles sheaths. The conjunctiva and Tenon's capsule are retracted in one piece towards the fornix.

Conjunctival incisions made more distant from the limbus are necessary in specific circumstances, such as reoperations, aphakic eyes with conjunctival scars, and eyes with filtering blebs. In eyes previously operated on for retinal detachment, difficulties encountered in the performance of the conjunctival incision depend on the location(s) of the previous conjunctival incision(s) and the care taken during the previous operation(s) in the performance and suturing of the conjunctival incision(s). When a juxtalimbal incision was made and properly sutured in a previous operation, a conjunctival incision is easy to perform. It is made 1mm posterior to the previous scar. The conjunctiva and Tenon's capsule can usually be freed and retracted in one piece towards the fornix, without excessive bleeding. In contrast,

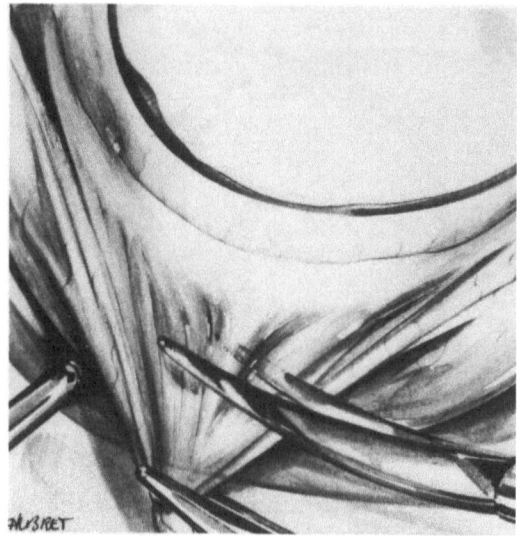

Figure 31. Anterior extensions of Tenon's capsule are cut close to the conjunctiva to avoid damage to episcleral vessels.

great difficulties may be encountered when the conjunctiva and Tenon's capsule were seriously damaged and poorly sutured during a previous operation(s). Dense adhesions with excessive amounts of scar tissue, symblepharon, or posterior retraction of the conjunctival flap are the most common causes of lengthy and difficult exposure of the sclera at reoperation. During reoperations great care should be taken when opening Tenon's space to expose the sclera. The sclera may be seriously damaged from a previous operation(s) and blind opening of the scissors blades to part cicatricial adhesions in Tenon's space may result in scleral perforation. Tissue dissection should be carried out under constant visual control. Careful hemostatsis should be performed as dissection of scar tissue is done.

Suture of the Conjunctiva

At the end of the operation Tenon's capsule and the conjunctiva are replaced on the sclera in one piece (Fig. 33). Suture of Tenon's capsule is unnecessary since the anatomical connections between the conjunctiva and Tenon's capsule are undamaged when proper tissue dissection has been done. Suture of the conjunctiva can be done using either absorbable sutures or 0–8 virgin silk. Absorbable sutures, such as 0–7 vicryl, are used by most surgeons. The author uses by preference 0–8 virgin silk, which gives less postoperative reaction. In most cases the suture is spontaneously eliminated after 2 or 3 weeks and suture removal is rarely required. The radial incisions as well as the juxtalimbal incision are tightly sutured.

Suture of the juxtalimbal incision has the advantage of permitting postoperative examination of the fundus with the contact lens on the very first postoperative days without any risk of separating the conjunctiva. Posterior slippage of the conjunctival flap is a common complication of the limbal incision secured with only one interrupted suture at each end. This complication can be avoided by performing a juxtalimbal incision and suturing the entire length of the incision. Interrupted sutures or a continuous suture are used to close the juxtalimbal incision. When suturing the relieving incisions, much care is taken to clearly identify both cut edges of the

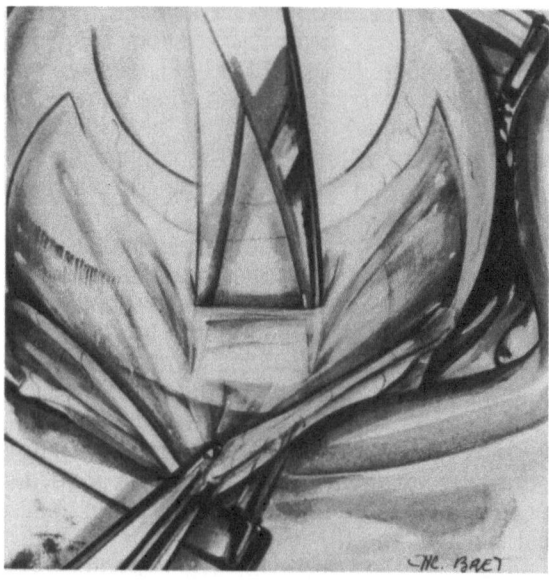

Figure 32. Tenon's capsule is opened between two recti muscles insertions with blunt scissors. The scissor blades are spread aside under visual control to avoid inadvertent tissue damage.

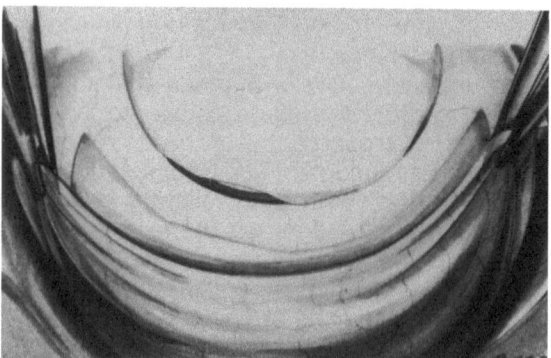

Figure 33. Two Bonn forceps are used to hold the conjunctiva and Tenon's capsule, which are replaced in one piece at their normal position.

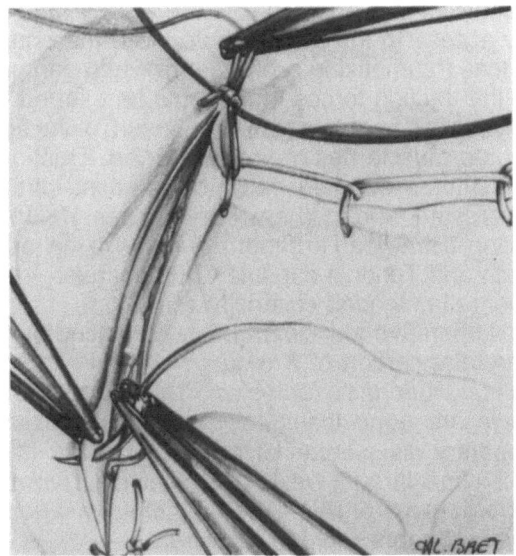

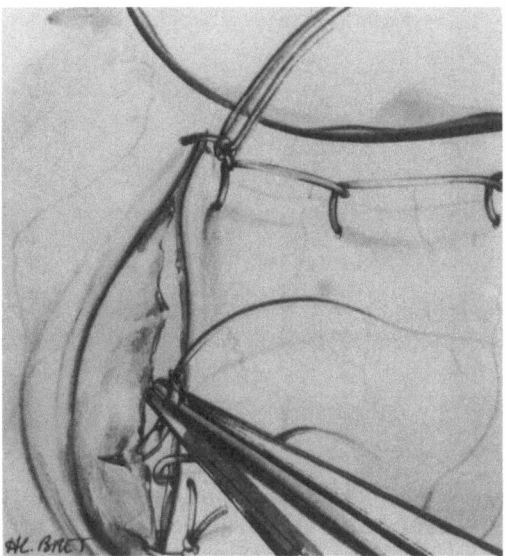

Figure 34. Correct suture of the conjunctival incision. The juxtalimbal incision has been secured using a continuous suture. One of the relieving incisions is being sutured from the fornix to the limbus. The end knot of the juxtalimbal incision is pulled by the assistant using Bonn forceps to stretch the cut edges of the relieving incision. This maneuver makes identification of the cut edges of the conjunctiva easier.

Figure 35. Error to avoid in suturing the relieving incisions. The cut edges of the conjunctival incision have not been stretched, making their identification difficult. Tenon's capsule protrudes through the conjunctival incision. It is being sutured in error to one cut edge of the conjunctival incision.

conjunctival incision (Fig. 34). If a cut edge of the conjunctiva is sutured to Tenon's capsule in error (Fig. 35), this will result in prolapse of Tenon's capsule and delayed healing. Poor apposition of the conjunctival edges may also result in a postoperative conjunctival cyst. Interrupted sutures or a continuous suture can be used to close both radial incisions.

Special care is taken when suturing the conjunctiva in reoperations. Owing to the sequelae of the previous operations and the difficulties encountered in tissue dissection, the conjunctiva may be in poor condition. Interrupted sutures rather than a continuous suture are used in such cases.

ISOLATION, DISINSERTION, AND REPOSITIONING OF THE EXTRAOCULAR MUSCLES

Isolation of the Recti Muscles

Bridle sutures placed in the recti muscles insertions are used in retinal detachment surgery with two main purposes: (1) to rotate the eye so as to obtain satisfactory exposure of the sclera and (2) to prevent rotation of the eye during localization and cryotreatment of the retinal breaks.

The number of bridle sutures to be placed for proper exposure of the sclera depends on the number of scleral quadrants to be exposed for scleral buckling. Two sutures placed in the adjacent muscles are sufficient to expose one scleral quadrant, and three sutures suffice to expose two scleral quadrants. Four bridle sutures are necessary when scleral buckling has to be performed in three or all quadrants. In most cases three bridle sutures are required to immobilize the eye in the straight ahead position during localization and cryotreatment of the retinal breaks. When only two bridle sutures are necessary for proper exposure of the sclera, the third bridle suture for proper immobilization of the eye is placed transconjunctivally to avoid unnecessary tissue dissection.

The muscle insertion is isolated using a squint hook with a short handle. Care is taken not to unnecessarily damage Tenon's capsule and the muscle sheath. The muscle is tagged with 0–4 black suture that can easily be identified during surgery. The squint hook and needle are passed close to the scleral insertion of the muscle.

These maneuvers, which are the simplest in pri-

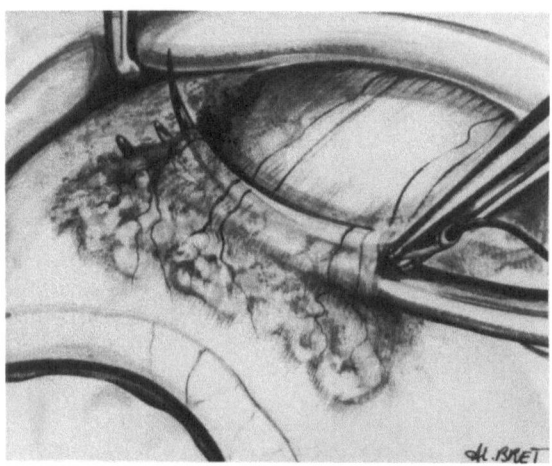

Figure 36. Placing a bridle suture after previous surgery for retinal detachment. A funnel has been made with Castroviejo scissors under the anterior part of the muscle tendon. The scissor blades are used as a guide for needle insertion beneath the muscle tendon.

mary operations, may be hazardous in reoperations. The forceful passage of a squint hook under a muscle in eyes that have had previous surgery for retinal detachment may result in scleral perforation. Therefore, a squint hook is not used to isolate the muscles in such eyes. A funnel under the anterior part of the muscle tendon is created using blunt Castroviejo scissors. The scissor blades should be held in a plane strictly parallel to the muscle insertion. The convex side of the scissors blades is directed toward the sclera. When the cicatricial adhesions have been freed along the entire width of the muscle tendon, the needle is inserted between the scissor blades and the muscle tendon (Fig. 36). This maneuver also permits avoiding inadvertent damage to vortex veins that may have been dragged anteriorly by cicatricial adhesions. At the end of the operation a piece of gelfilm is placed under the anterior part of any rectus muscle that has been tagged with a bridle suture. This will avoid cicatricial adhesions between the muscle and the sclera.

Temporary Disinsertion and Repositioning of a Rectus Muscle

INDICATIONS

Temporary disinsertion of a rectus muscle is carried out more often in microsurgical management of retinal detachment than in conventional surgery.[14] Disinsertion of a rectus muscle will provide excellent exposure of the sclera under the muscle and give easy access to the sclera posterior to the equator. It is less traumatizing a procedure when compared with the traction forces that should be exerted onto bridle sutures to obtain similar exposure of the sclera when no muscle has been disinserted. Traction on bridle sutures is a major cause of increased intraocular pressure and corneal edema (see p. 54). In addition, it may lead to serious damage to the muscle sheath and Tenon's capsule with secondary development of extended cicatricial scars.

Postoperative muscle imbalance induced by temporary disinsertion of a rectus muscle is most uncommon when disinsertion and repositioning of the muscle are done using microsurgical techniques. Temporary disinsertion of a rectus muscle should not be considered a waste of time, since it will make the basic steps of retinal detachment management easier and more rapid to perform.

Disinsertion of a rectus muscle is indicated (1) when the retinal break is located under the rectus muscle and (2) when access to the sclera, posterior to the equator is required. Disinsertion of two recti muscles is very rarely required. Disinsertion of three recti muscles must never be performed so as not to severely compromise the blood supply to the anterior segment. Disinsertion of the lower oblique muscle is required to give access to the posterior pole when a patch pocket is performed to buckle a macular hole (see p. 226). Disinsertion of the upper oblique muscle should never be performed owing to the high risk of postoperative diplopia.

Surgical Technique

Muscle Disinsertion. In primary operations the muscle insertion is isolated with a squint hook. No traction is exerted on the muscle so as not to induce increased intraocular pressure. A radial cut of Tenon's capsule is made at each border of the muscle tendon. The radial cuts of Tenon's capsule are approximately 2mm in length and will make placing of the muscle sutures easier. Then two lateral stitches are placed in the muscle 1mm from its scleral insertion using 7–0 absorbable suture. The stitches take up the whole thickness of the muscle and its unopened sheath. The needle is passed from the scleral side of the muscle towards its superficial side. It perforates the muscle inside the lateral vessels so that the vessels tightened by the stitch will bleed less when the myotomy is performed (Fig. 37). Two muscle bites are done for each suture. The sutures are secured with two double knots. Both sutures will be used to reinsert the muscle at the end of the procedure. Then the muscle tendon is severed close to the sclera with blunt Castroviejo scissors.

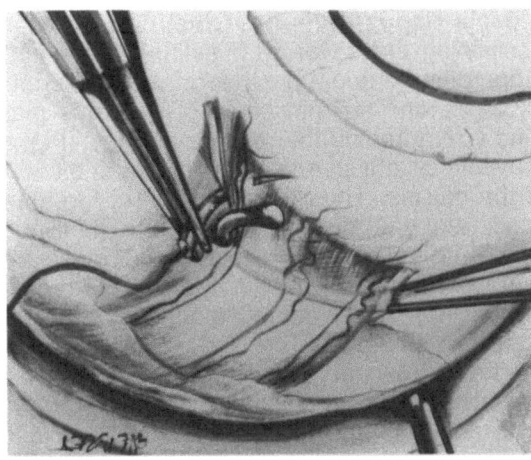

Figure 37. Disinsertion of a rectus muscle. The needle for the preplaced suture is inserted through the entire muscle thickness and the muscle sheaths. It perforates the muscle inside the lateral vessels to avoid bleeding.

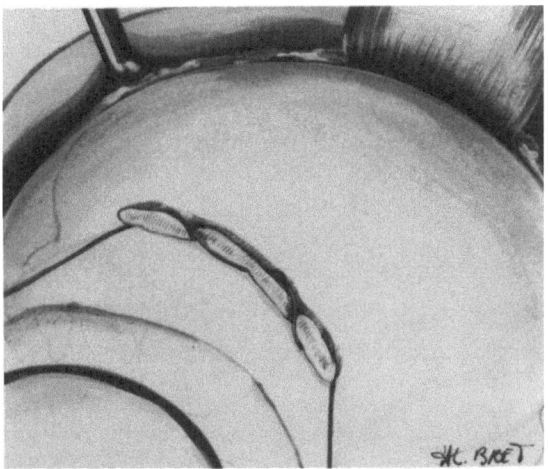

Figure 39. Disinsertion of a rectus muscle: both extremities of the traction suture, inserted in the sclera at the muscle insertion, are kept independent for easy maneuvering of the marker and the cryoprobe along the sclera.

The convex sides of the scissor blades are directed towards the sclera so as to avoid inadvertent cutting of the sclera (Fig. 38). The cut ends of bleeding vessels are closed with diathermy. Then the severed muscle is permitted to retract with Tenon's capsule and the conjunctiva. The muscle keeps its normal anatomic relationship with the latter since the muscle sheath and its ligament extensions have been kept untouched. A traction suture is placed along the entire length of the scleral insertion of the muscle. A 0–5 colored thread is used. It will be easily distinguished from the white sutures used for scleral buckling. Three scleral bites are made. The needle is inserted into half the thickness of the sclera. It is inserted in a radial direction from the posterior edge toward the anterior edge of the muscle insertion. Both extremities of the traction suture are kept independent (Fig. 39). Light hemostatic forceps are placed at each extremity of the traction suture. Keeping the two components of the traction suture independent makes it easier to shift the marker and the cryoprobe along the sclera when

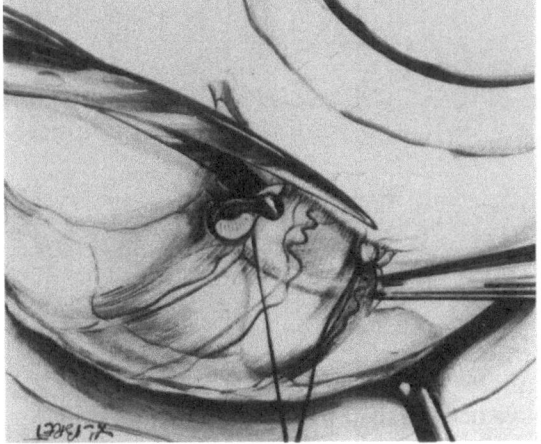

Figure 38. Disinsertion of a rectus muscle: correct tenotomy. The convex sides of the scissor blades are directed towards the sclera to avoid inadvertent damage to the sclera.

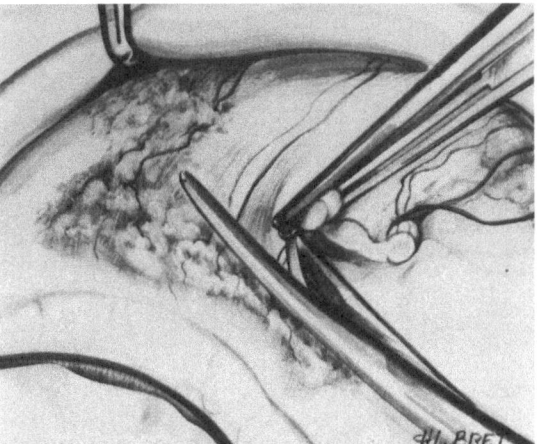

Figure 40. Correct disinsertion of a rectus muscle in reoperation: Squint hook is not used to isolate the muscle insertion to avoid difficulty and potential complications.

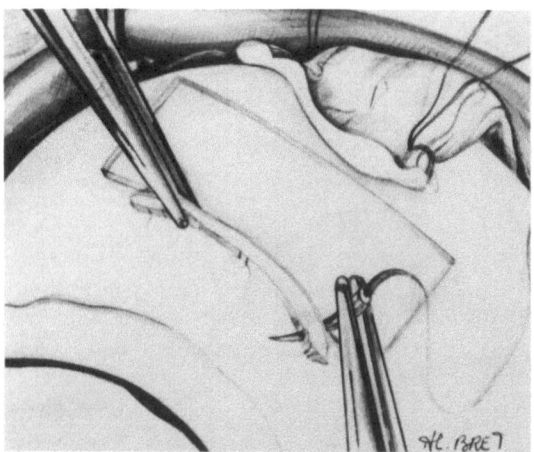

Figure 41. Muscle repositioning: A piece of gelfilm is placed behind the muscle insertion to avoid cicatricial adhesions between the muscle and the sclera.

the retinal break is located under the muscle that has been severed.

In reoperations a squint hook should not be used to isolate the muscle insertion, owing to scar adhesions and the potential risk of scleral perforation. The muscle insertion is isolated using forceps. A lateral suture is placed in the muscle 1mm distant from its scleral insertion. Then half of the muscle insertion is severed with Castroviejo scissors (Fig. 40). A medial suture is placed in the muscle. Then the other half of the muscle insertion is severed and the other lateral suture is placed. Scar adhesions between the muscle and the underlying sclera are freed under visual control with Castroviejo blunt scissors.

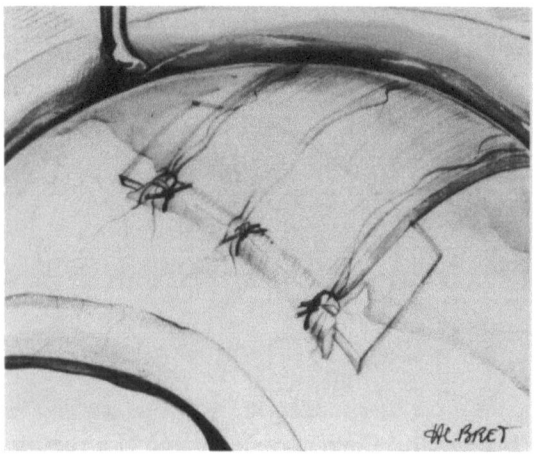

Figure 42. Muscle repositioning: Muscle suture has been completed using three interrupted stitches.

Muscle Repositioning. Great care is taken in repositioning the severed muscle(s) at the end of the operation to avoid postoperative muscle imbalance. A 13mm × 7mm piece of gelfilm is placed on the sclera behind the muscle insertion (Fig. 41). It prevents cicatricial adhesions between the sclera and the muscle. Thus modifications of the muscle contact arc and disturbance of eye motility are avoided. In addition, dissection of the muscle and sclera will be easier when reoperation is required. The muscle should be sutured along the whole length of its scleral insertion. The latter is easily identified under the microscope. The suture is completed using both stitches placed in the muscle before performing the myotomy. First, the lateral stitches are placed at each extremity of the scleral insertion. Then muscle suturing is completed with interrupted sutures (Figs. 42 and 43) or a continuous suture. The sutures should take the entire thickness of the muscle and both the anterior and posterior cut edges of the muscle sheath (Fig. 44). Sutures that involve only the anterior muscle sheath leaving the muscle fibers free is a common error of beginners. This error will result in serious muscle imbalance, especially when a vertical rectus muscle has been disinserted. The medial muscle fibers tend to retract posteriorly within the muscle sheath (Fig. 45). Spreading the anterior cut edge of the muscle sheath with forceps makes it easy to identify the muscle fibers and take them in the needle bite.

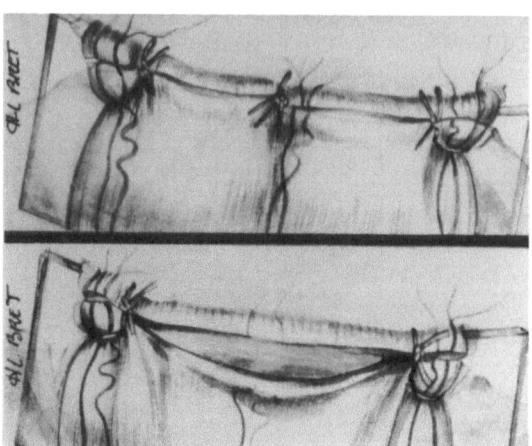

Figure 43. (A) Correct suturing of a rectus muscle: the cut edges of the muscle tendon have been placed into close apposition along the whole length of the muscle insertion. (B) error to avoid: The medial part of the muscle has not been sutured. The gap in the medial part of the muscle may result in poor muscle healing and postoperative muscle imbalance.

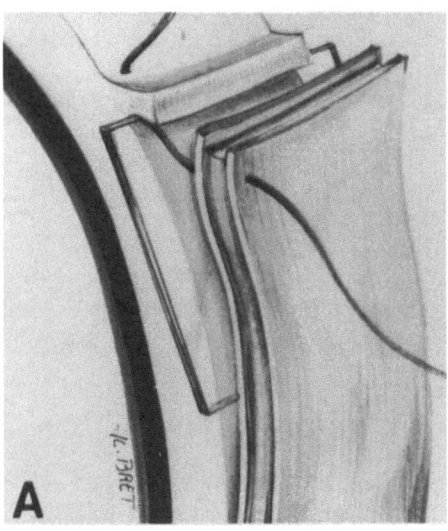
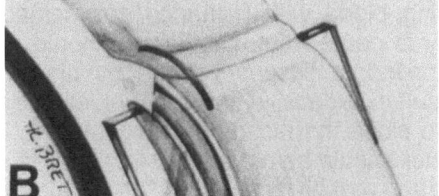

Figure 44. Correct suturing of a rectus muscle: (A) The suture takes the entire thickness of the muscle and both the anterior and posterior muscle sheaths. (B) Both the muscle and its sheath are replaced into normal position after suture tightening.

HEMOSTASIS

Proper hemostasis is a mandatory requirement of any microsurgical procedure. It is especially important in microsurgical management of retinal detachment since intraoperative bleeding will result in poor visualization of the outer surgical fields and, most

importantly, of the ocular fundus. Therefore, any bleeding vessel should be closed as the consecutive surgical steps are carried out. However, measures used to stop bleeding should not result in compromised blood supply to the extraocular and/or intraocular tissues.

Management of extraocular bleeding includes: (1) careful tissue dissection to avoid unnecessary damage to the extraocular vessels, in particular episcleral

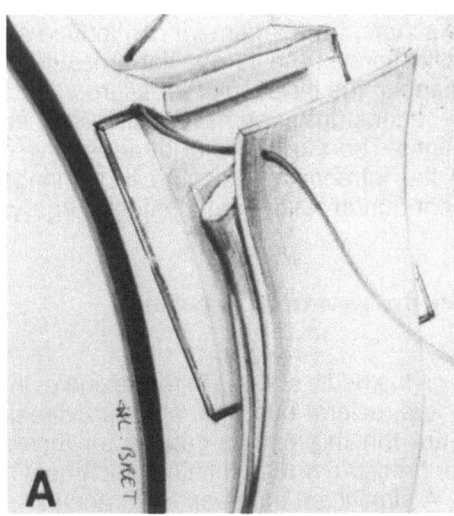
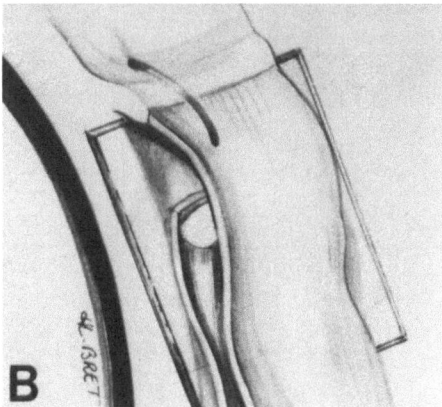

Figure 45. Error to avoid in muscle repositioning (A) Only the anterior muscle sheath has been taken by the suture (B) After suture tightening, muscle fibers will retract and reinsert on the sclera posterior to the normal muscle insertion. The error will result in postoperative muscle imbalance.

vessels (see p. 55) and vessels of the extraocular muscles (see p. 58), (2) accurate hemostasis using superficial diathermy, and (3) monitoring the blood pressure.

Accurate hemostasis of the bleeding vessels should be performed with a high quality diathermy unit. The Mira diathermy unit is one of the available units that perfectly fulfils microsurgical requirements. Diathermy coagulations should be strictly restricted to the cut ends of the bleeding vessels. Identification of the cut ends of the bleeding vessels is ensured by washing blood with balanced salt solution as diathermy is carried out. Diathermy should not be blindly applied to tissues flooded by blood. This would result in excessive tissue coagulation and an inability to close the bleeding vessel(s). The diathermy power should be preset at a low level to avoid unnecessary vessel destruction, which may result in permanent compromise of the blood supply. A low diathermy power is requried to efficiently close the cut ends of most extraocular vessels that may bleed intraoperatively. Diathermy for extraocular hemostasis should induce contraction of the vessel walls (Fig. 46) rather than heavy tissue coagulation (Fig. 47). Following such light diathermy applications, the bleeding vessels, which are efficiently closed during surgery, will again become patent postoperatively and ensure adequate blood supply to the ocular tissues.

Monitoring the patient's blood pressure is helpful in decreasing extraocular bleeding during surgery. Whenever possible the anesthesiologist lowers the patient's blood pressure within safe limits. Lowering the blood pressure by 2 cm of mercury is sufficient

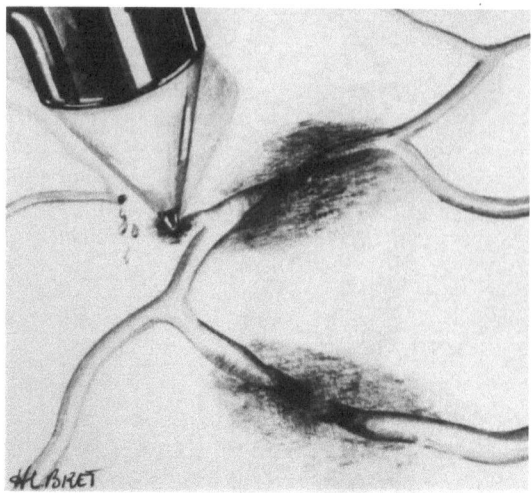

Figure 47. Error to avoid in hemostasis: Excessive diathermy has resulted in coagulation of the vessels and damage to surrounding tissues.

to stop diffuse bleeding from small extraocular vessels in most cases. (For management of intraocular bleeding during vitreous surgery see p. 143).

MONITORING THE INTRAOCULAR PRESSURE

A number of surgical maneuvers carried out during retinal detachment management can induce significant modifications of the intraocular pressure. Such modifications of the intraocular pressure can in turn result in serious intraoperative difficulties and/or complications. Therefore careful intraoperative monitoring of the intraocular pressure is a mandatory requirement during retinal detachment surgery.

Increased Intraocular Pressure

Pulling on the bridle sutures to rotate and/or immobilize the eye, scleral buckling, and intravitreal gas injection are the three main causes for increased intraocular pressure during retinal detachment management. A significant increase in intraocular pressure will result in immediate corneal clouding and arrest of the ciliary and/or retinal blood circulation. A transient increase in intraocular pressure can be sufficient to result in exfoliation of the corneal epithelium and permanently compromise visualization of

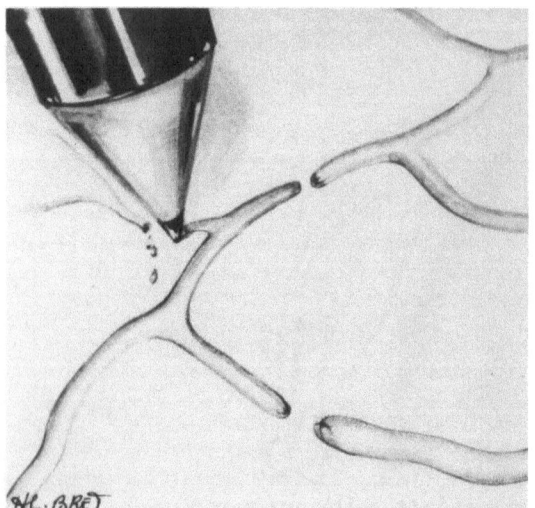

Figure 46. Proper hemostasis of bleeding vessels: Light diathermy induces contraction of the cut ends of the bleeding vessels.

the fundus throughout the operation. A prolonged increase in intraocular pressure can result in ciliary artery occlusion and/or optic atrophy.

Measures to prevent a dangerous increase in intraocular pressure include (1) care not to exert excessive and prolonged traction on the extraocular muscles, (2) surgical maneuvers to create intraocular space for scleral buckling and intravitreal gas injection, and (3) systemic agents to soften the eye.

GENTLE MANIPULATION OF THE EXTRAOCULAR MUSCLES

An abrupt and severe increase in intraocular pressure is likely to occur when the surgeon or assistant pulls an extraocular muscle with a squint hook. Isolation of the recti muscles should be most gentle. The squint hook should never exert forceful traction on the muscle insertion. Conversely, traction on the bridle sutures to rotate or immobilize the eye should be most gentle. When significant traction on the bridle sutures cannot be avoided for proper exposure of the sclera, transient relief of traction should be repeated.

CREATING INTRAOCULAR SPACE

A series of surgical maneuvers make it possible to create intraocular space and avoid increased intraocular pressure. They include: (1) paracentesis of the anterior chamber, (2) aspiration of fluid from the vitreous cavity or the retrovitreal space, and (3) subretinal fluid drainage. Choice of the maneuver to be used in any given case depends on the amount of intraocular space that should be created and the anatomical status of the eye.

Nonvitrectomized Eye. In nonvitrectomized eyes, choice of the measures to be used depends on whether the eye is phakic, aphakic, or pseudophakic.

In phakic eyes paracentesis of the anterior chamber is the maneuver used by preference to create intraocular space. It is sufficient in most cases. It is performed with a straight needle, such as the Kuhnt-Bregeat needle for cataract discision. The needle is inserted through the limbus in a plane strictly parallel to the iris plane. The needle is directed toward the meridian located at approximately 60° of the entry site. The needle tip is positioned at approximately half of the arc length between the entry site and the aiming meridian at 60° from the entry site. The needle must always be kept in front of the iris. The sharp side of the needle is directed anteriorly so as to avoid inadvertent iris damage (Fig. 48). Then a gentle rotating motion of the needle,

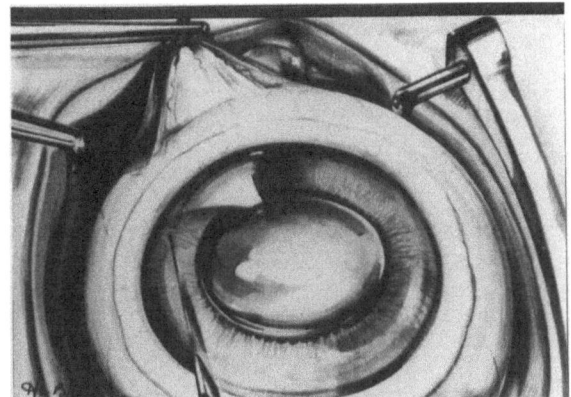

Figure 48. Anterior chamber paracentesis in a phakic eye. The bridle suture opposite the entry site of the knife is firmly held using forceps to immobilize the eye and induce increased intraocular pressure during aqueous humour leakage. The discision needle is held in front of the iris to avoid lens damage. The needle's sharp side is directed anteriorly to avoid iris damage.

which should not exceed 90°, is done. It produces leakage of aqueous humour through the tiny limbal incision. The needle is withdrawn from the eye before complete flattening of the anterior chamber. If the anterior surface of the iris becomes adherent to the inner side of the needle track, gentle massage is done on the cornea with a spatula so as to avoid permanent anterior synechiae. A proper technique and use of the operating microscope are most important to control anterior chamber paracentesis and to avoid inadvertent damage to the iris and/or lens by the needle. Paracentesis of the anterior chamber provides nearly 0.2ml intraocular space. In eyes with significant liquefaction of the vitreous gel, such as highly myopic eyes, fluid percolates from the vitreous cavity, through the zonula, and the anterior chamber reforms soon after the paracentesis. In such eyes paracentesis of the anterior chamber can be repeated.

The most severe complication that may occur during paracentesis of the anterior chamber is damage to the anterior lens capsule from the needle tip. This complication results from improper technique (Fig. 49). It is likely to occur when the needle tip is directed towards the pupillary area. Such a mistake can easily be avoided. Anterior chamber paracentesis may not provide enough intraocular space when high and broad scleral buckles and/or a large intravitreal gas bubble are necessary to reattach the retina. This event is more likely to occur in eyes with viscous vitreous, since repeated paracenteses of the anterior chamber are impossible in such eyes. In such cir-

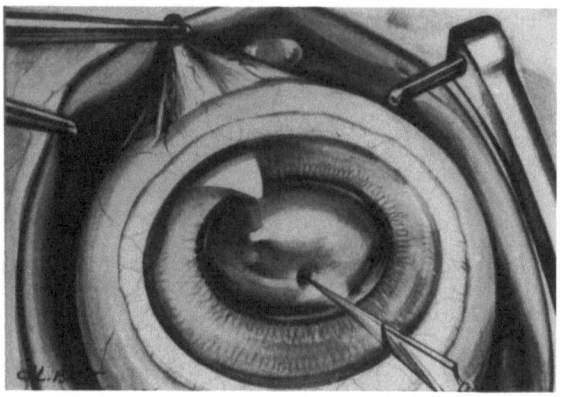

Figure 49. The needle tip has been incorrectly directed towards the pupil, an error to avoid in anterior chamber paracentesis. Damage to the anterior lens capsule occurs.

cumstances systemic agents to soften the eye are helpful. When systemic agents are ineffective and/ or contraindicated, subretinal fluid is drained off.

In aphakic eyes, paracentesis of the anterior chamber should not be performed because of the likelihood of vitreous fibril incarceration into the limbal wound. However, uneventful release of aqueous humour is occasionally performed by experienced microsurgeons. An intact anterior vitreous face is a mandatory requirement. Aqueous humour release

through the limbus is performed with a 30-gauge sharp needle and a syringe. The needle is inserted into the anterior chamber in a plane parallel to the iris plane. The needle tip is held in front of the iris and close to the cornea. The entry of the bevel edge is oriented anteriorly (Fig. 50). Aqueous humour is aspirated with the syringe. The syringe plunger is moved very slowly and gently while observing the position of the anterior vitreous face. Use of the slit lamp in conjunction with coaxial illumination provides accurate control of the anterior chamber depth and position of the anterior vitreous face. Aspiration with the syringe should be stopped when the anterior chamber depth is decreased by two-thirds.

Incarceration of vitreous fibrils into the limbal wound is a most serious potential complication of aqueous humour release through the limbus in aphakic eyes. Therefore, aqueous humour release through the limbus must never be performed when the anterior vitreous face is open and/or vitreous gel is protruding into the anterior chamber (Fig. 51). In spite of its potential complications, release of subretinal fluid should be performed, rather than aqueous humour release through the limbus, by beginners who have limited expertise in microsurgery.

When a large intraocular space is required to safely complete scleral buckling and/or gas injection in aphakic eyes, subretinal fluid release should be performed. Aspiration of fluid from the retrovitreal

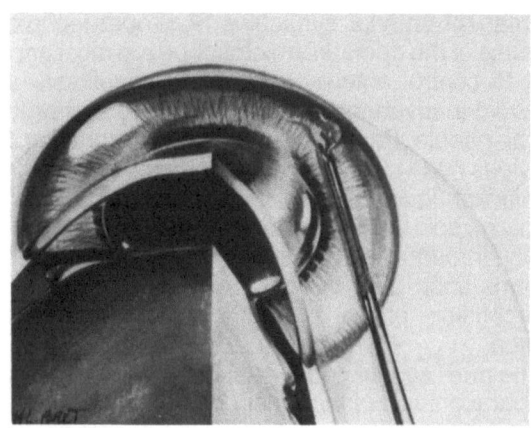

Figure 50. Anterior chamber paracentesis is occasionally performed in aphakic eyes when the anterior vitreous face is intact. Aqueous humour is gently aspirated using a 30-gauge sharp needle and a syringe. Position of the anterior vitreous face is carefully monitored during aqueous humour release. The entry of the bevel edge is in front of the iris. It is directed anteriorly.

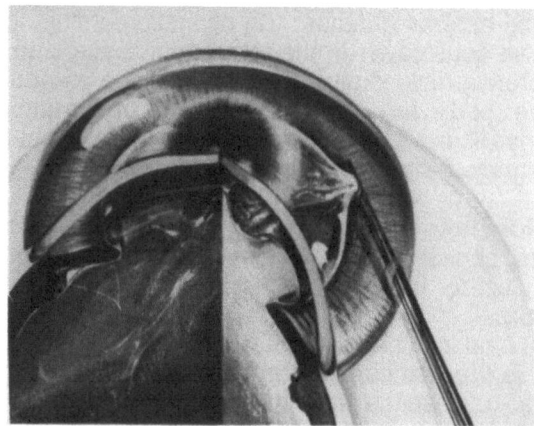

Figure 51. Serious error to avoid in anterior chamber paracentesis: The anterior vitreous face of an aphakic eye is open and vitreous gel protrudes into the anterior chamber. Anterior chamber paracentesis will result in vitreous incarceration into the limbal wound. Aqueous humour release through the limbus must never be performed in eyes with vitreous gel protruding into the anterior chamber.

space to obtain intraocular space is a hazardous procedure in most eyes. This maneuver should be used as a last resort in the rare cases where all other measures to lower the intraocular pressure have failed. Aspiration of fluid from the retrovitreal space is made through the pars plana with a 30-gauge needle. It is done under visual control using a planoconcave contact lens and the slit illumination. The needle tip is directed toward the optic disc. Fluid aspiration with the syringe should be most gentle. It should be withdrawn immediately when the surgeon discloses vitreous fibrils moving towards the needle tip.

In pseudophakic eyes, paracentesis of the anterior chamber must never be performed owing to the risk of permanent endothelial damage from the intraocular lens. In such eyes, systemic agents to lower intraocular pressure and/or release of subretinal fluid should be used.

Vitrectomized Eyes. Creating intraocular space for scleral buckling and/or gas injection is easy to achieve in most vitrectomized eyes.

When the eye is phakic, repeated paracenteses of the anterior chamber are performed. They provide sufficient intraocular space in most cases. However, in a few cases, fluid from the vitreous cavity does not migrate toward the anterior chamber. This occurs when a significant amount of viscous vitreous has been left in the retrolental space. In such eyes intraocular space can be obtained by either subretinal fluid release or drainage of fluid from the vitreous cavity through the pars plana. Choice between the two techniques is determined according to specific characteristics of any given case. Subretinal fluid release is performed by preference when the retina is highly detached. However choroidal edema and dilation of the choroidal vessels are common following a lengthy vitrectomy procedure and the likelihood of choroidal hemorrhage is increased. When the retinal detachment is rather shallow, intravitreal fluid rather than subretinal fluid is drained. Intravitreal fluid drainage is performed with a blunt 27-gauge needle and a syringe. The needle is inserted into the vitreous cavity between the sutures securing one of the pars plana incisions. The position of the needle tip in the posterior vitreous cavity is monitored using the planoconcave lens and the slit lamp. Care should be taken not to aspirate an excessive amount of intravitreal fluid so as to avoid collapse of the eye.

When the vitrectomized eye is aphakic, intraocular fluid is aspirated through the limbus with a 30-gauge needle. The needle tip is placed in the pupillary area during fluid aspiration.

In pseudophakic vitrectomized eyes intraocular fluid should not be removed from the anterior chamber. Subretinal fluid release or aspiration of intravitreal fluid through the pars plana is performed.

SYSTEMIC AGENTS

Intravenous administration of agents that dehydrate the vitreous gel and/or decrease aqueous humour secretion by the ciliary processes, is a helpful adjunct to avoid increased intraocular pressure during retinal detachment surgery.

The association of a carbonic anhydrase inhibitor and a hyperosmotic solution, such as a 20% mannitol solution, is commonly used. In an 80 kilo adult patient, 500mg of diamox are administered intravenously. The amount of 20% mannitol to be given is 1ml per kilo. Intravenous administration of mannitol solution should be completed within approximately 8–10 minutes for maximal efficacy. Administration of hyperosmotic agents and/or acetazolamide is contraindicated in selected patients. In particular acetazolamide should not be used in diabetic patients.

Decreased Intraocular Pressure

A severe decrease in intraocular pressure is much less frequent a problem as compared to increased intraocular pressure during retinal detachment surgery. However, a severe decrease in intraocular pressure may occur in specific circumstances. Abrupt and massive drainage of subretinal fluid is the most common cause of severe intraocular pressure decrease (see p. 69). Decreased intraocular pressure may also occur during a lengthy vitrectomy procedure. It is caused by leakage through the pars plana incisions, which tend to enlarge as the intraocular instruments are moved (see p. 148). Leakage of intraocular fluid through the pars plana incisions can also occur after completion of the vitrectomy procedure when the pars plana incisions have not been tightly secured.

Decreased intraocular pressure is one of the major causes of folds in Descemet's membrane and miosis that will prevent adequate visualization of the fundus. A severe decrease in intraocular pressure with collapse of the eye may also result in choroidal edema and choroidal hemorrhage.

A severe decrease in intraocular pressure during retinal detachment repair can be avoided by proper surgical technique in most eyes. If a technical error is made and results in collapse of the eye, the leaking incision(s) should be immediately secured by watertight suturing, and balanced salt solution or gas is injected into the vitreous cavity.

PROTECTION AGAINST LIGHT DAMAGE TO THE RETINA

Damage to the retina and pigment epithelium from light has been clinically documented in cataract surgery and reproduced experimentally with various extraocular sources including an intraocular fiberoptic source.[15–22] Therefore, the surgeon should be concerned about potential light damage to the retina and pigment epithelium during retinal detachment microsurgery. However, photic retinopathy due to prolonged exposure to the coaxial light of the operating microscope has not been observed in retinal detachment microsurgery. This is likely due to the fact that a shield is placed on the cornea during the surgical steps requiring use of coaxial illumination (see p. 52). Photic retinopathy from the intraocular fiberoptic probe is unlikely to occur during vitrectomy for retinal detachment repair because the retina is detached. The surgeon, however, should keep in mind that light damage to the macula from the fiberoptic probe may occur during lengthy preretinal membrane stripping on the posterior pole. The potential for light damage from the intraocular fiberoptic probe can be minimized by: (1) positioning the fiberoptic probe at some distance from the retina, (2) avoiding warming of the infusion fluid[23] since the threshold for light damage is lowered by increasing the body temperature,[15,16] and (3) avoiding keeping the fiberoptic probe in the same position for more than five minutes.[21]

SUBRETINAL FLUID DRAINAGE

Drainage of subretinal fluid is avoided in microsurgical management of most retinal detachments. Whenever possible, subretinal fluid release is avoided owing to two major reasons: (1) subretinal fluid drainage is unnecessary to permanently reattach the retina,[24–26] and (2) subretinal fluid drainage is the surgical step of conventional retinal detachment management that carries the highest risk of serious surgical complications.

Rationale for Subretinal Fluid Release

Subretinal fluid drainage is unnecessary to achieve permanent retinal reattachment in most retinal detachments, including reoperations[27] and retinal detachments associated with proliferative vitreoretinopathy,[28] provided all retinal breaks are sealed and tractions on the retina are relieved. Following proper scleral buckling procedures, subretinal fluid will spontaneously absorb within two days in approximately 50% of eyes and a week in approximately 75% of eyes.[29] In only 20%[7] to 25%[29] of these cases will complete absorption of subretinal fluid take longer than a week. Subretinal fluid absorption time is not related to the patient's age, refractive error, or the extent of the retinal detachment.[29] In certain circumstances subretinal fluid may persist for an unusually long period of time in spite of adequate sealing of all retinal breaks. The surgeon should be familiar with factors associated with delay in complete subretinal fluid absorption to avoid unnecessary reoperation. Delay in complete absorption of subretinal fluid, beyond 6 weeks after surgical repair, can be anticipated in longstanding retinal detachments with demarcation lines and subretinal proliferation.[29,30] Delayed absorption of subretinal fluid may be related to the high protein concentration of subretinal fluid in retinal detachments of long duration.[31] The probability for delayed absorption of subretinal fluid should not lead the surgeon to drain subretinal fluid in longstanding retinal detachments. Early retinal reattachment will not improve the visual results when the macula has been detached for longer than 2 weeks. Release of subretinal fluid carries a high risk of serious intraoperative complications in a number of long standing retinal detachments, particularly in retinal detachments associated with small atrophic holes in lattice and desinsertion at the ora serrata, owing to the fact that the detachment is shallow in most cases. Delayed absorption of subretinal fluid in retinal detachments of long duration does not mean that the detachment remains unchanged during the first several weeks following surgery. In most eyes, subretinal fluid absorption begins on the very first postoperative day but it is slow. When all retinal breaks have been adequately sealed, subretinal fluid will continue to absorb and total reattachment will occur within a few weeks in most eyes and within several months in infrequent cases. Slit lamp examination of the fundus repeated every few days can detect the slow decrease in the extent and height of the detachment. Ultrasonography can also be used to measure small changes in the detachment height[32] and thereby relieve the surgeon's anxiety. It is, however, unnecessary in most cases.

Since it is unnecessary to permanently reattach the retina intraoperatively, in most cases, subretinal fluid release has only one major advantage: to create intraocular space, so as to make the performance of certain surgical steps, mainly scleral buckling and intravitreal gas injection, safer and easier.

Indications

Intraocular space is required for the performance of scleral buckling and intravitreal gas injection without inducing increased intraocular pressure. To a lesser degree intraocular space is also required for the performance of proper and accurate cryotreatment of the retinal break(s) in certain bullous retinal detachments, since approximation of the pigment epithelium to the highly detached retina during cryoapplication requires heavy scleral depression with the cryoprobe. In most cases, specific measures make it possible to create the intraocular space required and to avoid increased intraocular pressure.

Indications for subretinal fluid release are restricted to two main circumstances: (1) when associated lesions make it likely that the eye will not tolerate a moderate increase in intraocular pressure and (2) when the other measures to lower intraocular pressure and to create intraocular space have failed or are contraindicated.

Subretinal fluid release is often necessary in eyes with recent cataract surgery, retinal vascular disorders, particularly in diabetic patients, eyes with deficient ciliary circulation, glaucoma, and staphylomatous sclera.

Subretinal fluid release should also be carried out when scleral buckling or intravitreal gas injection results in the arrest of blood circulation on the optic disc.

Surgical Technique

The main concern in the performance of subretinal fluid drainage is to avoid complications. Prophylaxis of potential complications depends on two parameters: (1) proper selection of the site for drainage and (2) proper surgical technique.

SELECTING THE DRAINAGE SITE

In selecting the most appropriate site for subretinal fluid drainage, four parameters are taken into account: (1) the site of subretinal fluid and the clinical characteristics of the detachment, (2) the site of large choroidal vessels, (3) the site of the retinal break(s), and (4) the anatomical status of the eye wall.

Site of Subretinal Fluid and Clinical Characteristics of the Retinal Detachment. Subretinal fluid is drained off in an area where the retina is highly detached. Examination of the fundus in an optical cross section using the slit beam and contact lens allows accurate evaluation of topographical variations in the depth of subretinal fluid. This examination is done intraoperatively with scleral depression, and the site for drainage is marked off on the sclera with the scleral marker used for the localization of retinal breaks. Intraoperative evaluation of the site where subretinal fluid is deep is important since the intraoperative subretinal fluid topography may be somewhat different from what it was preoperatively. In particular, in long standing retinal detachments with tiny breaks, subretinal fluid may shift from the peripheral lower fundus to the posterior pole. In such cases surgical access to the shifting subretinal fluid may be most hazardous and drainage should be avoided. In eyes with peripheral star-shaped fixed folds, release of subretinal fluid is performed preferably in the area of fixed folds, since the stiff retina will not tend to flatten against the pigment epithelium and incarcerate in the perforation site.[33,34]

Site of Large Choroidal Vessels. The site of choroidal puncture should be away from the vortex veins and their major tributaries, as well as the long posterior ciliary arteries. The 12 o'clock and 6 o'clock meridians as well as the meridians at the lower and upper borders of the horizontal recti muscles are relatively avascular areas. They are choosen preferably for the drainage site.

Site of the Retinal Breaks. Drainage should not be performed in areas of large retinal breaks, owing to the risk of vitreous gel shifting through the break and incarceration of formed vitreous into the choroidal perforation.

Anatomical Status of the Eye Wall. Subretinal fluid drainage should not be performed in very thin sclera, in particular beneath the most anterior part of the recti muscles, as well as in sclera damaged by previous surgery or a spontaneous staphyloma. Placing the scleral suture to close off the drainage site would be hazardous or impossible in such areas.

Areas that have just been treated with cryoapplication should also be avoided for the drainage site because cryotreatment results in dilatation of choroidal vessels and increased risk of choroidal hemorrhage.

SURGICAL TECHNIQUE

Both the scleral incision and the choroidal puncture are performed under very high magnification (X 20).

The scleral incision is oriented radially. It should be approximately 2mm in length to allow good visualization of the underlying choroid. A mattress suture with 8–0 nylon monofilament or 8–0 polyglycolic-acid suture is placed on the edges of the sclerotomy before performing the incision of the inner layers of the sclera. This preplaced suture will enable the surgeon to control subretinal fluid escape and immediately close the sclerotomy when an adequate amount of subretinal fluid has been drained. Before being cut, the deep scleral fibers are slightly raised by traction exerted on one edge of the sclerotomy with Bonn forceps. They are cut with the tip of a sharp cataract needle. The underlying choroid is exposed along a length of 1mm, prolapse of the choroid in the sclerotomy is induced by gently traction on both edges of the sclerotomy using the Bonn forceps. Then the choroidal knuckle is examined under the highest magnification provided by the surgical microscope so as to determine whether a large choroidal vessel is present in the choroidal knuckle. Transillumination can be combined with observation through the microscope to see large choroidal vessels in the choroidal knuckle. If a large choroidal vessel is visible in the choroidal knuckle, the sclerotomy is secured and another site for drainage is selected. When no large choroidal vessels are visible in the choroidal knuckle, puncture of the choroid can be performed. Diathermy can be applied on the knuckle before performing the puncture to reduce the potential risk of choroidal hemorrhage. However, diathermy may be ineffective to prevent bleeding from a large choroidal vessel. Diathermy is unnecessary in most cases, provided the site for drainage has been properly selected. The choroidal knuckle is perforated using a discision needle. The needle should be very thin so as to make a tiny perforation and very sharp for easy perforation of the choroidal tissue, which is rather elastic. A needle that is not sharp enough and with a somewhat blunt tip will push the elastic choroidal tissue and a full thickness choroidal puncture will be difficult to complete without inducing hemorrhage. The status of the needle tip should be verified under the microscope just before choroidal puncture. The needle tip is inserted into the posterior part of the choroidal knuckle, its sharp edge being orientated outward. The needle is moved into the choroid in a direction tangential to the eye surface (Fig. 52). The needle tip is inserted into, and withdrawn from, the choroidal knuckle with a rapid and precise motion so as to create a very small and clean choroidal puncture.

When draining subretinal fluid, care has to be taken with both the rate and amount. The drainage rate should be monitored to avoid a severe decrease in intraocular pressure and/or retinal incarceration into the drainage site. Controlled subretinal fluid escape is ensured by the tiny choroidal puncture. In most cases, the opening of the choroid is so small that subretinal fluid does not leak unless pressure is exerted on the eye wall. Thus, the necessary

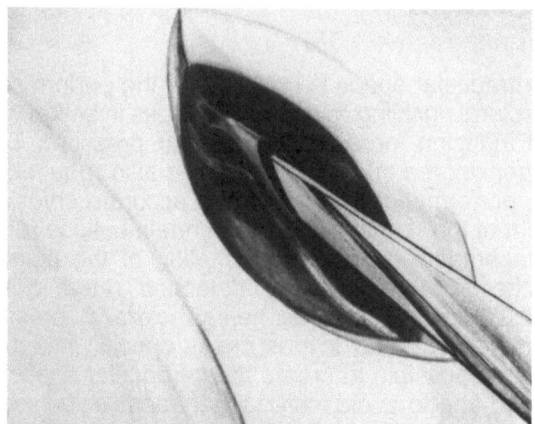

Figure 52. High magnification of the choroidal incision for subretinal fluid drainage. The sharp edge of the discision needle is orientated outward. The choroidal incision is made distant from a small choroidal vessel visible in the exposed choroid. The preplaced mattress suture to secure the sclerotomy is not represented.

amount of subretinal fluid is drained off each time the surgeon ties a scleral suture for scleral buckling.

Similarly, the total amount of subretinal fluid that is drained is controlled by the small size of the choroidal incision and the preplaced scleral suture. The suture of the sclerotomy is tightened as soon as the drainage is judged to be sufficient. The amount of subretinal fluid to be drained depends on the volume of intraocular space to be created for scleral buckling and/or intravitreal gas injection. When drainage is carried out to allow proper and accurate cryotreatment, a small amount of fluid should be released. Likewise release of a small amount of subretinal fluid is usually sufficient to manage increased intraocular pressure with arrest of the blood circulation on the optic disc.

COMPLICATIONS

Intraoperative complications of subretinal fluid drainage include failure to achieve fluid escape, failure to monitor fluid escape, choroidal hemorrhage, retinal damage, and vitreous gel incarceration.

Some of these complications, in particular retinal perforation with vitreous gel incarceration, may play a role in the development of proliferative vitreoretinopathy, and failure to reattach the retina.

The most severe complications of subretinal fluid release, such as massive choroidal hemorrhage and retinal perforation with vitreous gel prolapse, are most infrequent with microsurgical techniques. However, the potential hazards of subretinal fluid drainage have not been totally eradicated by microsurgery.

Failure to Drain. Failure to obtain subretinal fluid escape through the choroidal puncture can result from two distinct causes: (1) improper selection of the drainage site and (2) improper choroidal puncture.

Improper selection of the drainage site can be avoided by evaluation of the subretinal fluid depth using biomicroscopic examination just before selecting the drainage site. Such a precaution is mandatory in retinal detachments with shifting subretinal fluid.

Improper choroidal puncture can occur when the surgeon uses a needle or knife that is not perfectly sharp. Due to the elasticity properties of the choroidal tissue, the choroidal knuckle is pushed inward by the blunt instrument tip and a full thickness choroidal incision cannot be achieved.

When there is no subretinal fluid escape following the choroidal puncture, the fundus should be observed using the three-mirror contact lens before any repeated attempt to perforate the choroidal knuckle. When failure to obtain subretinal fluid escape is due to improper selection of the drainage site, the choroidal incision is visible at fundus examination under high magnification. There is a tiny whitish line in the choroid. A small choroidal hemorrhage and/or a small retinal perforation may be present. In such cases the sclerotomy should be secured and cryotreatment is performed on the perforation site. When failure to obtain subretinal fluid escape is due to the inability to perforate the choroid, the tiny choroidal incision cannot be detected. The choroidal incision is, however, clearly visible through the subretinal fluid when a full thickness puncture has been done. In such circumstances, a second attempt to perforate the choroidal knuckle is done, using a sharper instrument.

Occasionally, subretinal fluid escape ceases before an adequate drainage has been achieved. The inner aspect of the drainage site is observed using the three-mirror contact lens and the slit lamp. If the retina appears to be flattened in the area of the drainage site, the sclerotomy is secured and it is determined by fundus examination whether more fluid can be drained from another site. If 1mm or more fluid depth overlies the drainage site, cessation of subretinal fluid escape is likely due to spontaneous closing of the choroidal puncture. Both lips of the sclerotomy are gently lifted using two Bonn forceps. This will result in reopening of the choroidal incision and subretinal fluid escape when gentle pressure is applied on the eye.

Failure to Monitor Fluid Escape. If the choroidal incision is too large, sudden and massive subretinal fluid flow will occur. This can result in immediate collapse of the eye. Choroidal hemorrhage and postoperative choroidal detachment may develop. When subretinal fluid escape occurs too rapidly following the choroidal incision, the mattress suture preplaced on the sclerotomy is temporarily tightened to prevent more fluid escape. When subretinal fluid is associated with scleral buckling, the buckle sutures are rapidly tightened until normal intraocular pressure is restored. If more intraocular space is required to properly tighten all buckle sutures, the drainage site suture is slightly undone and the additional amount of subretinal fluid is released.

When subretinal fluid is associated with intravitreal gas injection, the mattress suture of the drainage site is loosely tightened to permit fluid escape during gas injection. The meridian for gas injection through the pars plana and the position of the eye are determined so that the intravitreal gas bubble does not push the retina against the drainage site during the injection.

When massive subretinal fluid escape and collapse of the eye occur before tightening of the drainage suture, the eye wall is indented using a cotton-tip applicator immediately after securing the drainage site, so as to restore a nearly normal intraocular pressure. Scleral depression by the cotton-tip applicator is gradually relieved by the assistant while the surgeon tightens the buckle sutures or completes gas injection.

Choroidal Hemorrhage. Choroidal hemorrhage is a most serious complication of subretinal fluid drainage. The incidence of this complication is significantly decreased by microsurgical techniques.[35,36,37] However, the potential risk for this complication should be kept in mind.

Choroidal bleeding can occur during choroidal incision or subretinal fluid escape. Bleeding during choroidal incision results from damage to a large choroidal vessel and/or improper choroidal puncture.

Bleeding can occur before the subretinal space has been entered. It is most likely to occur when the instrument used for choroidal puncture is not sharp enough or when the incision is carried out in an area that has just been treated by cryoapplication. In such circumstances blood accumulates in the sclerotomy. It does not enter the subretinal space. Diathermy is applied on the choroidal knuckle; the sclerotomy is sutured; and another drainage site is selected.

Bleeding can occur when the subretinal space has been entered. It is a most serious complication. Blood will leak into the subretinal space. Blood in the subretinal space is likely to spread to the posterior pole intraoperatively, owing to the fact that the posterior pole is the most dependent part of the eye in a supine patient. Subretinal hemorrhage involving the macular area is likely to permanently compromise the visual result of the operation.[38] There is no efficacious treatment to stop bleeding that results from damage to a large choroidal vessel. This complication should be avoided by proper surgical technique (see above).

Diffuse choroidal bleeding may result from too rapid a drainage with collapse of the eye. Choroidal bleeding caused by acute hypotony is more likely to occur when extensive cryotreatment has been applied or in patients with high blood pressure. This most severe complication can be avoided by proper surgical technique.

Retinal Damage. Retinal perforation during choroidal incision can be avoided by proper selection of the drainage site (see p. 67). When a mistake has been made and the retina is perforated, the sclerotomy should be secured and cryotreatment applied to the perforation site. Scleral buckling of the perforation site is necessary if vitreous gel is incarcerated in the drainage site.

Retinal incarceration into the drainage site can result from three main causes: (1) poor control of fluid escape with massive flow of fluid through a large choroidal incision, (2) drainage in an area of shallow detachment, and (3) increased intraocular pressure induced by tightening of the buckle sutures or gas injection.

Retinal incarceration is likely to occur when there is an abrupt cessation of subretinal fluid escape or increased intraocular pressure. In such circumstances the outer aspect of the drainage site is examined under high magnification. A knuckle of whitish translucent tissue indicates a large retinal incarceration. Tiny retinal incarcerations are invisible in most cases. However, the retinal incarceration is always visible by fundus examination. Tiny stellate retinal folds are centered by the perforation site (Fig. 53).

No attempt should be made to disengage the incarcerated retina. Any surgical maneuver will fail to disengage the retina and may end up in retinal perforation and vitreous gel prolapse. A tiny retinal incarceration that can be detected only by fundus examination requires no specific treatment except for tight suturing of the sclerotomy. When the retinal incarceration is visible within the sclerotomy at external examination, cryotreatment is applied after suturing the sclerotomy. However, the necessity and value of cryotreatment in this specific indication have not been established. Retinal incarceration complicated by retinal perforation and vitreous prolapse is a most severe complication. Vitreous traction is likely to develop postoperatively. It can result in failure to reattach the retina or in recurrent traction detachment. Management of retinal incarceration with vitreous prolapse should include freezing of the prolapsed vitreous gel, tight suturing of the scleral

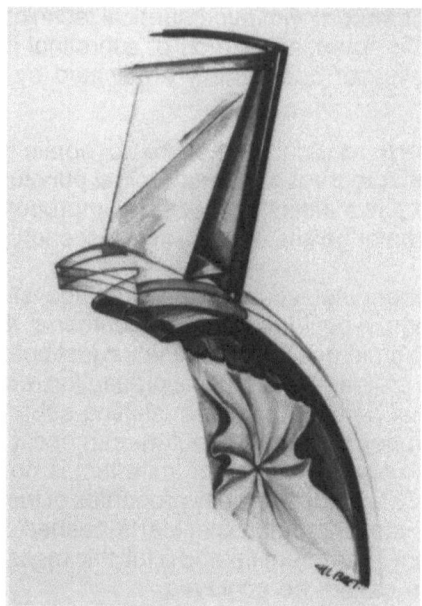

Figure 53. Retinal incarceration at a drainage site recognized by fundus examination using the three-mirror contact lens and microscope slit-lamp.

wound, cryotreatment of the surrounding choroid and retina, and segmental scleral buckling.

REFERENCES

1. Van Rij G, Renardel de Lavalette JGC, Baarsma GS, Jansen JTG: Effect of oxybuprocaine 0.4% in preventing surgically induced miosis. British J Ophthalmol 68:248–251, 1984
2. Duffin RM, Camras CB, Gardner SK, Pettit TH: Inhibitors of surgically induced miosis. Ophthalmology, 89:966–979, 1982
3. Keulen-de-vos HCJ, Van Rij G, Renardel de Lavalette JCG: Effect of indomethacin in preventing surgically induced miosis. British J Ophthalmol 67:94–96, 1983
4. Hull DS, Chemotti MT, Edelhauser HF, et al: Effect of epinephrine on the corneal endothelium. Am J Ophthalmol 79:245–250, 1975
5. Edelhauser HF, Hine JE, Pederson H, et al: The effect of phenilephrine on the cornea. Arch Ophthalmol 97:937–947, 1979
6. Michels RG: Vitreous surgery. St Louis, C.V. Mosby Company, 385–387, 1981
7. Landers MB, Robinson D, Olsen KR, Rinkoff J: Slit-lamp fluid-gas exchange and other office procedures following vitreoretinal surgery. Arch Ophthalmol 103:967–972, 1985
8. Van Horn DL, Edelhauser HF: Effects of glutathione and adenosine on the corneal endothelium. J Cell Biol 1973 59 (2 Pt 2) 351 a (Abstract)
9. Edelhauser HF, Van Horn DL, Miller P, Pederson HJ: Effect of Thioloxidation of glutathione with diamide on corneal endothelial function, junctional complexes, and microfilaments. J Cell Biol 68:567–78, 1976
10. Edelhauser HF, Van Horn DL, Schultz RO, Hyndiuk RA: Comparative toxicity of intraocular irrigation solutions on the corneal endothelium. Am J Ophthalmol 81:473–81, 1976

11. Edelhauser HF, Gonnering R, Van Horn DL: Intraocular irrigating solutions; a comparative study of BSS plus and lactated Ringer's solution. Arch Ophthalmol 96:516–520, 1978

12. Benson WE, Diamond JG, Tasman W: Intraocular irrigating solutions for pars plana vitrectomy; a prospective, randomized, double-blind study. Arch Ophthalmol 99,6:1013–1015, 1981

13. Rosenfeld SI, Waltman SR, Olk RJ, Gordon M: Comparison of intraocular irrigating solutions in pars plana vitrectomy. Ophthalmology 93:109–115, 1986

14. Chignel AH: Retinal detachment surgery. New York, Springer-Verlag, 112, 1980

15. Kuwabara T, Gorn RA: Retinal damage by visible light. An electron microscopic study. Arch Ophthalmol 79:69–78, 1968

16. Kuwabara T: Retinal recovery from exposure to light. Am J Ophthalmol 70:187–198, 1970

17. Tso MO, Fine BS, Zimmerman LE: Photic maculopathy produced by the indirect ophthalmoscope. I-Clinical and histologic study. Am J Ophthalmol 73:686–699, 1972

18. Hochheimer BF, D'Anna SA, Calkins JL: Retinal damage from light. Am J Ophthalmol 88:1039–1044, 1979

19. Parver LM, Auker CR, Fine BS: Observations on monkey eyes exposed to light from an operating microscope. Ophthalmology 90:964–972, 1983

20. Irvine AR, Wood I, Morris BW: Retinal damage from the illumination of the operating microscope. An experimental study in pseudophakic monkeys. Arch Ophthalmol 102:1358–1365, 1984

21. Fuller D, Machemer R, Knighton RW: Retinal damage produced by intraocular fiber optic light. Am J Ophthalmol 85:519–437, 1978

22. Robertson DM, Feldman RB: Photic retinopathy from the operating room microscope. Am J Ophthalmol 101:561–569, 1986

23. Rinkoff J, Machemer R, Hida T, Chandler D: Temperature dependent light damage to the retina. Am J Ophthalmol 102:452–462, 1986

24. Custodis E: Bedented die Plombenaufnahung auf die Sklera einen Fortschritt in der operativen Behandlung der Netzhautablösung? Ber Deutsch Ophthal Ges 58:102–105, 1953

25. Lincoff HA, Baras I, McLean J: Modifications to the custodis procedure for retinal detachment. Arch Ophthalmol 73:160–163, 1965

26. Chignell AH: Retinal detachment surgery without drainage of subretinal fluid. Am J Ophthalmol 77:1–5, 1974

27. Leaver PK, Chignell AH, Fison LG, Pyne JR, Saunders SH: Role of nondrainage of subretinal fluid in reoperations for retinal detachment. Brit J Ophthalmol 59:252–254, 1975

28. Bonnet M, Santamaria E, Mouche J: Intraoperative pure C3F8 as an adjunct to vitreoretinal microsurgery in the management of retinal detachments associated with proliferative vitreoretinopathy. Graefes Arch. Clin Exp Ophthalmol 225:299–302, 1987

29. Leaver PK, Chester GH, Saunders SH: Factors influencing absorption of subretinal fluid. Brit J Ophthalmol 60:557–560, 1976

30. Chignell AH, Talbot J: Absorption of subretinal fluid after nondrainage retinal detachment surgery. Arch Ophthalmol 96:635–637, 1978

31. Robertson DM: Delayed absorption of subretinal fluid after scleral buckling procedures. Am J Ophthalmol 87:57–64, 1979

32. Freyler H, Kutschera E: Echoikulometrie bei Amotiooperationen ohne subretinale drainage. Klin Mbl Augenheilk 169:442–444, 1976

33. Schepens C: Retinal detachment and allied diseases. Philadelphia, W. B. Saunders, Vol. 1, 409–416, 1983

34. Chignell AH: Retinal detachment surgery. New York, Springer-Verlag, 1980, 123–127

35. Bonnet M: Microsurgery of retinal detachment (vitreous surgery excluded). Developments in ophthalmology, Karger, Basel, Vol 1, 53–59, 1981

36. Gartner J: Release of subretinal fluid with the aid of the microscope. Report of 100 cases. Mod Probl Ophthalmol, 15:127–133, 1975

37. Draeger J: The microscope as a tool in the management of the sclera. Dev Ophthalmol 2:202–207, 1981

38. Bonnet M, Lenail B: Prophylaxie des complications maculaires du décollement de la rétine par microchirugie, J Fr Ophthalmol 3, 2:83–88, 1980

9
Inducing a Retinochoroidal Scar

RATIONALE FOR INDUCING A RETINOCHOROIDAL SCAR

Since Gonin,[1] chorioretinal irritation in the area of the retinal breaks has been accepted as the basic principle of rhegmatogenous retinal detachment management. The main goal of the induced chorioretinal scar is to seal the retinal break and prevent intravitreal or retrovitreal fluid to leak through the break towards the subretinal space.

INDICATIONS

Retinochoroidal irritation in the area of the retinal break(s) should be performed in all rhegmatogenous retinal detachments, except for selected retinal detachments associated with macular holes (see p. 221).

The possibility of successfully treating selected rhegmatogenous retinal detachments without inducing a retinochoroidal scar has been demonstrated.[2-3] In selected cases retinal reattachment can be achieved only by relieving vitreous traction with either scleral buckling[2] or vitrectomy.[3-4] However, vitrectomy without inducing a retinochoroidal scar in the retinal break area has been successful in reattaching the retina in only a few cases of retinal detachments associated with macular holes (see p. 222). In addition, when it fails to reattach the retina, the detachment is aggravated. Scleral buckling of peripheral retinal breaks without any chorioretinal irritation cannot be recommended. It can provide a high initial reattachment rate in selected cases,[2,5-7] but the risk of late redetachment is very high.[6-8]

METHODS FOR INDUCING A RETINOCHOROIDAL SCAR

In the past many techniques were used to create chorioretinal irritation. Currently, cryotreatment, diathermy, and photocoagulation treatment are the only methods used. In the future, other means such as N-butyl-2-cyano acrylate[9-11] or other tissue glue, may be used to seal retinal breaks in selected cases.

Cryotreatment

Cryosurgical treatment of retinal detachment was initially developed by Bietti in the 1930s.[12] However, owing to the limitation of the instrumentation, the technique had not been used until it was reintroduced and popularized by Lincoff in the 1960s.[13] At present cryotreatment is the technique most commonly used to produce a retinochoroidal irritation in the retinal break area.

Histological studies have demonstrated that chorioretinal irritation by cryotreatment can induce a firm chorioretinal adhesion.[14-19]

ADVANTAGES—DISADVANTAGES

Cryotreatment can be used either through the sclera or through the vitreous cavity.

Endocryotreatment of retinal breaks in the vitrectomized eye has important disadvantages. It is rarely used in microsurgical management of retinal detachment (see p. 144).

Transscleral cryotreatment is the preferred method in both vitrectomized and nonvitrectomized eyes. It has two main advantages compared to transscleral diathermy: (1) it causes virtually no permanent damage to the sclera and the surrounding Tenon's capsule, and conjunctiva; and (2) it is effective when applied to a wet surface, therefore, it is easily performed under simultaneous control of the fundus.

Cryotreatment, however, also has several disadvantages compared to diathermy and photocoagulation. In particular it produces dilatation of the choroidal vessels. Thus extensive cryotreatment, when required for treating multiple and/or large breaks, may predispose to choroidal hemorrhage. The retinochoroidal adhesion induced by cryotreatment develops more slowly than that produced by argon laser photocoagulation and diathermy.[20] In addition cryotreatment is likely to stimulate the development of preretinal membranes in predisposed eyes (see p. 234). Therefore, cryotreatment is rarely used in the management of giant retinal tears and in eyes with a high risk of proliferative vitreoretinopathy postoperatively.

SURGICAL TECHNIQUE

Transscleral cryotreatment is performed with simultaneous biomicroscopic observation of the fundus, in all circumstances. Cryotreatment with outside control of scleral freezing[21] is never used. Outside control of scleral freezing is unreliable, since multiple factors such as scleral thickness and pressure exerted on the sclera greatly influence the intensity of the cryolesion produced in the choroid and the retina.[22]

Advantages of Biomicroscopic Control of Cryotreatment. The main advantages of cryotreatment with simultaneous biomicroscopic examination of the fundus were initially emphasized by Hilsdorf.[23–24] Simultaneous biomicroscopic observation of the fundus during cryoapplication offers a degree of accuracy that no other control technique can provide. Indeed, freezing of the tissues can be controlled, not only in terms of surface, but also, and even more importantly, in terms of depth. Freezing is strictly limited to the area of the retinal break. Overtreatment of either the pigment epithelium or of the neurosensory retina, as well as freezing of the internal limiting membrane and the vitreous body, can be avoided in nearly all cases. Thus treatment of retinal breaks by means of cryoapplication is almost as accurate as treatment with argon laser photocoagulation. Such accuracy is possible because the progression of the ice ball is observed in an optical cross section of the tissues.

Surgical Technique. The contact lens is held on the cornea by the left hand and the cryoprobe by the right. The cryoprobe handle must be tilted outward in order to avoid pressure against the contact lens (Figs. 54, 55, and 56)

For cryopexy the magnification of the microscope should be higher than for the locating of the retinal break. It should be at least 13.4 × (zoom factor 1.5 with 12.5 eyepieces). A magnification of over 20 × is recommended for greater accuracy.

Biomicroscopic observation of the fundus is performed using a narrow slit beam for better stereopsis. Use of the cryoprobe especially designed for microsurgery is mandatory (see p. 35). Cryoprobe function is confirmed under the microscope before performing the first cryoapplication. Variations of freezing and thawing speed with the same apparatus and cryoprobe are common. They depend on many factors, in particular room temperature and tank nitrous oxide pressure. These variations are taken into account to determine when pressure on the foot pedal should be released to avoid overtreatment.

Control of the Cryoapplication Surface. As with photocoagulation treatment, cryoapplication is strictly limited to the area of the retinal break. Thus, it is mandatory that the limited area of the choroid and the retinal pigment epithelium, which are frozen, will correspond exactly to the retinal break when close apposition of the neurosensory retina and the

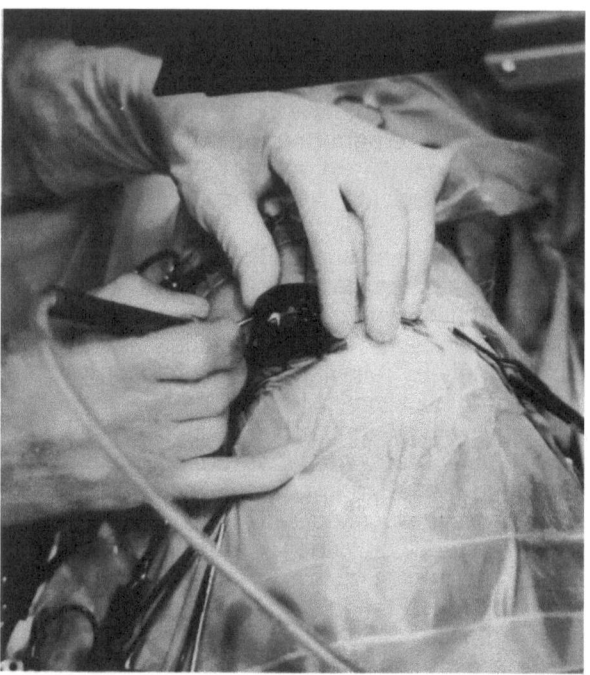

Figure 54. Position of the cryoprobe when the surgeon is seated in front of the retinal quadrant in which the retinal break is located.

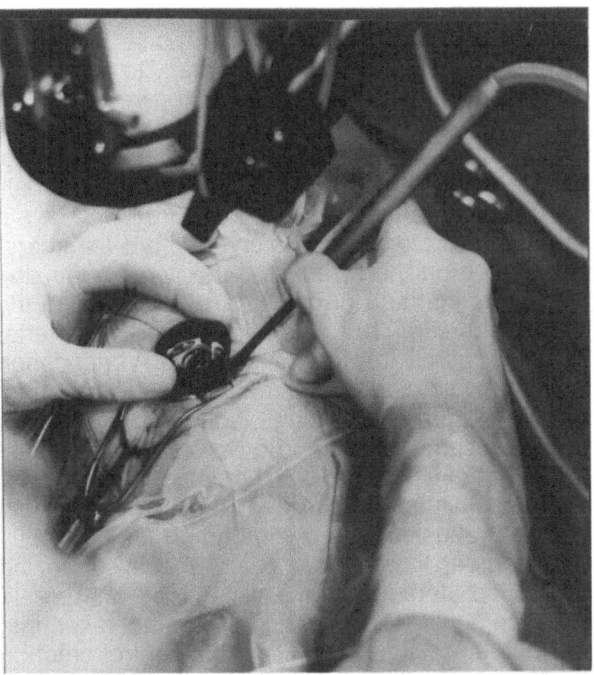

Figure 55. Position of the cryoprobe when the surgeon is seated at the opposite side of the retinal quadrant in which the retinal break is located. In both cases the cryoprobe is tilted outward so as to avoid pressure against the contact lens.

pigment epithelium has been achieved by means of scleral buckling. In fact, if subretinal fluid remains between the retinal pigment epithelium and the neurosensory retina during cryoapplication, the surgeon cannot be sure that the very limited area of the retinal

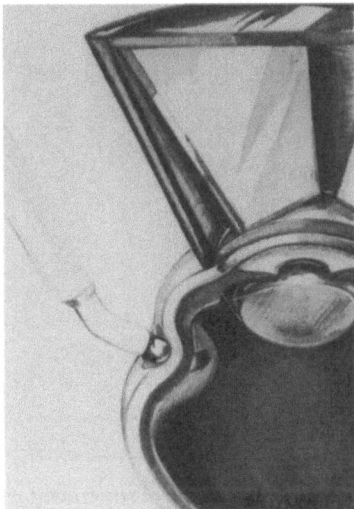

Figure 56. Diagram of correct positioning of the cryoprobe handle during cryotreatment with simultaneous biomicroscopic control of the fundus.

pigment epithelium being treated will correspond exactly to the retinal break after positioning of the scleral buckle.

In bullous and/or very prominent retinal detachments, it is advisable to manipulate the cryoprobe with the same technique as the marker during localization of the break (Fig. 57). The tip of the cryoprobe should not be initially placed on the scleral projection of the slit beam centered on the retinal break, since this projection is in fact too posterior. The tip of the cryoprobe is placed in front of the ora serrata in the meridian of the break. The choroidal indentation produced by the tip of the cryoprobe that depresses the sclera is observed through the microscope and the contact lens. Then with biomicroscopic control of the fundus, the cryoprobe is shifted backward pushing the choroid against the retina. When the choroidal indentation produced by the tip of the cryoprobe reaches the retinal break both areas of the choroid and of the retina, which are placed in contact by the cryoprobe, correspond to the areas that will be put in apposition after scleral buckling. This technique of shifting the cryoprobe backward under biomicroscopic control of the fundus is mandatory in bullous retinal detachments; it is, indeed, a necessary step to ensure that treatment is accurate.

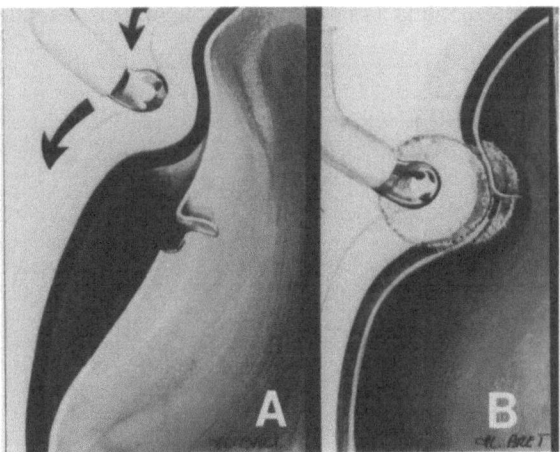

Figure 57. Cryotreatment of the retinal break with simultaneous biomicroscopic observation of the fundus in a bullous retinal detachment. (A) The cryoprobe tip has to be placed in front of the ora serrata on the meridian of the retinal tear. It is then gently shifted backward pushing the choroid against the retina (B) When the choroidal indentation produced by the cryoprobe tip reaches the retinal tear, the area of the choroid that is to be frozen corresponds to the area that will be put into contact with the retinal tear by further scleral buckling.

Control of the Cryoapplication Depth. Experimental studies have shown that a firm retinochoroidal adhesion is more likely to be obtained when the detached retina is involved in the freezing process.[17] However, cryolesions should spare the internal limiting lamina to avoid stimulation of preretinal membrane formation. To achieve this goal, freezing of the cryoprobe is begun only when the pigment epithelium and the edges of the retinal break have been placed in close apposition by the indentation of the cryoprobe, no subretinal fluid remaining between them. If close apposition of the pigment epithelium and the retinal break (without subretinal fluid remaining between them) cannot be obtained by scleral depression with the cryoprobe, paracentesis of the anterior chamber or subretinal fluid release are carried out. Release of intraocular fluid and decreased intraocular pressure allow for higher scleral depression.

The appearance of the ice ball in the choroid and its progression toward the neurosensory retina are controlled in the optical cross section of the tissues. Choroidal and pigment epithelium freezing shows a faint yellowish appearance. Retina freezing shows a conspicuous white color, just like an iceball. Freezing is ceased as soon as the iceball reaches the neurosensory retina (Fig. 58). The iceball must not reach the internal limiting lamina (Fig. 58). It may be difficult for beginners to accurately locate the internal limiting lamina in the optical cross section

owing to the thinness of the normal retina. The retinal vessels can be used as a landmark to locate the internal limiting lamina (Fig. 59). When freezing does not involve the retinal vessels, the surgeon can be certain that the internal limiting membrane has not been reached by the iceball. After thawing the iceball, the outer retina that has just been frozen shows a faint gray discoloration. The cryoprobe is then carefully shifted on the sclera and the same controlled freezing is carried out on the area adjacent to the first area treated. The posterior edge and the anterior edge are entirely treated, step by step. A brief period of time should elapse after each cryoapplication so that the cryoprobe is no longer adherent to the sclera when the surgeon shifts it to an adjacent position. Treatment of a medium-sized retinal break can usually be completed with no need to remove the contact lens and reposition the cryoprobe on the sclera.

Of course, the number of consecutive freezing applications depends on the size of the retinal break. For each application, freezing time is not taken into account, since it is not a valuable control criterion of choroidal and retinal freezing. In fact, the time required for proper freezing of the choroid and retina depends on many factors, in particular, the scleral

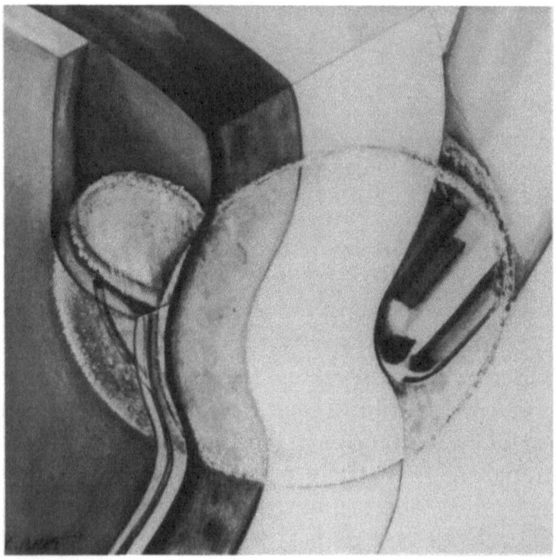

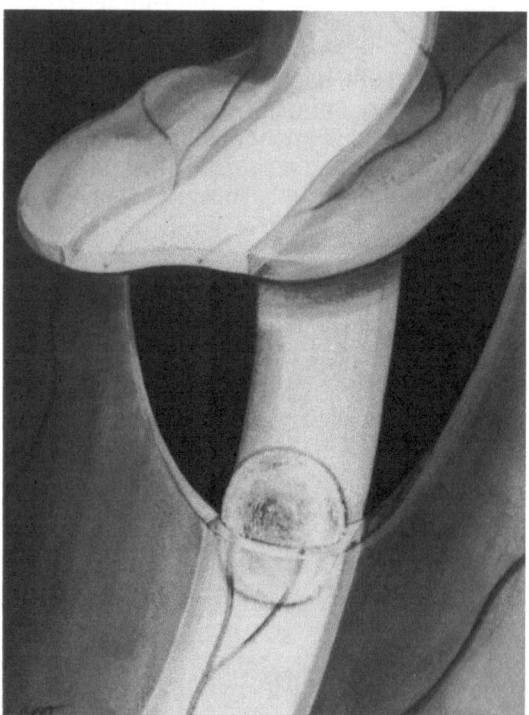

Figure 58. Correct cryotreatment of a retinal break. Pigment epithelium and neurosensory retina are placed into close apposition by scleral depression produced by the cryoprobe tip. Freezing involves the choroid and the outer third of the neurosensory retina.

Figure 59. Correct cryotreatment of a retinal break. Retinal vessels are used as a landmark to avoid freezing of the internal limiting lamina. Tissue freezing must not involve the retinal vessels.

thickness that may show variations in the retinal break area.

Errors to Avoid. To obtain the nearly perfect accuracy that can be expected from cryoapplication performed under biomicroscopic observation of the fundus, the surgeon has to operate with great care. The major errors to be avoided are as follows:

Errors in the Positioning of the Cryoprobe on the Sclera. Four errors should be avoided in the positioning of the cryoprobe on the sclera. The first error is incorrect inclination of the cryoprobe shaft. The cryoprobe shaft should be tilted outward as far as the orbit wall allows. Indeed, if the cryoprobe shaft is tilted toward the cornea and the contact lens, it applies strong pressure on the sclera. The resulting excessive deformation of the eyeball may lead to the passage of air and blood between the contact lens and the cornea.

The second error is improper orientation of the tip of the cryoprobe; such as when the tip of the cryoprobe has not been placed perpendicular to the sclera; it has been turned either laterally or even toward the orbit cavity. The resulting effect will be either excessive freezing of the sclera or freezing of the conjunctiva and Tenon's capsule instead of a well-controlled freezing of the sclera and the choroid. This error can easily be avoided by using the point of reference on the cryoprobe handle. The tip of the index finger is put on the reference point before placing the tip of the cryoprobe on the sclera. The orientation of the surgeon's finger, which must not move during cryopexy, indicates the exact orientation of the cryoprobe.

In the third error, the tip of the cryoprobe is initially placed in too posterior a position. In the case of a very bullous retinal detachment, the frozen choroidal area will not correspond exactly to the margin of the retinal break after scleral buckling (Fig. 60).

The final and most obvious error is easy to avoid. The cryoprobe has been shifted too far backward without control of the fundus. When the surgeon looks at the retinal tear through the contact lens and sees what is believed to be the choroidal indentation caused by the tip of the cryoprobe, this in fact has been caused by the cryoprobe shaft (Fig. 61). If the surgeon is unaware of this incorrect assumption, he or she will freeze a retinal territory that does not need treatment. Even worse, the sur-

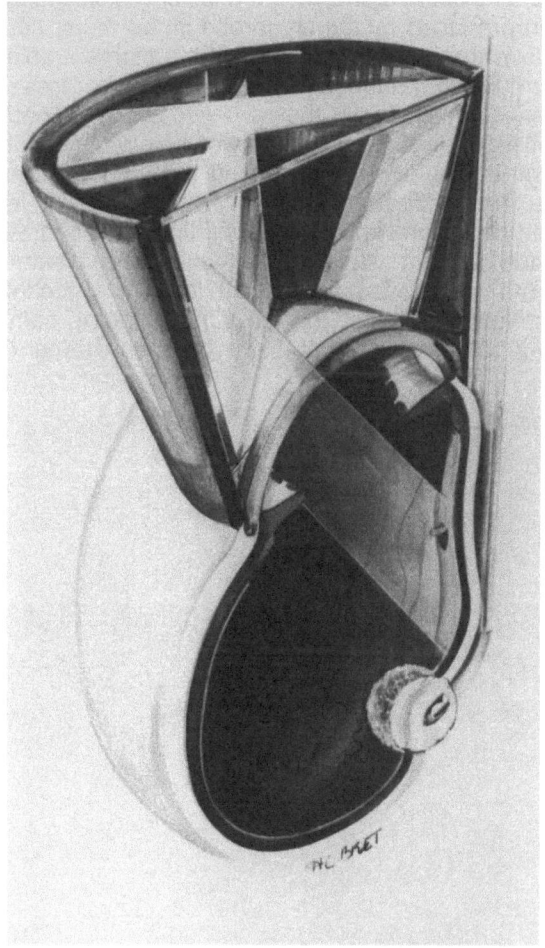

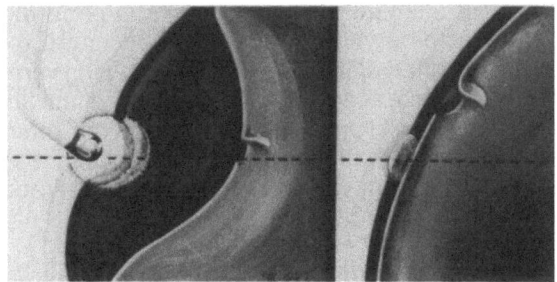

Figure 60. Error to avoid in cryotreatment in eyes with bullous retinal detachment (Left): The cryoprobe tip has initially been placed on the scleral projection of the slit beam centered on the retinal tear. This position is too posterior. (Right): Consequently, the area of the choroid that is frozen will not correspond exactly to the retinal tear after scleral buckling and subretinal fluid absorption.

Figure 61. Error to avoid in cryotreatment: The cryoprobe tip has been shifted too far posteriorly without simultaneous observation of the fundus. Scleral depression in front of the retinal tear is produced by the cryoprobe shaft. The surgeon unaware of the error freezes the posterior retina, which is out of the range of observation.

geon may freeze the internal limiting membrane and the vitreous body because the tip of the cryoprobe is out of the range of observation through the mirror of the contact lens. This most serious error can be avoided by the backward shifting technique under simultaneous control of the fundus.

Errors in the Dosage of Cryoapplication.   Excessive freezing is the most common error in cryoapplication. While this error is not always avoidable with other methods of cryoapplication control, it is more easily avoidable with biomicroscopic control of the fundus.

Overtreatment can affect either the pigment epithelium or both layers of the retina and the vitreous gel. Persistence of subretinal fluid between the margins of the retinal tear and the choroidal indentation produced by the cryoprobe is the major cause of overtreatment at the level of the pigment epithelium (Fig. 62). Indeed, in this case a longer freezing time is necessary for the ice ball to reach the neurosensory retina. Overtreatment of the pigment epithelium is visible when observing the fundus through the microscope: a cloud of pigment spreads from the frozen zone toward the subretinal fluid. Migration of the pigment can reach the macula. Overtreatment of the neurosensory retina with freezing of the internal limiting lamina and the vitreous gel is caused by a late shutting off of the cryoprobe freezing (Fig.

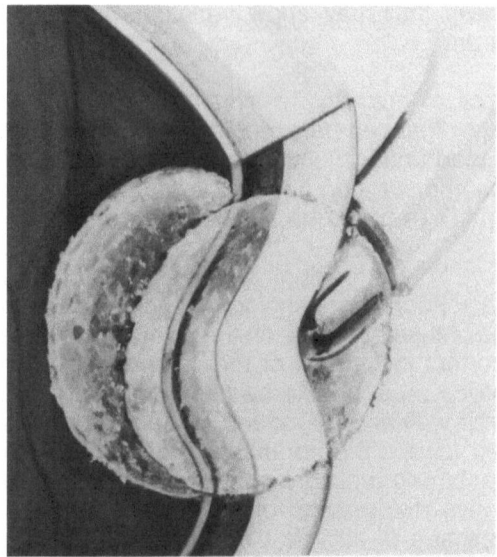

Figure 63.   Error to avoid in cryotreatment: excessively prolonged cryoapplication results in freezing of the inner retinal layers and vitreous gel.

63). Freezing of the internal limiting lamina and vitreous gel is recognized as feathery patterns of ice crystals. This is a serious intraoperative complication that may result in postoperative vitreous gel haziness or stimulation of preretinal membrane formation.

Control of the fundus in an optical cross section of the tissues during cryotreatment makes it easy to avoid the above mentioned errors in assessing the degree of cryotreatment necessary.

Cryotreatment in Eyes Managed with Vitrectomy.   When the surgical procedure includes vitrectomy, cryotreatment of retinal breaks is performed before vitrectomy whenever possible. Accurate cryotreatment is often difficult to achieve following vitrectomy due to increased choroidal and subretinal fluid thickness. In addition, when the vitrectomy procedure is performed after cryotreatment, pigment epithelial cells that may have spread into the vitreous cavity during cryotreatment are washed out.

Cryotretment in the Gas-Filled Eye.   Cryotreatment in the gas-filled eye should be avoided whenever possible owing to the high likelihood of overtreatment. Accurate visual control is difficult due to poor stereopsis through a gas bubble. In addition, progression of tissue freezing is more rapid in the gas-filled eye because of the thermal dynamic modification. Histopathology of transscleral cryopexy lesions in the gas-filled human eye have shown full-thickness retinal lesions with disruption of the internal limiting lamina.[25]

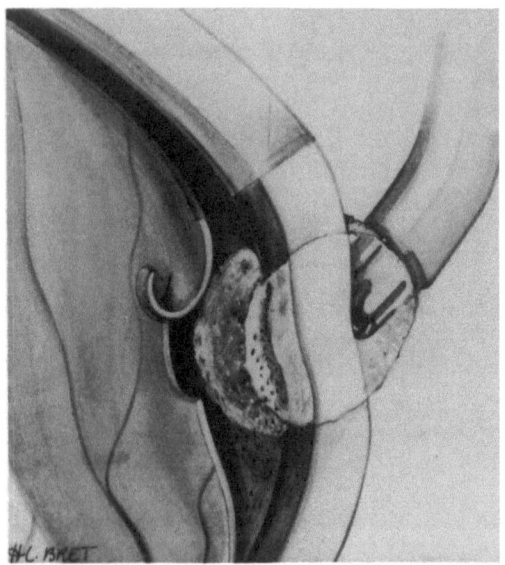

Figure 62.   Error to avoid in cryotreatment. Cryotreatment is performed through subretinal fluid. Prolonged tissue freezing results in excessive treatment of the choroid and pigment epithelium. Pigment epithelial cells are dispersed in the subretinal space.

COMPLICATIONS

Intraoperative Complications. Intraoperative complications of cryotreatment include: (1) inability to position the cryoprobe tip in front of the retinal break, (2) inability to obtain freezing of the choroid and/or retina, (3) increased intraocular pressure and corneal clouding, (4) scleral perforation, and (5) damage to a vortex vein.

Inability to Position the Cryoprobe Tip on the Sclera in Front of the Retinal Break. Proper placement of the cryoprobe tip at the ora serrata on the meridian of the break, and then shifting it backward up to the break, may be mechanically hindered by the eyelid speculum or the eyebrow. This difficulty is overcome by slightly rotating the speculum so that the cryoprobe can be shifted between the two speculum hooks. In addition a torsional rotation of the eye before fixing the bridle sutures to the surgical drapes is helpful to place the break meridian in the most accessible position (see p. 49)

Inability to Obtain Freezing of the Choroid or Retina in the Retinal Break Area. Inability to obtain freezing of the choroid or retina in the retinal break area can result from several causes: (1) malfunction of the cryoprobe, (2) improper positioning of the cryoprobe active tip, (3) tissue interposition between the cryoprobe tip and the sclera, (4) increased eye wall thickness by scar tissue, and (5) increased choroidal thickness.

Malfunction of the cryoprobe is easily recognized by slightly moving the cryoprobe along the sclera. If the cryoprobe can be moved during freezing this indicates that the cryoprobe actually is not freezing. Verification of cryoprobe function before use on the sclera is recommended so that time is not wasted with such problems.

Improper positioning of the cryoprobe active tip is easily avoided through proper technique (see above). The active tip of the cryoprobe should be placed on the sclera under visual control, using coaxial illumination of the microscope before placing the contact lens on the cornea. The point of reference on the cryoprobe handle is then used to monitor the position of the cryoprobe tip when the cryoprobe is moved along the sclera. The most serious error in positioning of the active tip of the cryoprobe is its placement posterior to the retinal break area. If the scleral depression produced by the cryoprobe shaft is misinterpreted as resulting from the cryoprobe tip, prolonged freezing applied to areas that are not in the field of observation may result in serious damage to the posterior retina or optic nerve. The backward shifting technique under fundus control makes it possible to avoid such a mistake.

Tissue interposition between the sclera and the cryoprobe tip can easily be avoided by proper opening of the conjunctiva and Tenon's capsule and by initially placing the cryoprobe tip on the sclera under visual control.

Increased eye wall thickness by scar tissue can be observed in reoperations. If the ice ball cannot reach the choroid and/or retina, dissection of scar tissue should be completed.

Increased choroidal thickness that prevents the ice ball from reaching the pigment epithelium layer and/or the neurosensory retina is observed when a choroidal detachment is associated with the retinal detachment or following lengthy vitrectomy procedures in severely diseased eyes. In such cases retinal breaks should be treated by argon laser photocoagulation. Argon laser photocoagulation treatment is carried out either intraoperatively using scleral depression to approximate the pigment epithelium layer and the neurosensory retina, or postoperatively after temporary sealing of the retinal break(s) by a gas bubble (see p. 81).

Increased Intraocular Pressure and Corenal Edema. Excessive scleral depression by the cryoprobe may result in increased intraocular pressure and corneal edema. The latter may compromise adequate visualization of the fundus. This complication is more likely to occur in bullous retinal detachments when deep scleral depression is required to obtain approximation of the pigment epithelium and the neurosensory retina. It can be avoided by performing paracentesis of the anterior chamber and by relieving scleral depression between each cryoapplication.

Scleral Perforation. Scleral perforation by the cryoprobe can occur when the sclera has been damaged by previous surgery or a staphyloma. This most severe complication can be avoided by reinforcing the damaged sclera with dura mater before performing cryotreatment. Scleral depression should be performed with great care in such eyes.

Damage to a Vortex Vein. Damage to a vortex vein from the cryoprobe can occur when the vein has been dragged anteriorly by scar tissue and/or when the retinal break is located in the area of the vortex vein. If the cryoprobe is moved before complete thawing, laceration of the outer part of the vein can occur when it is involved in the ice ball.

Postoperative Complications. Most postoperative complications of cryotreatment are probably related to improper or excessive application. Vitreous gel haziness, progression of premacular membranes and macular lesions are the main postoperative complications.

Postoperative vitreous gel haziness due to cryotreatment occurs when excessively prolonged cryoapplications have involved the inner surface of the retina and the vitreous gel. Corticosteroids are given in such cases, however, their therapeutic value in this specific indication has not been fully established. Postoperative vitreous haziness due to excessive cryotreatment can be avoided by proper control of cryoapplication in optical cross section of the fundus.

Cryotreatment may contribute to the development of proliferative vitreoretinopathy in predisposed eyes (see p. 234), and, therefore, cryotreatment should be avoided in such eyes whenever possible.

Cryotreatment can play a major role in the development of certain postoperative macular complications. Subretinal pigment migration to the macula (Fig. 64) is a specific complication of cryotreatment.[26–30] It is more likely to occur when more than 30 cryoapplications are performed and in bullous retinal detachments of the superior quadrants.[29] Subretinal pigment migration is caused by overtreatment of the pigment epithelium layer with subretinal fluid remaining between the choroid depressed by the cryoprobe and the neurosensory retina.[31–33] Although benign in most cases, pigment migration to the macula may compromise the visual result of the operation in a few cases.[30–34] This complication can be avoided through proper surgical technique in most cases.[33–35] Cryotreatment may contribute to the progression of premacular membranes.[8,17,33] This is probably related to overtreatment with freezing of the internal limiting lamina.[32,33] However, excessive cryotreatment is not the only cause of macular pucker after retinal detachment repair. Macular pucker has been observed in eyes managed without cryotreatment.[8] Cryotreatment is likely to induce a breakdown of the blood ocular barrier. However, no correlation has been found between the incidence of postoperative cystoid macular edema and the number of cryoapplications when performed with biomicroscopic control of the fundus.[36]

Argon Laser Photocoagulation

At present argon laser photocoagulation is the method that provides the most accuracy in the treatment of retinal breaks. However, owing to its limitations, argon laser photocoagulation can be used only in selected cases.

ADVANTAGES AND LIMITATIONS

Argon laser photocoagulation has several advantages compared to cryotreatment: (1) the laser burns remain clearly visible; therefore overtreatment due to overlapping of the lesions is easily avoided; (2) a firm retinochoroidal adhesion can be achieved with less risk of damage to the inner retinal layers; (3) the induced retinochoroidal adhesion is more rapid to develop;[20] and (4) argon laser photocoagulation is less likely to stimulate proliferative vitreoretinopathy. Argon laser photocoagulation has two major limitations in retinal detachment management: (1) close apposition of the neurosensory retina and pigment epithelial layer is a mandatory requirement to make photocoagulation treatment feasible; and (2) moderate haziness of the media may prevent transpupillary photocoagulation treatment.

INDICATIONS

The main indications for argon laser photocoagulation treatment in retinal detachment repair are as follows: (1) peripheral retinal break(s) with a shallow detachment, (2) macular holes in selected cases (see p. 223), (3) giant retinal tears in highly myopic eyes (see p. 207), (4) eyes with a high risk of postoperative proliferative vitreoretinopathy (see p. 233), and (5) iatrogenic retinal breaks during vitrectomy in selected cases (see p. 150).

Argon laser photocoagulation is also used by preference for prophylactic treatment of the other eye.

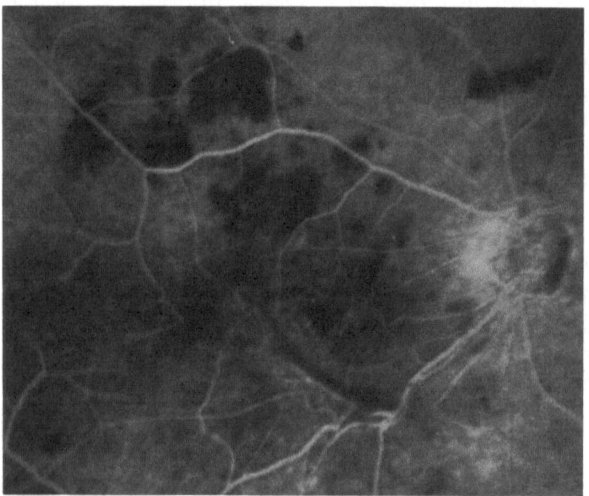

Figure 64. Subretinal pigment migration to the posterior pole in an eye that underwent four operations for retinal reattachment. Pigment migration is associated with a premacular membrane and cystoid macular edema. Central vision is 20/400.

SURGICAL TECHNIQUE

Depending on indications, argon laser photocoagulation is used preoperatively, intraoperatively, or postoperatively.

Argon laser photocoagulation treatment to close associated retinal breaks in attached retina and to destroy large areas of exposed pigment epithelial cells is performed preoperatively in most cases. Any argon laser device can be used, however, use of the argon laser attached to the surgical microscope is often advantageous when treating large areas of exposed pigment epithelial cells. The patient is more comfortable in the supine position when treatment is lengthy or when retrobulbar anesthesia is required to avoid ocular pain and eye movement.

Transpupillary[37] or endophotocoagulation[38–40] can be used intraoperatively. Endophotocoagulation during vitrectomy is used in selected cases. The main indications for transpupillary argon laser photocoagulation during retinal detachment surgery are as follows: (1) shallow retinal detachments with a high risk of proliferative vitreoretinopathy such as, in particular, retinal detachment with large horseshoe tear(s) and/or horseshoe tear(s) with a curled posterior edge, (2) iatrogenic retinal breaks in attached retina during vitrectomy, and (3) selected retinal detachments with macular holes and breaks of the posterior pole. When the retina is detached, argon laser photocoagulation is performed at the beginning of the surgical procedure. It is done with simultaneous scleral depression to approximate the pigment epithelium layer and the neurosensory retina. The cryoprobe is used as a scleral depressor in most cases When the break is peripheral and requires scleral buckling, argon laser photocoagulation can also be carried out after completion of the scleral buckle.

The main indications for postoperative argon laser photocoagulation through the pupil are as follows: (1) selected retinal detachments with peripheral retinal breaks managed by gas injection without scleral buckling,[41] (2) selected retinal detachments with macular holes managed by vitrectomy or gas injection (see p. 223), (3) selected retinal detachments with severe proliferative vitreoretinopathy managed by vitreous surgery and gas injection without revision of the scleral buckle performed at previous operation(s), (4) retinal detachments with giant tears in highly myopic eyes—postoperative photocoagulation of the tear edges is performed as an adjunct to preoperative ablation of exposed pigment epithelial cells (see p. 208), and (5) prophylactic treatment of the fellow eye in selected patients.

Postoperative argon laser photocoagulation in gas-filled eyes is performed with the slit lamp in a seated patient when the eye is phakic. When the eye is aphakic the treatment is easier to perform with the surgical microscope on a supine patient. In the latter case no contact lens is used. The high magnification provided by the surgical microscope is useful in clearly identifying retinal tear edges. Great care should be taken to avoid overtreatment during argon laser photocoagulation in the gas-filled eye. Owing to modifications of thermal dynamics, a laser burn of sufficient duration and power to provide a partial-thickness burn in the fluid-filled eye, is likely to produce a full-thickness retinal lesion in the gas-filled eye.[25] Uniform, cream-colored lesions should be obtained. Excessively heavy laser burns result in intraocular vapor formation.

In young children postoperative argon laser photocoagulation for prophylactic treatment of the fellow eye is performed under general anesthesia with the argon laser attached to the surgical microscope.[37]

COMPLICATIONS

Complications of argon laser photocoagulation used to seal retinal breaks are infrequent.[42]

Intraoperative Complications. Inability to completely seal the retinal break(s) and overtreatment are the two main intraoperative complications of argon laser photocoagulation.

Inability to completely surround the retinal break with uniform cream-colored retinal burns occurs when complete approximation of the pigment epithelium and neurosensory retina is not obtained by scleral depression. In such cases, intraoperative photocoagulation is withdrawn and cryotreatment, or postoperative photocoagulation, is performed.

Overtreatment, which may result in postoperative complications, is more likely to occur in the gas-filled eye.

Postoperative Complications. The precise role of argon laser photocoagulation in the development of postoperative complications after retinal detachment repair is uneasy to determine since a number of associated factors may contribute to the development of such complications.

Heavy and extensive argon laser photocoagulation treatment may contribute to the development of postoperative vitreous hemorrhage, inflammatory reaction, choroidal detachment, cystoid macular edema, macular pucker, and recurrent proliferative vitreoretinopathy. It may also contribute to the progression of preexisting lens opacities, in particular nuclear sclerosis.

Diathermy

At present diathermy is infrequently used to seal retinal breaks. Transscleral diathermy has two major disadvantages as compared to cryotreatment and photocoagulation treatment: (1) it induces permanent scleral damage[43–49] and (2) diathermy cannot be performed under simultaneous control of the fundus. The indications for transscleral diathermy are restricted to eyes with a high risk of severe proliferative vitreoretinopathy, such as eyes with giant tears, when opaque media prevent argon laser photocoagulation treatment. The Mira radiofrequency unit is used. The technique advocated by Schepens[50] is performed. Control of the fundus is done at regular intervals when diathermy is carried out to make certain that uniform mild retinal marks are obtained.

Endodiathermy can be used to seal retinal breaks during vitrectomy.[51–52] Argon laser photocoagulation is, however, more accurate and less hazardous as compared with endodiathermy. Transscleral cryotreatment with biomicrospic control of the fundus has nearly no limitations, therefore, the latter techniques are used in most cases, rather than endodiathermy.

REFERENCES

1. Gonin J: Le décollement de la rétine. Lausanne Switzerland Librairie Payot 1934
2. Zauberman H, Rosell FG: Treatment of retinal detachment without inducing chorioretinal lesions. Trans Am Acad Ophthalmol Otolaryngol 79:835–844, 1975
3. Gonvers M, Machemer R: A new approach to treating retinal detachment with macular hole. Am J Ophthalmol 94:468–472, 1982
4. Machemer R: The importance of fluid absorption, traction, intraocular currents and chorioretinal scars in therapy of rhegmatogenous retinal detachment. Am J Ophthalmol 98:681–693, 1984
5. Chignell AH: Retinal detachment surgery without cryotreatment. Trans Ophthalmol Soc UK 97:30–32, 1977
6. Axer-Siegel R, Yassur Y, Ben-Sira I: Surgical management of retinal detachment without cryopexy. Am J Ophthalmol 91:474–479, 1981
7. Fetkenhour CL, Hauch TL: Scleral buckle without thermal adhesion. Am J Ophthalmol 89:662–666, 1980
8. Chignell AH, Markham RH: Retinal detachment surgery without cryotherapy. Brit J Ophthalmol 65:371–373, 1981
9. Spitznas M, Lossagk H, Joussen F: Intraocular use of butyl-2-cyanoacrylate in retinal detachment surgery. Mod Probl Ophthalmol 12:183–188, 1974
10. McCuen BW, Hida T, Sheta SM, et al: Experimental transvitreal cyanoacrylate retinopexy. Am J Ophthalmol 102:199–207, 1986
11. Sheta SM, Hida T, McCuen BW: Experimental transvitreal cyanoacrylate retinopexy through silicone oil. Am J Ophthalmol 102:717–722, 1986
12. Bietti GB: Criocausticazioni episclerali come mezzo di terapia nel distacco retinico. Boll Oculist 13:576–617, 1934
13. Lincoff H, McLean J, Nano H: Cryosurgical treatment of retinal detachment. Trans Amer Acad Ophthalmol Otolaryngol 68:412–432, 1964
14. Curtin VT, Fujino T, Norton EW: Comparative histopathology of cryosurgery and photocoagulation. Arch Ophthalmol 75:674–682, 1966
15. Lincoff H, Long R, Marquardt J, et al: The cryosurgical adhesion. Trans Am Acad Ophthalmol Otolaryngol 72:191–202, 1968
16. Lincoff H, Kreissig I: The mechanism of the cryosurgical adhesion. IV Electromicroscopy. Am J Ophthalmol 81:823–832, 1976
17. Laqua H, Machemer R: Repair and adhesion mechanisms of the cryotherapy lesion in experimental retinal detachment. Am J Ophthalmol 81;833–846, 1976
18. Feman SS, Smith RS, Ray GS, Long RS: Electron microscopy study of cryogenic chorioretinal adhesions. Am J Ophthalmol 81:823–832, 1976
19. Lincoff H, Kreissig I, Jakobiec F, et al: Remodeling of the cryosurgical adhesion. Arch Ophthalmol 99:1845–1849, 1981
20. Brihaye M, Van Geertruyben M: Comparison between cryoapplication and argon laser photocoagulation. Dev Ophthal 2:303–307, 1981
21. Haut J, Limon S: Réflexions sur la rétino-cryopexie et sa technique. Arch Ophtalmol (Paris) 33:279–288, 1973
22. Brihaye M, Oosterhuis J: Extrinsic factors which influence cryolesion intensity. Mod Probl Ophthalmol 12:476–483, 1974
23. Hilsdorf C: Cryocoagulation rétinienne sélective et de dosage exact. Bull Mem Soc Fr Ophtalmol 84:120–124, 1971
24. Hilsdorf C: Retinocryopexy by three-mirror contact lens. Ann Ophthalmol 4:1077–1080, 1972
25. Johnson RN, Irvine AR, Wood ID: Endolasr, cryopexy, and retinal reattachment in the air-filled eye. Arch Ophthalmol 105:231–234, 1987
26. Shea M: Complications of cryotherapy in retinal detachment. Canad J Ophthal 3:105–115, 1968
27. Norton EW: Cryotherapy in retinal detachment surgery. Trans New Orleans Acad Ophthal 140–141, 1969
28. Metge P, Degabriel J, Chovet M: Valeur de l'angiographie fluorescéinique dans les suites des interventions pour décollement de rétine. Bull Soc Ophtalmol Fr 72:717–724, 1972
29. Hilton GF: Subretinal pigment migration following cryosurgical retinal reattachment. Mod Probl Ophthal Basel 12:64–70, 1974
30. Francois P, Bonnet M: La macula. Masson, Paris 446–447, 1976
31. Bonnet M: Les avantages de la chirurgie sous microscope du décollement de la rétine. Bull Soc Ophtalmol Fr 75:111–11, 1975
32. Bonnet M, Bonamour G: Les avantages de la microchirurgie du décollement de la rétine. Mod Probl Ophthalmol 18:373–376, 1977
33. Bonnet M, Lenail B: Prophylaxie des complications maculaires post-opératoires du décollement de la rétine opéré par microchirurgie. J Fr Ophtalmol 3:83–88, 1980
34. Theodossiadis GP, Kokolakis SN: Macular pigment deposits in rhegmatogenous retinal detachment. Brit J Ophthalmol 63:498–506, 1979
35. Bonnet M: Biomicroscopy of the ocular fundus during retinal detachment surgery. Ocular Therapy and Surgery, 1, 50–54, 1982
36. Bonnet M, Fernandez-Pastor D: Rupture de la barriére hémato-rétinienne après microchirurgie du décollement de la rétine. Ophtalmologie 1:29–31, 1988
37. Bonnet M: Adaptation du laser à l'argon sur le microscope opératoire. J Fr Ophtalmol 13:127–128, 1980
38. Michels RG: Vitrectomy techniques in retinal reattachment surgery. Ophthalmology 86:556–585, 1979
39. Peyman GA, Grisalono JM, Palacio MN: Intraocular photocoagulation with the argon-krypton laser. Arch Ophthalmol 98:2062–2064, 1980
40. Landers MB, Trese MT, Stefansson E, et al: Argon laser intraocular photocoagulation. Ophthalmology 89:785–788, 1982
41. Dominguez A, Fonseca A, Gomez Montana J: Traitement du décollement de la rétine avec insufflation répétée de gaz. Ophtalmologie 1:205–208, 1987
42. Zweng C, Little H: Argon laser photocoagulation. St. Louis, C. B. Mosby, 1977
43. Stallard HB: Histologic appearances of eye successfully treated by diathermy for retinal detachment. Brit J Ophthalmol 17:294–297, 1933
44. Coppez ML: Choroidites expérimentales pratiquées à l'aide de l'électro-de pyrométrique. Etude anatomique des lésions de l'oeil humain. Bull Mem Soc Fr Ophtalmol 47:327–338, 1934
45. Pischel DK: Diathermy operation for retinal detachment. Comparative results of different types of electrodes. Trans Am Ophthalmol Soc 42:543–547, 1944
46. Swan KC, Christensen L: Scleral changes induced by diathermy in retinal detachment. Trans Am Ophthalmol Soc 52:65–78, 1954
47. Oosterhuis JA, Brihaye M, Dehaan AB: A comparative study of experimental transscleral cryocoagulation by solid carbon dioxide

and diathermocoagulation of the retina. Ophthalmologica 156:38–76, 1968

48. Elzeneiry I, De Guillebon HF: Scleral damage in diathermy. Am J Ophthalmol 69:754–762, 1970

49. Wilson DJ, Green WR: Histopathologic study of the effect of retinal detachment surgery on 49 eyes obtained post mortem. Am J Ophthalmol 103:167–179, 1987

50. Schepens CL: Retinal detachment and allied diseases. W. B. Saunders, cie Philadelphia, Vol 1 pp. 296–299, 1983

51. Furiat M, Parent de Curzon H, Campinchi R: Retinopexie par endo-diathermo-coagulation. J Fr Ophtalmol 7:413–417, 1984

52. Ruellan YM, Roussat B: Oblitération des trous et déchirures postérieurs de la rétine par endodiathermie après vitrectomie. J Fr Ophtalmol 7:807–812, 1984

10

Retinal Break Localization

GOAL AND INDICATIONS

Localization of the retinal break(s) is required when scleral buckling of the breaks is necessary to achieve permanent retinal reattachment. Marking the scleral projections of the retinal breaks provides landmarks for accurate placement of the scleral buckles.

ADVANTAGES OF LOCALIZATION WITH THE SURGICAL MICROSCOPE

The advantages of localization of the retinal breaks under biomicroscopic observation of the fundus are rapidity, reliability, and accuracy.

Rapidity

The X/Y coupling system and the Zoom system make it possible to focus the beam on the retinal break within a few seconds, regardless of the situation or the size of the retinal tear.

Reliability

Observation of the fundus in an optical cross-section of the tissues, and under very high magnification when required, reveals minute lesions that are hardly visible, or even invisible with the indirect ophthalmoscope. Hence the smallest retinal breaks cannot escape the surgeon.[1,2,4,6,8] In addition, certain retinal lesions, such as microcysts and micro hemorrhages, which may simulate a retinal hole when observed under low magnification with the indirect ophthalmoscope, are easily differentiated from a hole when observed under high magnification with the slit lamp.

Accuracy

Observation of the fundus, placing the marker on the sclera and marking off the sclera are carried out by the surgeon. In addition, the backward shifting technique for placing the marker with simultaneous biomicroscopic observation of the fundus makes it possible to achieve accurate localization of retinal tears located in a highly detached retina.

SURGICAL TECHNIQUE

In most cases, localization of the retinal breaks is performed at the beginning of the surgical procedure, after exposure of the sclera. It can be done before or after cryotreatment. When the retinal detachment is associated with multiple breaks in different quadrants, cryotreatment and localization are done consecutively for each break. When the surgical procedure includes a vitrectomy, localization of the retinal breaks is carried out before the vitrectomy procedure whenever possible. Localization of the breaks after vitrectomy is often less accurate owing to the increased height of the detachment following vitrectomy. Multiple and large retinal folds, as well as decreased intraocular pressure after vitrectomy may make further localization of the breaks difficult and only approximate.

A right handed surgeon holds the three-mirror contact lens with the left hand and uses the right for maneuvering the marker along the sclera (Fig. 65).

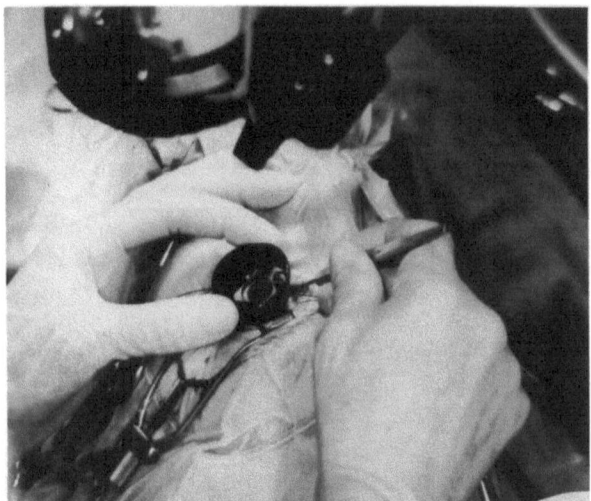

Figure 65. Localization of a retinal break using the microscope and the three-mirror contact lens (general view). Note that the marker handle is tilted outward so as to avoid pressure against the contact lens.

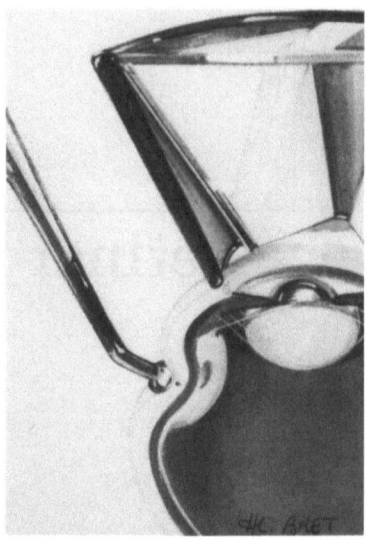

Figure 66. Correct inclination of the marker handle during retinal break localization with simultaneous use of the three-mirror contact lens.

With the X/Y coupling system, the slit beam is placed at the center of the chosen mirror to observe the area of the fundus where the retinal tear is located.

The microscope is then focused on the fundus. Next, with the combined operations of rotating the contact lens on the limbus and moving the biomicroscope with the X/Y coupling, the slit beam is centered on the tear. Magnification of the microscope is then increased; the magnification used for localization of the retinal breaks varies from 4.5 for the large tears to 17.9 for the smallest ones (zoom factor 0.5 to 2.0 with 12.5 × eyepieces).

When the surgeon is seated in front of the retinal quadrant in which the tear is located, he or she is able to see the projection of the slit beam through the sclera by observing the eye without the microscope. The tip of the marker is placed on the scleral projection of the slit beam. The surgeon then looks at the fundus once again through the microscope. The scleral depression produced by the marker is clearly visible. If the positioning of the marker is not perfectly accurate, the marker is gently shifted along the sclera under biomicroscopic control of the fundus. The marker handle must be tilted outward in order to avoid pressure against the contact lens (Figs. 65 and 66).

When seated at the opposite side of the retinal quadrant where the break is located, the surgeon is unable to see the scleral projection of the slit beam. Thus the meridian along which the marker should be shifted is determined by other means. This meridian is directly opposite the point of contact of the beam on the mirror through which the retinal

break can be observed. The tip of the marker is placed on this meridian; it must then be carefully shifted from the ora serrata to the retinal break.

When the position of the marker is considered to be accurate, slightly stronger pressure is applied on the sclera to fix the marker tip in the superficial layers of the sclera. The contact lens is then removed from the cornea. At the same time, the assistant removes both hemostatic forceps holding the bridle stitches to the surgical drapes. The eye can then be gently rotated to expose the zone where the tip of the marker is fixed. Next, the position of the retinal break is marked off on the sclera with superficial diathermy or China ink.

When the retinal break is large, the same localization and marking off is done for the posterior edge and both lateral anterior extremities. When the retinal tear is very large and irregular in shape, multiple markings on the sclera may be necessary. In oral dialysis, two scleral marks are made at each extremity and another mark is made at the center of the dialysis posterior edge.

When multiple breaks are present, marking of the scleral projection is carried out for all them.

When the retinal break is located in a bullous retinal detachment, it is pushed towards the center of the vitreous cavity and appears to be more posterior than it really is. With biomicroscopic control, the localizing error can be corrected as follows: The marker is not placed immediately on the scleral projection of the slit beam. It is placed at the ora serrata on the meridian of the break. Then it is gently shifted backward, pushing the choroid against the detached retina by scleral depression. When scleral depression produced by the marker tip is in front of the retinal break, the position of the marker corresponds exactly to what will be the scleral projection of the retinal break after completion of the scleral buckle (Fig. 67).

When the marker is shifted along the sclera, its sharp tip is directed laterally to avoid hooking the sclera (Fig. 67). When the blunt part of the marker tip is in front of the break, the marker handle is rotated by 90° to place the sharp tip in front of the sclera. Pressure exerted on the sclera to fix the marker tip should be moderate to avoid inadvertent scleral damage. Special care should be taken in eyes with a thin sclera and in reoperations to avoid inadvertent scleral perforation by the marker tip.

ERRORS TO AVOID

There are four main errors to be avoided during localization of the retinal break.

The first error is incorrect inclination of the marker handle (Fig. 68). The marker handle must be tilted outwards. In fact, if the marker handle is tilted toward the cornea and the contact lens, it applies pressure on the convexity of the sclera. The resulting deformation of the eye may lead to the passage of air bubbles or blood between the contact lens and the cornea.

The second error involves incorrect orientation of the marker tip (Fig. 69). The surgeon has to ensure that the tip of the marker has been orientated along

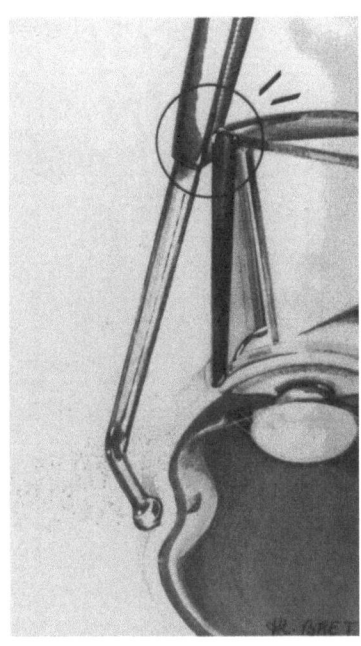

Figure 68. Error to avoid in retinal break localization: The marker handle has been tilted toward the contact lens. Consequently, maneuvering of the marker is difficult and the contact lens can no longer be kept well centered on the cornea.

the sclera and not toward the orbit before observing dynamic scleral depression resulting from the shifting of the marker through the microscope and the contact lens.

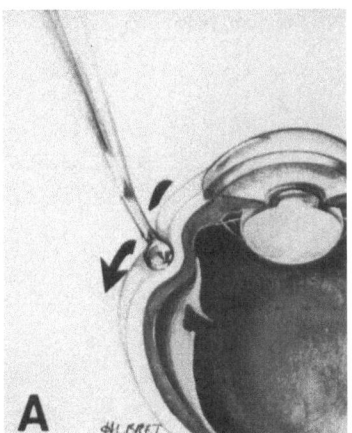 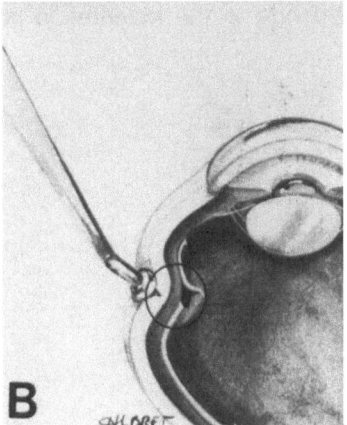

Figure 67. Retinal tear localization in a bullous retinal detachment. (A) The marker tip is initially placed in front of the ora serrata. It is then gently shifted backward, pushing the choroid against the detached retina. (B) The scleral projection of the retinal tear determined by the backward shifting technique corresponds exactly to what will be the scleral projection of the tear after scleral buckling.

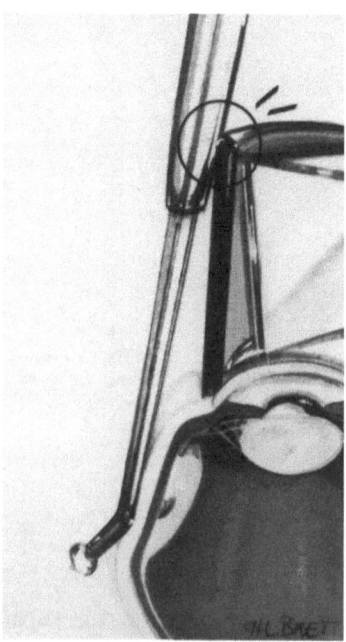

Figure 69. Error to avoid in retinal break localization: The marker tip has been orientated toward the orbit. As a result, scleral depression is produced by the marker stem. In addition, the marker handle applies pressure on the contact lens. Retinal tear localization will be difficult and inaccurate.

The third error occurs when the marker tip has initially been placed in an excessively posterior position. In fact, in this case, the scleral depression observed in the limited range of the microscope focused on the break corresponds to the indentation pro-duced by the shaft of the marker. This may be misinterpreted as the scleral depression produced by the instrument tip, which is actually in a more posterior position.

The fourth error possible occurs if the surgeon uses the scleral projection of the slit beam to localize a retinal tear in a bullous retinal detachment. The retinal tear is pushed toward the center of the vitreous cavity and the scleral projection of the slit beam reveals an image more posterior than the tear's actual position (Fig. 70). The backward shifting technique with simultaneous observation of the fundus must be used in such cases.[5–7]

REFERENCES

1. Bonnet M: Les avantages de la chirurgie sous microscope du décollement de la rétine. Bull Soc Ophtalmol Fr 75:1111–1112, 1975
2. Bonnet M, Bonamour G: Les avantages de la microchirurgie du décollement de la rétine. Mod Probl Ophthalmol 18:373–375, 1977
3. Bonnet M: Microsurgery of retinal detachment. in Boyd B (ed), Highlights of Ophthalmology, Silver anniversary edition 1:239–261, 1981
4. Urrets-Zavalia A: Retinal surgery under the microscope. Dev Ophthalmol 2:195–201, 1981
5. Bonnet M: Biomicroscopy of the ocular fundus during retinal detachment surgery. Ocular therapy and surgery 1, 50–54, 1982
6. Bonnet M, Nagao M: Microsurgery of aphakic retinal detachment. Ophthalmologica 186:177–182, 1983
7. Bonnet M: Biomicroscopie peropératoire du fond d'oeil dans la chirurgie du décollement de la rétine. Ann Instituto Barraquer 16:503–533, 1982–1983
8. Bonnet M: Microsurgery for retinal detachment repair. Dev Ophthalmol 14:5–10, 1987

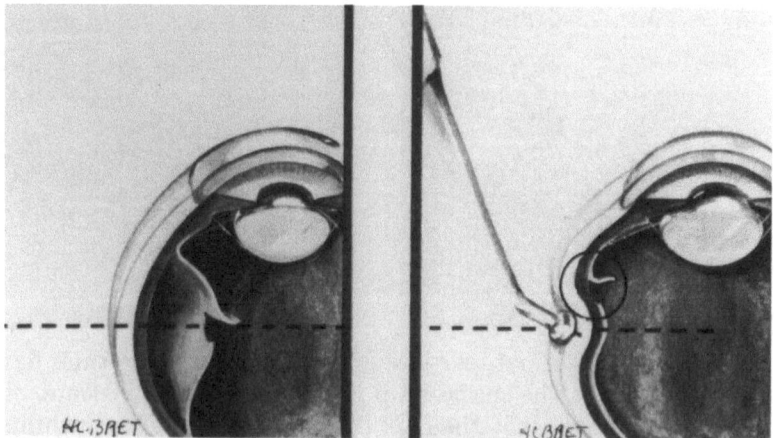

Figure 70. Error to avoid in localization of a retinal break in a bullous retinal detachment: The scleral projection of the slit beam has been used to place the marker tip. As a result, marking off on the sclera will be posterior to the retinal break position.

11
Scleral Buckling

In spite of the development of new techniques for retinal detachment repair during the last 15 years, scleral buckling remains the basic surgical procedure in the management of most rhegmatogenous retinal detachments.

RATIONALE FOR SCLERAL BUCKLING

The goals of scleral buckling in retinal detachment management are threefold: (1) to seal the retinal break(s) based on the long-established principles of Gonin,[1] Custodis,[2] and Schepens,[3] (2) to counteract ring contraction of the vitreous base in selected cases, and (3) to shorten the eye wall in eyes with a retina shortened by epiretinal membranes, which cannot be removed by vitreous surgery.

Sealing Retinal Breaks

Sealing retinal breaks is the main objective of scleral buckling in the vast majority of retinal detachments. Scleral buckling is used as an adjunct to choroidal irritation in the area of the retinal breaks. It has also occasionally been used as the only means to seal retinal breaks in selected cases.[4-6]

The mechanisms by which scleral buckling makes it possible to seal retinal breaks are threefold: (1) apposition of the pigment epithelium to the detached part of the retina containing the retinal break(s), (2) relief of vitreous traction on the retinal break, and (3) relief of traction exerted by epiretinal membranes on the retinal break(s).

PIGMENT EPITHELIUM APPROXIMATION TO THE RETINAL BREAK

Development of a firm retinochoroidal adhesion after choroidal irritation in the area of the retinal break(s) requires that the retinal break(s) and pigment epithelium be in close apposition. Surgical repair of mobile retinal detachments, without any significant and permanent vitreous traction, only requires choroidal irritation in the area of the retinal break and approximation of the retinal break to the pigment epithelium. In such detachments, retinal break approximation to the pigment epithelium can be achieved by either scleral buckling or retinal tamponade with gas. Intravitreal gas injection is more rapid a procedure to perform and less traumatizing compared to scleral buckling. Therefore, from a theoretical point of view, gas injection rather than scleral buckling should be used in the management of retinal detachments that are not associated with static vitreous traction, such as detachments due to oral dialyses, atrophic holes and operculated retinal tears. However, due to the limits and disadvantages of retinal tamponade with gas (see p. 118), scleral buckling is still performed in a significant number of easy detachments without static vitreous traction. Scleral buckling is used rather than gas injection in the management of most retinal detachments associated with oral dialyses and atrophic holes, because most dialyses and atrophic holes are located in the lower quadrants.

RELIEF OF VITREOUS TRACTION ON THE RETINAL BREAK

Relief of vitreous traction transmitted by the flap to the anterior edge of the tear(s) is required to achieve permanent retinal reattachment in a significant number of retinal detachments associated with horse shoe tears. Temporary relief of vitreous traction (until the development of a firm retinochoroidal adhesion) is sufficient to achieve permanent retinal reattachment in most eyes with horse shoe tears, which are subjected to only dynamic vitreous traction. In contrast, permanent, or at least prolonged, relief of vitreous traction is necessary to achieve

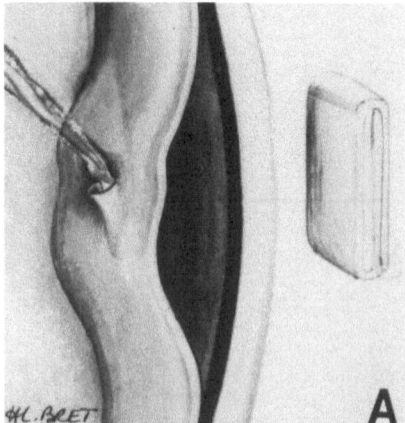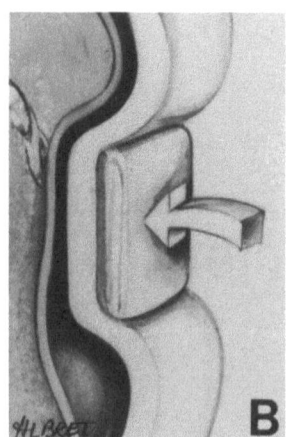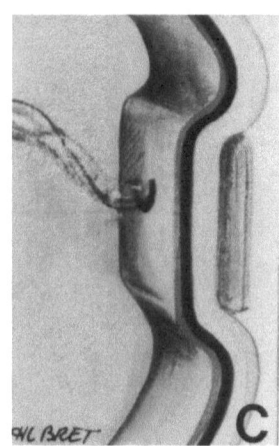

Figure 71. Relief of vitreous traction on the flap of a peripheral horseshoe tear by scleral buckling. (A) The tear flap is pulled anteriorly towards the vitreous cavity by vitreous fibrils. (B) Scleral buckling shortens the transverse diameter of the eye in the meridian of the tear. (C) Vitreous traction has been relieved. The tear flap is no longer pulled towards the vitreous cavity.

permanent retinal reattachment in eyes with horse shoe tear(s) that are under static vitreous traction. Surgical relief of vitreous traction on the retinal tear can be achieved by either scleral buckling or vitrectomy. At present, vitrectomy is the procedure of choice to relieve vitreous traction on the retinal breaks in eyes with tractional tears located posteriorly to the equatorial region (see p. 215). In such eyes vitrectomy is more rapid to perform and less traumatic compared with scleral buckling. In contrast, scleral buckling is the procedure of choice to relieve vitreous traction on the tear in eyes with horse shoe tears located in the periphery of the fundus (Fig. 71). In such eyes scleral buckling rather than vitrectomy should be used to relieve vitreous traction because it is more easy and less invasive a procedure than vitrectomy. The overwhelming majority of tractional tears are situated in the fundus periphery, therefore scleral buckling is used in the management of most retinal detachments with tractional retinal tears.

RELIEF OF EPIRETINAL MEMBRANE TRACTION ON THE RETINAL BREAK

In retinal detachments associated with proliferative vitreoretinopathy, scleral buckling is also used as an adjunct to vitreous surgery to relieve persistent traction exerted by epiretinal membranes on the retinal breaks. Because the inner eye wall is concave, the traction force exerted by epiretinal membranes includes a vector component that is perpendicular to the eye wall and directed towards the center of the vitreous cavity. A localized scleral buckle

changes the inner eye wall from concave to convex and reverses the direction of the vector force oriented perpendicular to the eye wall.[7] Therefore, after scleral buckling, the perpendicular vector component of the traction force exerted by epiretinal membranes pulls the retina towards the pigment epithelium and onto the scleral buckling instead of detaching the retina.[7]

Relief of Vitreous Base Traction

A 360° buckle provides permanent relief of vitreous traction in the plane of the encirclement by reducing the eye diameter (Fig. 72). An encircling scleral buckle is used to counteract permanent ring contraction of the vitreous base in selected cases, in particular retinal detachments with severe proliferative vitreoretinopathy (see p. 250)

Scleral Shortening

Shortening of the scleral wall may permit a retina shortened by limited epiretinal membranes to settle on the pigment epithelium (Fig. 73).

INDICATIONS FOR SCLERAL BUCKLING

At present scleral buckling is used in the management of most rhegmatogenous retinal detachments

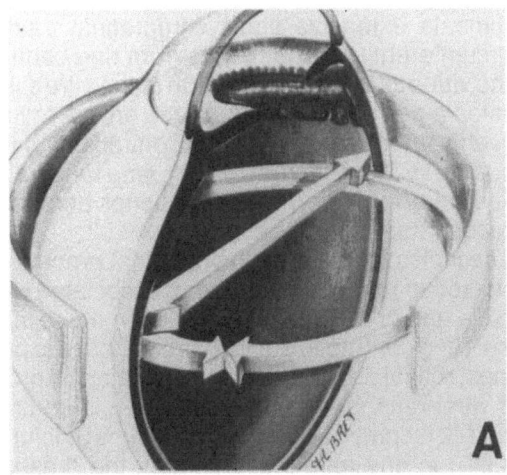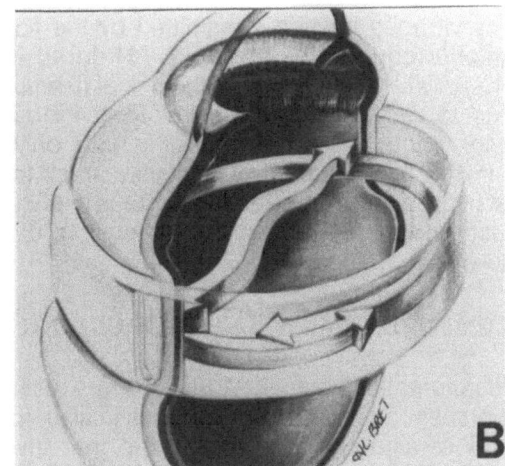

Figure 72. Relief of vitreous base traction by 360° scleral buckling. (A) Ring contraction of the vitreous base. (B) Reducing the transverse diameter of the eye anterior to the equator relieves traction produced by ring contraction of the vitreous base.

with peripheral retinal breaks. In most cases it is used as an adjunct to choroidal irritation to seal the retinal breaks. In selected cases scleral buckling and choroidal irritation are used as adjuncts to intra-vitreal gas injection and vitreous surgery.

The main indications for scleral buckling are as follows:

1. All peripheral retinal breaks located in the lower quadrants, in detached retina cases.
2. All peripheral horseshoe tears located in the upper quadrants over 30° in size or under static vitreous traction, in detached retina cases.

3. Ring contraction of the vitreous base.
4. Traction on the peripheral retina exerted by epi-retinal membranes that cannot be removed by vitrectomy.

METHODS FOR SCLERAL BUCKLING

Methods used for scleral buckling include segmental scleral buckles and encircling scleral buckling.

Segmental Scleral Buckling

Segmental scleral buckling of retinal breaks was developed by Custodis[2] and popularized by Lincoff.[8] Segmental scleral buckling has two main advantages compared with encircling scleral buckling. It is much less traumatic a procedure and subretinal fluid drainage is unnecessary in most cases.

The orientation of the scleral buckle is either parallel or perpendicular to the limbus. Both circumferential and radial scleral buckles have their own advantages and disadvantages. The choice of the direction of the buckle to be used in any given case is based on the type, size, and number of retinal break(s) as well as the relationship of one retinal break to another. Occasionally, a combination of circumferential and radial buckles should be used.

RADIAL SCLERAL BUCKLING

Radial scleral buckling is the most appropriate method to seal horseshoe tears.[9–11] A radial buckle

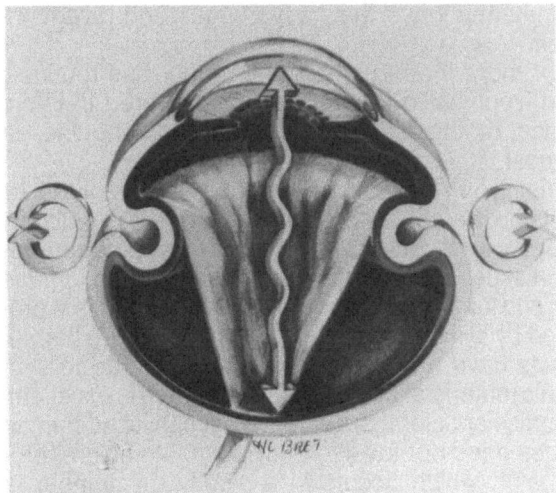

Figure 73. Scleral shortening reduces the axial diameter of the eye and may permit a retina shortened by limited epiretinal membranes to settle on the pigment epithelium.

relieves vitreous traction transmitted by the flap to the anterior edge of the tear (Fig. 71). In addition, it averts, or at least decreases, the risk of fishmouthing due to radial retinal folds involving the tear's posterior edge.[9–11] Radial buckling can only be used in the management of relatively small tears. Radial buckling of tears over 70° in size is impossible because the anterior-posterior dimension of the buckle would be too long.

CIRCUMFERENTIAL SCLERAL BUCKLING

Circumferential segmental buckles are used to seal horseshoe tears over 70 degrees in size, multiple and contiguous horseshoe tears that involve more than 70° of the eye circumference, multiple and contiguous holes, and oral dialyses regardless of their size.

The main disadvantage of circumferential scleral buckling in the management of retinal breaks is the tendency to induce radial retinal folds. When the radial fold(s) involve the tear's posterior edge, a fishmouth phenomenon develops.[11–13] The radial fold that extends from the posterior edge of the tear, over the buckle, toward the disc, allows fluid from the vitreous cavity to leak into the subretinal space (Fig. 74). The higher the buckle, the greater the tendency to radial folds and fishmouthing. Therefore, retinal breaks that involve more than 70° of the eye circumference are managed with circumferential buckles, which are rather shallow and retinal tamponade with gas (see p. 118).

Encircling Scleral Buckling

The encircling scleral buckle was introduced by Schepens.[14] Encircling procedures carry a higher incidence of postoperative complications as compared with segmental scleral buckling.[15–17] This is the reason a 360° scleral buckling procedure "to seal or wall-off undetected retinal breaks" is not used in microsurgical management of retinal detachment. Tiny retinal breaks may be difficult to identify in specific and infrequent circumstances. However, when the retina surgeon can spend enough time to conduct a thorough preoperative examination of the fundus with the three-mirror-contact lens and scleral depression, surgical failures after segmental scleral buckling related to undetected retinal breaks are most infrequent.[18]

The main objective of a 360° scleral buckling procedure is to permanently relieve static vitreoretinal traction involving more than 180° of the eye circumference. Relief of static vitreoretinal traction is achieved by reducing the diameter of the eye in the plane of the encirclement (Fig. 72). In the overwhelming majority of rhegmatogenous retinal detachments extensive static vitreoretinal traction in a circumferential plane results from ring contraction of the vitreous base. Contraction of the vitreous base creates a permanent pulling force on the retina and prevents retinal reattachment. Contraction of the vitreous base may increase with time and result in further tear formation at the posterior border of the vitreous base.

The indications for an encirclement procedure are restricted to retinal detachments associated with extensive and/or increasing contraction of the vitreous base. Ring contraction of the vitreous base is present in most retinal detachments complicated by proliferative vitreoretinopathy (see p. 250). It is common in retinal detachments after penetrating eye injury (see p. 294). In any retinal detachment the presence of multiple horseshoe tears at the posterior margin of the vitreous base is indicative of static vitreoretinal traction related to permanent and sometimes increasing contraction of the vitreous base. A circumferential retinal fold located at the posterior margin of the vitreous base is the first clinical sign indicating ring contraction of the vitreous base.

MATERIALS USED FOR SCLERAL BUCKLING

A large variety of materials have been used for scleral buckling, in particular polyviol implants,[2] Hard silicone implants,[19] soft silicone sponges,[8] absorbable gelatin implants,[20] implants made of teflon,[21–22] dexon[22] and polydioxanone,[22] and human tissues.[23] All materials have their advantages and disadvantages.

For more than 20 years the author has routinely used lyophylized human tissues prepared in Lyon, France, by the "centre de transfusion sanguine" of Beynost.[24]

Prior lyophylization has the same advantage as synthetic material in providing material immediately ready for use. Scleral buckling with lyophylized human tissues can produce choroidal indentations as high and long-lasting as[25] choroidal indentations produced by silicone sponges.[26–29] Lyophylized human tissues have a major advantage compared to synthethic materials: ocular tissue tolerance is excellent. In particular scleral buckling with lyophylized human tissues does not involve the risk of late scleral erosion,[30–31] which occurs in a significant number of eyes operated on with synthetical buckles.[32–37]

Three tissues are used: fascia lata, sclera, and dura mater.

Fascia lata is the most suitable material to fill a lamellar scleral pocket. Its malleability allows for an easy and accurate moulding of the implant to the

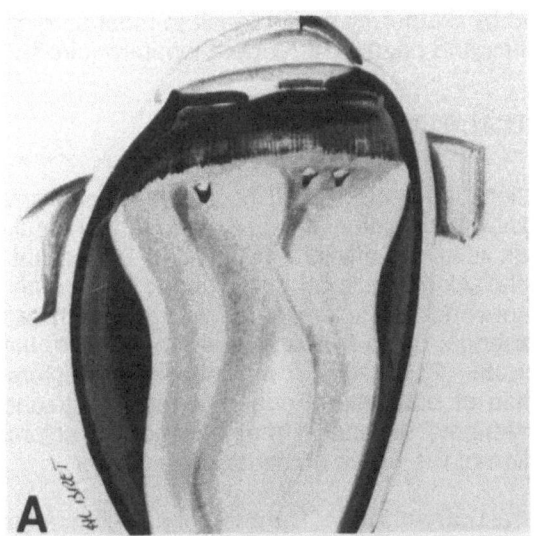

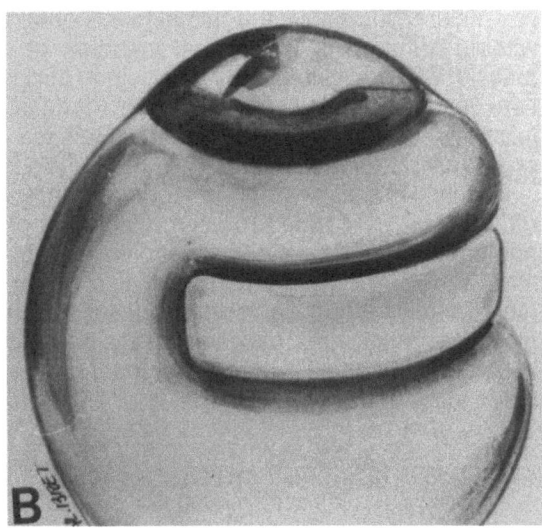

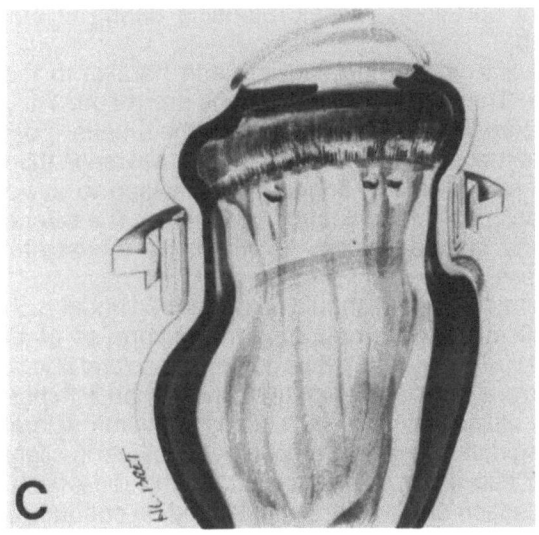

Figure 74. Radial retinal folds are the main disadvantage of circumferential scleral buckling. (A) Circumferential scleral buckling will be used to seal three horseshoe tears, each distant from the other. (B) Circumferential scleral buckling has reduced the eye wall circumference in the corresponding quadrants. (C) Reduction of the eye wall circumference has induced radial retinal folds and a fishmouth phenomenon.

retinal break. In addition, it can easily be placed beneath and behind a vortex vein that has been exposed.

Sclera is used in reoperations to repair the eye wall when the sclera has been eroded by previous scleral buckling with synthetic material.

Dura mater is the most suitable tissue for episcleral explant, since it easily permits the preparation of any explant, whatever its size and shape.

SURGICAL TECHNIQUE

Lamellar Scleral Pocket

Lamellar scleral pocket using the technique developed by Paufique[23] is the technique of choice for segmental scleral buckling when conditions allow.

ADVANTAGES

The advantages of the lamellar scleral pocket are as follows:

1. The implant is custom made in terms of its surface and height. Thus it can be adjusted to any given situation.
2. An accurately centered scleral buckling extending far posteriorly can easily be obtained when the location and/or posterior extension of the retinal break make it necessary. The only limit to the posterior dissection of a scleral flap is the scleral penetration of the short posterior ciliary arteries. Intrascleral undermining and implantation can be carried out behind a vortex vein without damaging the vein.
3. When the scleral projection of the retinal tear is in the area of the superior oblique muscle inser-

tion, scleral buckling of the retinal tear is obtained without damage to the scleral insertion of the muscle. When required, very high scleral buckling can be obtained without inducing a dangerous increase in intraocular pressure. Release of subretinal fluid is unnecessary in most eyes.

In eyes with a very high detachment, induced radial folds, which may result in fishmouth phenomenon, are less likely to occur with an implant than an explant. Radial folds are also easier to manage with a lamellar scleral pocket because pieces of fascia lata can selectively be placed into the pocket so as to achieve a higher choroidal indentation in front of the radial fold.

DISADVANTAGES AND LIMITS

The disadvantages, which have justly been attributed to scleral undermining, are as follows:

1. The procedure requires more time to perform than the suture of an episcleral explant.
2. Scleral dissection can involve specific complications, such as flap laceration or choroidal herniation.
3. The difficulties encountered in reoperations are greater after scleral undermining compared to explants.

INDICATIONS AND CONTRAINDICATIONS

The indications for scleral buckling by means of a lamellar scleral pocket are restricted as follows: (1) primary operation, (2) retinal detachment with a single retinal break or group of contiguous breaks involving 70° or less of the eye circumference, and (3) thick and undamaged sclera.

A lamellar scleral pocket should not be performed in reoperation unless the recurrent detachment is caused by a new break a distance from the area involved by the first operation. Scleral undermining should not be performed in areas involved by previous explant. In such eyes the sclera may appear undamaged. Actually the scleral tissue has lost its normal strength, due to compression by the explant, whatever the material previously used for scleral buckling. Therefore, intraoperative or postoperative laceration of the scleral flap is likely to occur.

Scleral undermining should not be performed as the primary operation in eyes with retinal breaks involving more than a quadrant and in eyes with retinal breaks whose scleral projections are located in thin sclera.

Finally, a lamellar scleral pocket should not be performed in conjunction with diathermy used to induce choroidal irritation. Damage to the scleral floor induced by diathermy would result in most surgical difficulties and hazards if reoperation is required.

SURGICAL TECHNIQUE

The location and size of the scleral pocket are dictated by the location and size of the retinal break.

To achieve an efficient buckling of the retinal break, the scleral pocket should extend (1) anteriorly, 2 mm beyond the scleral projection of the break anterior edge, or up to the scleral projection of the ora serrata, (2) laterally, 2 mm beyond the scleral projection of both lateral edges of the break, and (3) posteriorly, at least 4 mm beyond the scleral projection of the break posterior edge.

Scleral Dissection. The anterior and both radial borders of the pocket are drawn on the sclera with light and superficial diathermy (Fig. 75). This will prevent episcleral vessels bleeding during scleral incision.

The first scleral incision is made parallel to the limbus. Then, both radial incisions are made. They involve approximately two-thirds of the anterior-posterior dimension of the pocket. The posterior third of the pocket lateral edges is not incised to avoid the placing of scleral sutures posteriorly. The scleral incisions should involve two-thirds of the scleral thickness.

Scleral dissection should be performed under high magnification of the operating microscope so as to maintain visual control while cutting the scleral fibers. The sclera should constantly be moistened with balanced saline solution. Moistening prevents scleral thinning due to dessication and even results in slight scleral thickening, which facilitates the dissection.

Dissection of the scleral flap should be conducted between the outer two-thirds and the inner one-third of the sclera. This dissection depth will avoid immediate or late perforation of the flap. The floor is thick enough to prevent choroidal prolapse. In addition to this, the difference of the resistance to stretching between the thicker flap and the thinner floor will allow fascia lata pieces when placed in the pocket to push the floor toward the inside of the eye ball, rather than pushing the flap outward.

In the zones where the scleral thickness changes, in particular at the limit of the contact arcs of the recti muscles, great care should be taken to continue the dissection at the right depth. When dissection must be made under a rectus muscle, where the sclera usually is thinner, it should be done so at half the thickness of the sclera to avoid damage to the floor. In such cases the pocket flap will be strengthened with a piece of dura mater.

Scleral dissection is started where the anterior incision and one radial incision are joined (Fig. 75).

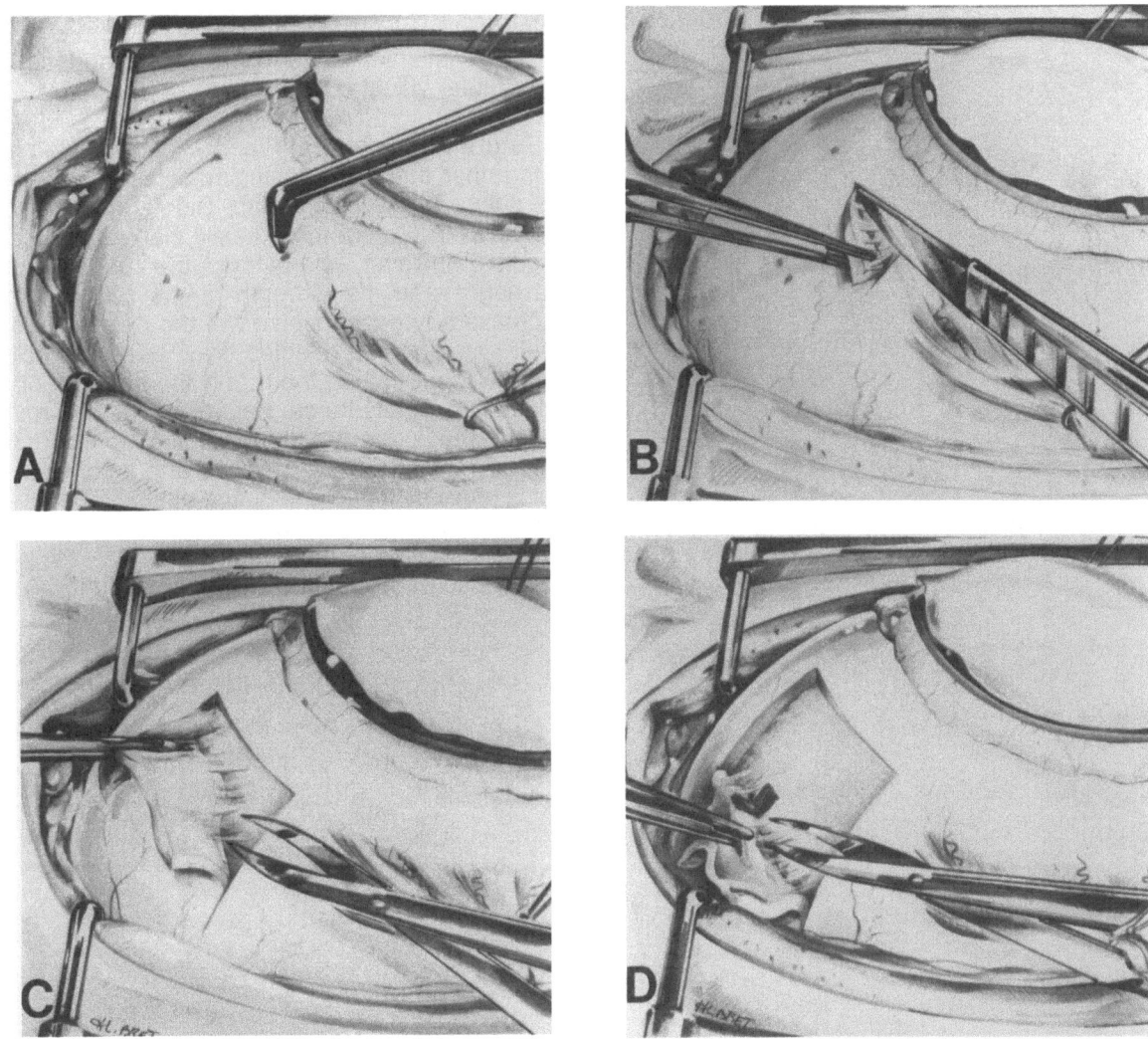

Figure 75. Lamellar scleral pocket: surgical technique. (A) Light and superficial diathermy is used to mark off the anterior and both radial edges of the scleral pocket. Two superficial diathermy landmarks on the sclera indicate the scleral projections of two contiguous tiny horseshoe tears to be buckled. (B) A knife is used to start scleral dissection where the anterior incision and one radial incision join. The blade's sharp side is directed outward. (C) Bonn forceps are used to hold the scleral flap and stretch the scleral fibers that are being cut using blunt corneal scissors. (D) Scleral fibers are being cut in close vicinity of a vortex vein.

A knife is used to start the dissection. When approximately 1 mm of the scleral flap has been dissected, blunt corneal scissors are used to undermine the sclera and cut the scleral fibers. Bonn forceps are used to raise the scleral flap and stretch the scleral fibers before cutting them (Fig. 75). The flap should be held with Bonn forceps near the dissecting angle stretching the fibers to be cut and avoiding excessive traction on the pocket flap. The scleral flap should be held very gently to avoid scleral laceration by the forceps' teeth.

When the scleral projection of the retinal break is located in the area of a vortex vein, it is possible to undermine the sclera and spare the vortex vein. The intrascleral part of the vortex vein is exposed in order to undermine the sclera posteriorly to the vien and place the intrascleral implant without damaging the vein. Under high magnification, the scleral fibers that encircle the vein are cut with the tip of the Lagrange knife, the Strampelli corneal dissector, or the blunt Vannas scissors (Fig. 75). The vein is lifted with a modified Tyrel blunt hook. Next, the

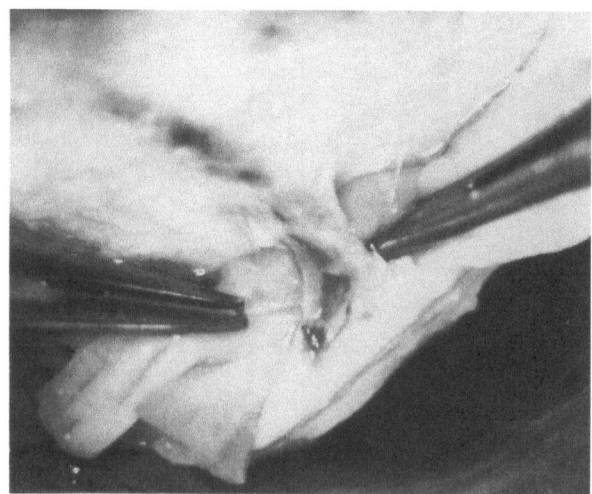

Figure 76. Placing small fascia lata pieces behind and beneath the intrascleral part of a vortex vein.

votex vein is raised with the flap. Finally, small pieces of fascia lata are placed behind and beneath the vein, under visual control (Figs. 76 and 77).

Suture of the Scleral Flap. Round-bodied needles rather than side-cutting needles are used for the suture of the scleral flap. Side cutting needles penetrate the sclera more easily than round-bodied needles. However, scleral fibers are cut by the needle edges and the strength of the scleral flap is decreased by each insertion of the needle. In contrast, round-bodied needles draw aside the scleral fibers without cutting them and the strength of the scleral flap is not altered. Scleral insertion of round-bodied needles is greatly facilitated by the use of a needle-holder with a concave and a convex jaw, which provides a firm grip on the needle. The needle should be inserted and moved into the sclera with a rotating motion of the needle-holder.

Nonabsorbable sutures should be used for suture

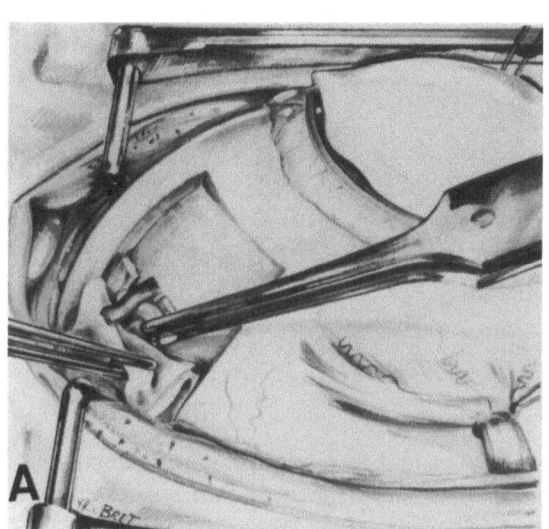

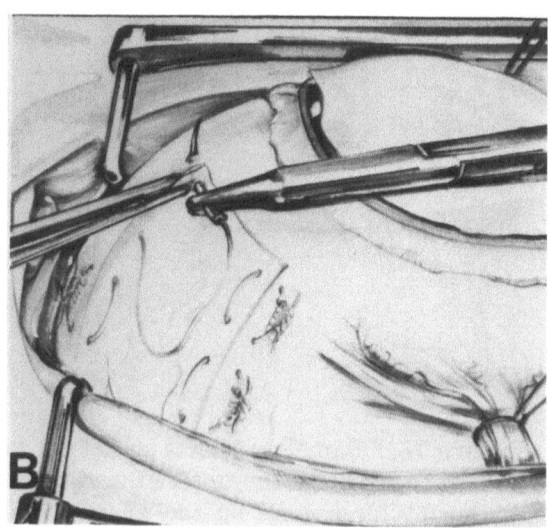

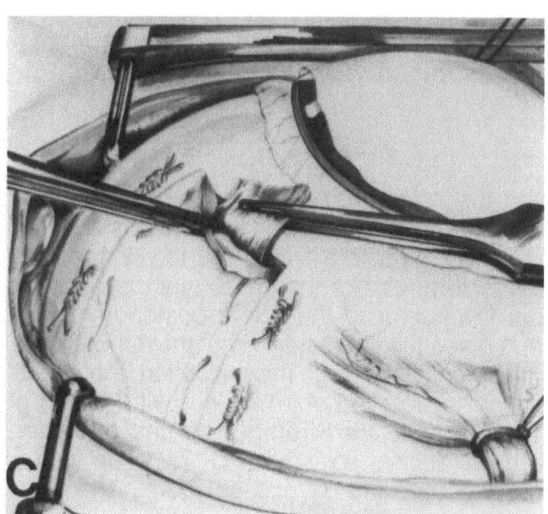

Figure 77. Lamellar scleral pocket: surgical technique. (A) The intrascleral part of a vortex vein has been exposed. Small pieces of fascia lata are being placed beneath the vein before suturing the scleral flap. (B) Both radial borders of the scleral pocket are sutured with interrupted mattress sutures. (C) Bonn forceps are used to insert pieces of fascia lata into the scleral pocket.

of a scleral pocket. Depending on the scleral thickness and the size of the scleral pocket, the author uses either 6–0 synthetic braided sutures of 8–0 nylon monofilament. The latter is used by preference for small-sized pockets or when the sclera is not very thick.

The needle is passed through the whole thickness of the flap and then at the joining of the outer two-thirds and the inner third of the nondissected sclera. When a piece of dura mater is used to reinforce the flap, the needle is passed through the scleral flap and the whole thickness of the dura mater. Suturing of the scleral flap is done in two stages. The radial borders are sutured first, with interrupted mattress sutures, the knot of which is placed on the side of the nondissected sclera (Fig. 77 and Fig. 78). The lateral edges of the anterior border are sutured before filling the pocket. The suture can be made either with interrupted sutures or two continuous sutures starting from each anterior corner of the pocket. A space is left between both continuous or interrupted sutures in order to allow for the filling

of the pocket. The suture is completed when the pocket has been filled.

Intrascleral Inclusion of Lyophylized Fascia Lata. Fascia lata is used by preference to fill the scleral pocket (Fig. 77). The strip of fascia lata is cut into pieces 3–10 mm long, depending on the pocket size, in order to make its manipulation easier (Fig. 79). Fascia lata are easier to handle in small pieces which must not touch the eyelids' margins in order to ensure perfect sterility of the implant. In addition, the fascia lata pieces are coated with penicillin powder.

Fascia lata is not rehydrated before inclusion in the scleral pocket. Rehydration will occur within the scleral pocket later and will increase the size of the implant and therefore the height of the buckle.

Insertion of the fascia lata pieces into the scleral pocket should be very progressive when subretinal fluid is not drained off. Great care should be taken to fill the most posterior part of the pocket as much as the anterior part. When a radial buckle extending

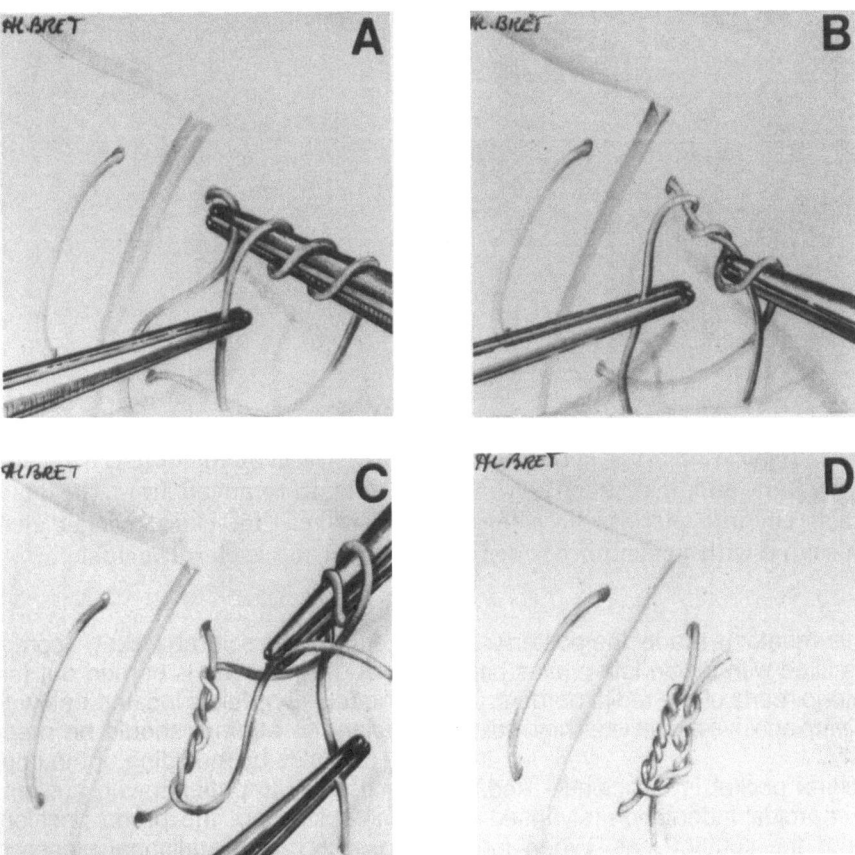

Figure 78. Tying scleral sutures of a lamellar scleral pocket. (A) A triple loop is made first. (B) The triple loop is pulled out on the sclera. (C) A second double loop is made. (D) The knot has been completed.

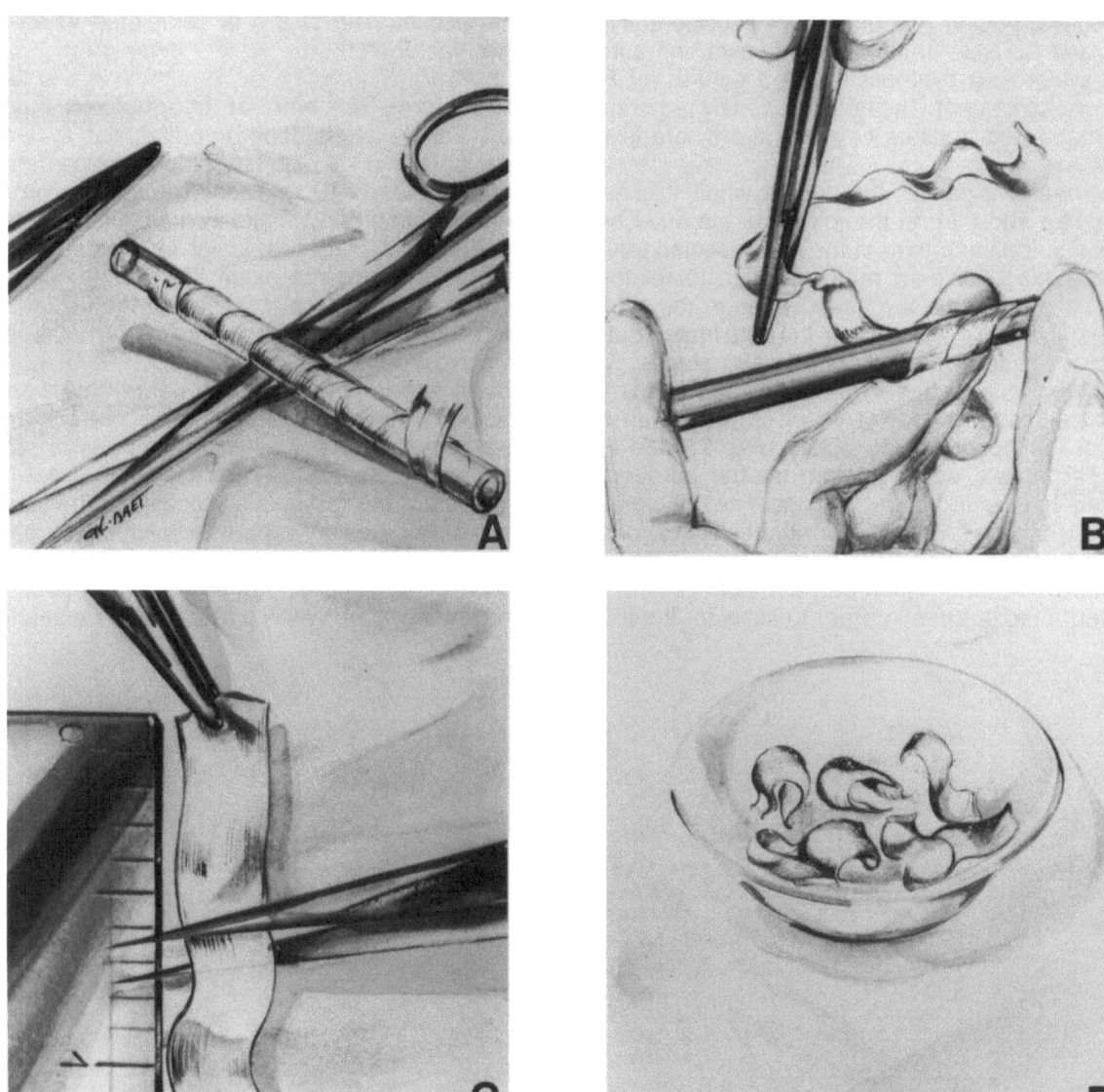

Figure 79.   Preparation of fascia lata pieces for intrascleral inclusion. (A) Ribbon of lyophilized human fascia lata and instruments. (B) Fascia lata is removed from the glass bobin. (C) Fascia lata is cut into pieces whose length is based on the scleral pocket size. (D) Fascia lata pieces coated with penicillin powder are ready for intrascleral inclusion.

posteriorly to the equator is made, the posterior part of the pocket is filled with fascia lata pieces before suturing the anterior parts of the radial borders. This will make it easier to achieve a buckle as high posteriorly as anteriorly.

When the scleral pocket is sufficiently filled, the position of the choroidal indentation is verified with the slit lamp and the contact lens. When fundus examination reveals a retinal fold involving the break or a fish mouth phenomenon, management technique depends on the break location. When the retinal break is located above the horizontal meridian,

suture of the scleral pocket is completed and intravitreal gas injection is carried out (see p. 118). When the retinal break is located below the horizontal meridian, an attempt should be made to manage the radial folds by moulding of the implant. This applies especially to patients who are not cooperative and will not accept the prone position postoperatively. In such cases additional pieces of fascia lata are inserted into the scleral pocket and placed in front of the radial fold. Increasing the buckle height until the retinal fold flattens on the indentation may require insertion of a large amount of fascia lata. Anterior chamber paracentesis, intravenous infusion of acetazolamide, and 20% Mannitol solution provide the necessary decrease in intraocular pressure in most cases. Release of subretinal fluid is rarely necessary.

Intraoperative Complications. Three main categories of intraoperative complications may be encountered in the performance of a lamellar scleral pocket.

Buckle Mispositioning. Mispositioning of the buckle may result from either improper localization of the scleral projection of the break, or improper scleral dissection. After inclusion of the implant, biomicroscopic examination of the fundus may show that one lateral edge of the break is too close to the radial edge of the buckle or not involved at all by the buckle. The complication has two main causes. First, the break size was underestimated and, second, the lateral edge of the pocket is not oriented in a radial direction. The error should be corrected. The scleral sutures are removed and the sclera is undermined 2–3 mm beyond the radial scleral incision. Insufficient scleral undermining posteriorly is the most common error in scleral buckling by means of a scleral pocket (Fig. 80). In most cases, the choroidal indentation height induced by a lamellar scleral pocket decreases gradually in the most posterior part of the pocket. The choroidal indentation height should be approximately the same at both the posterior and anterior tear edges, so as

to prevent subretinal fluid leakage at the posterior edge of the tear. Choroidal indentation produced by a lamellar scleral pocket should therefore extend at least 4 mm beyond the tear posterior edge (Fig. 81).

Complications During Scleral Dissection. Flap laceration, floor laceration with choroidal herniation, and damage to a vortex vein are three potential complications of scleral dissection.

Dissection of too thin a sclera, scleral dessication, use of forceps with sharp teeth, and excessive traction on the flap are the main causes of flap laceration. When the flap laceration is less than 1 mm in size and the sclera is of sufficient thickness, scleral undermining can be completed. The scleral flap will be reinforced with a piece of dura mater, which should be the same size as the entire scleral flap (Fig. 82). The dura mater is sutured with the scleral flap to the nondissected sclera (Fig. 82). When the flap laceration is over 2 mm in size, scleral buckling by means of a lamellar scleral pocket should be abandoned because there is a high risk of secondary implant extrusion in Tenon's space. The scleral flap is sutured with 8–0 nylon interrupted sutures and an explant is used for scleral buckling.

Too deep a scleral dissection, and thinning of the scleral floor due to dessication are the main causes of floor laceration. When the laceration is less than 0.5 mm in size, there is usually no choroidal herniation. The sclera should be moistened with balanced

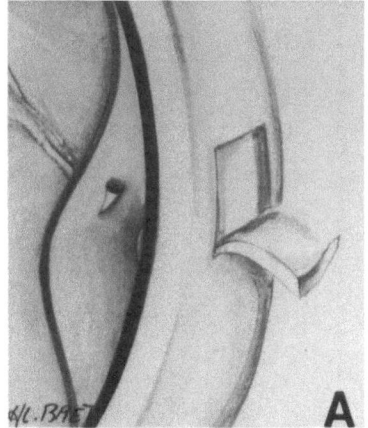 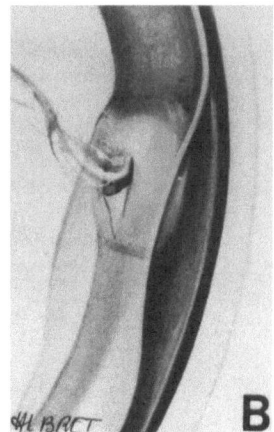

Figure 80. Error to avoid in the size of a lamellar scleral pocket: insufficient posterior scleral undermining. (A) Scleral undermining beyond the scleral projection of the tear posterior edge is insufficient. (B) Following fascia lata inclusion into the scleral pocket, vitreous traction on the tear flap has been relieved, but the choroidal indentation height is insufficient posteriorly, and the tear posterior edge has not settled on the pigment epithelium.

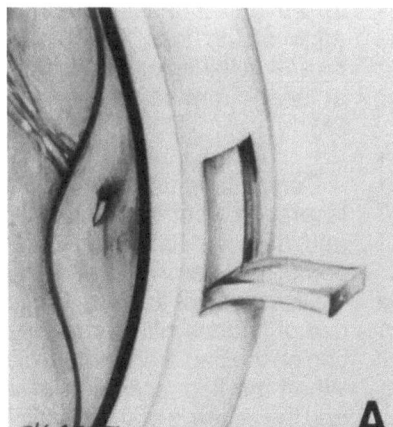 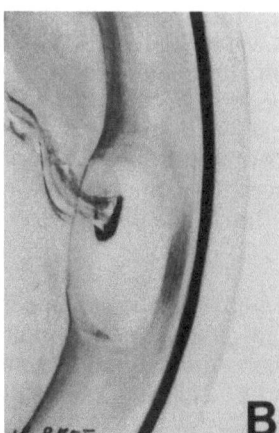

Figure 81. Correct extension of scleral undermining for scleral buckling by a lamellar scleral pocket. (A) Scleral undermining extends beyond the scleral projection of the tear posterior edge more than it does beyond the tear anterior edge. (B) Both the anterior and posterior edges of the tear have settled on the highest part of the choroidal indentation.

saline solution. Then dissection of the scleral fibers is conducted more superficially and the tiny scleral defect is covered with scleral fibers or a small piece of dura mater. When the floor laceration is over 0.5 mm in size and the choroid is exposed, scleral buckling by means of a lamellar scleral pocket should be abandoned, because there is a risk of immediate or secondary implant intrusion. The intraocular pressure is lowered to avoid a choroidal prolapse. The scleral flap is sutured to the nondissected sclera. An explant is used for scleral buckling.

Damage to the intrascleral part of a vortex vein may occur when dissection of the scleral fibers is not performed under visual control. Coagulation of the vein should be done to stop bleeding before completing scleral dissection.

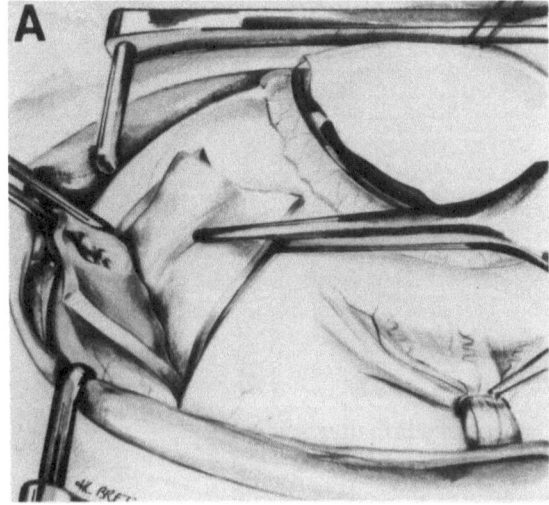 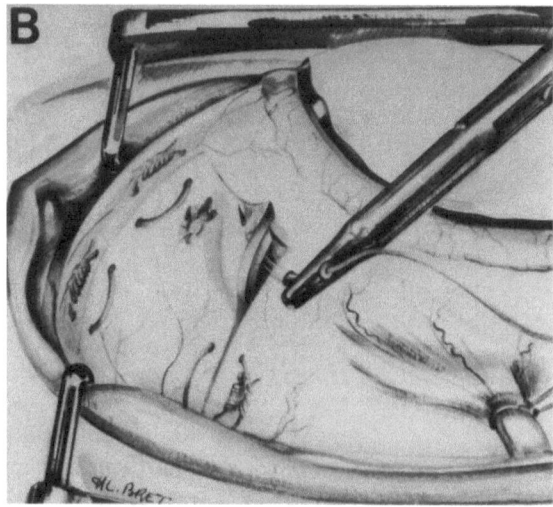

Figure 82. Management of a small laceration in the scleral pocket flap. (A) A small laceration has been inadvertently made in the anterior part of the scleral flap. A piece of dura mater, whose size is the same as that of the scleral flap, is being placed into the pocket to reinforce the scleral flap. (B) The piece of dura mater is sutured with the scleral flap to the nondissected sclera.

Complications During Scleral Suturing. Laceration of the scleral flap, choroidal damage with release of subretinal fluid, and difficulties in approximating the scleral flap to the nondissected sclera are the three main complications that may occur during scleral suturing. Laceration of the scleral flap most often results from the use of unsuitable needles. This complication can be avoided by the use of round-bodied needles. Choroidal damage with release of subretinal fluid is related to either poor insertion of the needle in the nondissected sclera or use of a reverse cutting edge needle. Such needles should not be used for scleral suturing. A suture that has resulted in choroidal damage or subretinal fluid release must be removed. Difficulties in the approximation of the scleral flap to the nondissected sclera may occur when the implant is too large. Excessive traction on the flap in an attempt to tighten the sutures may result in flap laceration (Fig. 83). Lowering the intraocular pressure should be done before tightening the sutures. This is achieved by paracentesis of the anterior chamber in phakic eyes or intravenous acetazolamide or mannitol solution. Release of subretinal fluid is unnecessary in most cases.

Explants

Episcleral explants rather than implants are used for scleral buckling in most cases. They have significant advantages and they also have, however, disadvantages as compared to implants. Therefore, in any given case, the surgeon should determine which of the two techniques is the most suitable.

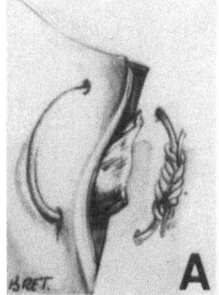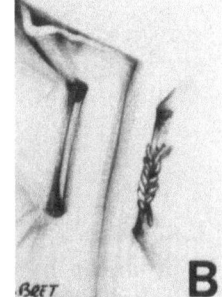

Figure 83. Two errors to avoid in suturing a scleral pocket. (A) The suture has not been sufficiently tightened. A piece of fascia lata protrudes outside the scleral pocket. (B) The suture has been excessively tightened. Traction on the scleral flap may result in further flap laceration.

ADVANTAGES

Scleral buckling with an explant is more rapid a procedure to perform as compared with a lamellar scleral pocket. The surgical technique is easy in most cases. Intraoperative complications are most uncommon. Most importantly the procedure induces no scleral damage. Therefore, when required, reoperation is much easier as compared with reoperation after scleral undermining.

Scleral buckling with explants is feasible in any circumstance, regardless of the condition of the sclera and the extent of the area to be buckled.

DISADVANTAGES AND LIMITS

There is no limit to the use of explants for scleral buckling. However segmental scleral buckling, especially with radial explants, may produce high degrees of astigmatism.[38–39] In contrast, refractive changes following trapdoor procedures are uncommon. In most cases refractive errors produced by explants diminish over 6 months postoperatively, and minor errors remain permanently. However, high degrees of permanent astigmatism following scleral buckling by radially oriented episcleral sponges have been observed.[38–39]

When the retina is highly detached, approximating the pigment epithelium to the retinal break is less easy to achieve with an explant compared with a lamellar scleral pocket. Persisting or induced retinal folds are not uncommon, even when radial explants are used. Therefore intravitreal gas injection to flatten the retinal folds should be used as an adjunct to scleral buckling in a significant number of eyes operated with explants.

When a very posterior choroidal indentation is required, placement of the scleral sutures posteriorly to the equator is uneasy, especially in highly myopic eyes. This technical difficulty can be overcome with a special technique, however.

INDICATIONS

Explants are used for scleral buckling in all circumstances by surgeons who are not familiar with scleral dissection or who may not have the time to perform a more sophisticated procedure.

For surgeons expert in the technique of scleral undermining, the indications for explants are restricted as follows:

1. thin and/or damaged sclera
2. reoperations

3. retinal break, or group of breaks, extending beyond more than 70° of the eye circumference
4. difficult cases that require the adjunct of vitreous
   surgery, in particular, retinal detachments complicated by proliferative vitreoretinopathy.

SURGICAL TECHNIQUE

**Determining the Size and Height of the
Buckle.** The extent of the choroidal indentation
produced by an explant is approximately the size
of the explant (Fig. 84). The height of the buckle is
determined by the distance that separates the limbs
of the scleral sutures, which will be tied over the
explant (Fig. 85).

The size of the explant is mainly determined by
two parameters: (1) the size of the retinal break(s)
to be treated and (2) the presence or absence of
proliferative vitreoretinopathy.

In mobile retinal detachments the buckle should
extend 2–3 mm beyond the break posterior edge,
1.5 mm beyond the anterior edge—or up to the ora
serrata—and 1.5–2 mm beyond both radial edges
of the break (Fig. 86). The height of the buckle is
determined by the height of the detachment.

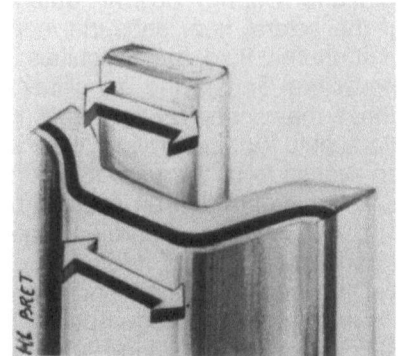

Figure 84. The extent of the choroidal indentation
produced by an explant is approximately the size
of the explant.

In most retinal detachments complicated by proliferative vitreoretinopathy, larger buckles are used
because precise localization of the scleral projection
of the tear involves a margin of error due to the
detachment height and fixed folds. In addition, high
buckles are often required in such eyes to counteract
traction caused by epiretinal membranes that may
remain after vitrectomy.

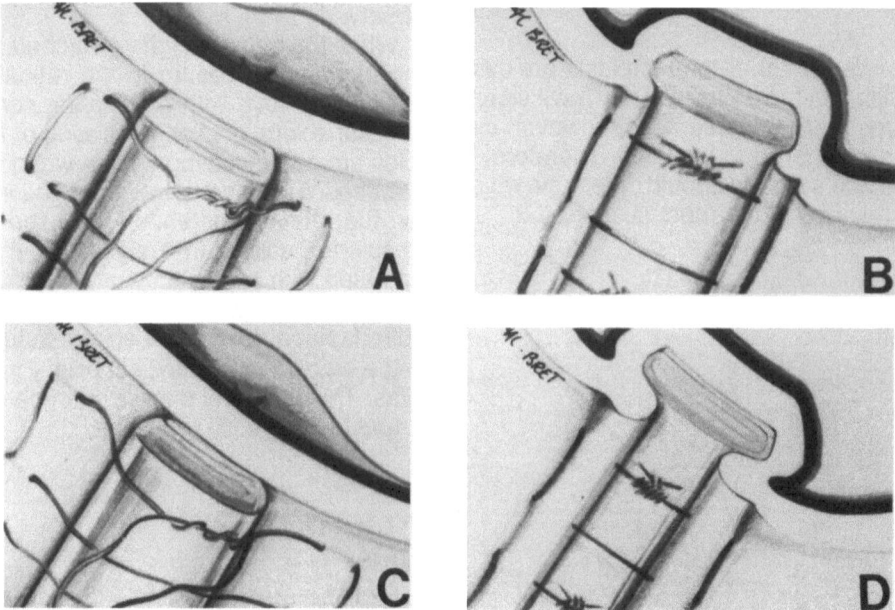

Figure 85. The choroidal indentation height produced by an explant is
determined by the distance that separates the limbs of the scleral sutures
rather than the explant thickness. (A) The distance that separates the
limbs of the scleral sutures is 1.5 times the explant width. (B) Following
suture tightening a moderate choroidal indentation is obtained. (C) The
distance that separates the limbs of the scleral sutures is twice as large
as the explant width. (D) Following suture tightening a high choroidal
indentation is obtained.

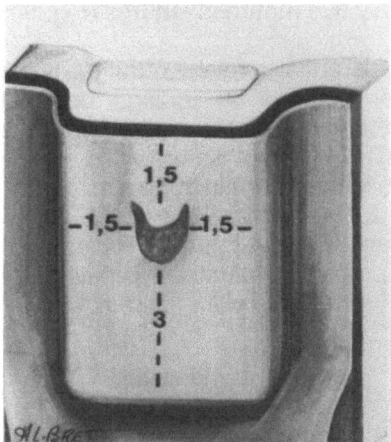

Figure 86. Size of a dura-mater explant to buckle a tear in mobile retinal detachment.

Preparation of the Explant. The explant is custom-made according to the size of the break(s). The precise size of the break is evaluated intraoperatively by measuring with a compass the width and length of its scleral projection.

The explant is prepared by the assistant while the surgeon places the scleral sutures. A piece of lyophylized dura mater is cut to the required dimensions (Fig. 87). It is folded to make an explant of 3–6 layers of dura mater. The layers are stuck together with cyanoacrylate glue. Dura mater must be kept dry to permit the adhesion effect of cyanoacrylate to develop. The explant is pressed hard with forceps for a few seconds after the placing of cyanoacrylate glue so that a firm adhesion develops between the explant layers. It is recommended that a very small amount of cyanoacrylate glue be used. One drop is usually sufficient to stick sufficiently 2 layers of dura mater 5 × 10 mm together. Larger amounts of cyanoacrylate glue are unnecessary to obtain a firm adhesion of the explant layers. Using large amounts of cyanoacrylate has two disadvantages: (1) the explant will be too hard or (2) cyanoacrylate glue will seep out the explant. When dry, the excessive amount of cyanoacrylate glue will form small sharp crystals on the outer surface of the explant. The crystals may cause subconjunctival irritation postoperatively.

Scleral Sutures. Mattress scleral sutures are used to hold the explant in place on the sclera and induce indentation of the eye wall. Indentation of the eye wall is produced by tightening of the sutures. The buckle height is determined by the distance between the intrascleral parts of the mattress sutures and the amount by which the thread is shortened when the sutures are tied over the explant. In most mobile detachments a distance between the limbs of the scleral mattress sutures 1.5 times the width of the explant will provide adequate buckle height. In most detachments complicated by proliferative vitreoretinopathy higher buckles are required. In such eyes the distance between the limbs of the scleral mattress sutures is 2 times the width of the explant (Fig. 85).

Adequate scleral sutures are most important to avoid intraoperative complications and to obtain prolonged scleral buckling.

Nonabsorbable sutures are used. A 5–0 synthetic thread is sufficiently resistant for buckle sutures. A braided thread is more suitable than a monofilament for buckle suturing because the knots prevent slippage and stay together.

At present the most suitable needles for buckle sutures have cutting surfaces confined to the tip. The sharp tip allows for easy intrascleral insertion of the needle at the proper depth, and damage to the scleral fibers is limited to a minimum.

The main advantage in using a microsope for placement of the buckle sutures is to provide improved control over the depth of the sutures. The suture track should be deep enough to avoid scleral laceration when the suture is tied, and yet still sufficiently superficial to avoid choroidal perforation by the needle. The depth of the suture is determined by the thickness of the sclera. When the sclera is thick, the needle is passed between the outer two-thirds and the inner one third (Fig. 97). When the sclera is thin, the needle is passed through one-half the thickness of the sclera.

The direction of the suture intrascleral tracks in relationship to the explant can be either parallel or perpendicular. Mattress sutures with intrascleral tracks parallel to the explant are anchored in the sclera by a single bite on each side of the explant (Fig. 88). The scleral bites should be 4–5 mm in length. Mattress sutures with intrascleral tracks perpendicular to the explant are anchored with two scleral bites on each side of the explant (Fig. 89). The bites are 2 mm in length and placed 4–5 mm apart on each side of the explant. Scleral mattress sutures with 4 intrascleral tracks perpendicular to the explant show less tendency to cut out the sclera when tied under tension. They are used by preference when high buckles are necessary or when the sclera is thin (Fig. 90). Mattress sutures with two intrascleral tracks parallel to the explant are used for radial buckles, which should be rather shallow and should extend posteriorly to the equatorial region. Proper passage of the needle into the sclera posterior to the equator is easier when the needle is oriented in a radial direction.

Placement of scleral sutures posteriorly to the equator may be difficult, especially in highly myopic eyes and on the nasal side of the eye. In such instances, the two-knot suture technique is helpful (Fig. 91). The needles are passed in the sclera in a backward radial direction. When both radial bites have been done, the needles are cut off. A double knot is made with the cut ends of the thread. Next, the thread is pulled anteriorly to place the posterior knot on the explant. The anterior loop is cut and both anterior cut ends are used to permanently tie the explant.

All scleral mattress sutures are prepared before placing the explant. In most cases a radial explant requires only two mattress sutures (Fig. 90 and Fig. 91).

A circumferential explant requires two mattress sutures per quadrant. In addition, both extremities of circumferential explants are sutured to the sclera (Fig. 92). The mattress sutures that fix the explant extremities to the sclera include a scleral bite, which is parallel to the explant extremity, and two bites in the explant, which are perpendicular to the explant extremities. The scleral bites are placed a distance of 2 mm from the explant extremities. Tightening

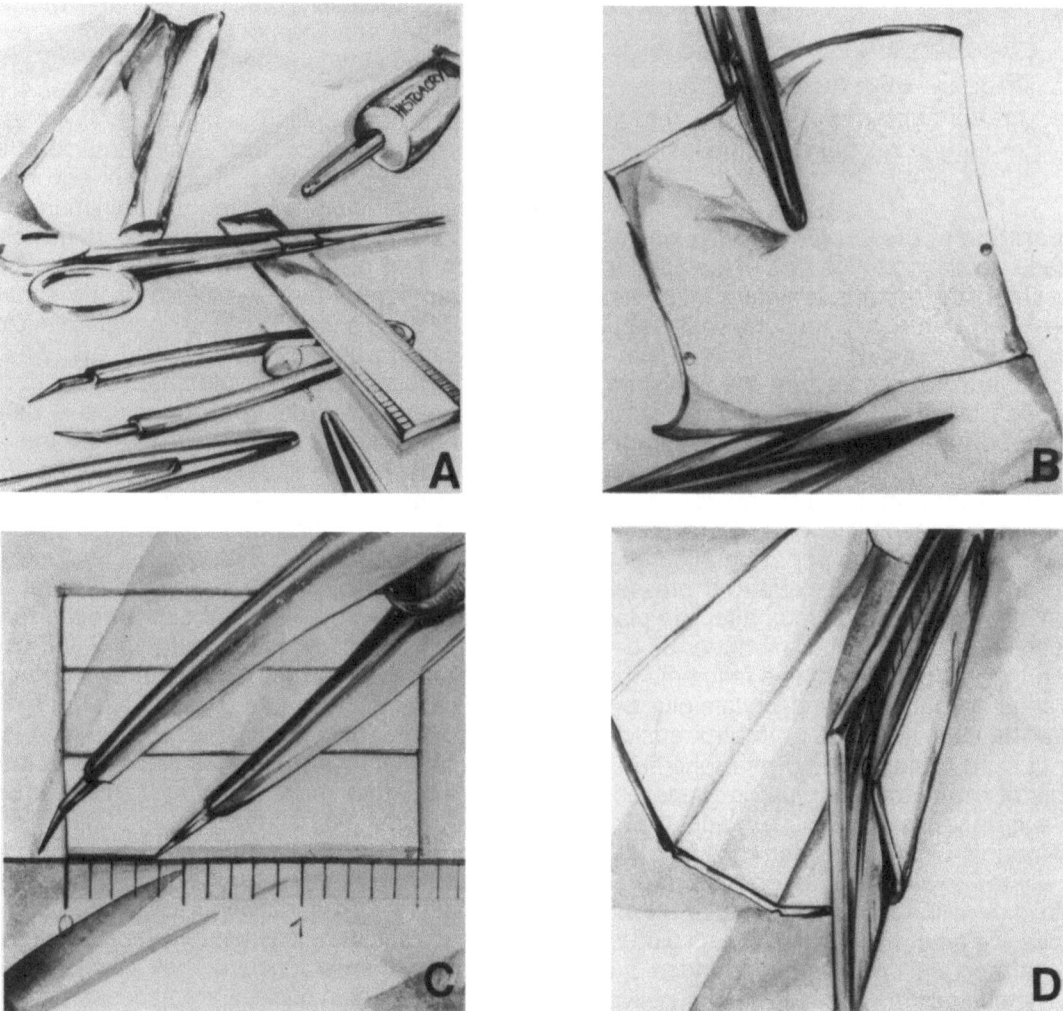

Figure 87. Explant preparation. (A) Piece of lyophilized human dura mater, cyanoacrylate glue, and instruments. (B) The piece of dura mater is cut at the explant length. (C) The width of the dura mater piece is determined to obtain the proper explant width after folding. The dura mater piece will be folded three times. A landmark is made with a compass to locate the places where the dura mater will be folded. The width of each outer layer is 0.5 mm larger in size than the inner layer. (D) Folds are made using the rule edge. (E) A small amount of cyanoacrylate glue is placed on the piece of dura mater. (F) The explant is pressed hard using forceps to stick together the explant layers.

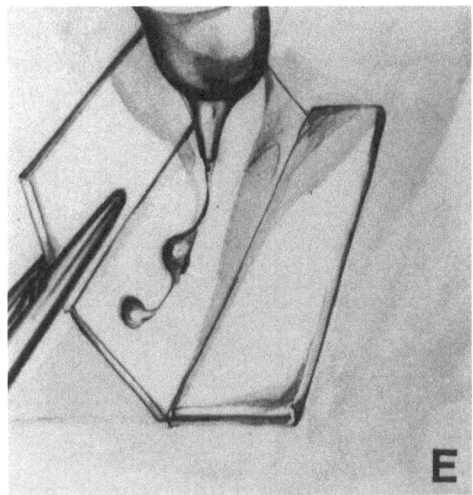 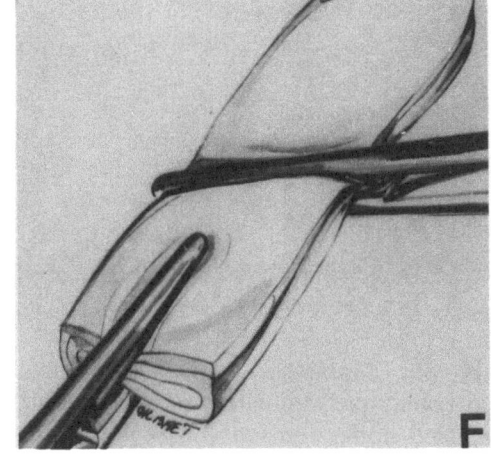

Figure 87. (Continued)

of these sutures will shorten the circumferential arc of the eye and induce a high buckling effect at both extremities of the explant (Fig. 92).

In microsurgical management of retinal detachment the indications for encircling procedures are restricted to the most severe retinal detachments, in particular, detachments complicated by proliferative vitreoretinopathy. In such eyes the encircling procedure is mainly used to counteract ring contraction of the vitreous base. The encircling procedure has two main objectives: (1) to decrease the transverse diameter of the vitreous cavity in the plane of the vitreous base and (2) to produce a high scleral buckle extending from the ora serrata beyond the posterior edge of the vitreous base. Decreasing the transverse diameter of the vitreous cavity in the plane of the vitreous base is obtained by shortening the length of the encircling explant (Fig. 72). Constriction should be limited to between 10% and 25% of the eye circumference to avoid anterior segment ischemia.[40] A high scleral buckle extending from the ora

serrata beyond the posterior border of the vitreous base is obtained by placing the scleral mattress sutures with the technique used for segmental circumferential scleral buckling (Fig. 93 and Fig. 94). Two scleral mattress sutures per quadrant are required. The limbs of the mattress sutures are placed twice as much apart as the width of the encircling explant. The anterior scleral bites are made on the scleral projection of the ora serrata. The site of the posterior scleral bites is determined by the width of the explant. In most cases explants 4–5 mm in width are used, and therefore, the posterior scleral bites of the mattress sutures are placed 8–10 mm posteriorly to the scleral projection of the ora serrata. When the encircling buckle is also used to seal retinal tear(s), the width and position of the encircling explant should be adjusted so that the scleral buckle extends 2–3 mm beyond the posterior edge of the retinal tear(s). When the detachment is associated with rather large horseshoe tear(s), radial explant(s) are used in combination with the encircling explant.

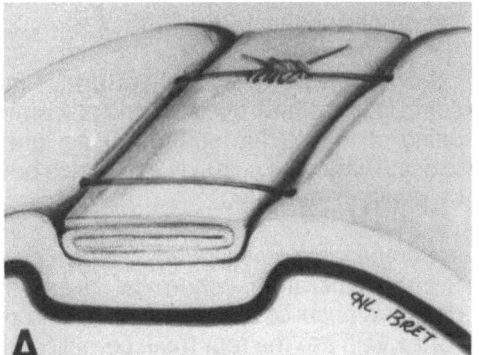 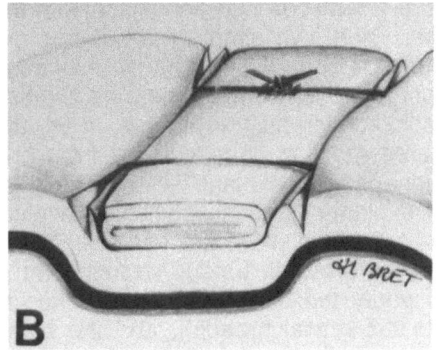

Figure 88. Mattress suture with intrascleral tracks parallel to the explant. (A) Suture properly tied. (B) Suture excessively tightened: the thread under excessive tension has cut through scleral fibers.

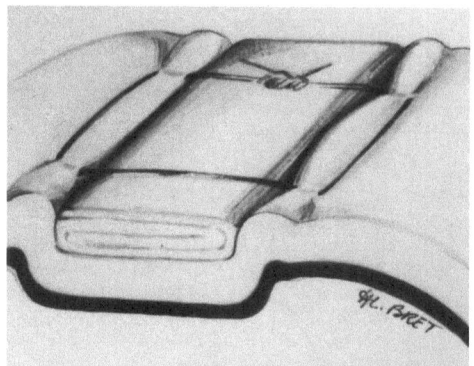

Figure 89. Mattress suture with four intrascleral tracks perpendicular to the explant. The suture tied under tension shows no tendency to cut out.

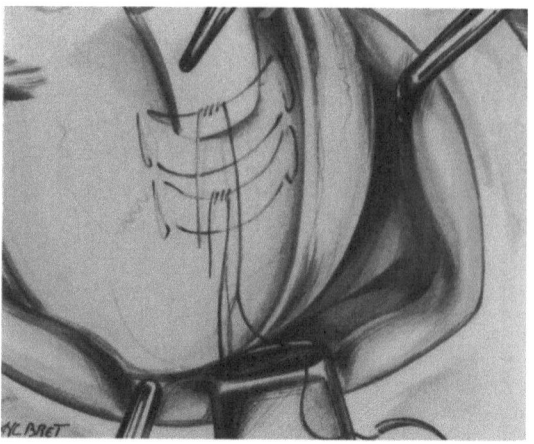

Figure 90. A single retinal tear at the 10 o'clock position is managed by segmental scleral buckling. The explant sutures are anchored in thin sclera beneath the lateral rectus muscle. Mattress sutures with four intrascleral tracks perpendicular to the explant are used rather than mattress sutures with two intrascleral tracks parallel to the explant.

Tightening of the Buckle Sutures. First, the explant is tied into place with temporary knots. Next, the fundus is examined to verify that the explant is correctly placed. Then, the sutures are permanently tied.

Tightening of the scleral sutures should not induce increased intraocular pressure. In phakic eyes, lowering the intraocular pressure is achieved by paracentesis of the anterior chamber. The anterior chamber paracentesis is carried out before tightening the sutures.

In aphakic eyes, lowering the intraocular pressure is obtained by intravenous administration of hyperosmotic solutions and/or 500 mg acetazolamide. However, a decrease in intraocular pressure may be insufficient to tighten the buckle sutures, especially when large or encircling explants have to be used. In such eyes subretinal fluid release is performed.

Gradual tightening of the buckle sutures is done with a triple throw first loop. The triple throw loop will not slip when the thread is under tension. Tightening is continued until both scleral limbs of the mattress suture are placed into apposition with the explant edges. Then, two simple throw loops are made to secure the knot. When a radial explant is used, the most posterior mattress sutures are tied first. When a circumferential explant is used, the mattress sutures are tied consecutively from one end to the other end of the explant. When a combination of radial explant(s) and an encircling explant are used, the radial explant(s) are tied first. When all buckle sutures are tied, fundus examination is performed to verify the buckle height, the buckle relationship to the retinal break(s), and the blood circulation on the optic disc. Insufficient height of a segmental scleral buckle is managed by placing small pieces of dura mater between the explant and the sclera. This usually increases the height of the

buckle. A significant amount of subretinal fluid, which remains between the buckle and the break and radial retinal folds, are managed by intravitreal gas injection. Arrest of the blood circulation on the optic disc should be managed immediately. When repeated paracentesis of the anterior chamber is not feasible or is inefficient, subretinal fluid should be released.

Mispositioning of the buckle may result from improper localization of the scleral projection of the retinal break. The most common errors in positioning of the scleral buckle are shown in Figures 95 and 96. In such cases the scleral sutures should be removed. The scleral projection of the retinal break(s) is determined again so as to place the explant in the proper position.

Intraoperative Complications. Intraoperative complications may occur during placement and tightening of the buckle sutures. They are more likely to occur when the sclera is thin or has been damaged by previous surgery.

Complications During Suture Placement. Scleral laceration, choroidal hemorrhage, accidental release of subretinal fluid, and damage to a vortex vein are the four main complications that may be encountered during placement of the buckle sutures. Such complications are most uncommon when proper needles are used. If needles with cutting surfaces confined to the tip are not available, side cutting

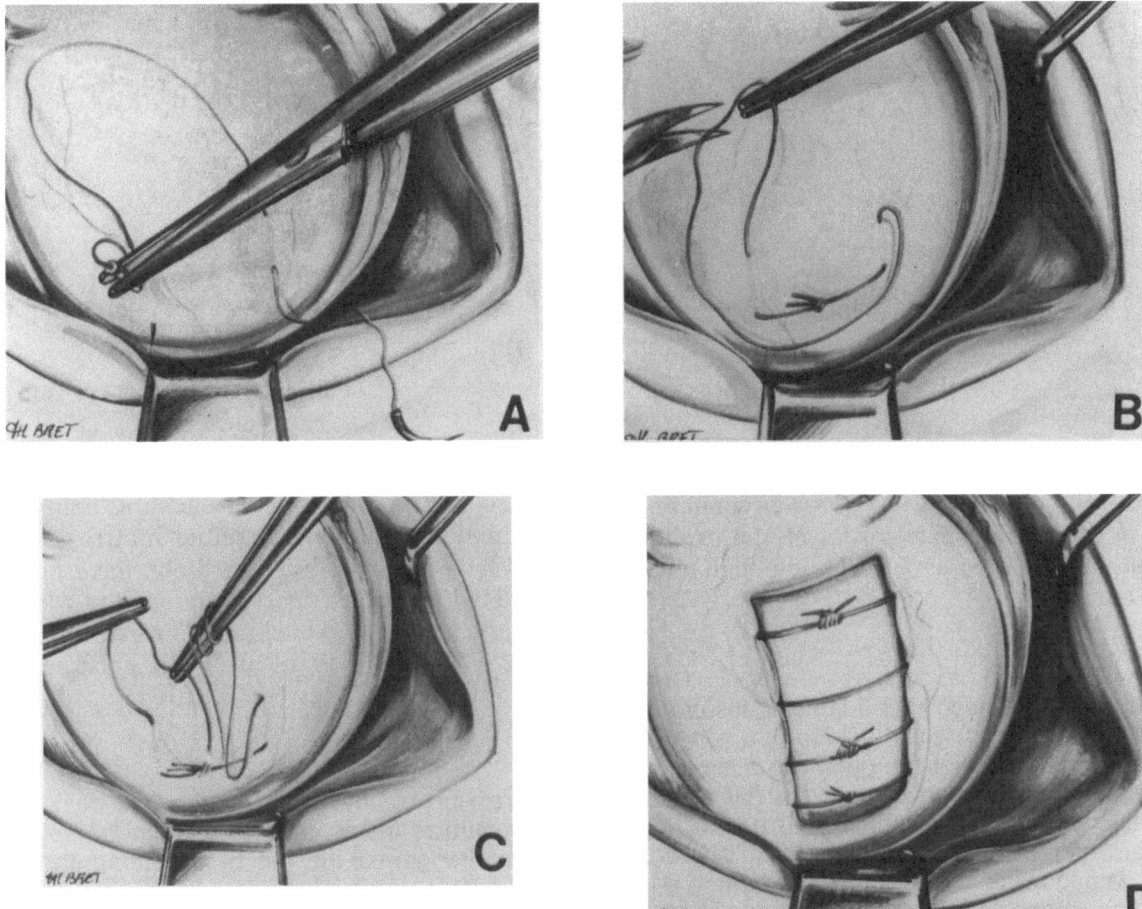

Figure 91. The two-knot suture technique for placement of a scleral suture posterior to the equator. (A) Both suture needles are inserted in a radial anterior posterior direction. (B) A posterior knot has been made with the cut ends of the thread. The anterior loop of the suture is cut. (C) A knot is being prepared with the cut ends of the anterior loop. (D) The explant has been secured by two mattress sutures. The posterior mattress suture shows two knots. The anterior knot was used to permanently tie the explant.

needles rather than reverse cutting edge needles should be used. Side cutting needles are the easiest to pass into the sclera, but they should be used with great care, since their lateral edges can cut through the outer or inner layers of the sclera when they are not inserted in a plane exactly parallel to the surface of the sclera. Reverse cutting edge needles should not be used for scleral sutures because their posterior cutting edge may damage the underlying choroid (Fig. 97).

When the scleral laceration involves 1 mm or more of the needle track, the scleral bite will become too weak and the suture must be removed with a new suture placed in undamaged sclera.

Choroidal damage from too deep a suture or from the cutting edge of a side cutting edge, or a reverse cutting edge needle, may result in severe choroidal

hemorrhage when a large choroidal vessel is hit. The suture must be removed and diathermy performed to stop choroidal bleeding.

Accidental perforation of the choroid with subsequent release of subretinal fluid is the most common complication encountered during buckle suture placement. The perforating suture should be removed. If subretinal fluid escape continues after suture removal, the leaking point should be sealed with an 8–0 nylon suture. Accidental release of subretinal fluid may result in severely decreased intraocular pressure and choroidal hemorrhage. The intraocular pressure must be restored by tightening the buckle sutures that have already been placed or with an intravitreal injection of balanced saline solution.

The intrascleral course of a vortex vein may be

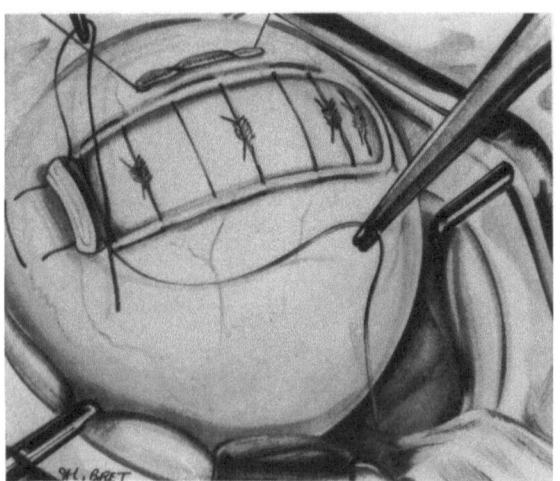

Figure 92. Scleral sutures for a circumferential explant: Both extremities of the explant are sutured to the sclera to obtain a high buckling effect.

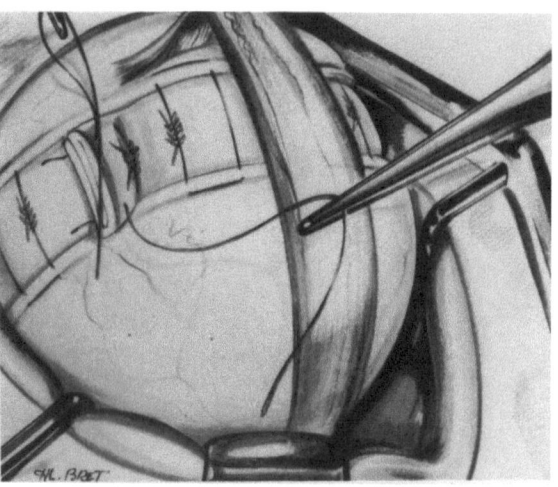

Figure 93. A 360° scleral buckling using a dura mater explant. The radial mattress sutures have been tied. Their limbs have been placed twice as much apart as the explant width to induce high scleral buckling. The extremities of the encircling explant are being sutured to each other by two mattress sutures.

damaged by the needle as it is being inserted into the sclera. The intrascleral course of a vortex vein is clearly visible under the operating miscroscope, therefore damage to a vortex vein during suture placement can be avoided. If poor control of the intrascleral passage of the needle results in vortex vein damage, the suture should be removed and bleeding stopped by compression of the vein or superficial diathermy.

Complications During Suture Tightening. The extrascleral course of a vortex vein may be dragged by the thread when the suture is being pulled. Vein

compression by the suture, when it is being tied, will jeopardize the blood circulation in the vein. To prevent dragging of the vein by the suture, the periocular fascia, which is adherent to the vein, are dissected with corneal blunt scissors. The vein is kept isolated from periocular fascia with surgical sponges while the buckle suture is pulled.

Scleral laceration from a suture as it is being tied may occur when the sclera is thin, the suture too superficial, or the sclera damaged by inadequate

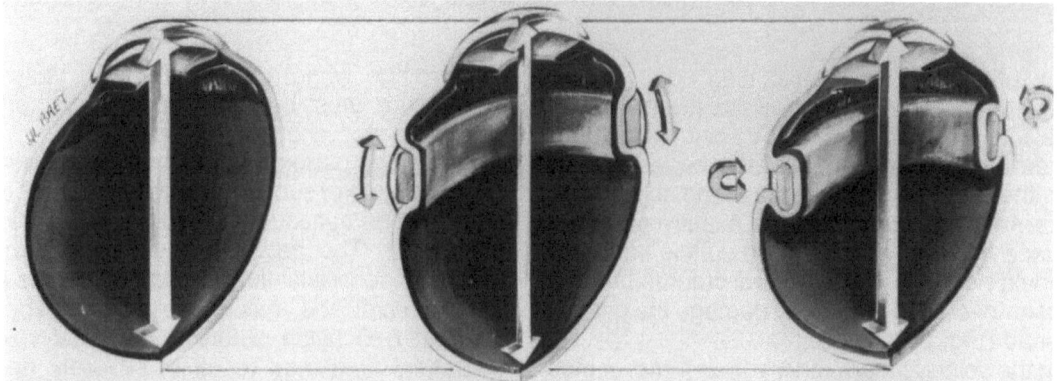

Figure 94. Mechanical effect of an encircling procedure using the 360° explant technique. (Left and center) Mere constriction of an encircling band reduces the transverse diameter of the eye and increases the axial length. (Right) Suturing the 360° explant with mattress sutures whose limbs are twice as much apart as the explant width provides high scleral buckle and avoids increased axial length.

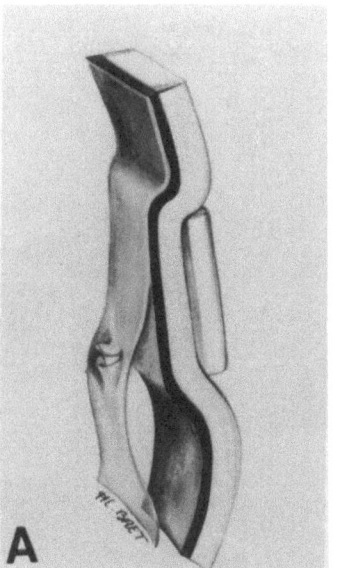 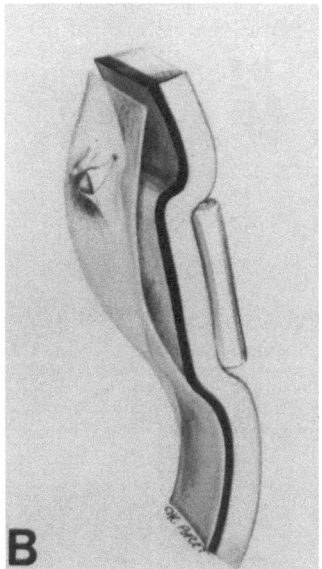

Figure 95. Errors to avoid in radial explant positioning. (A) The explant has been placed in too anterior a position. Subretinal fluid leaks at the tear posterior edge. (B) The explant has been placed in too posterior a position. Traction on the tear flap is not relieved, subretinal fluid leaks anteriorly.

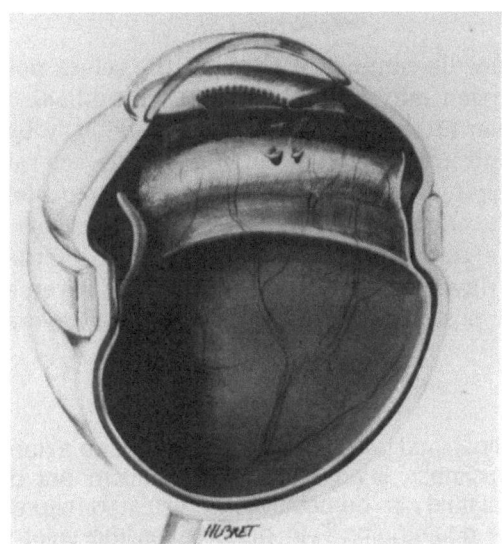

Figure 96. Error to avoid in positioning of an encircling explant. The 360° explant has been placed too posteriorly. The transverse diameter of the vitreous cavity is not reduced in the plane of the vitreous base and the tears are not supported by the buckle. Subretinal fluid leaks anteriorly and may result in recurrent detachment of the retina posterior to the buckle.

needles. The complication is more likely to occur when the intraocular pressure is raised. This complication should be avoided with proper technique for scleral sutures and by lowering the intraocular pressure before tightening the sutures. A suture that has cut out from the sclera should be removed and replaced with a new suture, even when the scleral bite is partially torn.

Increased intraocular pressure is the most common complication occurring during suture tightening. It will produce corneal edema and may prevent complete tightening of the sutures. A high increase in intraocular pressure will result in complete jeopardy of the blood circulation on the optic disc. The tension of the buckle sutures should be released without delay and subretinal fluid drained off. Subretinal fluid drainage should be performed after release of the buckle sutures to prevent too rapid a drainage and retinal incarceration into the drainage site.

Scleral Shortening

INDICATIONS

Scleral shortening is occasionally carried out in selected retinal detachments associated with prolif-

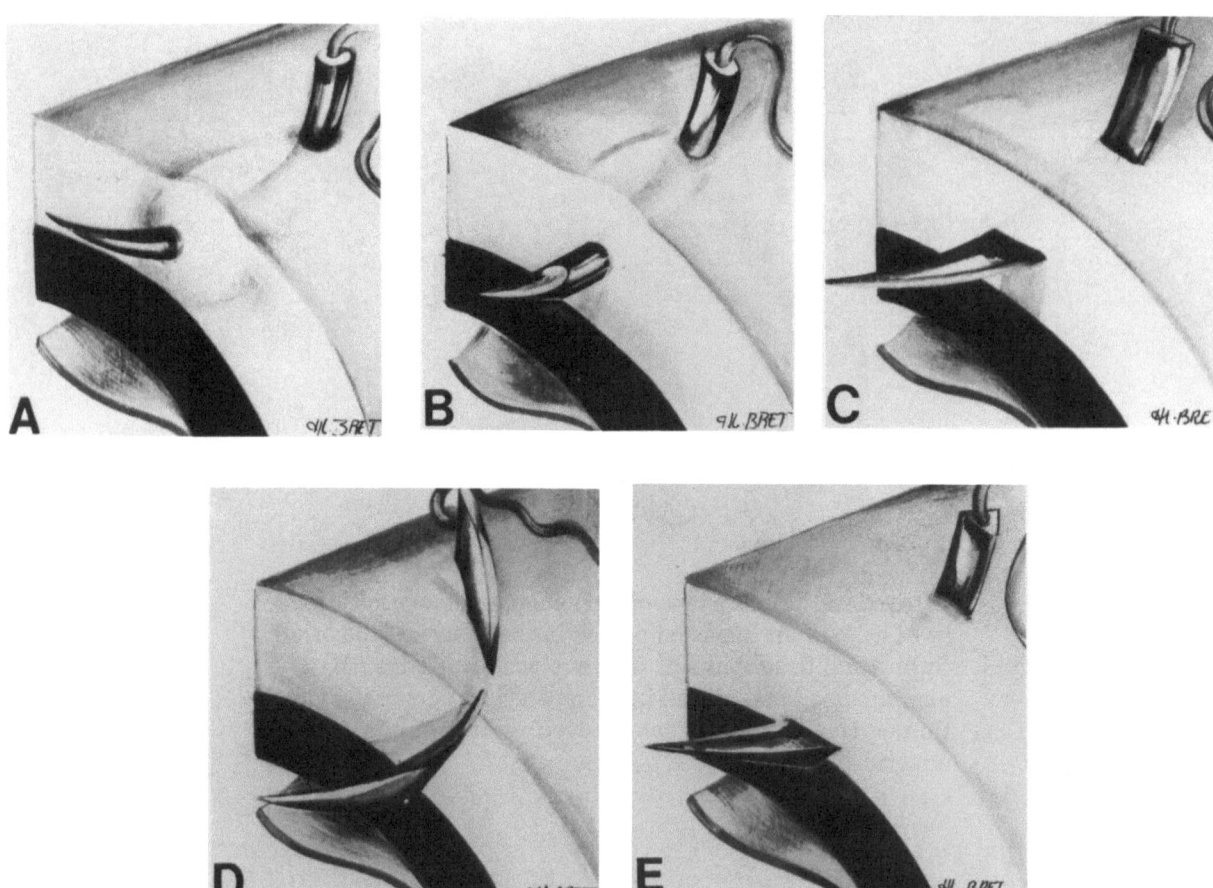

Figure 97. Needles for scleral suture. (A) Round-bodied needle cannot cut through the sclera nor damage the underlying choroid, however, intrascleral insertion may be difficult. (B) Round-bodied needle with cutting surfaces at the tip: intrascleral insertion at the proper depth is made easy by the sharp tip. Damage to scleral fibers is limited to a minimum. (C) Side cutting needle: scleral fibers are cut by the needle and scleral insertion is easy. Needle insertion should be strictly parallel to the scleral surface so as to avoid complications. The needle should not be used in dissected sclera. (D) When a side cutting needle is not inserted in a plane strictly parallel to the surface of the sclera, its edges can cut through the outer and the inner layers of the sclera. (E) use of reverse cutting edge needle should be avoided for scleral suture: the posterior edge may cut the inner layers of the sclera and damage the underlying choroid.

erative vitreoretinopathy of low-grade activity. The indications for scleral shortening in proliferative vitreoretinopathy are restricted to longstanding retinal detachments with fixed retinal folds that involve only the peripheral retina and are limited to one quadrant.[41] Scleral shortening can also be used as an adjunct to vitreous surgery to compensate retina shortening due to epiretinal membranes that cannot be removed.

SURGICAL TECHNIQUE

The length and the width of the scleral fold are determined by two main parameters: (1) the amount

of subretinal fluid to be drained off and (2) the extent of full thickness fixed folds. The total amount of subretinal fluid can be accurately calculated by preoperative oculometry.[42] In most cases the scleral fold involves 100° to 160° of the eye circumference, and the width ranges between 5 mm and 8 mm.

The position of the scleral fold is determined by the location of the retinal tear(s) and fixed folds. The position of the scleral fold in relationship to the ora serrata is determined so that at least one-half of the width of the scleral fold will overlap the tear posterior edge. The scleral fold is crescent shaped (Fig. 98). Its median part should be located in front of the retinal tear(s) and fixed folds. The scleral fold

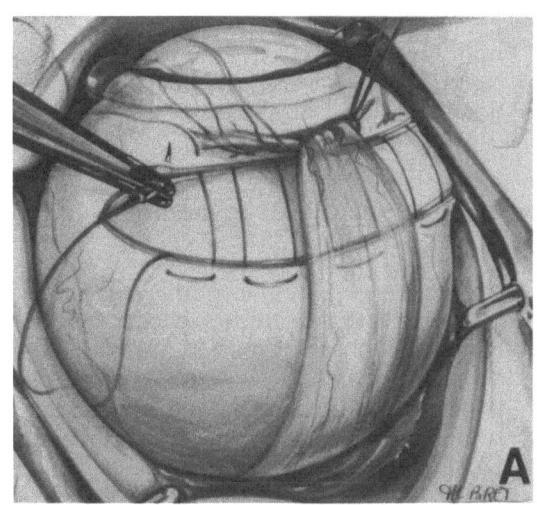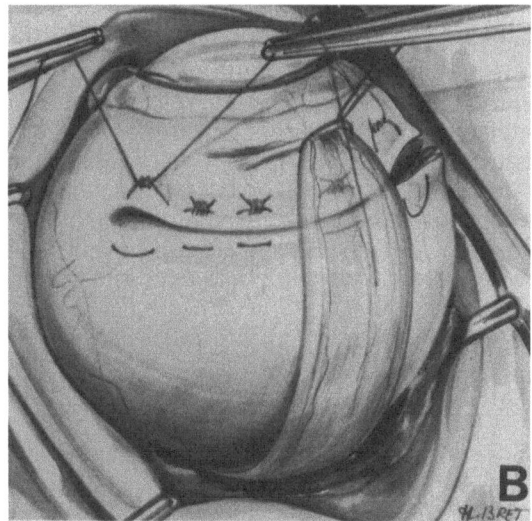

Figure 98. Surgical technique for scleral shortening by a scleral fold. (A) The mattress sutures are being placed. (B) The scleral sutures are tied.

is delineated by two superficial incisions of the sclera. No sclera is removed. Scleral mattress sutures are placed with double-armed sutures. 5–0 braided nonabsorbable sutures are used. The scleral bites are oriented in a radial direction. The posterior scleral bites are made first so that the knots of the stitches sit on the anterior edge of the scleral fold. The needle is engaged into the sclera 2 mm posteriorly to the posterior scleral incision, passed at half the sclera thickness, and exited out of the posterior scleral incision. For the anterior scleral bites scleral entry of the needle is in the anterior scleral incision and the exit 2 mm anteriorly to the incision (Fig. 98).

Scleral shortening requires subretinal fluid drainage. All scleral mattress sutures are placed before releasing the subretinal fluid. Next the sclerotomy for subretinal fluid drainage is done. The incision for subretinal fluid drainage is made in front of fixed retinal folds, since the retina is not likely to flatten in this area until nearly all subretinal fluid is released and all scleral sutures are tied. The choroidal incision should be tiny so that subretinal fluid will gradually escape during tightening of the mattress sutures.

INTRAOPERATIVE COMPLICATIONS

Complications that may occur during suture placement and tightening are the same as those of buckle suturing. Complications may also occur during subretinal fluid release (see p. 68). Inability to completely tighten all scleral sutures and achieve adequate scleral shortening occurs under the following circumstances: (1) The amount of subretinal fluid has been overestimated and the scleral fold is too

wide; and (2) complete release of subretinal fluid cannot be achieved. In such cases decrease in intraocular pressure by anterior chamber paracentesis or intravenous administration of acetazolamide and mannitol is helpful in completing tightening of the sutures.

POSTOPERATIVE COMPLICATIONS

Infection, extrusion, and intrusion are potential postoperative complications of all buckling procedures. Any buckling procedure can also induce refractive errors.

Anterior segment ischemia and closed angle glaucoma are potential complications that are more specific of encircling procedures.

Postoperative diplopia and buckle protrusion on the posterior pole are rare complications, more specific of radial buckling procedures.

Infection

Infection of explants made with lyophylized human tissues is most uncommon.[30] Infection may result from either improper sterilization of lyophylized human tissues or improper asepsis at surgery. The former cause of buckle infection has not been observed in human tissues prepared at the centre de transfusion sanguine in Beynost.

In most cases the course of buckle infection is

not modified by administration of local or systemic antibiotics; the buckle must be removed.

Prevention of buckle infection can be achieved by proper asepsis during surgery. In particular, dura mater explants and fascia lata pieces for implants must be handled with forceps rather than fingers. Great care should be taken not to touch the eyelid's margins when placing the explant or implant. In addition, the explant and implant are coated with penicillin powder before placing them onto or into the sclera.

Buckle Extrusion

Several months postoperatively, as the scleral mattress sutures tend to become loose, the explant may bulge beneath the conjunctiva and Tenon's capsule. In most cases the condition does not lead to any patient discomfort. It is discovered on routine eye examination. No treatment is required.

Buckle extrusion through the conjunctiva is most infrequent when lyophylized human tissues are used.[30] Predisposing factors to buckle extrusion are threefold; (1) improper buckle suturing, (2) low grade infection, and (3) improper dissection and suture of the conjunctiva and Tenon's capsule. Buckle extrusion is more likely to occur after reoperations, due to the difficulties encountered in tissue dissection and suturing when these surgical steps were poorly done at the previous detachment procedure(s).

Buckle extrusion through the conjunctiva requires buckle removal. The incidence of recurrent detachment following buckle removal shows a wide range of variation depending on the series.[16–37.] This has occurred in the author's experience less than 1% of her cases. The degree of vitreous traction at the time of the initial retinal detachment is a factor that has a statistically significant association with redetachment.[43]

Buckle Intrusion

Scleral erosion and buckle intrusion have not been observed when full thickness scleral buckles of lyophylized human tissues were made.

In contrast buckle intrusion may occur after intrascleral implantation of lyophylized human tissues. Four main factors predispose to implant intrusion: (1) too deep a scleral undermining, (2) inclusion of an excessive amount of fascia lata into the scleral pocket, (3) use of large pieces of dura mater as implant material, and (4) use of diathermy on the undermined sclera. In most cases intrusion of lyophylized human tissues does not lead to any clinical symptom. It is discovered upon fundus examination.

No attempt should be made to remove the buckle: complications caused by intrusion of lyophylized human tissue are most infrequent, whereas surgical removal would involve a high risk of severe complications.

Anterior Segment Ischemia

Anterior segment ischemia may develop after large buckling procedures, especially encircling procedures. It is recognized in the early postoperative course on flare of the anterior chamber and poor pupillary dilation. The latter involves the entire pupil in the most severe form of the syndrome, and a segment of the pupil in the least severe form. Iris atrophy and posterior synechiae will develop in the affected segment of the iris. Severe hypotony and subsequent cataract formation are associated with the most severe form of the syndrome.

Measures to decrease the incidence and severity of anterior segment ischemia following scleral buckling: (1) restrict the indications for encircling procedures to retinal detachments that cannot be successfully managed with segmental buckles, (2) limit constriction of the encircling buckle to less than 25% of the eye circumference,[40] (3) avoid damage to the vortex veins, and (4) avoid unnecessary muscle disinsertion to preserve the anterior ciliary arteries. If muscle disinsertion is necessary, it must be limited to one rectus muscle. Disinsertion of three recti muscles during the same operation must never be done.

Closed Angle Glaucoma

Encircling procedures may lead to closed angle glaucoma. This complication is most rare. It is due to an anterior shift of the lens iris plane[44] or compression of the vortex veins. It should be avoided by proper surgical technique.

Postoperative Diplopia

Postoperative diplopia related to the buckling procedure has not been observed after lamellar scleral pockets. In contrast it is occasionally observed after scleral buckling with explants when the explant is sutured on the superior oblique muscle insertion or beneath a vertical rectus muscle. In most cases diplopia spontaneously disappears within a few weeks and explant removal or muscle surgery for diplopia are unnecessary.

Buckle Protrusion on the Posterior Pole

Buckle protrusion on the posterior pole may occur when the anterior-posterior dimension of a radial buckle is excessive when the retinal break to be buckled is situated posteriorly to the equator. Distortion of the macular area by the buckle may delay recovery of central vision after retinal reattachment.

Refractive Errors

Encircling bands used in conventional surgery usually show a tendency to increase the axial length of the eye with a resultant shift towards myopia. In contrast deep encircling buckles, according to the technique described above (see p. 108), shorten the axial length of the eye with a resultant shift towards hypermetropia.

Deep radial buckles with explants, such as those usually made in proliferative vitreoretinopathy, may produce a high degree of postoperative astigmatism.

Scleral shortening with wide scleral folds may also produce high degrees of astigmatism.[41]

REFERENCES

1. Gonin J: Le décollement de la rétine. Pathogénie. Traitement Lausanne, Switzerland, 1934. Librairie Payot Edit.
2. Custodis E: Bedented die Plombenaufnahung auf die Sklera linen Fort-schritt in der operativen Behandlung der Netzhautablösung? Ber Deutsch Ophthal Ges 58: 102–105, 1953
3. Schepens CL, Okamura ID, Brockhurst RJ: The scleral buckling procedures: I Surgical techniques and management. Arch Ophthalmol 58: 797–811, 1957
4. Zauberman H, Rosell FG: Treatment of retinal detachment without inducing chorioretinal lesions. Trans Am Acad Ophthalmol Otolaryngol 79: 835–844, 1975
5. Chignell AH, Markham RH: Retinal detachment surgery without cryotherapy. British J Ophthalmol 65: 371–373, 1981
6. Theodossiadis: Traitement du décollement de la rétine consécutif à un trou maculaire sans application d'aucune forme d'énergie. J Fr Ophthalmol 5: 427–431, 1982
7. Michels RG , Thompson JT, Rice TA, Freund D: Effect of scleral buckling on vector forces caused by epiretinal membranes. Am J Ophthalmol 102: 449–451, 1986
8. Lincoff H, Baras I, Mc Lean J: Modifications to the custodis procedure for retinal detachment. Arch Ophthalmol 73: 160–163, 1965
9. Lincoff H, Kreissig I: Advantages of radial buckling. Am J Ophthalmol 79: 955–957, 1975
10. Goldbaum MH, Smithline M, Poole TA , Lincoff H A: Geometrical analysis of radial buckling. Am J Ophthalmol 79:958–965, 1975
11. Lincoff H: Mechanisms of failure in the repair of large retinal tears. Am J Ophthalmol 84:501–507, 1977
12. Pruett RC : The fishmouthing phenomenon. Arch Ophthalmol 95: 1777–1787, 1977
13. Birchall CM: The fishmouth phenomenon in retinal detachment: old concepts revised. Brit J Ophthal 63:507–510, 1979
14. Schepens CL, Okamura ID, Brockhurst RJ: The scleral buckling procedures. I Surgical techniques and management. Arch Ophthalmol 58: 797–811, 1957
15. Criswick VG, Brockhurst RJ: Retinal detachment, 360° scleral buckling as a primary procedure. Arch Ophthalmol 82: 641–650, 1969
16. Chignell AH: Retinal detachment surgery New York, Springer-Verlag, 1980, 77–86, 152
17. Bec P, Camezind M: Techniques d'indentation dans le décollement de la rétine. Année Thérapeutique Clinique Ophtalmol. 21: 145–152, 1970
18. Bonnet M: Microchirurgie du décollement de la rétine de l'aphake. An Inst Barraquer 16: 381–396, 1982–1983
19. Schepens CL: Retinal detachment and allied diseases. Philadelphia, W. B. Saunders Company, 1983, Vol. 1: 333–343
20. Jacklin FP, Freeman MK, Schepens CL, et al: Gelatin as an absorbable implant in scleral buckling procedures. Arch Ophthalmol 79:286–290, 1968
21. Deodati F, Bec P, Camezinf M: Utilisation du teflon comme matériel d'indentation dans la chirurgie du décollement de la rétine Bull Soc Ophtalmol Fr 71:69–71, 1971
22. Marti R, Burgues L, Gabarro I, Mariella V, Guix M: Explant synthétique absorbable de PDS pour le traitement du décollement de la rétine. J Fr Ophtalmol 9:373–379, 1986
23. Paufique L: Technique de compression intrasclérale. Le traitement moderne du décollement de la rétine, in Dufour R (ed), Probl Actuels Ophtalmol 3:152–153, 1965
24. Paufique L, Revol L, Charleux J, Tingault J, Denhaut X: Préparation de tissus humains conservés en ophtalmologie Ann Oculist 199:833–856, 1966
25. Jean-Louis B, Bievelez B, Bonnet M: An ultrasonographic study of choroidal indentation height after scleral buckling with lyophylized human tissues. Graefe's Arch Clin Exp Ophthalmol 222:158–161, 1985
26. Dominguez a: Ultrasonic control of ocular dimension and surgical indentations in retinal detachment. in, Onozeon E W, Dufour R, Gailloud C, Daicker B, (eds) Modern problems in ophthalmology. Turning points in retinal detachment surgery, 18, Karger, Basel, 77–81, 1977
27. Irvine AR, Stone RD: An ultrasonographic study of early buckle height after sponge explants. Am J Ophthalmol 92: 403–406, 1981
28. Kuroni S, Sakaue E: Ultrasonic biometry on scleral protrusion in the early course of retinal detachment surgery. Folia Ophthalmol (Japan) 32: 440–449, 1981
29. Stone RD, Irvine AR, Santos E: An ultrasonographic study of the persistance of buckle height three years after segmental sponge exoplants. Am J Ophthalmol 84: 508–513, 1977
30. Ravault MP, Belmont F: Indentation épisclérale par implants organiques lyophilisés dans la chirurgie du décollement rétinien. Arch Ophtalmol (Paris) 36: 579–594, 1976
31. Bacin F, Kantelip B, Lynch L: Décollement de Rétine opéré par cryoapplications et identation épisclérale par matériel biologique. Etude anatomoclinique après 2 ans. Bull Soc Ophtalmol Fr 83: 533–540, 1983
32. Colosi N J, Yanoff M: Intrusion of scleral implant associated with conjunctival epithelial ingrowth. Am J Ophthalmol 83: 504–507, 1983
33. Kurz GH, Ezrow L: Transscleral erosion of silicone band. Arch Ophthalmol 73: 183–188, 1965
34. Lindsey PS, Pierce LH, Welch RB: Removal of scleral buckling elements. Causes and complications. Arch Ophthalmol 101: 570–573, 1983
35. Smith ME, Zimmerman LE: Intraocular erosion of circling polyethylene tubing and silicone plate. Arch Ophthalmol 73: 618–622, 1965
36. Schwartz PL, Pruett RC: Factors influencing retinal redetachment after removal of buckling elements. Arch Ophthalmol 95: 804–807, 1977
37. Hilton GF, Wallyn RH: The removal of scleral buckles. Arch Ophthalmol 96: 2061–2063, 1978
38. Burton TC: Irregular astigmatism following episcleral buckling

procedure with the use of silicone rubber sponges. Arch Ophthalmol 90: 447–448, 1973

39. Goel R, Crewdson J, Chignell AH: Astigmatism following retinal detachment surgery. Brit J Ophthal 67:327–329, 1983

40. Lincoff H, Kreissig I, Parver R: Limits of constriction in the treatment of retinal detachment. Arch Ophthalmol 94: 1473–1477, 1976

41. Bonnet M, Dupuis L: Traitement chirurgical des décollements rétiniens idiopathiques avec rétraction rétinienne périphérique. Bull Soc Ophtalmol Fr 81: 973–979, 1981

42. Meyer-Schwickerath G, Gerke E, Mackensen D: Oculometry and detachment surgery. Mod Probl in Ophthalmology. New aspects of vitreoretinopathology. Karger, Basel 20: 202–204, 1979

43. Lindsey PS, Pierce LH, Welch RB: Removal of scleral buckling elements causes and complications. Arch Ophthalmol 101:570–573, 1983

44. Hartley RE, Marsh RJ: Anterior chamber depth changes after retinal detachment surgery. Brit J Ophthal 57: 546–550, 1973

12

Intravitreal Gas Injection

Internal tamponade of the retina by means of intravitreal gas injection antedates the basics of retinal detachment repair established by Jules Gonin in the 1930s. The first use of intravitreal air injection in retinal detachment management was reported by Ohm in 1911.[1] The following year Rohmer[2] reported 8 cases of retinal detachment in which intraocular air injection was attempted. Surgical success was achieved in two eyes. New interest in air injection arose in 1935 when Arruga mentioned the use of air as an adjunct to penetrating diathermy and encircling procedures in selected retinal detachments. Between 1938 and 1953 Rosengren[3,4] showed than an air bubble injected into the vitreous cavity was a useful adjunct to retinopexy and subretinal fluid drainage, especially in the management of poor prognosis cases. Rosengren also showed that intraocular air injection does not lead to any specific longterm complication,[4] however internal tamponade with air has a major limitation: the air bubble is frequently absorbed before a firm chorioretinal adhesion can form. Because of that major limitation, internal tamponade with air was supplanted by scleral buckling during the 1950s.

Since 1970 retinal detachment surgeons have shown renewed interest in the use of intraocular gas, due to the introduction of expansive and longlasting gases in ophthalmology.

Sulfur hexafluoride (SF6), which had already been used in medicine for intraperitoneal injection until the 1950s, was introduced in retinal detachment surgery by Norton in 1973.[5] The expansion of the gas and its longer persistence as compared with air appeared to be advantageous. Other gases that can expand and persist even longer in the vitreous cavity were sought.[6] In 1980 Lincoff et al.[7,8] introduced a family of straight chain perfluorocarbon gases with varying expansion properties and longevities. Some of them, especially perfluoropropane (C3F8) and perfluoro-n-butane (C4F10) appeared to have several advantages compared with sulfur hexafluoride in the management of selected retinal detachments.

In addition to this, the development of pars plana vitrectomy opened new avenues and brought new concepts in the management of complicated retinal detachments. Machemer[9] introduced SF6 as an adjunct to vitreous surgery for the management of complicated retinal detachments.

At present the ultimate role of intravitreal gases in retinal detachment repair is still incompletely determined. However, intravitreal gas injection already appears to be a major surgical adjunct in the management of selected retinal detachments.

GASES CURRENTLY USED IN RETINAL DETACHMENT REPAIR

Air

Air was the first gas used for retinal tamponade.[1] It has no known toxicity for the ocular tissues.[3,4] The only advantage of air is its availability at any time and no cost.

Unfortunately, the absorption of an air bubble in the vitreous cavity is very rapid and starts immediately after injection, although complete absorption of the air bubble may require 5–9 days, the volume of the air bubble often becomes too small to remain effective as early as the second day after injection.

In spite of its limitations related to nonexpansion of the bubble in the vitreous cavity and too rapid an absorption rate, air can be used for intravitreal injection in selected retinal detachments when an expanding gas such as SF6 is not available. In particular, air can be a valuable alternative to SF6 when the effectiveness of gas injection requires an internal tamponade of short duration. Such is the case in the treatment of fishmouth phenomenon when retinal detachment is not associated with clinical evidence of actual or impending proliferative vitreoretinopathy.

An air bubble can be as effective as any gas bubble for manipulating the inverted flap of a giant retinal tear.[10] However, air injection cannot be recommended in most retinal detachments associated with giant tears, since those eyes are at a high risk for developing severe postoperative proliferative vitreoretinopathy, which requires prolonged internal tamponade. When a long-lasting gas is not available, air injection has been a valuable alternative to long-lasting gas injection in recent giant retinal tears secondary to severe blunt trauma in emmetropic eyes that had no degenerative vitreous changes before the trauma. Air can be used in place of a long-lasting gas in specific cases when the detachment is recent, because the risk of proliferative vitreoretinopathy is significantly lower in those eyes as compared to highly myopic eyes with giant tears secondary to spontaneous vitreous liquefaction and retraction.[11]

Air can be used as an adjunct to scleral buckling to seal a retinal tear, however the effectiveness of the internal tamponade in this specific indication requires that the air bubble cover the whole retinal tear until a firm chorioretinal adhesion has developed. This requires at least 8–11 days.[12] Because of the rapid absorption of the intravitreal air bubble, use of air for the purpose of sealing a retinal tear should be limited to small tears involving less than 10° of the peripheral circumference of the fundus. A large amount of air should be injected in order to maintain a bubble large enough during the first postoperative week. The intravitreal injection of this large air bubble makes it necessary to drain the subretinal fluid.[13]

Expanding Gases

At present two expanding gases—sulfur hexafluoride (SF6) and perfluoropropane (C3F8)—have been used in microsurgical repair of retinal detachment.

Other gases may, however, be used in the future.

COMMON FEATURES OF EXPANDING GASES

Expanding gases currently used in microsurgical repair share common features, which have been established by experimental studies[7,8,14–17] and confirmed by clinical observations. They are inert nontoxic gases of high molecular weight, low water solubility, and low diffusion coefficient. The expansion and greater longevity of the gas bubble injected into the vitreous cavity are the two main advantages of expanding gases as compared to air. The expansion and the longevity of the bubble are related to the low water solubility and low diffusion coefficient of the gases.

Expansion. Three stages of gas dynamics occur after injection of a bubble of pure inert gas into the vitreous cavity.[15,18]

The first stage, or expansion period, is characterized by a rapid increase in volume of the intravitreal bubble. The rapid increase in volume of the gas bubble results from the high diffusion of carbon dioxide, oxygen, and nitrogen from the blood and surrounding tissues into the intravitreal gas bubble, and the low diffusion of the inert gas out of the vitreous cavity. The expansion period continues until the nitrogen diffusion into the bubble is equal to the diffusion of the inert gas out of the vitreous cavity.

The second stage, or transition period, is characterized by a slow decrease in volume of the gas bubble, which results from a continuing increase in nitrogen concentration and a continuing decrease in inert gas concentration.

The third stage or transfer period,[18] starts after the nitrogen pressure in the intravitreal bubble equilibrates with the nitrogen pressure in the blood. At this stage the composition of the intravitreal bubble remains constant and the bubble volume gradually decreases when all gases diffuse out of the vitreous cavity at a rate proportional to their concentration within the bubble.

The rate of expansion and the length of the expansion period are dependent on the rate of water insolubility of the inert gas. The more insoluble a gas is in water, the more extensive the expansion is, and the longer the expansion period lasts. However, the early rate of rapid expansion is independent of the type of inert gas, but largely dependent on convection currents of the surrounding fluid.[16] Variability in the convection and diffusion conditions of the eye accounts for the clinical variability of expansion and absorption of the gases. For example, convection currents in the vitreous cavity are increased by aphakia, vitrectomy, and eye movements. This may account for the more rapid rate of gas expansion and absorption in aphakic, rather than in phakic eyes, and in vitrectomized than nonvitrectomized eyes.[16] In addition, rapid changes in ambient atmospheric pressure can lead to secondary changes of the bubble volume.[19]

Longevity. The longevity of the gas bubble depends on the water solubility and diffusion coefficient of the gas. The lower the water solubility and diffusion coefficient of the gas, the greater the longevity of the bubble.

The disappearance rate of perfluorocarbon gases in the rabbit eye was found to be exponential and thus independent of the volume injected.[17] If it takes ten days for a gas bubble that completely filled the vitreous cavity to reach half volume, it will take 20 days to reach ¼ volume, 30 days to reach ⅛ volume, and 40 days to reach 1/16 volume. This exponential decay explains the common clinical observation that long periods of time are required for small bubbles to completely disappear.[17]

The total disappearance time of the gas bubble is not an adequate reflection of the therapeutic value of the gas because small bubbles remaining at the end of the absorption period are of little value, if any, for retinal tamponade. The half volume time, or half life, of the gas bubble, is a more valuable criteria for evaluation of the therapeutic value of the gas bubble.

The disappearance rate of the gas bubble may be affected by the size of the eye,[14] the presence or absence of formed vitreous, and aphakia. The disappearance rate is more rapid in aphakic than phakic eyes, and in vitrectomized more than non vitrectomized eyes, because the convection currents in the vitreous cavity are increased by aphakia and vitrectomy.[16] The disappearance rate may be increased in highly myopic eyes because the larger the eye, the greater the surface area available for gas diffusion.[14]

SPECIFIC CHARACTERISTICS OF EXPANDING GASES

Sulfur Hexafluoride (SF6). Experimental studies[14] have shown that sulfur hexafluoride (SF6) is nontoxic to intraocular tissues. Injected into the vitreous cavity, SF6 expands 2.0–2.5 times[20,21] the original bubble volume and persists twice as long as an air bubble of comparable initial size,[14] while the air absorbs in 5–6 days. SF6 completely absorbs in ten to eleven days.

Injected into the vitreous cavity of the owl monkey, pure SF6 was found to expand two times its original volume in the day; the bubble returned to its original size 5–6 days later; and the bubble was completely absorbed 10–11 days after the injection.[14]

Hence, the half life of a gas bubble of adequate volume to cover the retinal tear(s) is sufficient for a firm retinochoroidal adhesion to develop.

Perfluoropropane (C3F8). Perfluoropropane (C3F8) belongs to a family of straight chain perfluorocarbon gases with varying expansion properties and longevities. Experiments in animals[17] showed that the longer the chain of perfluorocarbon gas, the greater the expansion and longevity of the gas bubble. In the rabbit eye, the expansion of C3F8 was found to be 4–5 times.[15–17]

After injection of pure C3F8 in the vitreous cavity, maximum expansion occurs at day 3 or 4.[7,15,16]

When a volume of pure C3F8 expands to fill the vitreous cavity, the bubble persists for as long as 28 days in the rabbit eye[7] and 70 days in the human eye.[20] In the human eye the average half volume time for 1 ml of pure C3F8 injected in the vitreous cavity is 35 days.[8]

RATIONALE FOR INTRAVITREAL GAS INJECTION IN RETINAL DETACHMENT REPAIR

The mechanisms by which a gas bubble injected into the vitreous cavity can act in the management of retinal detachment are purely mechanical.

A gas bubble of sufficient volume acts as an internal tamponade. The gas bubble pushes back the detached retina towards the pigment epithelium. Hence gas injection can be used for flattening mobile retinal folds. Radial retinal folds involving a retinal tear that creates a fishmouth phenomenon are the main indications for flattening the retina with a gas bubble.

A large bubble of long-lasting gas maintains the retina in close apposition with the pigment epithelium during the active phase of proliferative vitreoretinopathy.

An intravitreal gas bubble that covers the whole area of a retinal tear isolates the retinal tear from the vitreous cavity and prevents passage of vitreous fluid into the subretinal space. Hence, gas tamponade can be used to seal a retinal tear, while the induced retinochoroidal adhesion is being made.

A gas bubble can also be used as a soft instrument that is maneuvered within the vitreous cavity from the outside by merely rotating the patient's head. This soft and nontraumatizing instrument can be used for unfolding the inverted posterior margin of a giant retinal tear.

In spite of the modifications of the vitreous body created by a large bubble of long lasting gas, intravitreal gas injection is not an alternative to vitrectomy. Gas injection into the vitreous body neither destroys vitreous strands nor creates a posterior vitreous detachment. Those clinical observations correlate well with experimental data on the monkey eye.[22] A perfluoropropane bubble injected into the vitreous body of monkey eyes creates a large cavity within the vitreous gel. However, posterior vitreous detachment does not occur.[22–24]

INDICATIONS FOR GAS INJECTION

The main indications for intravitreal gas injection in retinal detachment repair are as follows: (1) management of a fishmouth phenomenon, (2) manipulation of the inverted posterior margin of a large or giant retinal tear, (3) internal tamponade of the retinal break, and (4) internal tamponade of the retina during the active phase of proliferative vitreoretinopathy.

Fishmouth Phenomenon

Fishmouth phenomenon can be defined as a radial retinal fold that involves the posterior edge of a retinal tear after scleral buckling. The radial retinal fold behaves as a funnel through which fluid vitreous leaks into the subretinal space.

It has been estimated that approximately 10% of eyes with retinal detachment are at risk for developing a fishmouth phenomenon after scleral buckling.[25] In most cases the fishmouth phenomenon occurs in eyes with horseshoe retinal tears located in the equatorial region and associated with a bullous retinal detachment.

The factors that contribute to the development of a fishmouth phenomenon after scleral buckling are as follows:

1. Height of the detachment: the fishmouth phenomenon is more likely to occur in bullous retinal detachment.
2. Presence of preoperative radial retinal fold(s) involving the retinal tear(s). In many cases, scleral buckling fails to flatten such preoperative radial folds when the retina is highly detached.
3. Size of the retinal tear: The larger the retinal tear, the higher the risk of a fishmouth phenomenon induced by scleral buckling. The fishmouth phenomenon was one of the main causes of surgical failure when scleral buckling alone was used in the management of large retinal tears associated with bullous retinal detachments.[26]
4. Orientation of the scleral buckle: large circumferential buckles predispose to the development of the fishmouth phenomenon because they shorten the circumferential arc of the eye in front of the retinal tear. Large circumferential buckles tend to increase the redundancy of the posterior edge of the retinal tear and predispose to the formation of radial retinal folds.[25,26]
5. Height of the scleral buckle: when a fishmouth phenomenon develops, increasing the height of a circumferential scleral buckle results in an increased shortening of the circumferential arc, which augments the tendency of the posterior edge of the retinal tear to form radial folds.

Numerous techniques based mainly on modifications of the shape and orientation of the scleral buckle have been proposed for the management of fishmouth phenomenon.[25,27–29] The radial buckling approach is the most effective; however a radial buckle may fail when the detachment is very high. In addition, radial buckling is not possible when the retinal tear involves more than 70° of the eye circumference.[26]

Intravitreal gas injection is the most effective technique for eliminating surgical failures due to the fishmouth phenomenon. When a fishmouth phenomenon is likely to occur, the height of the buckle should be limited to the minimum necessary for counteracting vitreous traction, and gas injection is performed to push back the retinal tear against the pigment epithelium.

Gas injection virtually eliminates surgical failures due to fishmouth phenomenon.[21,30,31]

Manipulation of the Inverted Edge of a Large or Giant Retinal Tear

An intravitreal gas bubble is the least traumatic intravitreal instrument for manipulating the inverted posterior edge of a large or giant retinal tear.

Depending on the size of the retinal tear, the extent of retinal inversion, and the association or absence of preoperative proliferative vitreoretinopathy, gas injection is used either alone or in combination with vitreous surgery (see p. 202).

Internal Tamponade of Retinal Breaks

Internal tamponade of retinal break(s) is the most frequent indication for gas injection in retinal detachment repair. The goal of gas injection is to seal the retinal tear during the period of time necessary for formation of a firm retinochoroidal adhesion.

Internal tamponade with gas is used either as the sole procedure to keep the retina in apposition with the pigment epithelium or as an adjunct to scleral buckling.

GAS TAMPONADE WITHOUT SCLERAL BUCKLING

The indications for gas injection without scleral buckling remain controversial. High success rates have been published in a series of selected retinal detachments[32–36], however, the precise criteria for case selection remain to be established.

At present the author limits the indications for gas tamponade without scleral buckling to selected retinal detachments associated with retinal breaks that are not under permanent vitreous traction.

Basically, gas tamponade could be an effective alternative to scleral buckling in most retinal detachments associated with round atrophic holes, disinsertion at the ora serrata, or macular holes in highly myopic eyes. However, the majority of retinal detachments associated with round atrophic holes or a disinsertion at the ora serrata are still managed by scleral buckling rather than gas injection because those retinal breaks are most often inferiorly located. Gas tamponade without scleral buckling of such lesions would require a very large intravitreal gas bubble. This large gas bubble would be associated with a high risk of increased intraocular pressure, since the vitreous gel of such eyes is usually not liquefied. In addition, scleral buckling of inferior retinal breaks has the advantage over gas tamponade of making it possible for the patient to move around normally from the very first postoperative day.

In contrast to round atrophic holes and disinsertion at the ora serrata, most horseshoe retinal tears show biomicroscopic evidence of vitreous traction, which remains after posterior vitreous detachment. Vitreous traction on the tear flap may lead to late reopening of the retinal tear after gas absorption. Therefore, gas tamponade is used as the only surgical procedure to keep the retina in apposition with the pigment epithelium only in selected cases of horseshoe retinal tears (see p. 167).

GAS TAMPONADE AS AN ADJUNCT TO SCLERAL BUCKLING

The main indication for gas tamponade as an adjunct to scleral buckling are as follows: large or multiple contiguous retinal tears that can only be managed with circumferential buckle, retinal tear(s) associated with a bullous detachment, the fishmouth phenomenon, and any retinal tear whose flap remains under traction of the vitreous base after vitrectomy.

Internal Tamponade of the Retina During the Active Phase of Proliferative Vitreoretinopathy

At present internal tamponade with longlasting gases is currently used as an adjunct to vitreoretinal microsurgery in the management of retinal detachments associated with proliferative vitreoretinopathy. The use of gas is preferable to the use of silicone oil as the first vitreous substitute. Low toxicity and spontaneous absorption are the two main advantages of gas as compared to silicone oil.

Internal tamponade with gas is not an alternative to vitrectomy, since the gas bubble cannot flatten fixed retinal folds. Vitrectomy is required to free preretinal membranes and relieve vitreous traction. Then gas tamponade can mechanically flatten retinal folds that have been made mobile by vitreous surgery.

The main goal of gas injection in the management of retinal detachments associated with proliferative vitreoretinopathy is to maintain as much of the retina in apposition with the pigment epithelium until the proliferative process subsides. The duration of the active phase of proliferative vitreoretinopathy remains uncertain, therefore the optimal duration of retinal tamponade with gas remains to be determined. Internal tamponade with gas does not prevent the formation of sequential preretinal membranes, however a large intravitreal gas bubble may prevent the accumulation of fibrin deposits in the vitreous cavity and formation of sequential transvitreal strands.

Although at present gas injection is widely used as an adjunct to vitrectomy in the management of proliferative vitreoretinopathy, its mechanisms of action remain uncertain. The results are encouraging but far from excellent. The role of gas injection in the management of proliferative vitreoretinopathy in the future remains speculative.

SURGICAL TECHNIQUE

Choice of the Gas

Choice of the gas to be used in any given case is dictated by two main parameters: (1) the retinal lesion(s) to be managed and (2) the specific characteristics of the gases available (see above).

With regard to the choice of the most appropriate gas to be used, retinal detachments can be divided into two categories: retinal detachments without actual or potential proliferative vitreoretinopathy, as opposed to retinal detachments associated with actual or potential proliferative vitreoretinopathy.

Retinal tamponade with a gas bubble of rather short duration is efficacious in most retinal detachments that are not associated with clinical evidence of actual or potential proliferative vitreoretinopathy. In contrast, a prolonged retinal tamponade is required in retinal detachments associated with clinical evidence of proliferative vitreoretinopathy as well as in eyes that are at risk for developing severe proliferative vitreoretinopathy during the postoperative course.

MANAGEMENT OF THE FISHMOUTH PHENOMENON

Successful management of the fishmouth phenomenon can be achieved by gas tamponade of short duration. The effectiveness of the gas bubble is immediate, provided the gas bubble covers the retinal tear and the radial fold. Air can be used with success,[30] however, in most cases, SF6 rather than air is used.[3] SF6 provides an additional effect to the immediate flattening of the radial fold: the SF6 bubble provides an internal tamponade of the retinal tear until a firm retinochoroidal adhesion develops.

MANIPULATION OF THE INVERTED EDGE OF A LARGE OR GIANT RETINAL TEAR

Basically, manipulation of the inverted edge of a large or giant retinal tear can be performed with any of the gases available for intraocular use, since the mechanical effect of the retinal manipulation should be immediate. Repositioning of the rolled and inverted edge of a giant retinal tear can be achieved with air or SF6. At present, however, perfluoropropane (C3F8) or even longer lasting gases such as perfluoro-n-butane are used in the management of most retinal detachments associated with giant retinal tears.

Perfluoropropane is used rather than air or SF6 because manipulation of the inverted flap is not the only purpose of gas injection. In the management of large and giant retinal tears a gas bubble is injected into the vitreous cavity with 3 additional goals: (1) to prevent slipping of the posterior edge of the retinal tear in the early postoperative period, (2) ensuring internal tamponade of the whole area of the retinal tear until a firm retinochoroidal adhesion develops, (3) keeping most of the retina in close apposition with the pigment epithelium during the active phase of proliferative vitreoretinopathy, which is most frequent in large and giant retinal tears.

Hence, gas injection should provide a very large internal tamponade for a long period of time. At present, the optimal duration of the internal tamponade in eyes that are at high risk of developing active or recurrent proliferative vitreoretinopathy remains uncertain. However, clinical data would suggest that internal tamponade with a large gas bubble is required for a period of at least a month, and probably more in the most severe cases.

The expansion properties and the longevity of C3F8 make it possible, with a single injection, to unfold the inverted retinal flap with a small bubble and then insure retinal tamponade with a large gas bubble, for a long period of time.

INTERNAL TAMPONADE OF RETINAL BREAK

When the main or single goal of gas injection is to tamponade the retinal break, a gas bubble of sufficient volume should remain within the vitreous cavity until a firm retinochoroidal adhesion develops. Experimental data indicate that the retinochoroidal adhesion induced by cryo or photocoagulation reaches its maximum between day 8 and 11.[12] Thus, tamponade of the retinal tear should last at least 8 days. The expansion properties and the longevity of SF6 make it the gas of preference in this indication. Other gases, however can be used in certain circumstances. Air may be as efficient as SF6 to tamponade a very small retinal tear located in the superior quadrants when scleral buckling of the retinal tear is associated with internal tamponade. In contrast C3F8 is often used when internal tamponade with a large bubble of at least a week's duration is required. In particular C3F8 is often used rather than SF6 to tamponade (1) multiple retinal tears involving two or more quadrants (2) large retinal tears located in the inferior quadrants, and (3) in eyes at risk of developing proliferative vitreoretinopathy postoperatively. Injection of pure C3F8 is also recommended when there is not enough space in the vitreous cavity for injection of the volume of pure SF6 that would be required for effective tamponade of the retinal tear(s). In such cases injection of a small bubble of pure C3F8 makes it possible to achieve an intravitreal gas bubble of adequate volume with less risk of inducing increased intraocular pressure. Secondary displacement of vitreous fluid and absorption of subretinal fluid will provide the intraocular space necessary for gas expansion.

INTERNAL TAMPONADE OF THE RETINA DURING THE ACTIVE PHASE OF PROLIFERATIVE VITREORETINOPATHY

At present C3F8 is used in the management of retinal detachments associated with proliferative vitreoretinopathy. A long term tamponade with a large bubble that fills most of the vitreous cavity is probably necessary to maintain anatomical repositioning of the retina until the proliferative process subsides. The optimal duration for the internal tamponade remains uncertain. Clinical studies[37] have shown that long term tamponade with C3F8 improves the surgical results achieved by a single operation. Longer lasting gases may prove of greater benefit in this specific indication.

Volume of Gas to Be Injected

The optimal volume of pure gas to be injected must provide a bubble of therapeutic size that will last for the necessary length of time. The gas bubble must not induce complications, in particular increased intraocular pressure.

Three main parameters should be taken into account for calculation of the optimal volume of pure gas to be injected: (1) the expansion properties and longevity of the gas, (2) the goal of gas injection, and (3) the space available within the vitreous cavity. The surgeon also has to take into account associated factors that may affect tolerance by the eye of increased intraocular pressure. (For the expansion properties and longevity of the gas see above).

GOAL(S) OF GAS INJECTION

The optimal volume of the gas bubble depends on whether gas injection is performed for internal tamponade of the retinal break(s), manipulation of the inverted edge of a large retinal tear, or retinal tamponade during the active stage of proliferative vitreoretinopathy.

INTERNAL TAMPONADE OF THE RETINAL BREAK(S)

After expansion, the gas bubble must support a retinal arc large enough to cover the extent of the retinal break(s) and still allow the patient a latitude of movements. Parver and Lincoff[38] used a transparent model to demonstrate the configuration of gas bubbles in the vitreous cavity and a mathematical model to calculate bubble volumes. For clinically useful volumes, the base of the gas bubble in the vitreous cavity is flat. Table 2 lists the angular extent of the arc of bubble, retina contact, and bubble depth for bubbles volumes ranging from 0.25 to 2.4 cm3 in a vitreous cavity of 21 mm diameter, after Parver and Lincoff.[38]

The bubble volumes required to cover an arc of equal angular extent increase with the vitreous cavity volumes. Table 3 lists the bubble volumes required to cover a 90 degree arc of contact in vitreous cavities of increasing transverse diameters after Parver and Lincoff[38] and Lincoff and Kreissig.[39]

An increase in axial length of the eye causes only a linearly proportional increase in bubble volume required.[39] For example, a 10% increase in axial length alone would require only a 10% increase in gas volume to cover the same arc of contact. Parver

Table 2
Relationship of Bubble Volume to Angular Extent and Bubble Depth in a Vitreous Cavity of 21 mm Diameter (After Parver and Lincoff).[38]

Bubble Volume CM³	Arc of Bubble Retina Contact °	Bubble Height MM
0.25	88	2.9
0.50	106	4.2
1.00	132	6.1
2.00	168	9.1
2.40	180	10.5

and Lincoff[38] also published a simple formula to calculate the bubble volume for covering arcs extending from 90–180° (Table 4).

When the arc of bubble–retina contact required increases from 90 to 120, 150, or 180°, irrespective of the diameter of the vitreous cavity, the bubble volume necessary to produce these changes is equal to the volume for a 90 degree bubble multiplied by a factor of 2.7, 5.3, and 8.6 respectively. For example, the bubble volume required to cover an arc of 180° in an eye with a transverse diameter of 27 mm is 4.816 cc (0.560 × 8.6). In clinical practice

Table 3
Bubbles Volumes Required to Cover a 90 Degree Arc of Contact for Vitreous Cavities of Various Diameters (after Parver and Lincoff[38] and Lincoff and Kreissig).[39]

Transverse Diameter of the Vitreous Cavity MM	Bubble Volume CM³
19	0.208
20	0.243
21	0.280
22	0.320
23	0.369
24	0.420
27	0.560

Table 4
Relationship of Changes in Angular Extent to Changes in Bubble Volumes (after Parver and Lincoff).[38]

Change in the Arc of Contact °	Change in Volume
90 → 120	× 2.7
90 → 150	× 5.3
90 → 180	× 8.6

the majority of retinal breaks for which gas tamponade is indicated can be managed with relatively small volumes of gas. Only large and giant retinal tears require retinal tamponade with large volumes of gas, especially in the highly myopic eye.

MANIPULATION OF THE INVERTED EDGE OF A LARGE RETINAL TEAR

Surgical repair of large retinal tears usually requires retinal tamponade with a large volume of gas for a prolonged period of time. Manipulation of the inverted edge of a large retinal tear, without vitrectomy and use of a rotating table, is more easily achieved by primary injection of a relatively small amount of gas.

There are 3 main factors that determine the appropriate size of the gas bubble for unfolding the inverted posterior edge of a large retinal tear:[40] (1) the shape and volume of the bubble, (2) the angle at which the meniscus of the bubble touches the edge of the overhanging retina, and (3) the degree of folding of the retinal flap.

When rotated against the inverted edge of a large tear, a small gas bubble (1 cc or less in size) can pass as a thin wafer beneath the retinal flap. In contrast, a large gas bubble, because of the large arc of contact with the retina and the bubble thickness, tends to pass over and compress the flap. If the angle at which the bubble meniscus meets the edge of the inverted flap is greater than 90 degrees, the bubble will probably slide under the flap and unfold it. In contrast, if the angle is less than 90 degrees, the bubble tends to ride over the flap and compress it.

Retinal flaps that are severely folded are the most difficult to manipulate. Unfolding of the retinal flap may be achieved more easily with gas bubbles less than 1 cc.[40]

Use of longlasting and expanding gases, such as C3F8 and C4F10, make it possible, with a single injection of pure gas, to unfold the inverted retina with a small bubble and subsequently, tamponade the retinal break with a large bubble.

RETINAL TAMPONADE DURING THE ACTIVE PHASE OF PROLIFERATIVE VITREORETINOPATHY

The optimal therapeutic volume of gas to be used in retinal detachments associated with severe proliferative vitreoretinopathy remains speculative. Clinical experience indicates that retinal tamponade with a large bubble (approximately 80% of the vitreous cavity volume) for at least a one month period improves the anatomical success rate.[37] However, the mechanisms by which large and prolonged retinal tamponade may be efficacious in the management of severe proliferative vitreoretinopathy remain undetermined.

The main goal of the gas bubble is to maintain anatomical repositioning of the retina until the proliferative process subsides. Gas tamponade does not however, prevent subsequent cell proliferation. It is not known whether the gas bubble should cover only the retinal tear(s) or most of the surface of the retina. At present large bubbles, which cover most of the retinal surface, are used in severe proliferative vitreoretinopathy. It is not certain, however, that such large bubbles are necessary when there are no inferior retinal breaks.

SPACE AVAILABLE WITHIN THE VITREOUS CAVITY

To calculate the volume of pure gas that will fill the greatest part of the vitreous cavity after gas expansion, the surgeon will take into account three parameters: (1) the volume of the vitreous cavity, (2) the presence or absence of aphakia, (3) and the reduction of vitreous cavity volume due to the buckles. Those parameters are used to determine the space available for further expansion of the gas bubble.

Vitreous Cavity Volume. We used a mathematical model to calculate the vitreous cavity volumes of eyes with transverse diameters ranging from 22 to 34 mm and axial diameters ranging from 22 to 30 mm.[41] The relationship of changes in vitreous cavity volume to transverse and axial eye diameters are given in Table 5.

The transverse and axial diameters of the eye are measured before surgery with A-scan ultrasonography. Table 5 is used to determine the vitreous cavity volume.

Aphakia. Regardless of eye biometrics, the increase in intraocular space available for the gas bubble resulting from aphakia is 0.4 cc. The lens volume is 0.2 cc and the volume of the anterior chamber is 0.2 cc with small variations.[42]

Reduction of the Vitreous Cavity Volume Due to Buckles. High scleral buckles, which are commonly used in retinal detachments associated with severe proliferative vitreoretinopathy, result in reduction of the intraocular space available for the gas bubble. Thompson and Michels[43] developed a mathematical formula to calculate the volume displacement caused by a scleral buckle. The model is used to calculate volume displacement in the vitreous cavity as a function of buckle size, position, height, and circumference for a given axial length of the eye. For example, a single 5 mm radial sponge of moderate height displaces approximately 0.2 ml of fluid. Large circumferential tires of 7–10 mm in width displace 1.1–1.8 ml of fluid, depending on the height and configuration of the buckle.

To determine the precise reduction of the vitreous cavity volume due to the buckles, we collect all intraocular fluid removed from the eye for tightening the scleral sutures and maintaining normal intraocular pressure. The total volume of fluid removed from the eye is deducted from the volume of the vitreous cavity determined preoperatively.

TOLERANCE BY THE EYE OF INCREASED INTRAOCULAR PRESSURE

Increased intraocular pressure induced by bubble expansion is the most severe complication that may result from internal tamponade with gas (see p. 130). It is common in PVR cases with a gas bubble that fills almost the entire vitreous cavity. Therefore, in determining the optimal volume of pure gas to be injected, the surgeon should also keep in mind the factors that may affect the tolerance by any given eye of increased intraocular pressure. The optimal volume of pure gas for therapeutic effect, should be decreased 20–30% in eyes with compromised retinal or choroidal circulation, especially in senile or diabetic patients, eyes with severe myopia, or a clinical history of glaucoma. Such eyes may not tolerate a transient rise in the intraocular pressure, even moderate.

Surgical Technique

ANESTHESIA

Gas injection can be performed under general or local anesthesia. When it is performed under general anesthesia, it is recommended to cut off ventilation with nitrous oxide 20 minutes in advance. Experimental studies have confirmed that ventilation with nitrous oxide during gas injection results in an abrupt increase in bubble volume,[44] which may lead to a dangerously increased intraocular pressure. For the same reason it is recommended to avoid using nitrous oxide if a patient requires general anesthesia after gas injection.

When gas injection is the only surgical procedure to be performed, it is usually done under local anesthesia. Topical anesthesia is usually sufficient in aphakic eyes. Retrobulbar anesthesia is recommended in phakic eyes to prevent any eye movement that may result in lens damage by the needle tip during injection.

GAS PREPARATION

Gas is transferred from the high pressure tank into a 5 cc syringe through a sterile 0.22 μm millipore filter. The millipore filter is removed for gas injection. The syringe cannula should be held in its uppermost position to avoid an air–gas mixture before entering the eye. The excess of gas aspirated from the tank is withdrawn and only the volume of gas required is kept in the syringe.

GAS INJECTION

Intraocular space should be created before gas injection to avoid increased intraocular pressure. (For techniques to create intraocular space and avoid increased intraocular pressure see p. 63).

A 30-gauge needle is used for gas injection. In the aphakic vitrectomized eye, the injection can be performed through either the limbus (Fig. 99) or the pars plana. In the phakic eye the injection is performed through the pars plana 3.5 mm–4 mm from the limbus (Fig. 100). The injection can be performed on any meridian, except for the 3 and 9 o'clock positions, to avoid the long posterior ciliary arteries and nerves. The optimal meridian for needle insertion depends on the localization of the detachment and surgeon's preference. The meridians where the retina is highly detached should be avoided to prevent inadvertent retinal damage by the needle tip, or even gas injection into the subretinal space.

The patient's head and eyeball are positioned to make the injection site uppermost. The needle tip is introduced 3–4 mm posteriorly to the limbus. The needle tip must be kept close to the eye wall during injection. With this technique, the gas bubble that is created at the needle tip will stay at the injection

Table 5
Eye Axial Length

Eye Transverse Diameter at the Equator	21.5	22	22.5	23	23.5	24	24.5	25	25.5	26	26.5	27
22	3.6	3.7	3.8	3.9	4.1							
22.5	3.7	3.8	4	4.1	4.2	4.4	4.5	4.6	4.8			
23	3.9	4	4.2	4.3	4.4	4.6	4.7	4.8	5	5.1	5.3	5.4
23.5	4.1	4.2	4.3	4.5	4.6	4.8	4.9	5.1	5.2	5.4	5.5	5.6
24	4.2	4.4	4.5	4.7	4.8	5	5.1	5.3	5.4	5.6	5.7	5.9
24.5		4.6	4.7	4.9	5	5.2	5.3	5.5	5.7	5.8	6	6.1
25				5.1	5.2	5.4	5.6	5.7	5.9	6.1	6.2	6.6
25.5							5.8	6	6.1	6.3	6.5	6.6
26								6.2	6.4	6.6	6.7	6.9
26.5									6.6	6.8	7	7.2
27										7.1	7.3	7.6
27.5												7.7
28												
28.5												
29												
29.5												
30												

site and a single large bubble rather than multiple fish-egg bubbles will be obtained. As the needle is withdrawn from the eye, the needle track is immediately covered with a cotton-tipped applicator to prevent loss of gas. Then, the patency of the central retinal artery is monitored. Observation of the fundus is made using the microscope slit lamp. No contact lens is required in the aphakic eye. In the phakic eye, observation of the fundus through the gas bubble requires the use of a biconcave lens or indirect ophthalmoscopy with the microscope. If gas injection has resulted in an increased intraocular pressure and arrest of the retinal circulation, paracentesis of the anterior chamber is repeated in the phakic eye. When paracentesis of the anterior chamber is not feasible, or when it fails to reestablish central retinal artery patency, a small volume of gas should be aspirated.

POSTOPERATIVE CARE

Monitoring of Intraocular Pressure

Careful monitoring of intraocular pressure is mandatory during the first five hours after gas injection, when the bubble expands rapidly. Then intraocular pressure is measured by applanation tonometry daily for four days if SF6 was used and eight days if C3F8 was injected.

When the intraocular pressure is over 22 mm Hg 0.25% or 0.5% topical timolol is administered. If the intraocular pressure is 30 mm Hg or over, carbonic anhydrase inhibitors such as diamox or hyperosmotic agents, such as intravenous mannitol and oral glycerin, are administered.

27.5	28	28.5	29	29.5	30	30.5	31	31.5	32	32.5	33	33.5	34
5.5													
5.8	5.9	6.1											
6	6.2	6.3	6.5	6.6	6.8								
6.3	6.4	6.6	6.8	6.9	7.1	7.2							
6.5	6.7	6.9	7	7.2	7.4	7.5	7.7	7.9					
6.8	7	7.2	7.3	7.5	7.7	7.8	8	8.2	8.3	8.5			
7.1	7.3	7.4	7.6	7.8	8	8.1	8.3	8.5	8.7	8.8	9	9.2	9.4
7.4	7.5	7.7	7.9	8.1	8.3	8.5	8.6	8.8	9	9.2	9.4	9.6	9.7
7.6	7.8	8	8.2	8.4	8.6	8.8	9	9.2	9.4	9.5	9.7	9.9	10.1
7.9	8.1	8.3	8.5	8.7	8.9	9.1	9.3	9.5	9.7	9.9	10.1	10.3	10.5
		8.6	8.8	9	9.2	9.4	9.6	9.9	10.1	10.3	10.5	10.7	10.9
					9.6	9.8	10	10.2	10.4	10.6	10.8	11.1	11.3
						10.1	10.4	10.6	10.8	11	11.2	11.5	11.7
								10.9	11.2	11.4	11.6	11.8	12.1
									11.5	11.8	12	12.3	12.5

Patient Head Positioning

Maintenance of proper head position is essential for efficacy of the gas bubble and prevention of complications.

The patient is instructed not to lie on the back in order to avoid dessication cataract in the phakic eye and pupillary bloc in the aphakic eye.

On the other hand, head position is specified to keep the retinal break(s) uppermost and insure optimal tamponade effect of the gas bubble. Information concerning the retinal tear(s) localization and the mechanism of action of the gas bubble given to the patient is essential for optimal cooperation. Patients who are not likely to cooperate or who are unable to maintain the required head position should not be treated by gas injection.

The therapeutic head position depends on the size of the retinal break(s) and the volume of the gas bubble. Broadly speaking, the patient head position should be as follows:

1. For retinal breaks located between 11 and 1 o'clock, the patient is instructed to sit or stand up with a normal head position. The patient is allowed to move around normally.
2. For retinal breaks located between 2 and 4 o'clock and 8 and 10 o'clock the patient is instructed to lie on the opposite side of the break.
3. For retinal breaks located between 5 and 7 o'clock and macular holes, the patient's head must be in the prone position.

A greater latitude of movement is given to the patient when the bubble volume allows for this. The therapeutic head position should be followed 14 hours a day for 5–6 days in retinal detachments

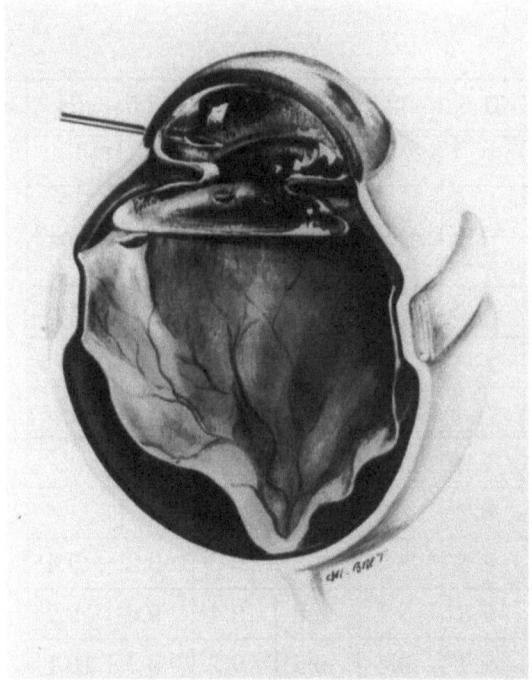

Figure 99. Gas injection in the vitrectomized aphakic eye. Gas is injected through the limbus with a 30-gauge sharp needle.

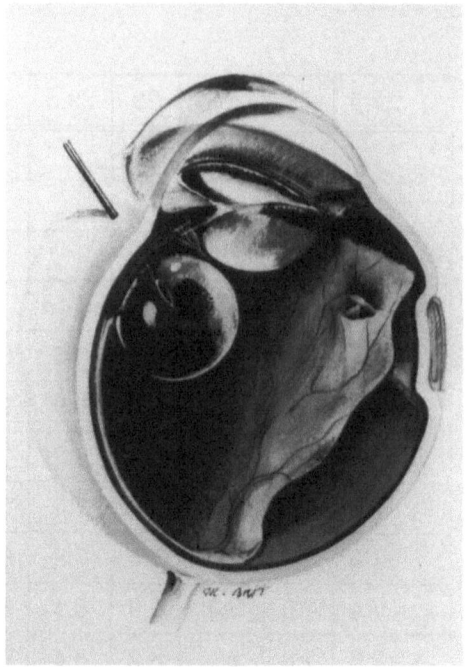

Figure 100. Gas injection in the phakic eye. Gas injection is performed through the pars plana. The needle tip is directed toward the optic disc. It is kept close to the eye wall so as to create a single intravitreal bubble. In this case gas injection is performed to manage a fishmouth phenomenon induced by scleral buckling.

without proliferative vitreoretinopathy and 10–15 days in retinal detachments associated with proliferative vitreoretinopathy. The patient is allowed to have a normal head position for washing and meals. The patient should sleep on his side, preferably the side opposite the retinal break. The patient must never lie on his back as long as the gas bubble has not disappeared. Patients with intravitreal gas bubble of 1ml or more should be instructed to avoid air travel, as well as ground transportation to high altitude.

Eye Examination

In addition to intraocular pressure monitoring, the patient should be monitored closely for the status of the anterior segment, the status of the retina, and the volume of the gas bubble. The first slit lamp examination is performed the first postoperative day. Fundus examination is performed through the gas bubble without any corneal contact lens in the aphakic eye, and with a three-mirror-contact lens in the phakic eye. The position of the bubble meniscus in the seated position is the best indicator of the latitude of movements that the patient may be allowed.

Then eye examination is repeated every other day for six days, weekly for 2 weeks. Further eye examination depends on the specific characteristics of any given case, especially the presence or absence of proliferative vitreoretinopathy as well as the nature and volume of gas used for retinal tamponade.

COMPLICATIONS

Intraoperative Complications

Fish-egg bubbles, increased intraocular pressure with arrest of the blood circulation in the central retinal artery, lens damage, retinal damage, and placing of the gas bubble in the subretinal space are five main intraoperative complications of gas injection.

FISH-EGG BUBBLES

When the injection site is not uppermost and the needle tip is too deep in the vitreous cavity, the gas injected tends to move upward and away from the needle tip. This results in multiple small bubbles within the vitreous cavity (Fig. 101).

In most circumstances fish-egg bubbles are an irritation rather than a complication. They only prevent visualization of the fundus before the end of the surgical procedure. The small bubbles will spontaneously coalesce into a single large bubble within a short period of time, and fundus examination through the gas bubble will be possible the first postoperative day.

Fish-egg bubbles may be a true complication, however, in the following circumstances: (1) when gas injection produces a significant increase in intraocular pressure and the surgeon cannot monitor central retinal artery patency, (2) when argon laser photocoagulation or cryoapplication was planned immediately after gas injection, and (3) when the retinal detachment is associated with a large retinal tear. Some of the small bubbles may pass through the retinal tear into the subretinal space (Fig. 102).

To avoid fish-egg bubbles it is recommended to

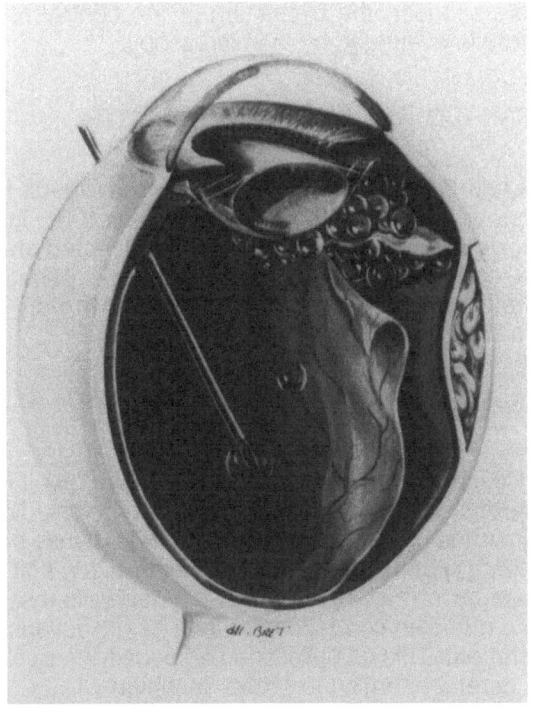

Figure 102. Error to avoid in gas injection: Fish-egg bubbles in an eye with a large retinal tear. Some of the small gas bubbles have migrated into the subretinal space through the large tear.

use a dry syringe, position the patient's head so that the injection is made in the uppermost part of the eye, keep the needle tip close to the eye wall, and perform the injection quite rapidly so that the needle tip remains within the bubble until the injection is completed.

INCREASED INTRAOCULAR PRESSURE WITH ARREST OF THE BLOOD CIRCULATION IN THE CENTRAL RETINAL ARTERY

Methods for avoiding increased intraocular pressure and arrest of blood circulation in the central retinal artery have been previously described (see p. 63). In any case if a simple maneuver, such as paracentesis of the anterior chamber, fails to restore the central retinal artery patency, some of the gas bubble should be removed from the eye. In the aphakic eye the gas is aspirated using a 30-gauge needle through the limbus. In the phakic eye, gas is aspirated through the pars plana. Gas aspiration is performed under biomicroscopic observation of the fundus, to avoid inappropriate positioning of the needle tip. Generally, removal of 0.1–0.3 ml of gas will sufficiently lower intraocular pressure. After

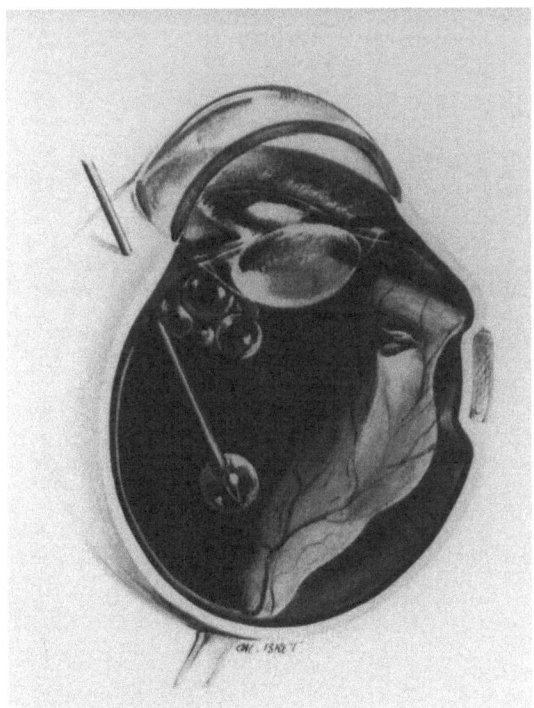

Figure 101. Error to avoid in gas injection: Fish egg bubbles. The needle tip has been inserted too deeply into the vitreous cavity; small gas bubbles move upward and away from the needle tip.

gas aspiration the circulation in the central retinal artery is evaluated by biomicroscopy.

LENS DAMAGE BY THE NEEDLE TIP

Lens damage by the needle tip may result from improper direction of the needle (Fig. 103). In the phakic eye the needle tip should be directed toward the optic disc. The surgeon should be especially careful when inserting the needle into a very soft eye (Fig. 103).

RETINAL DAMAGE

Retinal damage by the needle tip can result from improper technique. It occurs when the needle tip is inserted posteriorly to the ora serrata. It may occur when: (1) gas injection is administered in a soft collapsed eye (Fig. 103) and (2) the needle is inserted on a meridian corresponding to a highly bullous detachment. This complication can usually be avoided by careful attention to proper technique.

GAS BUBBLE IN THE SUBRETINAL SPACE

Gas bubble in the subretinal space may result from (1) mispositioning of the needle tip (Figs. 104,

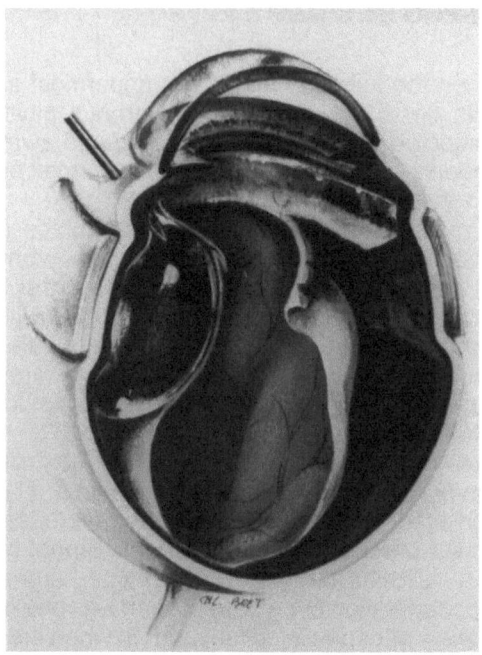

Figure 104. Error to avoid in gas injection: gas injection in the subretinal space. The needle tip has been inserted into the eye in a quadrant where the retina is highly detached.

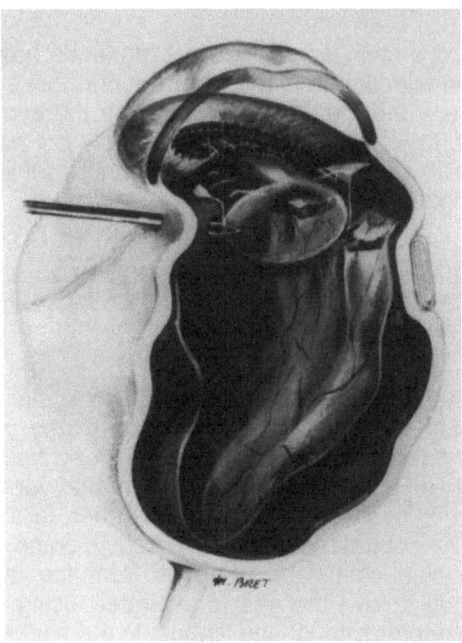

Figure 103. Error to avoid in gas injection: lens damage by the needle tip. This complication results from improper direction of the needle tip inserted into a soft collapsed eye.

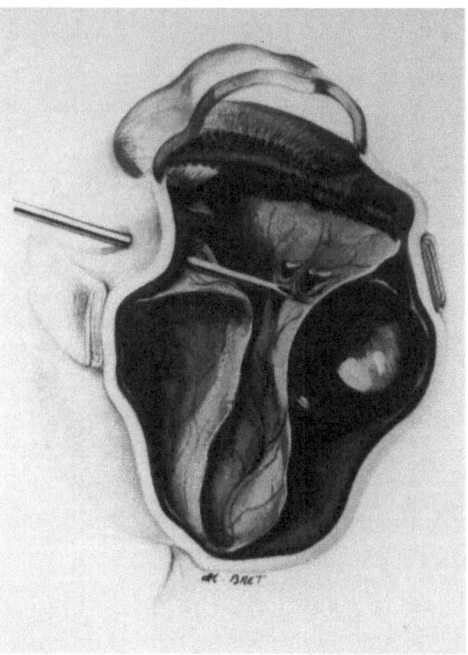

Figure 105. Error to avoid in gas injection: gas injection in the subretinal space. The needle tip has been inserted into the subretinal space through the highly detached retina in a soft collapsed eye.

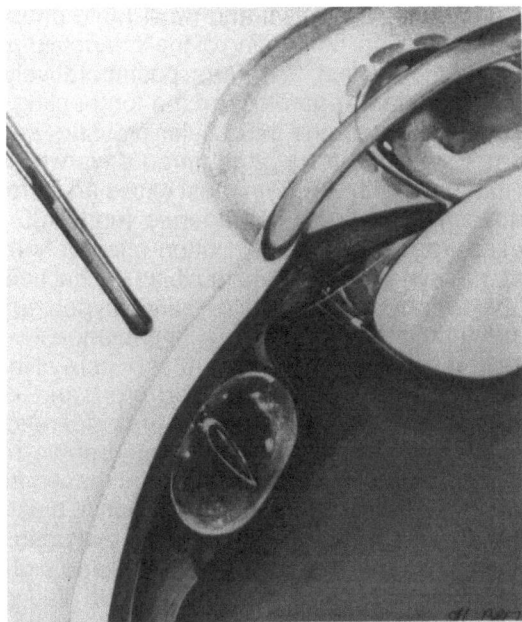

Figure. 106. Error to avoid in gas injection: gas injection beneath detached ciliary epithelium. The retinal detachment is associated with detachment of the ciliary epithelium. The needle tip has been inserted on a meridian of detached ciliary epithelium and kept improperly close to the eye wall.

105, and 106) and (2) migration of small bubbles from the vitreous cavity to the subretinal space through a large retinal break in a highly detached retina (Fig. 102). Mispositioning of the needle tip in the subretinal space resulting from internal puncture through the detached retina can be avoided with proper technique. Mispositioning of the needle tip and gas injection into the subretinal space may also occur when the retinal detachment is associated with detachment of the ciliary retina (Fig. 106). In such eyes the needle should be inserted on a meridian where the ciliary retina is not detached. If 360° of the ciliary retina are detached, the needle tip should be pushed under visual control through the ciliary retina before gas injection.

A bubble of pure gas, even very small, must not be left in the subretinal space. Removal of the gas bubble is performed through the choroid (Fig. 107). The same choroidal incision for subretinal fluid release is performed (see p. 68). The patient's head and eye are then rotated to place the choroidal incision in an uppermost position. Scleral depression on the opposite side will induce transient increased intraocular pressure and gas escape through the choroidal incision. Internal removal of subretinal gas through a retinal break is occasionally performed in aphakic vitrectomized eyes (Fig. 108). It is done using a 27-gauge blunt needle.

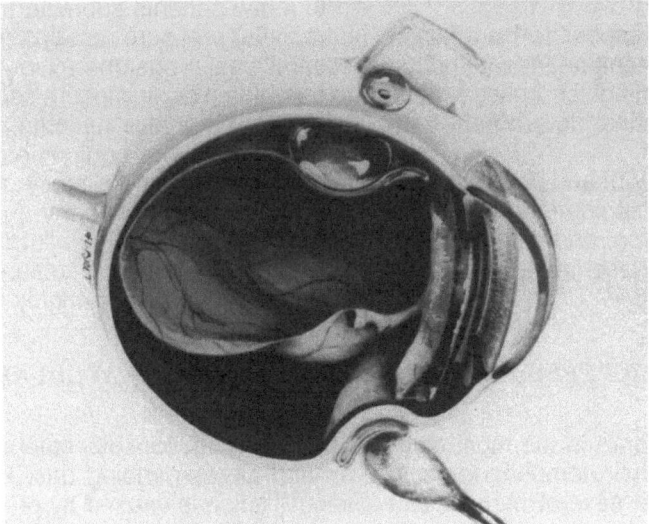

Figure 107. External removal of subretinal gas: The eye has been rotated so as to place the choroidal incision uppermost. Increased intraocular pressure induced by the cotton-tip applicator results in gas escape through the choroidal incision.

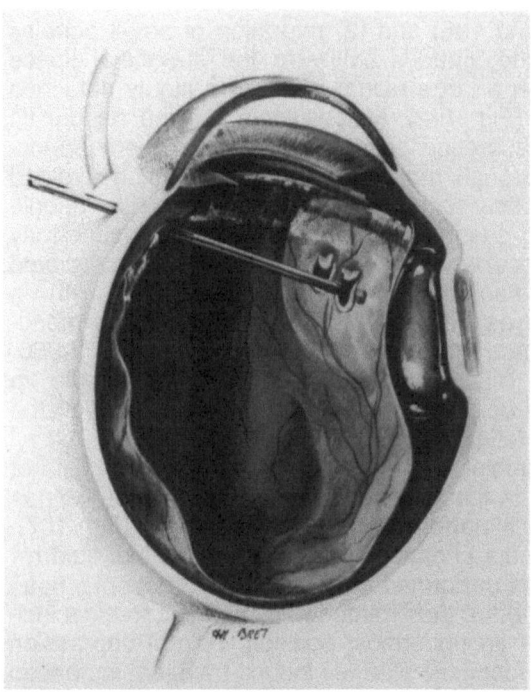

Figure 108. Internal removal of subretinal gas through a retinal break in an aphakic vitrectomized eye.

Postoperative Complications

Postoperative complications of retinal tamponade with gas are more related to physical properties than toxicity.

Retinal function does not appear to be affected adversely by prolonged gas tamponades, although it is somewhat difficult to distinguish between loss of function caused by the retinal detachment from the possible effects of gas.[20]

Increased intraocular pressure and posterior subcapsular cataract are the most common complications. Intraocular inflammation and infection are probably related more to surgical maneuvers than gas.

INCREASED INTRAOCULAR PRESSURE

Increased intraocular pressure is the most common complication of retinal tamponade with gas.[20,21,31,39,45–47] There are several causes that may lead to increased intraocular pressure after gas injection. The most common cause is related to gas expansion. Increased intraocular pressure occurs when the rate of expansion exceeds the fluid outflow from the eye or when the expanded volume exceeds the capacity of the vitreous cavity. The most critical

period is during the initial and most rapid phase of bubble expansion. Monitoring of the intraocular pressure during the first 24 hours postoperatively, is equally important regardless of the long-acting gas used. Monitoring of the intraocular pressure should then be continued for at least three days with SF6 and four days with C3F8. In most cases an increase in intraocular pressure is moderate (under 35 mm Hg) and transient. It is most often effectively managed with hypotensive drugs such as topical timolol, carbonic anhydrase inhibitor, and hyperosmotic agents administered orally or intravenously. An increased intraocular pressure 40 mm Hg or more may lead to vascular occlusion and optic atrophy.[21–47] When the intraocular pressure reaches 40 mm Hg or more, part of the gas bubble must be immediately aspirated. Severely increased intraocular pressure related to bubble expansion can be avoided in most cases by accurate evaluation of the space available for gas expansion (see p. 122). Great care should be taken in patients with glaucoma or vascular diseases, especially diabetic, senile, and myopic patients.

Increased intraocular pressure can also result from a pupillary block in aphakic patients (Fig. 109). The importance of the face down position should be stressed to the patient to reduce the risk of pupillary block and angle closure glaucoma.

Increased intraocular pressure can also be induced by rapid changes in ambient atmospheric pressure.[19–48] Patients with an eye containing 1 cc or more of expansible gas should be advised to avoid air travel as well as ground transportation to high altitude.

In a few patients submitted to C3F8 injection the intraocular pressure remains or becomes increased several weeks postoperatively. This can be related to permanent angle closure secondary to early pupillary bloc in aphakic patients, persisting intraocular inflammation, or corticosteroids. Prolonged increased intraocular pressure, even when moderate, may result in optic atrophy and visual loss, in spite of successful management of the retinal detachment. Prolonged intraocular pressure monitoring is especially recommended in highly myopic patients.

POSTERIOR SUBCAPSULAR CATARACT

Posterior subcapsular cataract has been seen with air and any expanding gas. Posterior subcapsular vacuolization is caused by prolonged contact of the gas bubble with the posterior lens capsule. Lens opacities are more likely to occur when the gas bubble remains in contact with more than two-thirds of the posterior lens capsule.[20] Early posterior subcapsular opacities are reversible, but they become irreversible when the gas bubble remains in contact

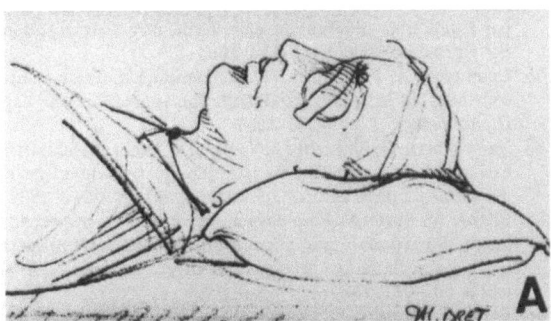 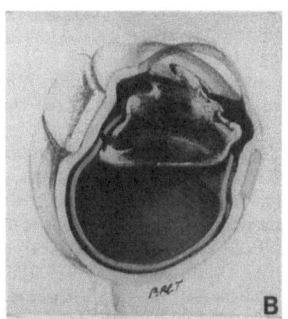

Figure 109. Error to avoid in patient head positioning after gas injection. (A) The patient lies on his back. (B) As a result, the aphakic eye develops pupillary block and increased intraocular pressure.

with the lens for a prolonged period of time. Some patients with early and reversible early posterior lens opacities develop subsequent nuclear sclerotic cataracts, which may require lens extraction. Early posterior subcapsular cataract can be avoided by adequate positioning of the patient's head to avoid prolonged contact of the gas bubble with the posterior lens capsule.

OCULAR INFLAMMATION

Some degree of ocular inflammation is common after gas injection. It is more frequent in PVR cases where aqueous flare may persist several months after gas disappearance. It is difficult to differentiate between surgical trauma and intraocular inflammation due to the gas bubble from inflammation related to the vitreoretinal disease.

OCULAR INFECTION

Postoperative intraocular infection may occur after gas injection just as after any intraocular procedure. A few cases have been reported in the literature.[49] Endophthalmitis should be avoided by proper surgical technique and gas transfer from the tank through a millipore filter.

SEQUENTIAL RETINAL TEARS ATTRIBUTED TO INTRAOCULLAR GAS

Sequential retinal tears attributed to intravitreal gas injection develop two or three days after gas injection.[34,50,51] They are located in an inferior quadrant and related to either islands of lattice degeneration[34] or the posterior margin of the vitreous base.[50] Early development of sequential tears sug-

gests that they are likely related to vitreoretinal traction induced by the gas bubble in eyes with incomplete posterior vitreous detachment.

REFERENCES

1. Ohm J: Uber Die Behandlung der Netzhautablösung durch operative Entleerung der subretinalen Flüssigkeit und Einspritzung von Luft in den Glaskörper. Graefes Arch Ophthal 79: 442–450, 1911
2. Rohmer M: Effets des injections d'air stérilisé dans le vitré contre le décollement de la rétine: Arch Ophtalmol 32 :257–274, 1912
3. Rosengren B: Results of treatment of detachment of the retina with diathermy and injection of air into the vitreous. Acta Ophthalmol 16: 573–579, 1938
4. Rosengren B: 300 cases operated upon for retinal detachment. Methods and results. Acta Ophthalmol 30: 117–122, 1952
5. Norton EWD: Intraocular gas in the management of selected retinal detachments. Trans Am Acad Ophthalmol Otolaryngol 77: 85–98, 1973
6. Peyman G, Vygantas C, Benett T, et al: Octafluorocyclobutane in vitreous and aqueous humour replacement. Arch Ophthalmol 93: 514–517, 1975
7. Lincoff H, Mardirosian J, Lincoff A, et al: Intravitreal longevity of three perfluorocarbon gases. Arch Ophthalmol 98: 1610–1611, 1980
8. Lincoff A, Haft D, Liggett P, Reifer C: Intravitreal expansion of perfluorocarbon bubbles. Arch Ophthalmol 98: 1646–1649, 1980
9. Machemer R, Aaberg TM: Vitrectomy. 2nd ed. Orlando FL: Grune & Stratton, 124–144, 1979
10. Norton EWD, Aaberg T, Fung W, Curtin VT: Giant retinal tears. I—Clinical management with intravitreal air. Am J Ophthalmol 68: 1011–1021, 1969
11. Fleury J: Traitement des décollements de la rétine associés à une déchirure géante. Thèse université Lyon, 1986
12. Bloch D, O'Connor P, Lincoff H: The mechanism of cryosurgical adhesion. III statistical analysis. Am J Ophthalmol 71: 666–673, 1971
13. Chawla HB, Coleiro JA: Retinal detachment treatment with intravitreal air: an evaluation of 241 cases. Brit J Ophthalmol 61: 588–592, 1977
14. Fineberg E, Machemer R, Sullivan P, et al: Sulfur hexafluoride in owl monkey' vitreous cavity. Am J Ophthalmol 79: 67–76, 1975

15. Peters MA, Abrams GW, Hamilton LH, et al: The nonexpansible, equilibrated concentration of perfluoropropane gas in the eye. Am J Ophthalmol 100: 831–839, 1985

16. Crittenden JJ, De Juan E, Tiederman J: Expansion of long-acting gas bubbles for intraocular use. Arch Ophthalmol 103:831–836, 1985

17. Lincoff H, Maisel OM, Lincoff A: Intravitreal disappearance rates of four perfluorocarbon gases. Arch Ophthalmol 102: 928–929, 1984

18. Tenney SM, Carpenter FG, Rahn H: Gas transfers in a sulfure hexafluoride peritoneum. J Appl Physiol 6: 201, 1953

19. Aronowitz JD, Brubaker RF: Effect of intraocular gas on intraocular pressure. Arch Ophthalmol 94: 1191–1196, 1976

20. Lincoff H, Coleman J, Kreissig I, Richard G, Chang S, Wilcox L: The perfluorocarbon gases in the treatment of retinal detachment. Ophthalmology 90: 546–551, 1983

21. Sabates WI, Abrams GW, Swanson DE, Norton EW: The use of intraocular gases. The results of sulfur hexafluoride gas in retinal detachment surgery. Ophthalmology 88: 447–454, 1981

22. Miller B, Miller H, Ryan SJ: Experimental vitreous syneresis. Arch Ophthalmol 103: 1385–1388, 1985

23. Lincoff H, Horowitz J, Kreissig I, Jakobiec F: Morphologic effects of gas compression on the cortical vitreous. Arch Ophthalmol 104: 1212–1215, 1986

24. Faulborn J, Bowald S: The vitreous after C3F8 gas instillation: long-term histologic findings after spontaneous reabsorption of the gas in rabbit eyes. Graefe's Arch Clin Exp Ophthalmol 225: 99–102, 1987

25. Pruett RC: The fishmouth phenomenon. II—wedge scleral buckling Arch Opthalmol 95: 1782–1787, 1977

26. Lincoff H, Kreissig I, Lafranco F: Mechanisms of failures in the repair of large retinal tears. Am J Ophthalmol 84: 501–507, 1977

27. Pruett RC: The fish mouth phenomenon. I—Clinical characteristics and surgical options. Arch Ophthalmol 95: 1777–1781, 1977

28. Lincoff H, Kreissig I: Advantages of radial buckling. Am J Ophthalmol 79: 955–957, 1975

29. Goldbaum MH: Geometric analysis of radial buckling. Am J Ophthalmol 79: 958–965, 1975

30. Birchall CH: The fishmouth phenomenon in retinal detachment: old concepts revisited. Brit J Ophthalmol 63: 507–510, 1979

31. Bonnet M: Apport des injections intravitréennes de gaz dans la microchirurgie du décollement de la rétine. J Fr Ophtalmol 6: 139–144, 1983

32. Dominguez DA: Cirurgia precoz y ambulatoria del desprendimiento de retina. Arch Soc Esp Oftal 48: 47–54, 1985

33. Hilton GF, Grizzard WS: Pneumatic retinopexy. A two-step out patient operation without conjunctival incision. Ophthalmology 93: 626–641, 1986

34. Constantinides G, Aracil P: Traitement chirurgical des décolle-ments de la rétine par cryocoagulation et indentation ab interno par C3F8 sans indentation épisclérale. Premiers résultats. Bull Soc Ophtalmol Fr 86: 411–444, 1986

35. Dominguez A, Fonseca A, Gomez-Montana J: Traitement du dé-collement de la rétine par insuflation répétée de gaz expansifs. Ophtalmologie 1: 205–208, 1987

36. Van effentere G, Abirached J, Vachet JM, Khairallah M: Utilisation exclusive d'une injection de gaz dans le traitement de certains décollements de la rétine. Ophtalmologie 1: 209–212, 1987

37. Bonnet M, Aracil P, Pecoldova K, Dacol E: Les gaz expansifs de-longue durée dans le traitement des décollements rétiniens rhegma-togènes associés à une prolifération vitréo:rétinienne. J Fr Ophtal-mol 8: 607–611, 1985

38. Parver LM, Lincoff H: Geometry of intraocular gas used in retinal surgery. Mod Probl Ophthalmol 18: 338–343, 1977

39. Lincoff H, Kreissig I, Brodie S, Wilcox L: Expanding gas bubble for the repair of tears in the posterior pole. Graefe's Arch Clin Exp Ophthalmol 219: 193–197, 1982

40. Lincoff H: A small bubble technique for manipulating giant retinal tears. Annals Ophthalmol 13: 241–243, 1981

41. Jean-Louis B, Bievelez B, Bonnet M: Evaluation du volume de la cavité vitréenne avant tamponnement interne avec un gaz expansif. J Fr Ophtalmol (to be published)

42. Delmarcelle Y, Francois J, Goes F: Biométric oculaire clinique. Bull Soc Belge Ophtalmol 1976, 197–230

43. Thompson JT, Michels RG: Volume displacement of scleral buckles. Arch Ophthalmol 103: 1822–1824, 1985

44. Wolf GL, Capvano C, Hartung J: Effect of nitrous oxide on gas bubble volume in the anterior chamber. Arch Ophthalmol 103: 418–419, 1985

45. Chang S, Coleman DJ, Lincoff H, Wilcox LM, et al: Perfluoropropane gas in the management of proliferative vitreoretinopathy. Am J Ophthalmol 98: 180–188, 1984

46. Chang S, Lincoff HA, Coleman DJ et al: Perfluorocarbon gases in vitreous surgery. Ophthalmology 92:651–656, 1985

47. Abrams GW, Swanson DE, Sabates WI, Goldman AL: The results of sulfur hexafluoride gas in vitreous surgery. Am J Ophthalmol 94: 165–171, 1982

48. Dieckert JP, O'Connor PS, Schacklett DE, Tredici TJ et al: Air travel and intraocular gas. Ophthalmology 93: 642–645, 1986

49. Landers MB, Robinson D, Olsen KR, Rinkoff J: Slit lamp fluid-gas exchange and other office procedures following vitreoretinal surgery. Arch Ophthalmol 103: 967–972, 1985

50. Dreyer RF: Sequential retinal tears attributed to intraocular gas. Am J Ophthalmol 102: 276–278, 1986

51. Poliner LS, Grand MG, Schoch LH, et al: New retinal detachment after pneumatic retinopaxy. Ophthalmology 94: 315–318, 1987

13

Vitreous Surgery

The first attempts to use vitreous surgery to relieve vitreoretinal traction[1,2] antedate recognition of the role of retinal breaks in the pathogenesis of retinal detachment by Gonin.[3] During the 1960s vitreous surgery had occasionally been used by retina surgeons to cut intravitreal bands and membranes associated with retinal detachment.[4,5] Due to the limits of the available instrumentation, however, and fear of creating iatrogenic lesions, attempts to relieve vitreoretinal traction using intravitreal surgery had been most infrequent until the development of closed vitrectomy though the pars plana by Machemer[6] in the U.S.A. and Klöti[7] in Europe in the early 1970s. The basic principles and techniques of modern vitreous surgery were established by Machemer. During the last 15 years many surgeons have contributed to the development of the instrumentation and methods currently used today.[8–25] Modern vitreous surgery has made desperate and hopeless retinal detachments amenable to surgical management. It has, therefore, been rapidly included in the armentarium of most retinal detachment surgeons. Closed vitreous surgery through the pars plana is the most significant advance in the management of retinal detachment during the last 15 years.

OBJECTIVES OF VITREOUS MICROSURGERY

The objectives of vitreous microsurgery in retinal detachment management are twofold, optical and mechanical.

Optical Objectives

Closed vitrectomy provides the ability to remove intraocular opacities, such as dense vitreous hemorrhage and dense pupillary membranes, which prevent fundus examination.

Mechanical Objectives

Mechanical objectives of vitreous microsurgery in retinal detachment management are threefold: (1) Relief of vitreoretinal traction, (2) creating intravitreal space for retinal tamponade with gas, and (3) direct manipulation of the inverted flap of a giant tear.

In most cases, relief of vitreoretinal traction is the main objective of vitreous surgery in retinal detachment management. Removal of vitreous bands and sheets, and segmentation and peeling of epiretinal membranes make it possible to relieve tractions that prevent the retina from settling against the pigment epithelium (Fig. 110).

INDICATIONS

The indications for vitreous surgery in the management of retinal detachment can be divided into three distinct categories.

In the first group of indications, vitreous surgery is the only approach that may be successful in the management of the detachment, and no surgical adjunct to vitrectomy is required. This group of indications includes most tractional retinal detachments located posteriorly to the vitreous base, and not associated with a rhegmatogenous component.

In the second group of indications, vitreous surgery is an adjunct to scleral buckling. This group of indications includes a large variety of complicated rhegmatogenous retinal detachments, such as detachments associated with dense intraocular opacities, nontraumatic giant tears, or proliferative vitreoretinopathy. Vitreous surgery has dramatically

133

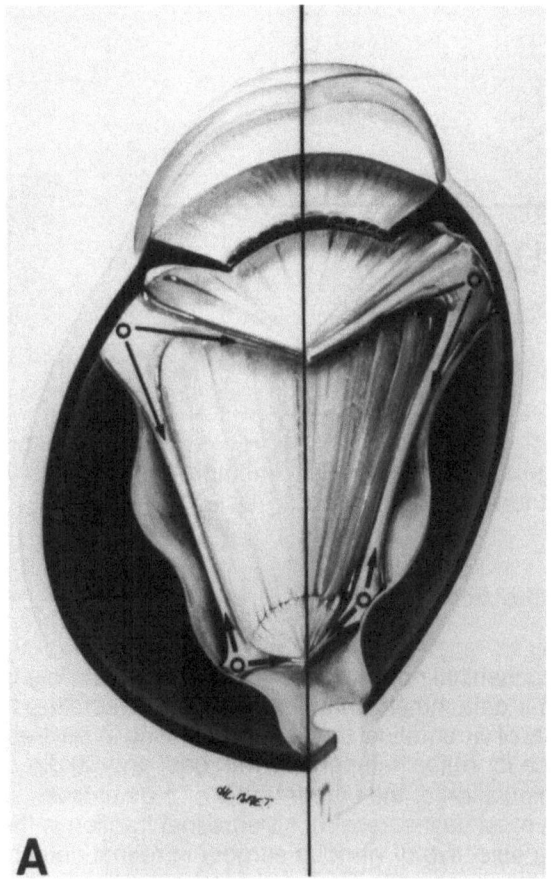

A

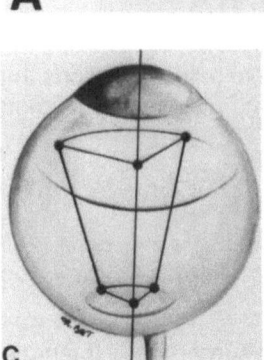

C

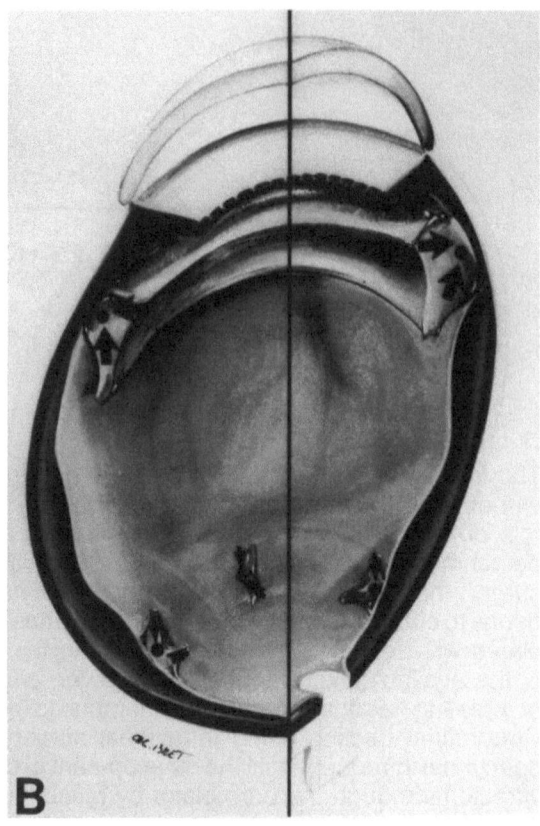

B

Figure 110. Mechanical objectives of vitreous surgery in retinal detachment management. (A) Traction forces exerted on the retina by vitreous changes. (B) Removal or segmentation of the condensed posterior vitreous face relieves anterior posterior and tangential traction on the retina. Removal of the condensed anterior vitreous face relieves anterior traction on the vitreous base. (C) Corresponding cross-section of the eye.

improved the surgical results achieved in such complicated detachments. In most cases, however, scleral buckling as an adjunct to vitrectomy is necessary to permanently reattach the retina.

In the third group of indications, vitreous surgery is an alternative to scleral buckling. This group includes selected retinal detachments associated with retinal breaks located posteriorly to the equator. Vitreous surgery has also been used as an alternative to scleral buckling in the management of selected retinal detachments associated with peripheral retinal breaks.[26] However, the advantages of vitrectomy as compared to scleral buckling in this specific indication remain to be fully established.

At present the indications for vitreous surgery in retinal detachment management include (1) most traction retinal detachments, (2) retinal detachments complicated by proliferative vitreoretinopathy, (3) retinal detachments associated with dense vitreous hemorrhages, (4) retinal detachments associated with postequatorial retinal breaks, (5) nontraumatic giant tears, and (6) selected retinal detachments associated with macular holes in highly myopic eyes.

Traction Retinal Detachments

Traction retinal detachments that may benefit from vitreous surgery include (1) retinal detachments complicating neovascular proliferative retinopathies, such as diabetic retinopathy, Eale's disease, retinal vein occlusion, sickle cell retinopathy, retinopathy of prematurity, and hereditary proliferative vitreoretinopathy; (2) retinal detachments after penetrating eye injury; (3) retinal detachments following cataract extraction complicated by vitreous incarceration in the corneal wound; and (4) retinal detachments due to idiopathic fibrosis of the posterior vitreous face and incomplete posterior vitreous detachment in senile eyes.

Traction retinal detachments result from static and an increasing vitreoretinal traction. Vitreoretinal traction is secondary to cell proliferation on the vitreous gel scaffold and contraction of the sheets of proliferative tissue. In most cases, in particular, neovascular proliferative retinopathies and idiopathic fibrosis of the posterior vitreous face, vitreoretinal traction results from cell proliferation on the posterior vitreous face and an incomplete posterior vitreous detachment. Vitreoretinal traction is exerted on areas where the posterior vitreous face remains adherent to the retina. Contraction of the posterior vitreous face between areas of vitreoretinal adhesion induces tangential retinal traction.

In other instances, such as after penetrating eye injury and cataract extraction complicated by vitreous gel incarceration in the wound, vitreoretinal traction is oriented in an anteroposterior direction or a frontal direction.

The main objective of vitreous surgery in traction retinal detachments is to relieve vitreous traction that drags the retina towards the vitreous cavity. Vitreous surgery makes it possible to relieve tangential traction exerted by the posterior vitreous face and anteroposterior traction resulting from intravitreal fibrovascular ingrowth, or vitreous incarceration in a corneal wound. Vitreous surgery does not, however, allow to relieve traction resulting from contraction of the vitreous base. Therefore, in eyes with tractional retinal detachment associated with ring contraction of the vitreous base, vitrectomy is associated with scleral buckling of the vitreous base. The goal of scleral buckling is to counteract ring contraction of the vitreous base.

Retinal detachment may be purely tractional. However a significant number of traction retinal detachments are associated with a rhegmatogenous component. Retinal breaks result from vitreoretinal traction. They develop in areas of strong vitreoretinal adhesion or predisposing retinal weakness. Any retinal break associated with traction retinal detachment requires specific management to achieve permanent reattachment of the retina. The surgical approach to treat the retinal breaks varies depending on the break location and the persistence or absence of vitreoretinal traction after vitrectomy. Any retinal break that remains under traction in spite of vitrec-

tomy is managed by scleral buckling. In contrast scleral buckling is unnecessary when complete relief of vitreoretinal traction has been achieved by vitrectomy.

Retinal Detachments Complicated by Proliferative Vitreoretinopathy

Vitreous surgery is indicated in most retinal detachments complicated by proliferative vitreoretinopathy (see p. 241). Relief of tangential traction exerted on the retina by epiretinal membranes is the main goal of vitreous surgery. Relief of tangential traction can be achieved by epiretinal membrane delamination and segmentation.

Vitrectomy is required, but it is not sufficient in the management of most retinal detachments complicated by proliferative vitreoretinopathy. In most cases vitreous surgery is only a step of a more complicated surgical procedure that includes scleral buckling of the retinal breaks and the vitreous base.

The objectives of surgery in proliferative vitreoretinopathy are purely mechanical. Epiretinal membranes recur in a significant number of eyes. Recurrence of epiretinal membranes may be stimulated by heavy surgery, which is required in the management of most retinal detachments complicated by proliferative vitreoretinopathy.

Retinal Detachments with Dense Vitreous Hemorrhage

Dense vitreous hemorrhage may be associated with rhegmatogenous and/or traction retinal detachment.

RHEGMATOGENOUS RETINAL DETACHMENT

In rhegmatogenous retinal detachment associated with vitreous hemorrhage, the main objective of vitrectomy is to clear the media and make identification of the retinal tear(s) possible. Dense vitreous hemorrhage that prevents fundus examination and identification of the retinal breaks is infrequent, however, in nontraumatic rhegmatogenous retinal detachment (see p. 165). Therefore, removal of vitreous blood for optical reasons is a rare indication for vitrectomy in primary rhegmatogenous retinal detachment.[27,28]

Intravitreal blood is probably a stimulating factor in epiretinal membrane formation.[29] Severe proliferative vitreoretinopathy is more likely to develop after scleral buckling in eyes with vitreous hemorrhage (see p. 234). In addition, clinical evidence of moderate proliferative vitreoretinopathy, preoperatively, is common in eyes with vitreous hemorrhage.[28] Therefore early vitrectomy to remove stimuli of cell proliferation and the vitreous gel scaffold may be indicated to prevent the development of severe proliferative vitreoretinopathy in eyes with moderate vitreous hemorrhage, which do not prevent identification of the retinal breaks. The value of vitrectomy in this specific indication remains to be established.

Recurrent vitreous hemorrhage after conventional treatment of a horseshoe tear with a bridging vessel is also an indication of vitrectomy (see p. 168).

TRACTION RETINAL DETACHMENT

Vitreous hemorrhage is common in eyes with traction retinal detachments secondary to neovascular proliferative retinopathies and after penetrating eye injury. In a significant number of eyes the vitreous hemorrhage is dense and prevents fundus examination. In such eyes the diagnosis of retinal detachment is made by ultrasonography.

Vitrectomy is indicated in most cases, regardless of the degree of vitreous hemorrhage. Treatment of traction retinal detachment is the main objective of vitrectomy.

Retinal Detachments Associated with Postequatorial Retinal Breaks

Vitrectomy is a most valuable alternative to scleral buckling in the management of retinal detachments associated with retinal breaks located posteriorly to the equatorial region.

Most postequatorial retinal breaks are observed in two distinct types of retinal detachments: (1) Primary rhegmatogenous retinal detachments in highly myopic eyes (see p. 213) and (2) retinal detachments secondary to neovascular proliferative retinopathies, in particular, diabetic retinopathy and retinal vein occlusion (see p. 269). In both instances the retinal breaks are due to vitreous traction. In most cases relief of vitreoretinal traction is required to permanently reattach the retina.

Due to the location of the retinal breaks, relief of vitreoretinal traction is easier to achieve by vitrectomy as compared to scleral buckling. In addition, vitrectomy has two main advantages compared to scleral buckling in the management of such retinal breaks: The surgical procedure is more rapid to perform and it is less traumatic.

Retinal Detachments Associated with Macular Holes

Vitrectomy is indicated in selected retinal detachments associated with macular holes in highly myopic eyes. The pathogenesis of such retinal detachments is not yet fully understood. It may not be uniform in all cases. Relief of vitreoretinal traction is probably the key to achieve permanent retinal reattachment in selected cases.[30,31] Vitrectomy, however, is not required in all retinal detachments associated with macular holes. A significant number of cases are successfully managed merely by intravitreal gas injection.[32] At present we restrict the indications for vitrectomy as follows: (1) eyes that failed to reattach after two consecutive attempts to reattach the retina with gas injection, and (2) associated ocular or systemic conditions that make it necessary to create intravitreal space for injection of a large bubble of gas (see p. 222).

SURGICAL TECHNIQUE

Vitreous surgery techniques have been extensively described in numerous publications, especially outstanding books[16,23-25] that are the basic references for any microsurgeon of the posterior segment of the eye. In this chapter we shall restrict ourselves to the techniques currently in use for retinal detachment management. Points of special importance in this specific field of vitreous surgery will be emphasized.

Pars Plana Sclerotomies

INCISIONS

At present the 3-incision technique is used in retinal detachment management. The pars plana incisions are made parallel to the limbus. They are made 3.5–4 mm posteriorly to the limbus.

Sclerotomies are not performed in the meridians of the rectus muscle insertions to avoid damage to the anterior ciliary vessels. In eyes with detachment of the ciliary epithelium, the sclerotomies are performed in areas where the ciliary epithelium remains attached. Insertion and withdrawal of the instruments through detached ciliary epithelium may result in laceration of the detached retina at, or posteriorly to, the ora serrata.

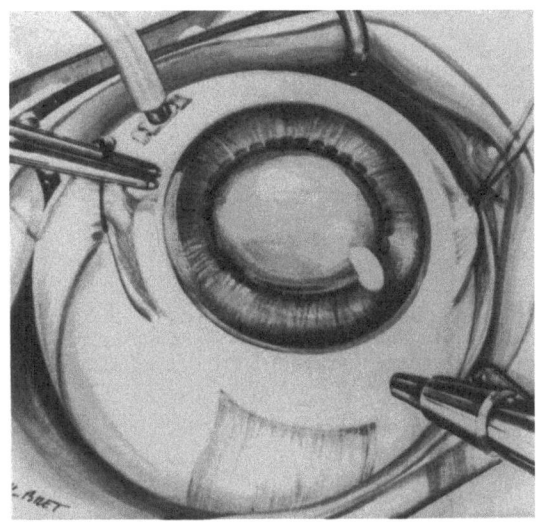

Figure 111. Pars plana sclerotomies (Right eye) The infusion cannula has been placed in the lower nasal quadrant. The bridle suture in the medial rectus muscle is used to immobilize the eye during insertion of the trocar to enlarge the incision of uveal tissue in the supero temporal sclerotomy. Using the bridle suture rather than the muscle to hold the eye avoids bleeding.

In most cases the sclerotomy for the infusion cannula is made in the lower nasal quadrant and each of the two other sclerotomies is made in a superior quadrant (Fig. 111). In specific circumstances, however, when most of the vitreoretinal pathology is situated in the nasal quadrants, two sclerotomies made in the superior and inferior temporal quadrants make intraocular maneuvers easier to perform. In such instances the surgeon is seated on the lateral side of the patient's head. The sclerotomies used for introduction of the vitrectomy probe and fiberoptic probe are made approximately 150° apart. An increased distance between the sclerotomies makes it easier to perform bimanual intraocular maneuvers.

Each sclerotomy is the size of the instrument shaft to minimize fluid escape through the sclerotomies during intraocular surgery. Sclerotomies are made using a sharp knife the size of the vitrectomy instruments. The knife is directed toward the optic disc. The knife thrust creates a scleral incision of adequate size. Due to elasticity of the uveal tissue, however, the opening of the uveal tissue is smaller in size than the scleral incision (Fig. 112). Incision of the uveal tissue is enlarged and made circular in shape with a trocar (Fig. 112). Pars plana incision, especially incision of the uveal tissue, are difficult to perform properly when the eye is very soft. Injection of balanced saline solution into the anterior chamber to increase the intraocular pressure prior to the performance of the pars plana incisions is helpful when the eye is very soft. Bridle sutures, preplaced in the medial and lateral recti muscles, are used to

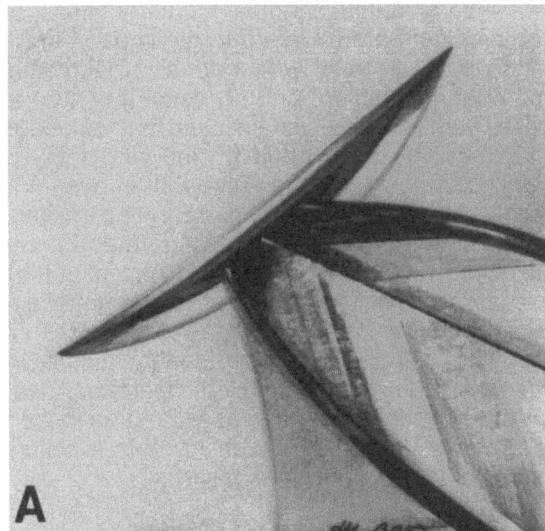

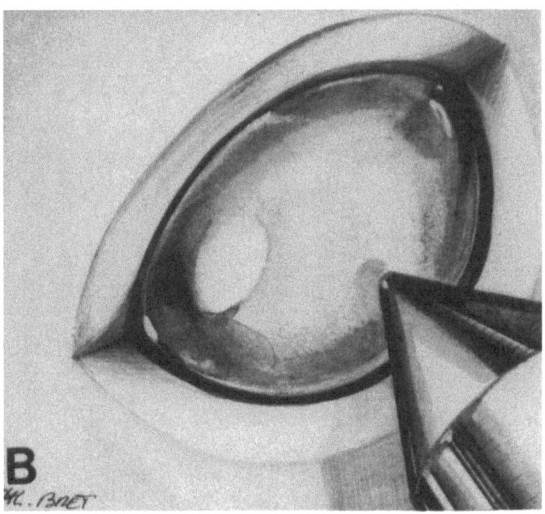

Figure 112. Pars plana sclerotomy. (A) Owing to elasticity of uveal tissue, the incision of uveal tissue is smaller in size than the scleral incision. (B) Incision of the uveal tissue has been enlarged and made circular in shape by the trocar.

stabilize the eye during the sclerotomies. In soft eyes, gentle traction on the bridle suture used to hold the eye increases the intraocular pressure and makes sclerotomies easier to perform. Use of bridle sutures to immobilize the eye avoids bleeding due to vessel damage when the eye is directly held with forceps. Bridle sutures are also used to rotate and immobilize the eye during suture of the sclerotomies (Fig. 111).

The infusion cannula is introduced into the eye before performing the other sclerotomies. It is sutured to the sclera with a mattress suture. Viewing the tip of the infusion cannula after its insertion through the pars plana is an essential step. It is done by slit lamp biomicroscopy using the three-mirror contact lens. If the tip of the cannula is covered by pars plana tissue (Fig. 113), the cannula is withdrawn, the sclerotomy revised, and the cannula reinserted into the vitreous cavity. If the cannula tip does not penetrate completely through the pars plana tissue, infusion fluid will flow under the ciliary epithelium or into the subchoroidal space (Fig. 114).

When the surgeon has made certain that the infusion cannula has properly penetrated the pars plana uveal tissue, the two additional sclerotomies are completed. Rapid escape of liquefied vitreous gel through superior sclerotomies is common in eyes with retinal detachment. Decreased intraocular pres-

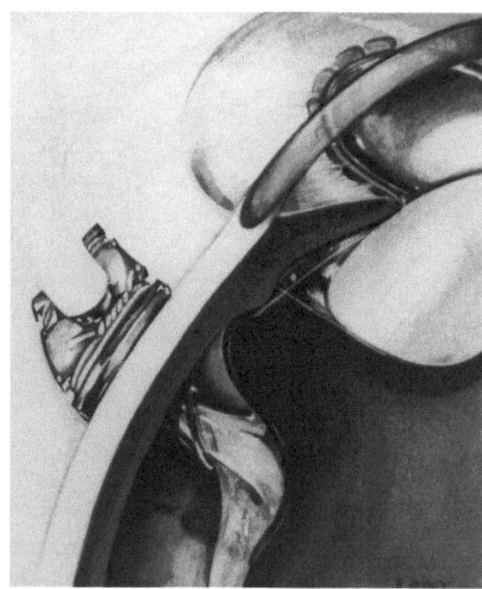

Figure 114. Error to avoid in placing the infusion cannula. The tip of the infusion cannula was not monitored after insertion. Uveal tissue has not been perforated. Infusion fluid flows into the subchoroidal space.

sure with collapse of the eye and difficulties in completion of the sclerotomies are avoided by automated fluid infusion, monitored by a computer (see p. 38).

USE OF A PILOT TUBE

A scleral guide cannula for introduction of the working instruments into the eye is used in two instances: (1) in eyes with extensive detachment of the ciliary epithelium and (2) when it can be anticipated from complexity of the case that various instruments will be substituted for the vitrectomy probe during the course of the operation. In eyes with extensive detachment of the ciliary epithelium, the sclerotomies are necessarily performed in areas of detached ciliary epithelium. Use of a pilot tube decreases the risk of laceration of the peripheral retina during introduction and withdrawal of the instruments (Fig. 115). When it is anticipated that multiple instruments will be used during the operation, use of a pilot tube decreases the surgical trauma in the vitreous base. The scleral guide cannula is sutured to the sclera with a mattress suture.

TEMPORARY CLOSURE OF THE SCLEROTOMIES

Plugs are used to temporarily close one or both sclerotomies during the course of the operation in

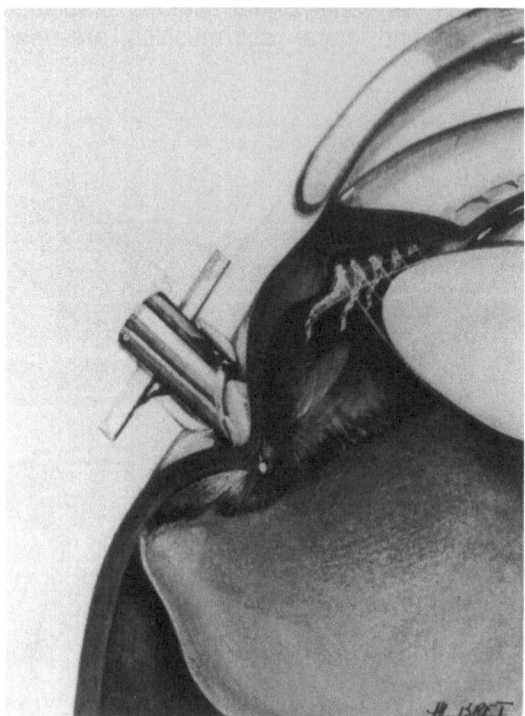

Figure 113. The tip of the infusion cannula is covered by uveal tissue. The cannula must be withdrawn and the sclerotomy revised.

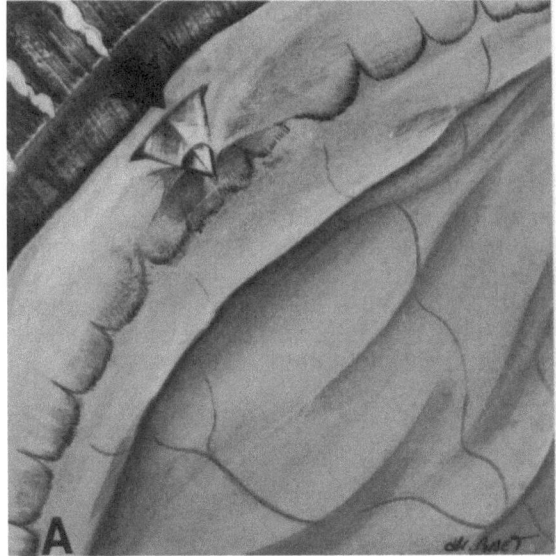 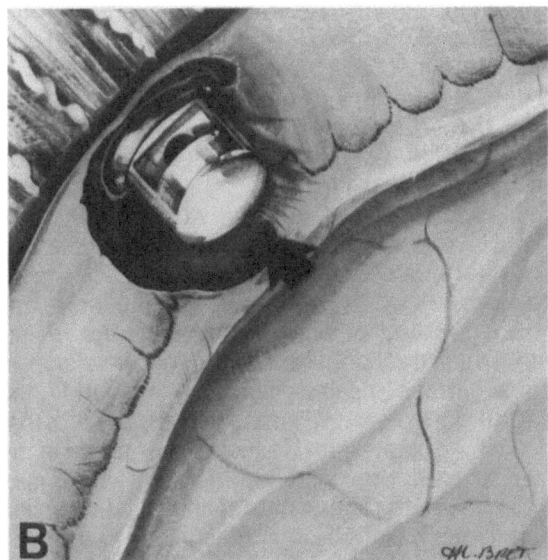

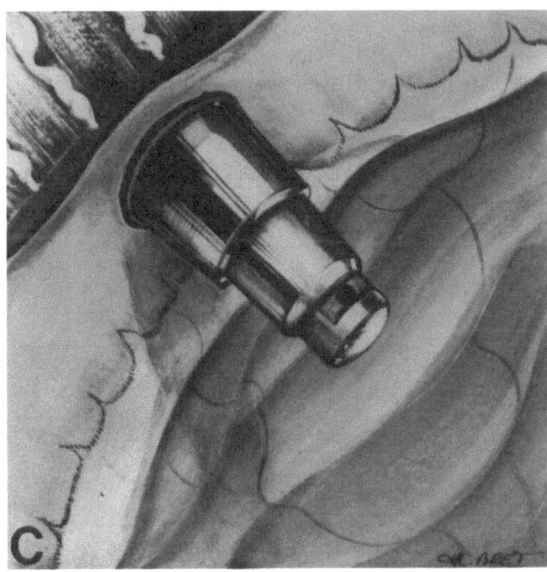

Figure 115. Pars plana incision through detached ciliary epithelium. (A) Knife insertion into the detached ciliary epithelium. (B) Laceration of the detached ciliary epithelium is enlarged by insertion and withdrawal of the vitrectomy instrument. Laceration has extended posteriorly to the ora serrata. The detached retina is being incarcerated into the sclerotomy by instrument withdrawal from the eye. (C) Use of a pilot tube avoids extension of the ciliary epithelium hole to the retina during insertion and withdrawal of instruments.

several circumstances. One sclerotomy in particular is closed with a plug during the surgical steps requiring use of a single instrument, especially those selected surgical steps in the anterior segment of the eye. During these steps, adequate illumination of the surgical field is provided by combination of coaxial and slit lamp illumination of the operating microscope. Temporary closure of a sclerotomy with a plug is occasionally done during specific surgical maneuvers in the posterior segment. In particular, it is done when the three-mirror contact lens and slit lamp are used for viewing the peripheral fundus during surgical maneuvers in the area of the vitreous base, such as radial cuts of fibrous tissue on the vitreous base. When the vitrectomy procedure has been completed, both sclerotomies are temporarily closed with plugs, and thorough examination of the peripheral fundus is routinely performed with the three-mirror contact lens and the slit lamp before suturing the sclerotomies.

SUTURE

Examination of the sclerotomy using high magnification of the surgical microscope is carried out before placing the scleral sutures to close the wound. Lowering the intraocular pressure before withdrawal of the instruments decreases the likelihood of vitreous gel or retinal incarceration into the sclerotomy. However, vitreous strands are commonly present within the wound. They are excised using Bonn forceps and Vannas scissors. No traction is exerted on the vitreous strands during excision to avoid further vitreous gel or retinal incarceration.

Scleral sutures are placed when the internal aspect of the sclerotomy is free of any vitreous gel and intraocular fluid freely escapes through the wound (Fig. 116).

Retinal incarceration into the wound may occur during withdrawal of the instruments or excision of vitreous gel incarcerated in the sclerotomy. It is more likely to occur when the intraocular pressure has not been lowered before withdrawal of the instruments, when traction is exerted during excision of vitreous strands incarcerated in the wound, and when the sclerotomy is located in an area of detached ciliary epithelium. Retinal incarceration in the wound, when not recognized or left untreated, may result in failure to reattach the retina or late traction detachment. The intraocular pressure is lowered and the incarcerated retina is gently pushed back with a blunt spatula. The inner surface of the sclerotomy is then examined using the slit lamp and 3-mirror contact lens. If the retina remains incarcerated in the wound, further attempts to disengage the retina from the wound are performed; they may, however, remain unsuccessful. In most instances the incarcerated tissue is the detached ciliary epithelium with a portion of the retina of the oral region or the flap of a large tear. When those tissues cannot be disengaged from the wound, they are resected and cryotreatment is performed on the iatrogenic tear after suturing the sclerotomy. Each sclerotomy is closed with two interrupted sutures or a running suture using 8–0 nylon monofilament or a long-term absorbable material such as PDS (polydioxanone). The sutures are placed at the join of the two outer thirds and the inner third of the scleral wound (Fig. 116) so as to ensure close apposition of the wound edges and avoid late complications such as fibrous ingrowth and rupture of the wound.

Vitreous Gel Removal

Vitreous gel removal is made using the aspirating and cutting vitrectomy probe. The port of the probe should be under direct visualization at all times. Low levels of suction force are used. The port of the vitrectomy probe is positioned adjacent to the vitreous gel to be cut. Strong suction force to pull the vitreous gel towards the probe port should be avoided. Visualization of the vitreous gel during excision is best achieved through retroillumination using the fiberoptic probe.

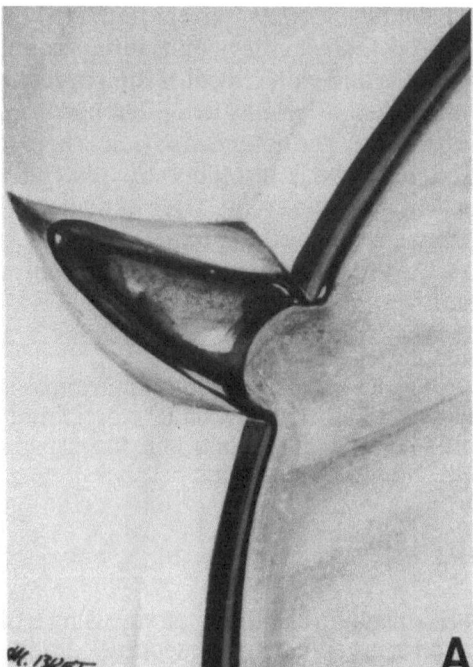 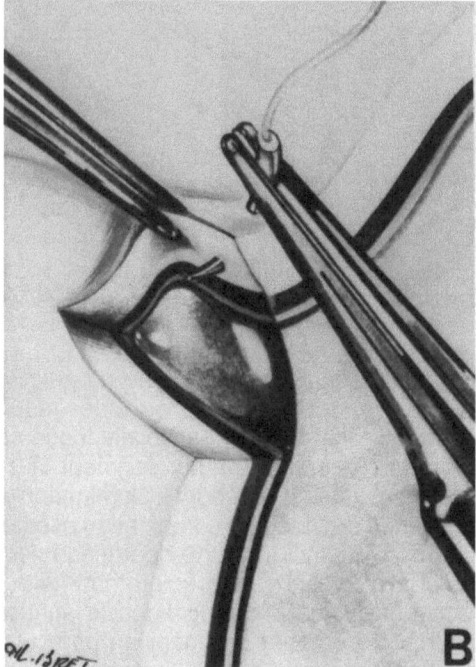

Figure 116. Suture of a pars plana sclerotomy. (A) The internal aspect of the sclerotomy is examined using high magnification of the surgical microscope to ensure that no vitreous gel is present in the scleral wound. (B) The edge of the scleral wound is lifted using Bonn forceps to avoid vitreous gel incarceration during needle insertion.

Excision of the vitreous gel includes three consecutive steps: excision of the anterior vitreous face, removal of the central vitreous gel, and excision of the posterior vitreous face.

EXCISION OF THE ANTERIOR VITREOUS FACE

Indications for excision of the anterior vitreous face are based upon careful biomicroscopic examination of the anterior vitreous gel performed preoperatively. The anterior vitreous face should be excised when slit lamp examination discloses clinical evidence of condensation or contraction of the anterior vitreous gel. In contrast, excision of the anterior vitreous gel is unnecessary when slit lamp examination shows that the anatomy and mobility of the anterior vitreous remain normal.

Excision of the anterior vitreous face is required in most traction retinal detachments after penetrating wound of the ciliary region (see p. 291), aphakic retinal detachments associated with vitreous gel incarceration in the corneal wound (see p. 258), nontraumatic giant tears (see p. 203), retinal detachments complicated by proliferative vitreoretinopathy, grade C3 to D3 (see p. 241), and pseudophakic retinal detachments associated with dense pupillary membranes.

Excision of the anterior vitreous face is unnecessary in most other retinal detachments, particularly in traction retinal detachment complicating diabetic retinopathy, retinal detachments associated with a macular hole or postequatorial retinal breaks, and retinal detachments complicated by proliferative vitreoretinopathy, grades C1 and C2.

In phakic eyes, lens removal is required to achieve complete excision of the anterior vitreous face in most cases. Only in a few cases can proper excision of condensed anterior vitreous gel be completed while leaving the clear lens untouched. (For the surgical techniques to be used for lens removal see p. 145).

Visualization of the anterior vitreous face during excision is best achieved by retroillumination using the fiberoptic probe combined with slit lamp illumination using a narrow slit beam. No contact lens is used during excision of the anterior vitreous gel.

In aphakic eyes, the port of the vitrectomy probe is positioned at the center of the pupil. The port is directed anteriorly. Suction is first activated to aspirate the anterior vitreous face into the port. Then cutting is activated. A hole is made at the center of the anterior vitreous face. Next the hole is enlarged toward the periphery in all directions. Dense pupillary membranes cannot be aspirated into the port. In such cases the membrane is incised using a sharp knife. Then the vitrectomy probe is used to excise

the pupillary membrane. During excision of the anterior vitreous face, great care is taken not to touch the iris to avoid pupillary constriction due to iris trauma or iris aspiration into the port. In eyes with pupillary membranes, iridovitreal adhesions at the pupillary margin are common, and they are freed before excision of the anterior vitreous face. Weak adhesions are freed using a blunt spatula. Strong adhesions are freed using a discision knife. The instrument tip is inserted behind the iris between two synechiae, gently lifted anteriorly, and then moved circumferentially on 360° of the pupil.

In phakic eyes it is possible to excise the anterior vitreous gel when the anterior vitreous face remains elastic, leaving a clear lens untouched. The slit lamp illuminator, with a quite narrow slit beam, is used for precise localization of the posterior lens capsule. Fiberoptic endoillumination is used simultaneously for visualization of the vitreous gel. The vitreous probe is conducted parallel to the posterior lens capsule until the tip is close to the optical axis of the eye. The port probe should not be oriented towards the lens. It is oriented at 90° from the lens in the surgeon direction. Linear aspiration is applied to aspirate the anterior vitreous gel. When the anterior vitreous face is engaged into the port, the cutting blades are activated. Then the hole in the anterior vitreous face is enlarged. This maneuver is ineffective when the anterior vitreous is condensed. In such cases the lens should be removed.

EXCISION OF THE CENTRAL VITREOUS ARCHITECTURE

Excision of the central vitreous architecture is the first step of the vitrectomy procedure in retinal detachments that do not require removal of the anterior vitreous gel, and the second step in retinal detachments that require excision of the anterior vitreous face. Use of a contact lens is required for visualization of the vitreous architecture in all cases.

When the anterior vitreous gel has been excised, the vitrectomy is continued in a posterior direction from the center towards the periphery.

When the anterior vitreous gel is left untouched, the vitrectomy probe is positioned in the optical axis of the eye at the join of the anterior third and the two posterior thirds of the vitreous cavity. A central hole is made. Then the hole is enlarged laterally up to the posterior edge of the vitreous base and posteriorly up to the posterior vitreous face.

Excision of the vitreous gel involves various difficulties depending on the vitreous gel changes and the presence or absence of posterior vitreous detachment. In a significant number of retinal detachments that require vitrectomy, the vitreous gel is liquefied and the posterior vitreous face is detached from the retina. In such eyes the vitrectomy procedure is most rapid and easy to perform. However, care is taken to excise the viscous vitreous gel that has collapsed in the lower part of the fundus. In eyes with complicated retinal detachments, such as retinal detachments with severe proliferative vitreoretinopathy, traction retinal detachments in proliferative diabetic retinopathy of recent onset in young patients, or retinal detachments after penetrating eye injury, the vitreous gel remains highly viscous and the posterior vitreous face is not detached or partially detached. In such eyes excision of the vitreous gel requires great care and takes more time to be completed. A low suction force, which is just supra-liminal is used. The port of the vitrectomy probe is directed opposite the detached retina. Movements of the underlying detached retina during vitreous gel excision indicate persisting vitreoretinal adhesions and too high a suction force.

Dense vitreous strands and sheets cannot be excised using the vitrectomy probe. They are cut with automated scissors. Due to relief of tissue contraction, a wide gap usually develops immediately between the cut ends of the vitreous band or sheet.

EXCISION OF THE POSTERIOR VITREOUS FACE

Excision of the posterior vitreous face to relieve tangential vitreoretinal traction is the most important step of the vitrectomy procedure in most retinal detachments requiring vitrectomy.

Surgical difficulties and hazards in excision of the posterior vitreous face show a wide range of variations depending on the status of the posterior vitreous gel and the presence and extent or absence of posterior vitreous detachment.

When the vitreous gel is extensively detached posteriorly, such as in most senile rhegmatogenous retinal detachments, the posterior vitreous face is easily identified during vitrectomy and excised from the prepapillary ring towards the periphery, using the vitrectomy probe. The port is positioned towards the vitreous cavity.

When the posterior vitreous detachment is incomplete, difficulties encountered in the excision of the posterior vitreous face depend mainly on the extent of the persisting vitreoretinal attachments and the anatomy of the posterior cortical vitreous. In a significant number of rhegmatogenous retinal detachments managed with vitrectomy, the posterior vitreous detachment is incomplete. However, the persisting vitreoretinal adhesions are weak. They are frequently freed by supraliminal suction force used during central vitrectomy. In such eyes excision of the posterior vitreous face is easily completed. When the partially detached posterior vitreous face is dense and somewhat fibrous, such as in most

traction retinal detachments complicating proliferative diabetic retinopathy, it is easily identified during vitrectomy. In areas of posterior vitreous detachment, the posterior vitreous face is excised with the vitrectomy probe or cut with automated scissors to isolate each island of firm vitreoretinal adhesion. In areas where the posterior vitreous face remains adherent to the underlying retina, a cleavage plane can usually be achieved between the fibrous posterior vitreous face and the retina. Delamination is carried out wherever it can be done without excessive traction. It is performed using the hooked blunt fiber optic. Then the islands of fibrous posterior vitreous face are cut with scissors to relieve tangential traction. When the partially detached posterior vitreous face remains viscous and elastic, such as is common in rhegmatogenous retinal detachments complicated by severe proliferative vitreoretinopathy and traction retinal detachments of recent onset in young patients, excision of the posterior vitreous face may involve great difficulties. In such eyes a cleavage plane between the posterior vitreous face and the retina should be created before attempting to excise the posterior vitreous face. The cleavage plane is done using the hooked fiber optic. It is often difficult to complete due to elasticity of the posterior vitreous cortex. Areas of firm vitreoretinal attachment are left untouched. The posterior vitreous face is excised using the vitrectomy probe or cut with scissors in areas where delamination has been completed.

When the posterior vitreous face has not detached, such as in a number of recent onset proliferative vitreoretinopathy cases, early traction detachment after penetrating injury, and nontraumatic giant tears, the cortical posterior vitreous gel is hardly distinguished from the retina. The posterior vitreous face is engaged with the hooked fiber optic probe in areas where it can be identified, gently lifted from the retina, and tangential traction is applied to separate it from the retina. Traction exerted by the hooked fiber optic probe should be most gentle. Excessive traction on areas of firm vitreoretinal adhesion will result in iatrogenic retinal breaks. Total delamination of the posterior vitreous cortex cannot be achieved in most cases. The posterior vitreous cortex is cut with scissors in areas where a cleavage plane has been achieved. In most cases areas where a cleavage plane can be achieved are located between two large retinal folds. Delamination and cutting of the posterior vitreous face are conducted from the posterior pole towards the equatorial region.

Endosurgery in the Vitreous Base Region

Scleral depression combined with decreased intraocular pressure can be used for visualization of the vitreous base in aphakic eyes.[33] The eyewall is indented with a cotton-tip applicator. Scleral depression pushes the vitreous base into the pupillary area and tissue excision or radial cuts in fibrous anterior ring can be carried out. Excessive scleral depression and decreased intraocular pressure may result in iris root bleeding. Due to the risk of lens damage, this technique should not be used in phakic eyes.

In phakic eyes the vitreous base and the pars plana can be visualized with the three-mirror contact lens. However use of the three-mirror contact lens during vitrectomy has three disadvantages: (1) the surgeon should hold the lens and only unimanual intraocular maneuvers can be carried out, (2) only the slit lamp can be used for illumination of the surgical field, and (3) the peripheral mirrors of the lens provide an indirect image of the surgical field.

Use of a prismatic planoconcave lens is an alternative to the use of the three-mirror contact lens, however, visualization of the anterior part of the vitreous base is not possible.

Each of the three techniques for visualization of the vitreous base is used in selected circumstances. Scleral depression or the prismatic planoconcave lens are used when bimanual endosurgery is carried out in the peripheral fundus opposite to the entry sites of the instruments. The three-mirror contact lens is used in phakic eyes for selected unimanual maneuvers, such as radial cuts on the vitreous base.

For epiretinal membrane delamination and segmentation see p. 245.

Management of Vitreous Hemorrhage

Vitreous hemorrhage and intraoperative bleeding are infrequently encountered during vitreous surgery for retinal detachment repair (except for traction retinal detachments complicating proliferative retinopathies), particularly in diabetic retinopathy and early detachment after penetrating injury.

REMOVAL OF VITREOUS HEMORRHAGE

Removal of intravitreal blood is performed with the vitrectomy probe using a high speed cutting rate. It is started in the part of the vitreous cavity corresponding to areas of attached, or the least detached, retina. These areas have been determined by preoperative ultrasonography.

Nonclotted blood in the preretinal space usually swirls into the center of the vitreous cavity when the posterior vitreous face is incised. Nonclotted blood is removed either actively by using a linear suction force of the vitrectomy probe, or passively, by venting a flute needle to the atmosphere. The

port of the instrument is placed near the hole in the posterior vitreous face. The instrument port is positioned opposite the retina and a low-suction force is used to avoid engaging the retina.

MANAGEMENT OF INTRAOPERATIVE BLEEDING

Intraoperative bleeding may occur from new retinal vessels in retinal detachment complicating proliferative retinopathies, from an avulsed retinal vessel in rhegmatogenous retinal detachment and from fibrovascular ingrowth in retinal detachment after a penetrating eye injury. Bleeding occurs when the vessels are cut, or from traction on vitreoretinal adhesions. When active bleeding occurs, the intraocular pressure is temporarily raised to stop bleeding. The bleeding vessels are identified and coagulated with endodiathermy. The intraocular pressure is then lowered to determine whether the bleeding vessels have been closed by endodiathermy. In high risk eyes, intraoperative bleeding can be minimized by presetting the intraocular pressure at 30 mmhg, avoiding traction on areas of vitreoretinal adhesion, coagulation of new vessels before cutting vascularized sheets, and coagulation of the cut edges of fibrovascular tissue.

Endovitreal Methods to Induce Tissue Scarring

Endodiathermy, endophotocoagulation, and endocryotreatment are the three methods currently used to induce tissue scarring during vitrectomy. Additional methods may be available in the near future.

ENDODIATHERMY

The indications for bipolar endodiathermy during vitrectomy for retinal detachment management are as follows: (1) coagulation of bleeding vessels in fibrovascular proliferative tissues, (2) coagulation of a retinal vessel that bridges a retinal tear and bleeds, (3) creating a retinal landmark that will make further localization of a small tear through a gas bubble easier, and (4) retinal coagulation to prevent bleeding during a retinotomy. Endodiathermy is rarely used to seal a retinal break because it is associated with excessive damage to retinal tissue.

A bipolar coaxial microprobe is used for endodiathermy (see instrumentation p. 39).

Tissue coagulation is begun at low intensity. The intensity is gradually increased until slight shrinkage of vessels to be closed off, or blanching of the retina, is achieved. When using endodiathermy on the retina, special care is taken to avoid excessive intensity level that would result in shrinkage of the retina and coagulative adhesion between the retina and the instrument tip.

ENDOCRYOTREATMENT

Endocryotreatment has been advocated to seal retinal breaks and induce tissue destruction in proliferative retinopathies.[24] It is performed using a straight 0.9 mm diameter cryoprobe.

The technique is rarely used in retinal detachment management because it is associated with excessive damage to the retina compared to retinal damage associated with photocoagulation treatment or transscleral cryotreatment performed with biomicroscopic control of the fundus. Indications for endocryotreatment are restricted to eyes in which intraoperative bleeding is likely to prevent visualization required for further transscleral cryotreatment or photocoagulation treatment after closure of the pars plana sclerotomies. Great care should be taken not to move the cryoprobe before it is fully defrosted. Moving the cryoprobe while it is still adherent to the retina will result in severe retinal laceration and bleeding.

ENDOPHOTOCOAGULATION

Endophotocoagulation can be used to seal the retinal breaks and treat areas of hypoxic retina. In most rhegmatogenous retinal detachments including retinal detachments complicated by proliferative vitreoretinopathy, subretinal fluid drainage is not carried out, since it is unnecessary to permanently reattach the retina. Therefore, intraoperative treatment of retinal breaks by means of endophotocoagulation is not possible in most cases. Producing a retinochoroidal scar in the retinal break area is achieved by using either transscleral cryotreatment or transpupillary photocoagulation. The latter technique is carried out postoperatively through the expanded gas bubble after spontaneous absorption of subretinal fluid.

The most frequent indication for intraoperative endophotocoagulation is ablation of hypoxic retina in traction retinal detachments complicating proliferative retinopathies, such as diabetic retinopathy. Endophotocoagulation treatment is applied to attached hypoxic retina. Endophotocoagulation is carried out as the last step of the vitrectomy procedure. Photocoagulation through the pupil, or transscleral cryotreatment performed after closing the sclerotomies, are alternative methods to treating hypoxic retina. Poor clarity of the media, however, may prevent performance of the latter techniques.

Endophotocoagulation treatment is performed using the argon laser attached to the surgical microscope (see p. 41). The probe, which is 0.89 mm in diameter, is entered into the vitreous cavity through any of the pars plana sclerotomies. The distance of the probe tip from the retina determines the coagulation size. Coagulations are begun using a low power level. The power is then increased until proper whitening of the retina is obtained.

Fluid-Gas Exchange

Intravitreal gas injection is used as an adjunct to vitreoretinal microsurgery in most rhegmatogenous retinal detachments managed by vitrectomy. Intravitreal gas injection is associated with removal of intraocular fluid so as to avoid increased intraocular pressure.

Several techniques have been developed to perform fluid-gas exchange.[23,24,34,35]

Partial fluid gas exchange without subretinal fluid drainage is the technique that we performed in most cases at our clinic.

This technique has two advantages: (1) no special instrumentation, such as a pump, is required and (2) the procedure is most rapid to perform. Sequential fluid gas exchange is performed after closing the sclerotomies. An amount of intraocular fluid equal to the volume of pure gas to be injected is first evacuated.

In most cases withdrawal of intraocular fluid is performed through the limbus. In the vitrectomized eye, fluid percolates from the vitreous cavity to the anterior chamber through the zonula. Therefore, withdrawal of the proper amount of intraocular fluid can be obtained by anterior chamber paracentesis in most cases. However, when the anterior vitreous gel has not been removed by vitrectomy, fluid may not percolate through the zonula. In such eyes fluid is removed from the vitreous cavity through the pars plana. A blunt tip 30 gauge cannula is used. Position of the cannula tip is monitored using a planoconcave lens and the slit lamp. During fluid aspiration, the eye wall is gently indented with a cotton-tip applicator to avoid collapse of the eye. Then pure gas is injected. Gas injection is performed through the limbus in aphakic eyes and the pars plana in phakic eyes.

Vitrectomy Techniques in the Anterior Segment

Surgical management of complicated retinal detachments may require microsurgery of the anterior segment as an adjunct to vitrectomy.

In selected cases, microsurgery of the anterior

segment is performed through the pars plana as the initial step of the vitrectomy procedure. Surgery of the anterior segment through the pars plana in retinal detachment management includes lens removal, iridectomy, removal of pupillary membranes, and section of anterior synechiae.

LENS REMOVAL

The indications for lens removal, as an adjunct to vitreoretinal microsurgery in retinal detachment management are as follows:

1. Heavy contraction of the vitreous base, which will be managed by radial cuts.
2. Heavy densification and contraction of the anterior vitreous gel or a cyclitic membrane on the anterior vitreous face.
3. Preexisting lens opacities which prevent fundus examination.

Most indications for lens removal are encountered in retinal detachments after penetrating eye injury, retinal detachments complicated by severe proliferative vitreoretinopathy and retinal detachments with nontraumatic retinal tears 180° and over in size.

Whenever possible lens removal is combined with the surgical procedure for retinal detachment management, since delay in retinal surgery may worsen the prognosis. However, when a cataractous lens with advanced nuclear sclerosis requires lens extraction through a limbal incision in an eye with proliferative vitreoretinopathy, grade D, lens surgery is carried out as an independent procedure 2 weeks before retinal detachment surgery.

Choice of the surgical technique for lens removal depends on the patient's age and biomicroscopic characteristics of the lens. A hard lens with advanced nuclear sclerosis is removed using either phacoemulsification or conventional intracapsular extraction through the limbus. Soft lenses in patients under 40 years of age are removed through the pars plana using the vitrectomy probe.

Several techniques have been developed for lens removal through the pars plana.[23,24,34] Whatever the surgical details, which may vary depending on the surgeon's preference, three major rules should be followed: (1) removal of the lens material should be completed as an intracapsular procedure, (2) removal of both the anterior and posterior capsules should be as complete as possible, and (3) iris trauma should be avoided.

Following these basic rules is of primary importance in avoiding intraoperative complications. Inadvertent opening of the posterior capsule during lens aspiration may result in loosing lens fragments into the vitreous cavity. Premature opening of the anterior capsule will result in collapse of the anterior chamber

due to the fact that aqueous humor is more easily aspirated than lens fibers. Iris trauma by the vitrectomy probe will lead to pupillary contraction, difficulty in proper lens removal and further vitreoretinal surgery.

The surgical technique that we use in most cases is as follows: the vitrectomy probe is entered into the eye through the supero temporal pars plana incision. This location is chosen preferably as the entry site of the vitrectomy instrument to hold the instrument in a frontal plane parallel to the iris plane. When the vitrectomy probe is inserted through a supero nasal pars plana incision, it cannot be orientated in a frontal plane strictly parallel to the iris plane because of the orbit and nose prominence in adult patients. Entering the vitrectomy instrument through the supero temporal incision in a left eye requires that the surgeon use either the left hand or is seated at the lateral left side of the patient's head. Coaxial illumination of the surgical microscope is used for illumination of the surgical field. The slit illuminator with a narrow slit beam is used in combination with coaxial illumination for better visualization of the lens capsule. During lens removal the fiberoptic probe is used to stabilize and rotate the eye rather than to provide illumination (Fig. 117). The port of the vitrectomy probe is positioned against the lens capsule at the equator. Suction is activated to aspirate the capsule into the port (Fig. 117). The cutting function is then activated to make a small hole in the capsule of just sufficient size to insert the vitrectomy probe into the capsular bag. Opening of the capsule at the equator can also be performed with the knife used for the pars plana incision. The lens material is hydrated and mechanically disrupted before aspiration with the vitrectomy probe. Hydration softens the nucleus and facilitates its removal. It is performed using a 28 gauge blunt cannula, which is pushed between the nucleus and cortex and moved laterally in a frontal plane while gently injecting balanced saline solution into the capsular bag. When disruption and softening of the lens fibers have been obtained, lens material is aspired using the vitrectomy probe. The nucleus is first aspirated using suction (Fig. 117). The cutting function of the probe is used intermittently at a low speed rate to fragment hard nuclear material. When nucleus aspiration has been completed, the cortex fibers are removed using only aspiration. The cortex fibers are aspirated near the equator and stripped from the capsule using only suction, while slowly moving the vitrectomy probe radially in a centripetal direction. During this maneuver the port of the vitrectomy probe is directed, laterally to avoid inadvertent aspiration of the lens capsule. When lens fiber removal has been completed, the posterior capsule is excised using a high speed cutting rate. Next, the anterior capsule is resected in the same fashion. In young patients the anterior lens capsule is often elastic

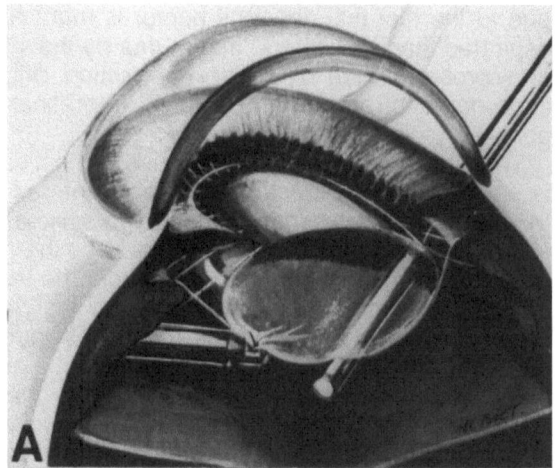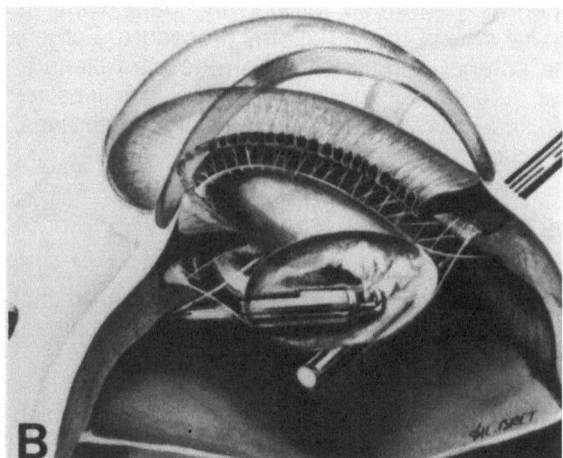

Figure 117. Lens removal through the pars plana using the vitrectomy probe. (A) A small hole is being made in the lens capsule at the equator. The fiberoptic probe is used to stabilize the eye rather than to provide illumination. (B) The nucleus is being removed using suction and cutting functions of the probe.

and resistant, and resection using the vitrectomy probe may be somewhat difficult. In such cases a cruciform opening of the anterior capsule is made with a discision knife to facilitate further excision by the vitrectomy probe. Excision of both the anterior and posterior capsules should be as complete as possible. The peripheral ring of capsule left in place should not exceed 2 mm in width. When pupillary dilation is poor, proper excision of the lens capsules may be difficult and hazardous due to iris trauma and risk of iris aspiration into the port. In such cases the anterior lens capsule is excised with the vitrectomy probe up to the pupillary margin. Then several radial cuts are made in the peripheral capsular ring behind the iris using scissors. Radial cuts in the capsular ring result in peripheral retraction of the capsular remnants, which roll up toward the equator.

IRIDECTOMIES

A superior sectorial iridectomy is made to facilitate further vitreoretinal observation in aphakic eyes with a small pupil. In most cases a sectorial iridectomy provides adequate visualization of the posterior segment. Superior sectorial iridectomy is performed rather than sphincterotomies or excision of portions of the pupillary margin, since the latter technique will result in a permanent wide pupil and postoperative dazzling. An inferior peripheral iridectomy is performed in aphakic eyes when a nearly total retinal tamponade with a long lasting gas is planned (Fig. 118). Inferior peripheral iridectomy is made to avoid postoperative pupillary block by the gas bubble,

which may occur when the patient's head is in the upright position (Fig. 119).

Both sectorial and peripheral iridectomies are made using the vitrectomy probe. The area of the iris to be excised is first aspirated using linear suction without activating the cutting function. The cutting function is activated only when the proper amount of iris tissue is engaged in the port. Iris tissue is easily aspirated into the vitrectomy probe. Therefore low levels of suction force are used to avoid excessive excision of iris tissue.

When a sectorial iridectomy is performed, iris excision is begun at the pupillary margin. It is continued in a peripheral direction. The iris root is left untouched because the section of the peripheral arterial circle of the iris may result in significant bleeding.

Inferior peripheral iridectomy is made between the iris sphincter and the iris root (Fig. 118).

The vitreous probe is positioned behind the iris, the port being orientated anteriorly. Proper position of the probe tip is monitored by tilting the probe tip anteriorly. Prominence of the iris tissue pushed by the probe tip makes it possible to determine the position of the port. When the probe tip is in the proper position, the suction force is activated. Iris tissue is aspirated without activating the cutting function until the anterior surface of the iris is engaged in the port (Fig. 118). Then the cutting function is activated. Suction force is released using the foot pedal as early as the probe tip is visible in the iris hole. Delayed release of the suction force will result in too large an iridectomy. Such a large iridectomy may result in postoperative diplopia and should be avoided. Iris excision should be large enough, however, to ensure a patent iridectomy.

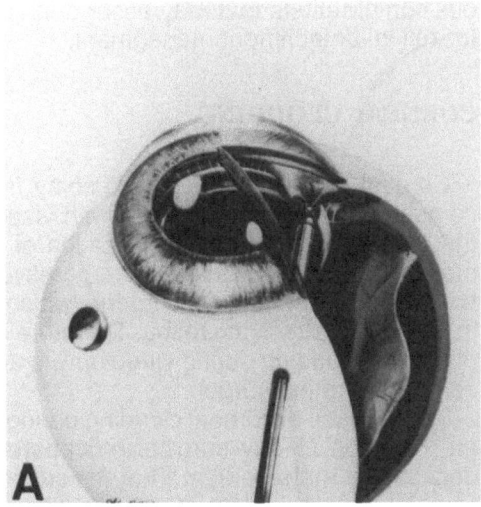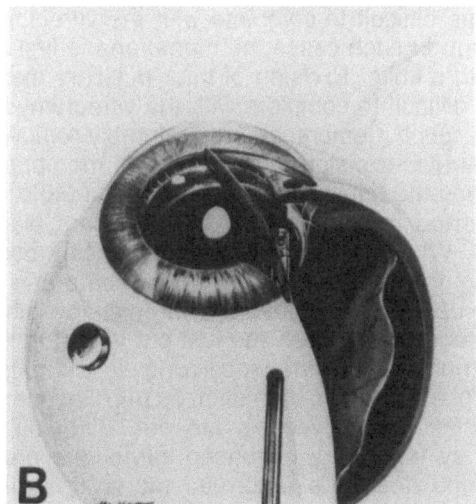

Figure 118. Inferior peripheral iridectomy using the vitrectomy probe. (A) iris tissue is being engaged into the port of the vitrectomy probe using only suction. (B) Peripheral iridectomy of proper size has been completed.

PUPILLARY MEMBRANE EXCISION

The technique for excision of pupillary membranes varies according to specific features of the membrane.

When posterior iris synechiae are associated with the pupillary membrane, they are freed as the initial step of the procedure in all cases. Sectioning of weak synechiae is done using a blunt spatula. Sectioning of strong iris synechiae is done using a disci-sion knife. The sharp edge of the knife is positioned in a frontal plane to avoid iris damage. Synechiae are cut with lateral movements of the knife in a plane parallel to the iris.

Excision of thin pupillary membranes is performed using the vitrectomy probe. A hole is made in the center of the pupil or at the thinnest portion of the membrane. Then the hole is enlarged up to the pupillary margin. A thin pupillary membrane may be resistant or elastic making the central opening of the

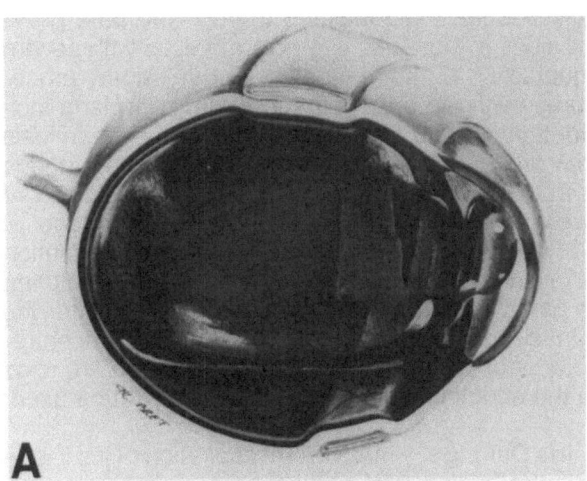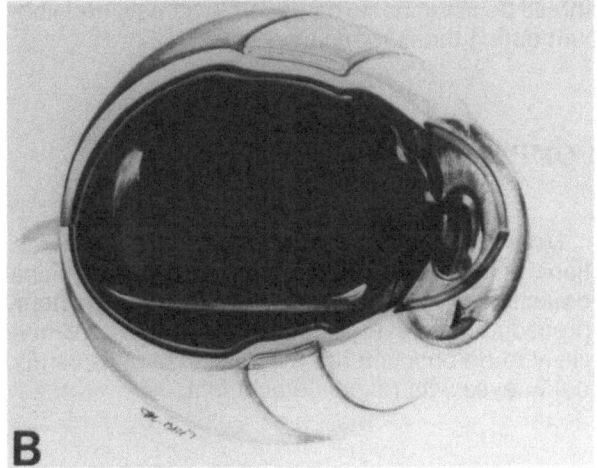

Figure 119. Prevention of pupillary block produced by a large gas bubble in aphakic eyes. (A) A large bubble of longlasting gas is used to seal a giant retinal break in an aphakic eye. When the patient's head is in the upright position, the gas bubble protrudes in the pupil and induces a pupillary block. (B) Inferior iridectomy allows fluid to flow from the posterior chamber to the anterior chamber and prevents increased intraocular pressure.

membrane difficult to complete with the vitrectomy instrument. In such cases the membrane is first incised with a knife. Excision of thick pupillary membrane is difficult to complete with the vitrectomy instrument. Such membranes are preferably removed using the bloc-excision technique. The membrane is cut along the pupillary margin using manual scissors inserted through one of the two pars plana incisions. When most of the membrane has been cut along the pupillary margin, the membrane is grasped using forceps inserted through the other pars plana incision. Then the last cut is performed and the membrane is removed in one piece through the pars plana incision. Vascularized pupillary membranes bleed when vessels are cut. Bleeding is stopped by temporary increased intraocular pressure; Endodiathermy is performed, thereby lowering intraocular pressure.

SECTION OF ANTERIOR SYNECHIAE

Iris or vitreous gel adhesions to corneal wounds may be present in eyes with retinal detachment after penetrating injury and retinal detachment after complicated cataract extraction. Such synechiae are cut using either a limbal approach or a pars plana approach. Choice between the two approaches is dictated by the location, extent, and thickness of the synechiae. Peripheral synechiae are often more easily managed via the limbus, whereas more central synechiae are easily cut using the pars plana approach. Iris synechiae are freed using a blunt spatula or a discision knife. Thin vitreous synechiae are excised with the vitrectomy probe. Thick vitreous synechiae are cut using automated scissors. Care should be taken not to damage the corneal endothelium during these maneuvers.

COMPLICATIONS

Most intraoperative and postoperative complications occurring in vitrectomy performed for retinal detachment repair are common to any vitrectomy procedure. However, certain complications are more likely to be encountered when vitrectomy is carried out in eyes with retinal detachment.

Intraoperative Complications

Corneal clouding, miosis, iris damage, lens damage, bleeding and retinal damage are the most serious complications that may occur during vitrectomy for retinal detachment managment.

CORNEAL CLOUDING

Corneal clouding during vitrectomy is a serious complication when it interferes with visualization of the ocular fundus. Poor visualization of the fundus may be the cause of severe intraoperative complications or improper retina surgery, which will result in failure to reattach the retina. Therefore, prevention of corneal clouding during vitrectomy is a major concern of the retina surgeon.

Most causes of corneal clouding during vitrectomy are common to any surgical procedure for retinal detachment management. (For the causes, prevention, and management of corneal clouding during retinal detachment surgery see p. 52.)

IRIS COMPLICATIONS

Iris complications during vitrectomy include miosis and iris damage by the vitrectomy instrument.

Miosis. Decreased intraocular pressure and iris trauma with the intraocular instruments are the two main causes of miosis during vitrectomy. Iris trauma may occur during lens removal through the pars plana. Iris trauma by the vitrectomy instrument can be avoided through proper technique (see p. 145). Intraocular fluid leakage through the pars plana incisions is the main cause of decreased intraocular pressure when the vitrectomy instrument is not equipped with automated regulation of the intraocular pressure. Fluid leakage through the pars plana incisions is more likely to occur in eyes with severe liquefaction of the vitreous gel or in lengthy procedures owing to enlargement of the pars plana incisions during the operation. In aphakic eyes, miosis that prevents adequate visualization of the fundus is managed by performing a sectorial iridectomy at twelve o'clock with the vitrectomy probe (see p. 146). In phakic eyes 1/10,000 epinephrine solution is injected into the anterior chamber. The solution is gently injected though the limbus onto the iris surface using a 30 gauge blunt needle. Concentrations of epinephrine stronger than 1/5,000 are toxic to the endothelium,[36] and they should not be used.

Iris Damage. Inadvertent aspiration of iris tissue into the cutting port may occur during removal of the anterior lens capsule, which can result in an iridectomy or an iridodialysis. This complication can be avoided with proper surgical technique (see p. 145). A low-suction force should be used during lens capsule excision and the cutting port should be directed in an opposite direction to the iris.

LENS DAMAGE

Mechanical trauma from the knife used for the pars plana incisions may occur when the knife is not oriented in the proper direction. This is more likely to occur when the pars plana incisions are performed on a soft collapsed eye. In very soft eyes the intraocular pressure should be raised before performing the pars plana incision for placement of the infusion cannula. The intraocular pressure is raised by injecting balanced saline solution into the anterior chamber. In eyes with severe vitreous gel liquefaction, rapid escape of intraocular fluid through the pars plana incision(s) may result in collapse of the eye and difficulty in the performance of proper pars plana incisions. In such eyes infusion fluid should be allowed to flow into the eye through the preplaced infusion cannula during performance of the two additional pars plana incisions.

Mechanical trauma to the posterior lens capsule from the vitrectomy instrument or light probe may occur during removal of retrolenticular vitreous gel. When removal of the anterior vitreous gel is required in phakic eyes, the posterior lens capsule should be kept in clear focus using the slit lamp illumination with a narrow slit beam.

When iatrogenic damage to the posterior lens capsule occurs, complete opacification of the lens is likely to develop in the early postoperative period in most cases. Therefore, lens removal is carried out during the same operation when visible damage to the posterior lens capsule is recognized intraoperatively.

INTRAOPERATIVE BLEEDING

Intraoperative bleeding is an infrequent complication during vitrectomy for retinal detachment repair, except for specific retinal detachments (see p. 277). It is a major complication when it results in poor visualization of the fundus. In most cases intraoperative bleeding is related to intravitreal new vessels (see p. 277). Such bleeding can be minimized by appropriate measures (see p. 277).

Bleeding at the pars plana incision(s) is rare and self limited in most cases. Iris bleeding may result from iris trauma and decreased intraocular pressure. In phakic eyes, bleeding in the anterior chamber or passage of blood cells from the vitreous cavity to the anterior chamber through the zonula, is a most serious complication because complete removal of blood from the anterior chamber through the limbus is difficult to achieve in most cases. Blood clots in the pupillary area that cannot be removed will make intraoperative visualization of the fundus very difficult or impossible.

RETINAL DAMAGE

Retinal damage is the intraoperative complication most likely to occur in vitrectomy procedures for retinal detachment repair. It is a most serious complication that will require specific management and may result in failure to reattach the retina. This potential complication of vitreous surgery should be kept in mind by the retina surgeon at all times during intravitreal surgery.

Intraoperative retinal damage includes mechanical damage and light damage.

Mechanical Damage. Full thickness retinal breaks and laceration of the inner retinal layers can occur during vitreous surgery for complicated retinal detachments.

Full Thickness Retinal Breaks. Retinal breaks can occur from excessive vitreoretinal traction during vitreous surgery or direct trauma from the instruments. Iatrogenic retinal breaks can occur during introduction and withdrawal of the instruments, removal of the vitreous gel and posterior vitreous face, and dissection of epiretinal membranes. Severe retinal damage can also occur as a complication of endodiathermy and endocryo treatment (see pp. 39 and 144).

Iatrogenic retinal breaks include three main groups: (1) peripheral retinal break in the meridians of the sclerotomies, (2) peripheral retinal breaks in other meridians, and (3) retinal breaks posterior to the equator.

Peripheral retinal breaks near a pars plana sclerotomy are most infrequent with the instrumentation and techniques currently used. Retinal breaks due to too posterior a sclerotomy and retinal breaks resulting from traction on the vitreous base during withdrawal of the instruments have been reported.[24] Retinal breaks in the meridians of the pars plana sclerotomies are likely to occur when the sclerotomies are performed in areas of detached ciliary epithelium. In such cases, laceration of the ciliary epithelium will enlarge during entry and withdrawal of the instruments. The laceration can enlarge posteriorly and involve the retina. Retinal breaks in the meridians of the sclerotomy are more likely to occur in eyes with retinal detachment after penetrating injury of the ciliary region when the retina is dragged anteriorly to the ora serrata by the fibrovascular ingrowth. In such eyes great care should be taken to perform all pars plana sclerotomies in meridians distant from the penetrating wound (see p. 290). Iatrogenic retinal breaks can also occur as a complication of retinal incarceration in the pars plana incision (see p. 138). Peripheral retinal breaks distant from the meridians of the sclerotomy are infrequent. They may occur in eyes with incomplete posterior vitreous detachment in areas of vitreoretinal lesions, such as lattice degeneration. They are caused by excessive traction on peripheral vitreoretinal attachments.[37] In eyes with incomplete posterior detachment special care should be taken to use low levels of suction force.

Thorough examination of the peripheral fundus is routinely performed immediately after completing the vitrectomy procedure. It is done using the slit lamp and 3-mirror contact lens, with scleral depression, before suturing the sclerotomies. The sclerotomies are temporarily closed with plugs and the infusion cannula is left in place during fundus examination.

Most iatrogenic retinal breaks occur posteriorly to the equator. Retinal breaks inadvertently created by the vitrectomy instrument or scissors are infrequent. Most retinal breaks posterior to the equator result from excessive traction on the retina during delamination of the posterior vitreous face or dissection of epiretinal membranes. Such retinal breaks occur in traction retinal detachment complicating proliferative retinopathies (see p. 277) and retinal detachments complicated by proliferative vitreoretinopathy (see p. 247). In traction retinal detachments complicating proliferative retinopathies, iatrogenic retinal breaks are more likely to occur when traction is exerted on areas of thinned, hypoxic retina. In retinal detachments complicated by proliferative vitreoretinopathy, most iatrogenic retinal breaks occur in the close vicinity of retinal vessels. The break is often very small. An iatrogenic break should be suspected when localized retinal bleeding occurs during dissection of epiretinal membranes. If it is not recognized and treated intraoperatively, the small break will enlarge postoperatively and may result in an intractable detachment.

Management of iatrogenic retinal breaks depends on the location of the break and the presence or absence of persistent vitreoretinal traction on the break.

Peripheral retinal breaks are managed by transscleral cryotreatment, a high segmental scleral buckle, and gas injection. Scleral buckling is required in peripheral breaks because such breaks are under traction of the vitreous base. Breaks located in a retina dragged anteriorly by fibrous ingrowth after penetrating injury of the ciliary region are often difficult to seal permanently, due to persistent vitreoretinal traction. Two rows of cryoapplications that involve at least 3 mm of the retina surrounding the break, and a very high scleral buckle are required in such cases.

Iatrogenic retinal breaks posterior to the equator are managed by intravitreal gas injection and transscleral cryotreatment or argon laser photocoagulation when complete relief of traction on the surrounding retina has been achieved by vitrectomy. Breaks that remain under traction after completion of vitrectomy are supported by a segmental scleral buckle.

Damage to the Inner Retinal Layers. Damage to the internal limiting membrane and inner retinal layers can occur during dissection of epiretinal membranes. It is more likely to occur during membrane delamination and peeling than segmentation. Bleeding of small retinal vessels during membrane peeling is indicative of excessive traction and probable damage to the internal limiting lamina. Damage to the inner retinal layers cannot be seen intraoperatively due to the limits of the instrumentation for intraoperative examination of the retina. Mechanical damage to the internal limiting lamina may play a role in recurrent epiretinal membranes and failure to reattach the retina.

Postoperative Complications

Any of the potential postoperative complications of vitrectomy can occur when the surgical procedure is performed for retinal detachment management. Severe intraocular inflammation, corneal dystrophy, late lens opacification, fibrovascular ingrowth in the sclerotomy wound, and recurrent retinal detachment are the most serious postoperative complications. Associated preoperative and intraoperative factors are likely to play an adjunctive role to the vitrectomy procedure in the development of most postoperative complications. In any given case it is often difficult to determine whether one, several of these factors, or the vitrectomy procedure was the main cause(s) for the development of the postoperative complication(s).

INTRAOCULAR INFLAMMATION

Postoperative intraocular inflammation is frequent. The degree and duration of intraocular inflammation show large variations. In most cases intraocular inflammation is mild; there is moderate flare of the vitreous cavity and the anterior chamber. In a few cases intraocular inflammation is severe with a lenticular exudate in the anterior chamber.

The degree and duration of postoperative intraocular inflammation are correlated with the amount of surgical trauma for retinal detachment management. The vitrectomy procedure is only part of the surgical trauma. Cryotreatment, scleral buckling, and intravitreal gas injection also play a major role in the development of postoperative intraocular inflammation. Severe postoperative intraocular inflammation is more likely to occur after repeated surgery and complicated surgical procedures that include difficult lens removal through the pars plana, lengthy dissection of epiretinal membranes, extensive cryotreatment, and 360° scleral buckling procedures. Intraocular inflammation is more frequent and severe when intraoperative complications occurred.

CORNEAL DYSTROPHY

Corneal dystrophy with recurrent epithelial erosion or permanent corneal edema are infrequent complications after vitrectomy for retinal detachment repair.

Corneal dystrophy with recurrent epithelial erosions has been observed only in diabetic patients. The complication is likely related to the loose adhesion of the corneal epithelium to the basement membrane in diabetic eyes.[24]

Permanent corneal edema due to endothelial cell loss may occur in aphakic and pseudophakic eyes. The potential for severe endothelial cell loss during vitrectomy in phakic and pseudophakic eyes can be minimized by taking specific measures (see p. 259).

LENS OPACIFICATION

Lens opacities, especially nuclear sclerosis, can develop several months or years after vitrectomy for retinal detachment repair. Late nuclear sclerosis following successful retinal reattachment surgery that included a vitrectomy, is more frequent in patients with preexisting lens opacities, patients over 60 years of age, diabetic patients, myopic eyes, and after severe retinal detachments that required complex surgical procedures. Intravitreal gas and vitrectomy are likely to play an important role in the development of late opacification of the lens. The potential for late nuclear sclerosis related to vitrectomy can be minimized by using enriched irrigating solution, minimal amounts of irrigating solution, and leaving the anterior vitreous gel intact.[24]

FIBROVASCULAR INGROWTH

Histopathologic examinations have shown that in experimental models, vitreous strands are almost always adherent to or incarcerated in the internal aspect of pars plana incisions.[38] This provides a scaffold for fibrous ingrowth and may lead to late complications. Histopathologic examinations have shown that some amount of fibrovascular ingrowth from a pars plana sclerotomy is not uncommon.[39-41] However, late complications related to fibrovascular ingrowth from the pars plana wound are very rare in eyes successfully operated on.[39,42] Fibrovascular ingrowth should be suspected when there are dilated subconjunctival vessels in the area surrounding a sclerotomy site. In such eyes the inner surface of the sclerotomy wound should be examined using the 3-mirror contact lens and scleral depression. Significant fibrovascular ingrowth may result in recurrent vitreous hemorrhage or traction retinal detachment. Most cases of fibrovascular ingrowth associated with late complications have been observed in diabetic eyes.[39,42] Fibrovascular ingrowth may be destroyed by cryotreatment using the multiple thaw-freeze cycle technique, however, the value of this treatment remains to be fully demonstrated.[43]

RECURRENT RETINAL DETACHMENT

Recurrent retinal detachment following vitrectomy for retinal detachment repair can relate to three distinct causes: (1) specific clinical characteristics of the initial retinal detachment, (2) improper surgical technique for the procedures associated with the vitrectomy procedure, and (3) complications of the vitrectomy procedure.

Most recurrent retinal detachments related to the initial detachment are due to recurrent proliferative vitreoretinopathy (see p. 251) and a few cases are of unknown pathogenesis.

Recurrent detachments related to improper surgery for the procedures associated with vitrectomy can be caused mainly by improper scleral buckling technique and inability to seal the retinal break(s).

Recurrent detachments directly related to the vitrectomy procedure can be either rhegmatogenous or tractional. Rhegmatogenous retinal detachment can be related to unrecognized iatrogenic retinal breaks, inability to seal a peripheral iatrogenic break (see p. 149), or sequential retinal breaks in areas remaining under traction after vitrectomy. Tractional retinal detachment is caused by either vitreous gel incarceration in the sclerotomy wound (Fig. 120) and subsequent fibrovascular ingrowth, or retinal incarceration in the wound (Fig. 121). Tractional retinal detachment related to incisional complications can be avoided by proper surgical technique (see p. 136).

Most recurrent retinal detachments in vitrectomized eyes spread very rapidly. They are characterized by a large amount of subretinal fluid (Fig. 121).

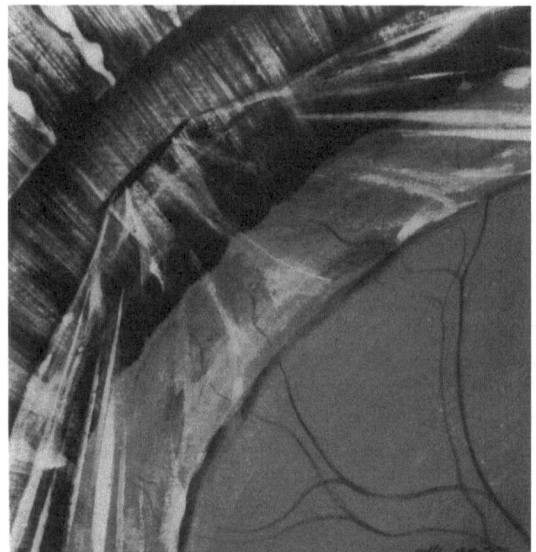

Figure 120. Vitreous gel incarceration into the pars plana sclerotomy has resulted in subsequent traction detachment of the peripheral retina.

This is likely due to the fact that there is no more retinal tamponade by the vitreous gel.

The indications for reoperation are based on the same criteria as in any recurrent detachment, mainly the probability for successful surgery and the condition of the other eye.

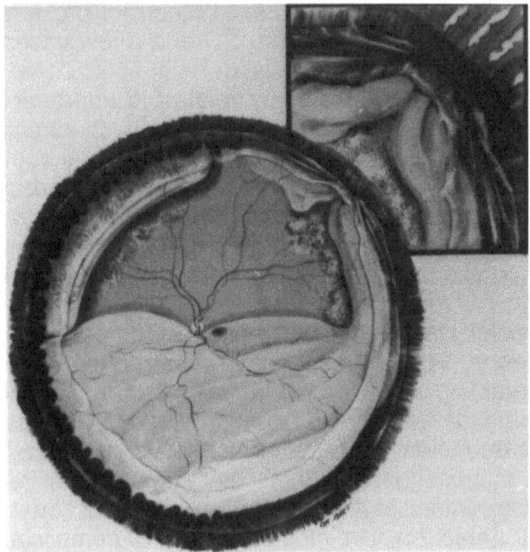

Figure 121. Traction retinal detachment after vitrectomy for retinal detachment repair. Retinal and vitreous gel incarceration into the pars plana sclerotomy has resulted in recurrent retinal detachment.

REFERENCES

1. Von Graefe AV: Ueber Operative Eingriffe in die tieferen Gebilde des Auges. Perforation von abelösten Netzhaüten und Glaskör-per-membranen. Albrecht Von Graefes Arch Klin Ophthalmol 9, 2:85–104, 1863
2. Deutschman R: Ueber ein neues Heilverfahren bei Netzhautahloesung. Cbl Augenheilkd, 176, 1895
3. Gonin J: Le décollement de la rétine. Pathogénie, traitement. Lausanne, Switzerland, Librarie Payot et co, 1934
4. Von Paque W, Meyer-Schwickerath G: Durchschneidung von Glasköerpersträengen bei Netzhautablösung Klin Monatsbl Augenheilkd 142:522–526, 1963
5. Cibis PA: Vitreoretinal pathology and surgery in retinal detachment St Louis, C. V. Mosby Company, 83–86, 1965
6. Machemer R, Parel JM, Buettner H: A new concept for vitreous surgery, 1—Instrumentation. Am J Ophthalmol 73:1–7 1972
7. Klöti R: Vitrectomie. Bull Mem Soc Fr Ophtalmol 86:251–253, 1973
8. Klöti R: Vitrecktomie:Ein neves instrument für die hintere Vitrecktomie. Albrecht von Graefes Arch Klin Ophthalmol 187:161–170, 1973
9. Kreiger AE, Straatsma BR: Stereotaxic vitrectomy. Mod Probl Ophthalmol 10:411–423, 1974
10. Parel JM, Machemer R, Aumayr W: A new concept for vitreous surgery, 4 improvements in instrumentation. Am J Opththalmol 77:6–12, 1974
11. Machemer R: A new concept for vitreous surgery, VII two instrument techniques in pars plana vitrectomy. Arch Ophthalmol 92:407–412, 1974
12. Tolentino F, Banko A, Schepens A, et al: Vitreous surgery: new instrumentation for vitrectomy Arch Ophthalmol 93:667–672, 1975
13. O'Malley C, Heintz RM: Vitrectomy with an alternative instrument system Ann Ophthalmol 7:585–594, 1975
14. Douvas NG: Microsurgical roto-extractor instrument for vitrectomy. Mod Probl Ophthalmol 15:253–260, 1975
15. Freeman HM, Schepens CL, Tolentino F: The current status of vitreous membrane surgery Mod Probl Ophthalmol 15:261–271, 1975
16. Machemer R, Aaberg TH: Vitrectomy, 2d Ed. Orlando FL, Grune & Stratton, 1979
17. Federman JL: The "Site" instrument (suction infusion tissue extractor), in New and controversial aspects in vitreoretinal surgery, McPherson A (Ed) St. Louis, C. V. Mosby, 184–189, 1977
18. Karlin D: Ultrasonic and laser techniques in vitreoretinal surgery. New and controversial aspects, in vitreoretinal surgery, McPherson A (Ed) St. Louis, C. V. Mosby, 274–280, 1977
19. L'Esperance F A: Vitreolysis. Mod Probl Ophthalmol 18:224–235, 1977
20. O'Malley C, Tripp RM, Heintz RM: Recent modifications in closed-eye intraocular surgery, in McPherson, New and controversial aspects of vitreoretinal surgery, edited by McPherson St. Louis, C. V. Mosby, pp 190–194, 1977
21. Spitznas M: New developments in instrumentation for vitreous surgery. Mod Probl Ophthalmol 18:201–204, 1977
22. Limon S, Offret H, Sourdille PH: Chirurgie du vitré. Bull Soc Ophtalmol Fr Annual Report 1978, Marseille, Ed Fueri Lamy, 1978
23. Charles S: Vitreous microsurgery. Baltimore, Williams and Wilkins, 1981
24. Michels RG: Vitreous surgery. St. Louis, C. V. Mosby Company, 1981
25. Peyman GA, Schulman JA: Intravitreal surgery, Principles and practice. Norwalk, Appleton Century Crofts, 1986
26. Escoffery RF, Olk RJ, Grand MG, Boniuk I: Vitrectomy without scleral buckling for primary rhegmatogenous retinal detachment. Am J Ophthalmol 99:275–281, 1985
27. Bonnet M: Indications de la vitrectomie dans le traitement des décollements rétiniens rhegmatogènes. Ophtalmologie 1:95–100, 1987

28. Fournier P, Bonnet M, Aracil P: Décollement rétinien rhegmatogène et déchirures rétiniennes, associés à une hémorragie du vitré. J Fr Ophtalmol 11:7–14, 1988

29. Ehrenberg M, Thresher RJ, Machemer R: Vitreous hemorrhage nontoxic to retina as a stimulator of glial and fibrous proliferation. Am J Ophthalmol 97:611–626, 1984

30. Gonvers M, Machemer R: A new approach to treating retinal detachment with macular hole. Am J Ophthalmol 94:468–472, 1982

31. Machemer R: The importance of fluid absorption, traction, intraocular currents and chorioretinal scars in therapy of rhegmatogenous retinal detachment. Am J Ophthalmol 98:681–693, 1984

32. Mikaye Y: A simplified method of treating retinal detachment with macular hole. Arch Ophthalmol 104:1234–1236, 1986

33. O'Malley C: Collapsing technique for removing vitreous base ocutome. Newsletter 2 (1), 1977

34. O'Malley C: Closed eye endomicrosurgery. Highlights of ophthalmology, Silver anniversary vol. 1, Boyd B (ed), 97–177

35. Michels RG: Vitrectomy techniques in retinal reattachment surgery. Ophthalmology 86:556–585, 1979

36. Hull DS, Chemotti MT, Edelhauser H, et al: Effect of epinephrine on the corneal endothelium. Am J Ophthalmol 79:245–250, 1975

37. Faulborn J, Conway BP, Machemer R: Surgical complications of pars plana vitreous surgery. Ophthalmology 85:116–125, 1978

38. Kreiger AE, Straatsma BR, Griffin JR: Stereotoxic vitrectomy. Mod Probl Ophthal 12:411–423, 1974

39. Kreiger AE, Straatsma BR, Foos RY: Incisional complications in pars plana vitrectomy Mod Probl Ophthal 18:210–223, 1977

40. Tardif Y, Schepens CL: Closed vitreous surgery, XV: fibrovascular ingrowth from the pars plana sclerectomy. Arch Ophthalmol 95:235–239, 1977

41. Tardif Y, Schepens CL, Tolentino FI: Vitreous surgery, XIV: complications from sclerectomy in 89 consecutive cases. Arch Ophthalmol 96:229–234, 1977

42. Bonnet M, Grange JD: Photocoagulation et vitrectomie dans les rétinopathies prolifératives neo-vasculaires. Bull Soc Ophtalmol Fr 11:1399–1406, 1986

43. Bonnet M: Treatment of retinal detachment after penetrating injury: heavy cryotreatment of the fibrous ingrowth remnants as an adjunct to vitreoretinal microsurgery Ophthalmologica 194:164–168, 1987

IV

Types of Retinal Detachment: Clinical Characteristics and Surgical Management

14

Retinal Detachment with Horseshoe Tears

The vast majority (approximately 85%) of primary rhegmatogenous retinal detachments are associated with horseshoe tears of the peripheral retina. Primary retinal detachments with horseshoe tears are a specific clinical entity that should be distinguished from retinal detachments due to atrophic holes and oral disinsertion. The major difference between the two groups is related to the fact that retinal detachments with horseshoe tears are always associated with some degree of vitreous pathology, whereas the vitreous body is normal or nearly normal in primary detachments due to atrophic holes and desinsertion at the ora serrata. Horseshoe tears are always due to vitreous traction, whereas primary retinal holes and dialyses are due to localized retinal lesions.

Nontraumatic retinal detachments with horseshoe tears have a more guarded surgical prognosis than that of detachments due to atrophic holes and oral desinsertion. Their surgical management may involve specific difficulties and, most importantly, the course of the disease may be complicated by the development of proliferative vitreoretinopathy.

ETIOLOGY

Myopia, aphakia, and the aging process are the three main predisposing factors to retinal detachments with horseshoe tears. Retinal detachments with horseshoe tears related to other predisposing factors are significantly less common.

Myopia

The important role of myopia in the development of primary rhegmatogenous retinal detachment has been well established.[1,2] In the Caucasian population, the incidence of myopia varies between 5% and 18%.[3] In the population of patients affected by primary retinal detachment, the incidence of myopia varies between 42%[1] and 46%.[4] Retinal detachments due to horseshoe tears of the peripheral retina account for approximately 63% of all primary rhegmatogenous retinal detachments in myopic patients.[5] Thirty-two of such patients have myopia lower than − 8 diopters spherical equivalent and 68% have myopia greater than 8 diopters.[5] Approximately 40% of the myopic patients with retinal detachment due to horseshoe tear(s) of the peripheral retina experience bilateral retinal detachment.[5] Patient ages range from less than 10 years to over 80 years. However most cases (75%) are observed in patients between 30 and 60 years of age.[5] Males account for 59% and females for 41% of the myopic patients affected with retinal detachment due to horseshoe tears

Aphakia

The important role of aphakia in the development of primary rhegmatogenous retinal detachment has been well established.[1,2,6–10] The proportion of aphakia found among patients with retinal detachment varies from 27%[4] to 42.7%.[6] The increasing life expectancy of the general population and the rising number of cataract extractions may account for the greater proportion of aphakia found among patients with retinal detachment in recent studies.[6,10]

Approximately 95%[4] of nontraumatic retinal detachments in aphakic eyes are associated with horseshoe tears. The mean age of patients with aphakic detachments is approximately 66 years.[1–6] The incidence of bilateral retinal detachment in bilateral aphakic patients observed for many years ranges from 36.8%[51] to 48%.[4]

Aging Process

The aging process accounts for approximately 30% of primary rhegmatogenous retinal detachments. The overwhelming majority of senile retinal detachments are associated with horseshoe tears that develop at the time of senile posterior vitreous detachment.

Uncommon Causes

Retinal detachments with horseshoe tears have been observed in eyes with previous peripheral uveitis and, as a late complication, in cicatricial retinopathy of prematurity. They are a common complication of congenital ectopia lentis. Infrequent hereditary vitreoretinal degenerations, such as Wagner's disease, are associated with a high incidence of retinal detachments with horseshoe tears.

Trauma

Horseshoe tears can develop after penetrating injury (see p. 289) or blunt trauma of the eye. Blunt trauma can produce horseshoe tears in emmetropic eyes with abnormal vitreoretinal adhesions. The horseshoe tears develop along abnormal posterior extensions of the vitreous base or at the posterior border of a meridional fold.[11] Horseshoe tears secondary to blunt trauma in healthy eyes are most uncommon as compared to oral dialysis with avulsion of the vitreous base.

Blunt trauma can also induce the formation of horseshoe tears in predisposed eyes.

CLINICAL CHARACTERISTICS

Retinal detachments with horseshoe tears have specific clinical characteristics. These specific clinical features are related to the constant association of some degree of vitreous liquefaction and posterior vitreous detachment.

In addition, retinal detachments with horseshoe tears may be complicated by proliferative vitreoretinopathy.

In the present chapter only clinical features of retinal detachments without proliferative vitreoretinopathy are dealt with. Retinal detachments associated with proliferative vitreoretinopathy are dealt with in chapter 20, (see p. 231).

Visual Symptoms

Most retinal detachments due to horseshoe tears show an acute onset. Light flashes, vitreous floaters, and sudden visual field defect are reported by most patients. Flashes indicate localized traction on the retina by the vitreous gel and accompany the formation of the horseshoe tears. They are often localized in one quadrant, which is opposite to the retinal quadrant where the horseshoe tear is situated. Vitreous floaters result from sudden posterior vitreous detachment that may be associated with vitreous hemorrhage. The visual field defect is due to the retinal detachment. All visual symptoms may develop either almost simultaneously or in a two step sequence. In the latter circumstance, the retinal detachment develop a few days, or less commonly, weeks after the posterior vitreous detachment and formation of horseshoe tears.

The localization of light flashes and the initial visual field defect are indicative of the area of the fundus where the retinal detachment has begun and at least one horseshoe tear is present. However these clinical signs have little value in terms of the management because additional tears may be present in other retinal quadrants and must be treated as well as the tear(s) located in the detached retina.

The progression of the visual field defect and the subsequent loss of the central vision are rapid in most retinal detachments with horseshoe tears. There is, however, a wide range of variations in the extent and progression of the visual defects with clinical cases. These variations are related to two main parameters: (1) the characteristics of the horseshoe tears and (2) the associated vitreous pathology.

— The location, size and number of horseshoe tears greatly influence the onset and extension of the retinal detachment and the visual defect. For example, most nontraumatic retinal detachments due to horseshoe tears located in the superior quadrants extend rapidly and involve the macula after a few days. In contrast detachments due to horseshoe tears located in the inferior quadrants often extend more slowly and loss of central vision may occur after several weeks.

— The progression and extent of the retinal detachment and visual field defect are greatly dependent on the associated lesions of the vitreous gel. The extent and severity of vitreous liquefaction and posterior vitreous detachment are determining factors in the progression of the retinal detachment. Most retinal detachments due to superior tears progress rapidly and become bullous because due to vitreous liquefaction and posterior vitreous detachment, there is no more tamponade of the superior retina by viscous vitreous. In contrast, many retinal detachments due to inferior tears extend rather slowly because the vitreous gel, which is collapsed within the lower part of the vitreous cavity acts as a tamponade on the lower retina and horseshoe tear(s). In eyes with extensive vitreous gel liquefaction, there is no retinal tamponade by viscous vitreous gel in the lower quadrants, and retinal detachment with inferior horseshoe tears spreads quite rapidly. In retinal detachments of recent onset, the extent of the visual field defect is one of the clinical features that reflects the severity of the vitreoretinal disease. The more rapid and extensive the visual field defect, the more severe the vitreoretinal disease. Eyes with retinal detachments due to horseshoe tears that still have normal central vision are considered as emergency cases that should be operated on very shortly before the macula become detached. Conservation of normal central vision is the reason for most rapid surgical management. However, the surgeon and the patient should be aware that early surgery applied to eyes with a macula still attached does not always guarantee conservation of normal central vision after retinal detachment repair. Conservation or restoration of a visual acuity equal to the visual acuity before the occurrence of retinal detachment depends on several parameters. A macula preoperatively attached is only one of those parameters and does not exclude the role of the other parameters. Postoperative macular complications, such as cystoid macular edema and macular pucker, may develop in eyes with a macula preoperatively attached. Therefore, the patient should be informed of the potential macular complications that may develop postoperatively, so as to avoid disappointment or law suits.

RETINAL DETACHMENT

Clinical Characteristics. Most nontraumatic retinal detachments with horseshoe tears that extend beyond the equator exhibit retinal folds. The retinal folds are mobile; they move freely with eye movements. Retinal fold mobility indicates that the retinal detachment is not associated with preretinal proliferation. The retinal folds are related to the absence of retinal tamponade by the vitreous gel that is most often deeply altered in front of the detached retina. Conversely, the height of the detachment is indicative of the degree of vitreous gel degeneration. Eyes with bullous detachment of the superior retina have extensive posterior vitreous detachment or vitreous liquefaction in the corresponding area.

In contrast, the infrequent superior detachments with horseshoe tears that develop after blunt trauma in otherwise healthy eyes do not exhibit retinal folds and remain rather shallow in most cases. These clinical features are indicative of a limited posterior detachment of the vitreous gel that remains normally viscous. Surgical management of such detachments is easy, regardless of the tear size, and prognosis for retinal reattachment is excellent in most cases. In contrast surgical management of nontraumatic bullous detachments may involve specific difficulties related to the detachment height.

Location and Extent of the Detachment. With regard to the clinical value of the location and extent of the detachment, one should distinguish detachments of recent onset from detachments that have been present for a month or more.

The location and extent of recent onset detachments associated with horseshoe tears depend on two parameters: (1) the location and number of tears and (2) the extent and degree of vitreous syneresis and posterior vitreous detachment. The latter parameter is the most important with regard to the extent of the detachment.

Guidelines have been given to localize the retinal tears according to the localization and extent of the detachment[2] (see p. 12). However, in recent onset detachments, these guidelines are of questionable value with regard to the treatment, since retinal tears may be present in attached retina.

When the retinal detachment is limited to one upper quadrant, this indicates that there is at least one tear located in the corresponding quadrant and that significant posterior vitreous detachment may be limited to this quadrant. However, careful examination of the entire fundus should be performed, since additional tears may be present in areas of attached retina. A recent onset detachment involving three or more quadrants often indicates that there are multiple tears in two or more quadrants. In eyes with extensive vitreous liquefaction, however, a retinal detachment due to a single horseshoe tear can spread to three quadrants within a few days.

A retinal detachment due to a single retinal tear, or group of small tears located in the same quadrant, may remain unnoticed or be neglected by the patient for weeks. Longstanding detachments due to a tiny horseshoe tear are common in aphakic eyes, particularly in elderly patients. In spite of the extensive detachment commonly present at initial presentation, there is no clinical evidence of proliferative vitreoretinopathy, and retinal reattachment can be achieved by localized surgery, limited to the small horseshoe tear(s). Because the tiny tear(s) may be difficult to disclose, some retina surgeons manage such eyes with cryoapplications on 360° of the peripheral retina and a 360° scleral buckling procedure.

Such heavy surgery is unnecessary to achieve permanent retinal reattachment. It may be associated with rather disappointing visual results due to excessive surgical trauma. In addition a 360° cryo and scleral buckling procedure may fail to reattach the retina when the tear is not sealed. Therefore, preoperative identification of the tiny tear(s) is most important. Preoperative examination using the surgical microscope (see p. 11) is helpful in difficult cases. In addition there are guidelines[2,12,13] that are useful in determining what part(s) of the peripheral fundus the retinal tear(s) should be searched for with the most tenacity. In most cases, the position of the retinal tear can be deduced from the shape of the detachment because subretinal fluid spreads in a predictable manner[12] (see p. 12).

A tiny horseshoe tear located in a lower quadrant may result in a gradual spread of subretinal fluid.[14] In such eyes the detachment is frequently recognized only when subretinal fluid reaches the macula. Such detachments exhibit signs of long duration. A tiny horseshoe tear located in an upper quadrant, although rarely, may result in a localized detachment of the same quadrant that remains subclinical for an extended period of time. The detachment remains subclinical, probably because posterior vitreous detachment is limited and retinal tamponare by viscous vitreous prevents subretinal fluid spread. Such detachments are often recognized at a later stage, when further extension of posterior vitreous detachment is followed by rapid subretinal fluid spread. In such cases fundus examination shows that the detachment consists of two distinct parts. The peripheral part of the detachment in the vicinity of the small tear exhibits signs of long duration. In contrast the posterior part of the detachment shows no sign of long duration. Such two-step detachments may be misinterpreted as retinal detachments complicating a retinoschisis (see p. 265).

Detachment of the Pars Plana Epithelium. Detachment of the nonpigmented epithelium of the pars plana is common in giant tears (see p. 197) and severe proliferative vitreoretinopathy (see p. 237). It may also be observed in mobile detachments with small horseshoe tears. It indicates a marked contraction of the vitreous base. Scleral buckling of the vitreous base is indicated in the management of such detachments.

Macular Detachment. Macular detachment is present at initial presentation in less than 50% of recent detachments due to horseshoe tears. Macular detachment is more frequent in aphakic eyes as compared to phakic eyes[1] and in eyes with horseshoe tears in the upper temporal quadrant. Surgery should be carried out as soon as possible in eyes with an attached macula to prevent extension of the detachment to the macula. Surgical management should also be considered as an emergency in eyes with a macular detachment of less than a week's duration.

Postoperative recovery of useful, or even normal, central vision may still be achieved in eyes with macular detachment of less than a week's duration.

Preoperative macular detachment is, by far, not, the only parameter that allows to predict the visual outcome after retinal reattachment. Macular complications, particularly cystoid macular edema and macular pucker, may develop postoperatively, regardless of preoperative macula status.

RETINAL TEARS

Site. Horseshoe retinal tears may be located in the equatorial region or the oral region. Equatorial horseshoe tears are much more common than oral horseshoe tears.

Equatorial Horseshoe Tears. Many equatorial horse-shoe tears are not related to any equatorial degeneration detectable by clinical examination. Approximately 38%[15] of horseshoe retinal tears develop along the posterior margin or at the extremity of an island of lattice degeneration (Fig. 122). The island of lattice degeneration may also be entirely within the flap. Equatorial horseshoe tears related to lattice degeneration are much more common in

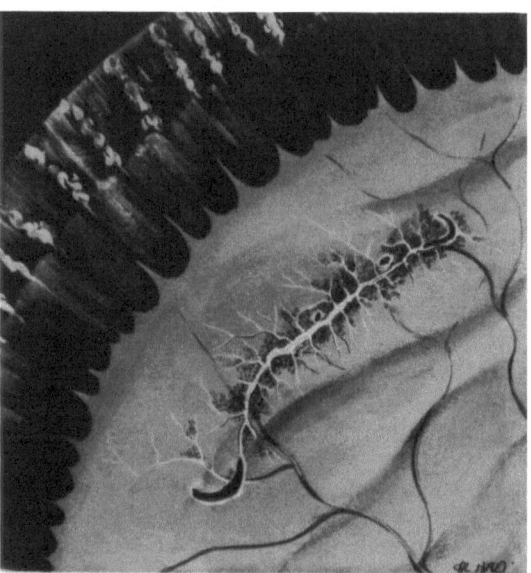

Figure 122. Horseshoe tears at both extremities of an island of lattice degeneration. Small holes are also present within the island of lattice degeneration.

phakic retinal detachments than in aphakic retinal detachments. According to Morse[15] 73% of retinal tears related to lattice degeneration are observed in phakic retinal detachments and 27% in aphakic retinal detachments.

Horseshoe tears related to lattice degeneration are significantly more common in the temporal than nasal quadrants. They are more frequent in the upper than lower quadrants.

Patients with retinal tears related to lattice have a younger age range than the nonlattice detachment patients. The average age of lattice retinal detachment patients is 51 years as compared to 62 years for the nonlattice detachment patients.[15] Twenty-four percent of patients with lattice retinal detachment are less than 40 years old with an average of 25.5 years.[15]

Approximately 25% of myopic eyes with retinal detachment and horseshoe tears related to lattice degeneration, also have small holes in lattice degeneration.[5]

The role of predisposing lesions to retinal tears, and particularly the role of lattice degeneration has been extensively studied,[1,2,15–19] and has brought about most useful information for selection of the indications for prophylactic treatment. However, in eyes that have already developed retinal detachment, the presence or absence of predisposing vitreo retinal degeneration has little clinical value in terms of preoperative evaluation and surgical management of the retinal detachment. Indeed retinal detachments with horseshoe tear(s) related to islands of lattice degeneration may also show additional retinal tears in areas without any detectable predisposing lesion. Therefore, thorough examination of the entire peripheral fundus must be performed in retinal detachments with horseshoe tears related to lattice, as in any rhegmatogenous retinal detachment. Eyes with lattice degeneration may develop retinal detachment with horseshoe tears that are distant from the islands of lattice degeneration. The approach for surgical management of the retinal tear(s) does not depend on the presence or absence of lattice degeneration in the area of the retinal tear(s). In addition islands of equatorial degeneration without retinal tear will not be subjected to any treatment.

Tractional retinal tears of the equatorial region may occasionally develop on cystic retinal tufts. Approximately 7% of phakic nontraumatic retinal detachments are related to tractional tears on cystic tufts.[18] Full-thickness retinal breaks associated with cystic retinal tufts are invariably of tractional origin. Two types of retinal tears related to cystic retinal tufts can be observed: (1) small horseshoe or crescent-shaped flap tears, which are the most frequent and (2) round tears with a free operculum. The cystic retinal tuft is present in the flap or the free operculum torn from the retina.

Oral Retinal Tears. Horseshoe retinal tears of the oral region are much less common than equatorial horseshoe tears. They are more frequent in aphakic than phakic retinal detachments. They are invariably very small. Oral horseshoe tears include two distinct groups: (1) tears related to anatomical variations of the ora serrata and (2) tears along the posterior edge of the vitreous base.

Horseshoe Tears Related to Anatomical Variations of the Ora Serrata. Horseshoe tears related to anatomical variations of the oral region are infrequent. They are generally observed in young individuals, usually very small, and often multiple. Horseshoe tears may be related to meridional folds or islands of granular tissue or cystic tufts. Vitreous traction on meridional folds may result in a crescentic tear at the posterior edge of the meridional fold (Fig. 123) or linear tear(s) along one or both sides of the fold. Most tears related to meridional folds are located in the nasal quadrants with a predilection for the upper nasal quadrant. Small horseshoe tears related to meridional folds are uncommon in the temporal quadrants. Approximately 10% of eyes with retinal detachment show unusual meridional folds.[2] However, the proportion of retinal detachments with tears related to meridional folds is less than 2%.

Vitreous traction on a cystic tuft may result in a small horseshoe or operculated tear. The granular tissue is present in the flap or the opeculum. The retinal tear is very small.

Horseshoe Tears at the Posterior Edge of the Vitreous Base. Most oral horseshoe tears are lo-

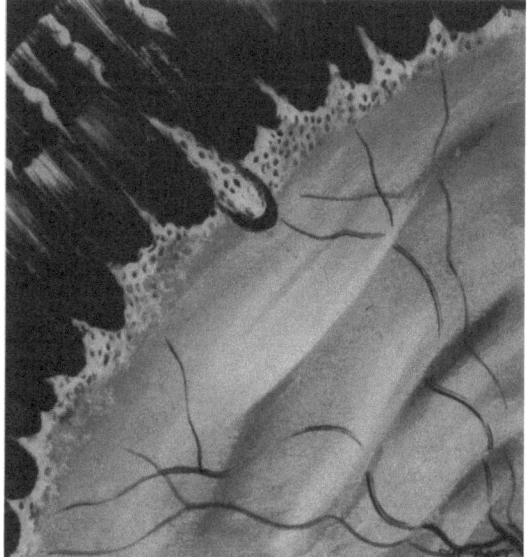

Figure 123. Small crescentic tear at the posterior edge of a meridional fold.

cated at the posterior edge of the vitreous base. The distance between the ora serrata and the tears varies, according to individual and age related variations in the situation of the vitreous base posterior edge. Horseshoe tears along the posterior edge of the vitreous base are more frequent in aphakic retinal detachments, invariably, very small, and often multiple (Fig. 124). They may be located in any retinal quadrant. The base of the small retinal flap is often continuous with a circular retinal fold that is adjacent to the posterior border of the vitreous base.

Associated Features of Clinical Significance. Associated features of clinical significance with regard to surgical management and prognosis include: (1) the retinal tear(s) size(s), (2) the number of retinal tears, (3) the number of quadrants involved by the retinal tears, (4) the clinical characteristics of the retinal tear flap, (5) the presence of a bridging vessel, and (6) the configuration of the posterior edge of the retinal tear(s).

Retinal Tear Size. Horseshoe retinal tears exhibit a wide range of variation in their size. They may be tiny or involve more than 180° of the eye circumference. Very small horseshoe tears may be difficult to identify, but their surgical management is easy in most cases. In contrast, large horseshoe tears are easy to identify, but their surgical management may involve technical difficulties.

Surgical management of retinal detachments as-

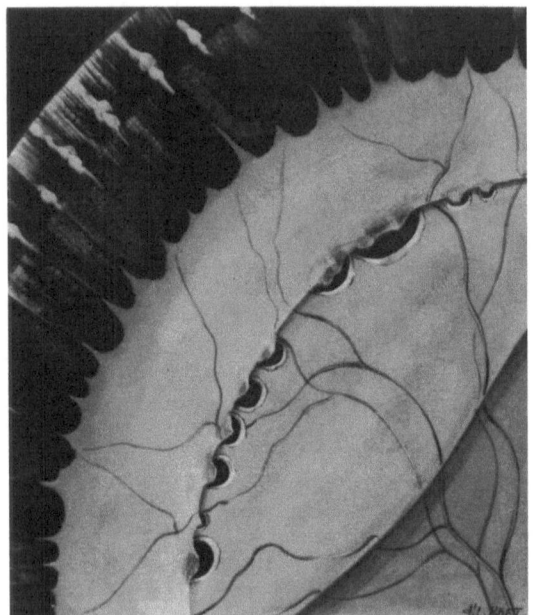

Figure 124. Multiple small horseshoe tears at the posterior edge of the vitreous base in an aphakic and myopic eye.

sociated with large horseshoe tears is fraught with two potential problems: (1) development or proliferative vitreoretinopathy and (2) mechanical difficulties to adequately seal the retinal tears. As a rule, the larger the horseshoe tears, the more complex the surgical management and the more guarded the prognosis. Difficulties that may be encountered to adequately seal large horseshoe tears are related to the size of the scleral buckles required and the frequent development of the fishmouth phenomenon. The guarded surgical prognosis is related to the potential for development of proliferative vitreoretinopathy postoperatively. The larger a horseshoe tear, the higher the risk of postoperative proliferative vitreoretinopathy (see p. 233).

Number of Retinal Tears. The number of retinal tears is one parameter of the severity of the retinal detachment. Most retinal detachments associated with a single horseshoe tear, that is less than 70° in size, have a good prognosis. In contrast, retinal detachments associated with multiple horseshoe tears have a more guarded prognosis. Inability to adequately seal all retinal tears, as well as severe and extensive vitreoretinal pathology responsible for the multiple horseshoe tears account for the guarded prognosis.

Retinal detachments associated with multiple horseshoe tears are more frequent than retinal detachments with a single horseshoe tear. In a unilateral nontraumatic retinal detachment series, which include cases of reoperation, Schepens and Marden[3] found a single retinal break in 27% of eyes, and multiple retinal breaks in 73%. In a recent series of retinal detachments,[20] from which giant tears and cases of reoperation were excluded, we found a single horseshoe tear in 30% of eyes and multiple tears in 70%. The number of multiple horseshoe tears ranged from 2 to 18.

The high incidence of retinal detachments with multiple horseshoe tears should be kept in mind to avoid unpardonable failures due to a missed retinal tear.

Number of Quadrants Involved by the Tears. In eyes with multiple horseshoe tears, the number of retinal quadrants involved by the tears is not by itself an important parameter for the prognosis, however this parameter will influence the choice of the surgical procedure.

As a rule, multiple horseshoe tears that are close to each other in the same quadrantic area, will be easier to manage surgically than multiple tears scattered in all four quadrants. Multiple retinal tears close to each others can be managed by segmental scleral buckling, whereas a 360° scleral buckling procedure is required in most eyes with multiple tears in all four quadrants.

Most retinal detachments with multiple horseshoe tears located above the horizontal meridian are easier to manage compared to retinal detachments with multiple tears in the inferior quadrants. In the former instance segmental scleral buckling and retinal tamponade with a relatively small gas bubble can provide retinal reattachment. In contrast, management of retinal detachments with multiple horseshoe tears in the lower quadrants may require high scleral buckling of the inferior tears or retinal tamponade with a gas bubble of more than half of the vitreous cavity volume.

Clinical Characteristics of the Tear Flap. When the flap has been torn away from the retinal tear and has become an operculum moving with the detached posterior vitreous cortex, the retinal tear is no longer under vitreous traction (Fig. 125).

Most horseshoe tears with an anterior flap remain under vitreous traction. Traction may be dynamic and related to the movements of the vitreous gel induced by rotation of the eye. Traction may be static and related to vitreous contraction.

A retinal flap under dynamic vitreous traction is usually slightly elevated. It shows slight movements induced by eye rotation. Dynamic vitreous traction on the anterior flap is common in equatorial horseshoe tears, in particular horseshoe tears related to lattice degeneration. Vitreous strands attached to the tear flap are visible in most cases. They are thin and show undulating movements with eye movements.

A retinal flap under static vitreous traction is usually significantly elevated. Its torn edge is pulled toward the anterior part of the vitreous cavity. Most often the flap is significantly smaller in size than the area of pigment epithelial cells exposed by the retinal tear (Fig. 126). The flap position is not modified by eye movements. Most horseshoe tears with a flap under static vitreous traction are located at the posterior edge of the vitreous base. The everted anterior flap may be associated with a rolled over and fixed posterior edge of the retinal tear. Such clinical findings are indicative of gradual contraction of the vitreous base and impending proliferative vitreoretinopathy (see p. 233).

Characteristics of the Posterior Edge of the Retinal Tear. Characteristics of the posterior edge of the retinal tear is one of the most important clinical findings with regard to the potential for severe proliferative vitreoretinopathy (see p. 233).

Horseshoe tears with a posterior edge rolled over and stuck to the underlying detached retina (Fig. 126) indicate that retinal detachment is already complicated by epiretinal membrane formation.

A rolled over and fixed posterior edge must be

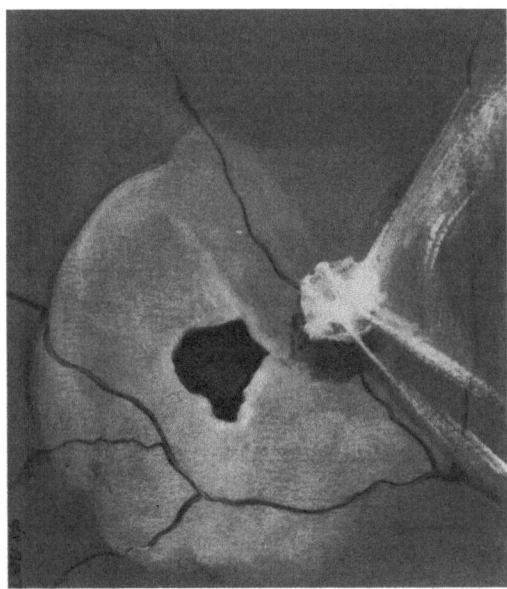

Figure 125. Operculated retinal tear. The tear flap has been torn away from the retina remaining adherent to the detached posterior vitreous cortex. The retina is no longer under traction. The retinal detachment is limited and shallow in spite of posterior vitreous detachment.

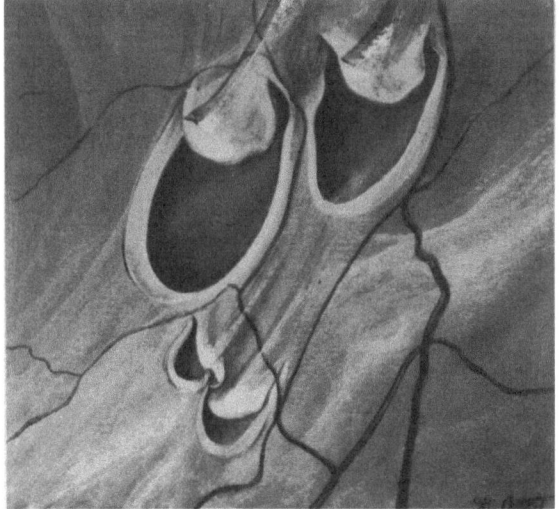

Figure 126. Group of horseshoe tears with a curled and fixed posterior edge. In addition, the anterior flaps are smaller in size than the area of exposed pigment epithelial cells. The anterior flaps are pulled towards the anterior part of the vitreous cavity by condensed vitreous strands. (Courtesy of BONNET M., Graefe's Arch Clin Exp Ophthalmol 226:201–205, 1988).

differenciated from a posterior edge, which is merely inverted towards the vitreous cavity and remains mobile. Large horseshoe tears that are located in the upper quadrants often show an inverted posterior edge. The inverted posterior edge remains mobile, however, and there is a free space between the inverted edge and the underlying detached retina. Such features are not indicative of incipient proliferative vitreoretinopathy. They are merely related to the large retinal tear size, are gravity dependent, and are also indicative of significant vitreous liquefaction and posterior vitreous detachment.

Horseshoe Tears with Bridging Vessels. Horseshoe retinal tears may be associated with one or, less commonly, several bridging vessels (Fig. 127). Most tears with bridging vessels are located in the equatorial region. The bridging vessel(s) may be partially torn and bleed. In such eyes the retinal detachment is associated with vitreous hemorrhage of variable degree. A bridging vessel may also cause recurrent vitreous hemorrhages in eyes with a retina that has been permanently reattached surgically.

VITREOUS BODY STATUS

Preoperative evaluation of retinal detachments with horseshoe tears must include thorough biomicroscopic examination of the vitreous body. Vitreous gel liquefaction and posterior vitreous detachment, as well as vitreous hemorrhage, are important clinical features with regard to surgical management and prognosis.

Vitreous Gel Liquefaction and Posterior Vitreous Detachment. Some degree of vitreous gel liquefaction and posterior vitreous detachment are constant clinical findings in eyes with nontraumatic horseshoe tears. There are, however, large variations in the degree and extent of both changes. Vitreous gel liquefaction and posterior vitreous detachment may be limited to the quadrant or area of the retinal tear, or may involve two or more quadrants (Fig. 128).

Total posterior vitreous detachment with collapse is most common in senile retinal detachments. The prognosis for permanent retinal reattachment after surgical repair is good in most cases.

In contrast, nontraumatic retinal detachments with horseshoe tear(s) and incomplete posterior vitreous detachment have a more guarded prognosis. Development of proliferative vitreoretinopathy postoperatively and sequential horseshoe tears are more frequent in such eyes. Incomplete posterior vitreous detachment is more common in highly myopic eyes and young patients. It is also more common in eyes with retinal tears which exhibit a curled and fixed posterior edge.[20]

The actual extent of posterior vitreous detachment may be difficult to determine in eyes with extensive vitreous gel liquefaction, such as highly myopic eyes. In the areas of large lacunae of the posterior vitreous body a thin layer of vitreous cortex is adherent to the retina and is clinically invisible in most eyes. Therefore, large lacunae due to vitreous liquefaction may be misinterpreted as areas of posterior vitreous detachment. At present there are no clinical tools to identify with certainty a thin layer of vitreous cortex remaining adherent to the internal limiting membrane in eyes with extensive vitreous gel liquefaction and incomplete posterior vitreous detachment. Clinical data obtained using the clinical means presently available, suggest that eyes with extensive vitreous gel liquefaction and incomplete posterior vitreous detachment are at an increased risk of recurrent retinal detachment due to postoperative proliferative vitreoretinopathy or sequential horseshoe tears. Sequential horseshoe tears and recurrent retinal detachment may develop days, weeks, or years later.

In most eyes the posterior edge of horseshoe tears is free from any vitreoretinal adhesion. The vitreoretinal adhesions that are responsible for the horseshoe tear formation are located on the anterior flap of the tear. They are easily identified by biomicroscopic examination with the 3-mirror contact lens.

In horseshoe tears with a curled and fixed posterior

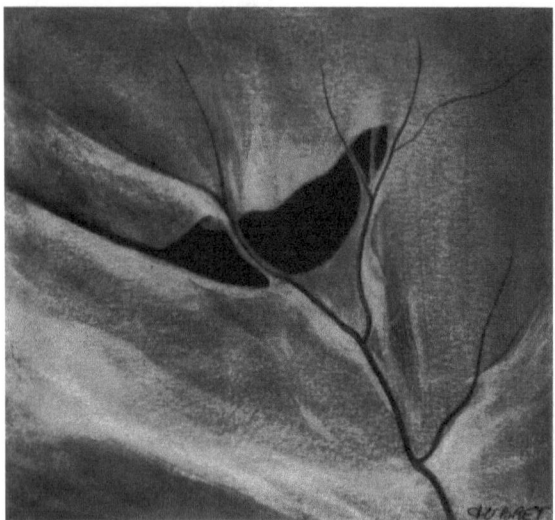

Figure 127. Horseshoe tear of the equatorial region with two bridging vessels. A vortex vein ampulla is visible through the exposed pigment epithelium. The tear posterior edge is neither inverted nor curled. The tear anterior flap is slightly elevated and mobile (Courtesy of BONNET M., Graefe's Arch Clin Exp Ophthalmol 226:201–205, 1988).

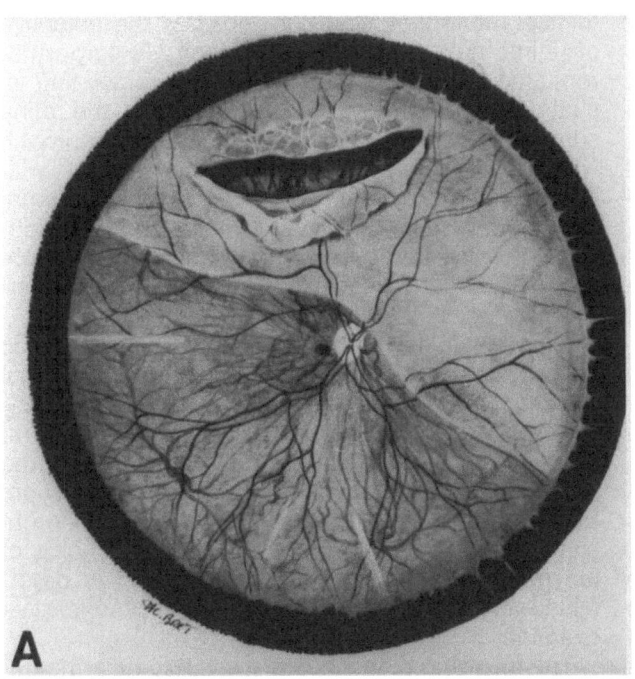
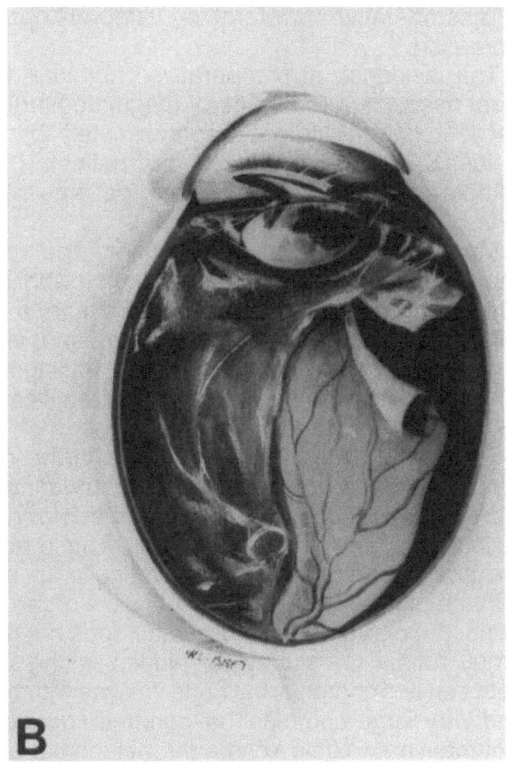

Figure 128. Retinal detachment associated with a large horseshoe tear in a myopic eye. (A) A large horseshoe tear developed at the posterior edge of an island of lattice degeneration. Owing to its large size, superior site, and association of posterior vitreous detachment, the tear shows an inverted posterior edge, however, the inverted retina is mobile. (B) Cross-section of the vitreous cavity. Retinal detachment is associated with posterior vitreous detachment. Owing to lack of retinal tamponade by viscous vitreous gel, the tear posterior edge is inverted.

edge, the membrane that sticks the inverted edge and the underlying retina together may be remnants of the cortical vitreous[2] rather than a newformed membrane due to pigment epithelial cell proliferation.

Vitreous Hemorrhage. Vitreous hemorrhage is most common in retinal detachments with horseshoe tears (approximately 25% of the eyes).[1] Bleeding occurs at the time of acute posterior vitreous detachment and retinal tear formation.

In most eyes the vitreous hemorrhage is minimal and does not interfere with detailed examination of the retina. In such eyes the presence of intravitreal blood will not modify the therapeutic approach for retinal detachment management.

Mild vitreous hemorrhages which are sufficient to prevent accurate examination of the inferior retina are uncommon in nontraumatic retinal detachments. In most cases intravitreal blood does not prevent identification of the retinal tear(s) because the tears are nearly always located in the upper quadrants,[2–3] and therefore, retinal detachment can be managed merely by scleral buckling. However, severe

proliferative vitreoretinopathy is more likely to develop postoperatively in eyes with vitreous hemorrhage.[20, 23] In addition, signs of moderate proliferative vitreoretinopathy are more common preoperatively in eyes with vitreous hemorrhage. The indications for vitrectomy, as part of the initial operation, are more frequent in eyes with mild vitreous hemorrhage compared to eyes with discrete or no vitreous hemorrhage.

Massive vitreous hemorrhage that prevents fundus examination and identification of the retinal tear(s) is most infrequent in nontraumatic retinal detachments (less than 1%).[23–24] Surgery should not be delayed. Vitrectomy is indicated and will be performed as the first step of the operation.

PREOPERATIVE CHOROIDAL DETACHMENT

Choroidal detachment present before any surgery for retinal reattachment is a sign of poor prognosis. Choroidal detachment will make surgical management of the retinal detachment uneasy, and the risk of postoperative proliferative vitreoretinopathy is increased.[25]

The incidence of preoperative choroidal detachment associated with primary rhegmatogenous retinal detachment is low. It is approximately 2%.[25] The incidence is increased in aphakic patients (3%) as compared to phakic (1.3%)[1] and patients who are over 60 years of age.

Most eyes with preoperative choroidal detachment show marked intraocular inflammation and severe hypotony. Folds in descemet's membrane, poor pupillary dilation, posterior synechiae, and vitreous body haziness are constant clinical findings. They make fundus examination difficult. Identification of all retinal tears may be arduous.

There are large clinical variations in the degree and extent of choroidal detachment. The most common and conspicuous variety is in the form of large balloons in three or four quadrants. These balloons are smooth and the overlying retina is in contact with the pigment epithelium. At the site of the vortex veins, the choroid is anchored and does not detach. Small retinal tears may be hidden in the valleys between two choroidal balloons. In eyes with a single and very large choroidal balloon, the choroidal detachment may mimic a choroidal melanoma. Ultrasonography allows differential diagnosis. The choroidal detachment may be limited to the region just posterior to the ora serrata and escape notice. However, severe hypotony associated with the detachment should alert the observer. Hypotony is due to detachment of the ciliary body, which is constant.

As a rule surgical management should be postponed for a few days in patients with choroidal detachment. During this period of time, corticosteroids are administered topically and systemically. The period of time for medical preparation should not exceed a few days owing to the risk of severe proliferative vitreoretinopathy. In eyes with extensive and bullous choroidal detachment that does not respond to corticosteroids, subchoroidal fluid should be drained off. Surgery for retinal detachment repair is performed at the same operation.

SURGICAL MANAGEMENT

Current surgical techniques make it possible to achieve permanent retinal reattachment in most eyes with mobile retinal detachments due to horseshoe tears. In a large series of retinal detachments operated on by experienced retina surgeons, the anatomical success rate is approximately the same regardless of the specific surgical approach

used by each surgeon.[26–29] A few cases, however, still fail to reattach with a single operation. In addition, restoration of useful vision, rather than solely anatomical reattachment of the retina, is the objective of retinal detachment repair. Excessive surgery or repeated operations may result in disappointing visual results. Therefore, in any given case, the retina surgeon should determine which surgical approach will provide the highest anatomical success rate with a single operation and the least surgical trauma. In most cases the operative protocol can be established preoperatively. In only a few cases, the preoperative protocol has to be modified according to operative findings.

In mobile retinal detachments, permanent sealing of the retinal tear(s) is the only goal of surgery, but requires that three objectives be fulfilled: (1) inducement of a retinochoroidal scar in the retinal tear(s) area, (2) approximation of the retinal tear to the pigment epithelium, and (3) relief of vitreous traction. Each of these objectives can be achieved by different surgical approaches. In any given case, choice of the most appropriate surgical approach is determined according to clinical findings at preoperative examination.

The following guidelines are given to help the beginner. These guidelines are related to four distinct groups of preoperative clinical findings: (1) the retinal detachment, (2) the retinal tears, (3) the vitreous body changes, and (4) the association of a choroidal detachment.

Retinal Detachment

Subretinal fluid is the clinical finding that makes surgical management mandatory. However, the extent, location, and height of a mobile detachment are the least relevant parameters in the choice of the surgical technique. There are only two clinical features related to the detached retina that should be taken into account when establishing the operative protocol: (1) bullous detachment of the superior retina, and (2) detachment of the pars plana epithelium.

BULLOUS DETACHMENT OF THE SUPERIOR RETINA

Release of subretinal fluid may be required to carry out efficient and accurate cryotreatment of the retinal tears (see p. 671).

In most eyes intravitreal gas injection will be necessary to achieve apposition of the retinal tear and pigment epithelium.

DETACHMENT OF THE PARS PLANA EPITHELIUM

Scleral buckling of the retinal tears should be associated with circumferential scleral buckling to counteract ring contraction of the vitreous base.

If vitrectomy is indicated, the pars plana incisions should be performed in the quadrants where the pars plana epithelium remains attached (see p. 138).

Retinal Tears

Clinical characteristics of the retinal tears are the most important parameters to be taken into account in the choice of the surgical approach.

RETINAL DETACHMENT WITH A SINGLE TEAR

Operculated Retinal Tear. Choroidal irritation and intravitreal gas injection is sufficient to achieve permanent retinal reattachment (Fig. 129).

Horseshoe Tear Involving 30° or Less of the Eye Circumference. Choroidal irritation and intravitreal gas injection can provide permanent retinal reattachment in eyes with small tears located above the horizontal meridian, provided the tear shows a mobile posterior edge and the retinal flap is not under static vitreous traction.

Scleral buckling of the retinal tear is necessary in the following circumstances: (1) the tear is located in a lower quadrant; (2) the tear is associated with a bridging vessel; (3) the posterior edge is curled and fixed; (4) the tear is located at the posterior edge of the vitreous base or the flap is under static vitreous traction. The scleral buckle should be orientated radially. The buckle size is determined according to the tear size. (see p. 102)

The optimal height of the buckle depends on the height of the retinal detachment and the degree of vitreous traction. A high scleral buckle is recommanded in tears with a curled posterior edge or an anterior flap under static vitreous traction or a bridging vessel.

Gas injection as an adjunct to scleral buckling may be required in eyes with a highly detached retina or a radial fold involving the retinal tear. The indication for gas injection will be made during surgery according to findings at fundus examination after scleral buckling.

Horseshoe Tear Involving More than 30° of the Eye Circumference. Retinal reattachment may be achieved merely by gas injection and choroidal irrita-

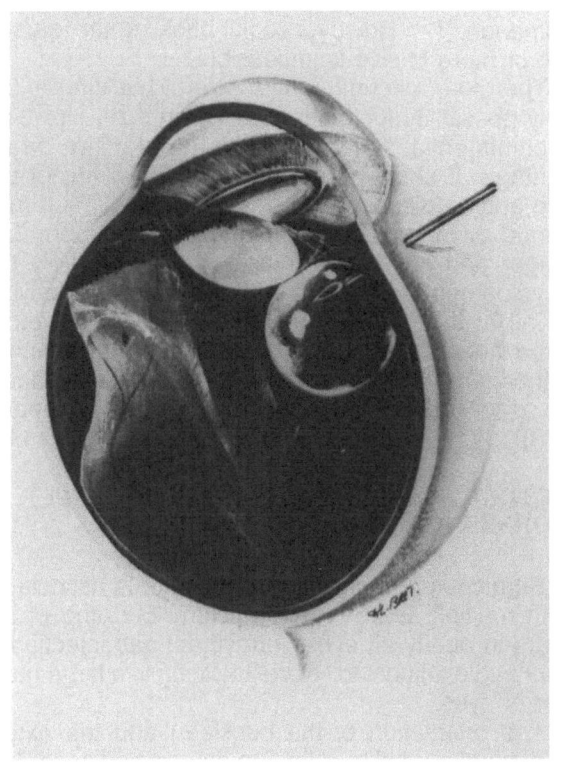

Figure 129. Retinal detachment associated with a small operculated tear of the superior quadrant. The retinal tear is no longer under vitreous traction. It is managed by localized choroidal irritation and intravitreal gas injection.

tion in retinal detachments with equatorial tears over 30° in size.[27,29] However, a significant number of eyes fail to permanently reattach after this surgical approach. Recurrent detachment is more severe than initial detachment in most cases. Therefore, relief of vitreous traction on the tear flap should remain one of the main objectives of surgical management. Scleral buckling and vitrectomy are the two possible approaches to relieve vitreous traction on the tear flap. However, complete relief of peripheral vitreous tractions by vitrectomy involves surgical difficulties and hazards, especially in phakic eyes. In contrast, scleral buckling of peripheral retinal tears is easy to perform and efficient in most cases. Late complications of scleral buckling are uncommon. Therefore, scleral buckling of the retinal tear(s) should still be considered as the basic and necessary surgical procedure in the management of retinal detachments with horseshoe tears of the peripheral retina.

Radial scleral buckling is the most appropriate technique to relieve vitreous traction on the anterior flap and avoid development of a fishmouth phenomenon.[30–32] However radial buckling for tears of 70° or more in size is impossible.

Therefore, circumferential scleral buckling is the only possibility for tears over 70° in size. However circumferential scleral buckling has a major disadvantage. It shortens the circumferential arc of the eye and predisposes to radial retinal folds.[33] It may create or increase a fishmouth phenomenon. The longer and higher the buckle, the more likely the development and degree of radial folds and leaking areas at the posterior edge of the tear. Therefore large horseshoe tears should be managed with a rather shallow choroidal indentation which should be associated with intravitreal gas injection (see p. 118).

RETINAL DETACHMENTS WITH MULTIPLE HORSESHOE TEARS

Surgical repair of retinal detachments associated with multiple tears requires scleral buckling of the tears in nearly all eyes. Intravitreal gas injection is a valuable adjunct to scleral buckling in a large number of eyes.

The orientation of the buckle(s) and the extent of circumferential buckles are determined according to the number, size, and location of the tears (Fig. 130).

Two small contiguous horseshoe tears can be managed by a single radial buckle.

Two tears located more than 90° apart are managed by two separate radial buckles.

Two or more contiguous tears that involve more than 70° and less than 200° of the eye circumference, are managed by a localized circumferential buckle and gas injection. Each extremity of the circumferential buckle should extend 3 mm beyond the tears. The circumferential dimension of the buckle should be increased in eyes with multiple tears located at the posterior edge of the vitreous base, because contraction of the vitreous base may increase postoperatively and sequential tears may develop.

Management of retinal detachments with multiple tears in 3 or all 4 quadrants requires a 360° circumferential buckling procedure. In a few cases one or two radial buckles may be required, in addition to the 360° circumferential buckle, to seal tears that extent more posteriorly.

In most eyes with a highly detached retina and multiple horseshoe tears, gas injection is required as an adjunct to scleral buckling. The goal of gas injection is to flatten radial folds at the posterior edge of the tears.

HORSESHOE TEARS WITH A CURLED AND FIXED POSTERIOR EDGE

Retinal detachment due to horseshoe tears with a curled and fixed posterior edge are associated with a high risk of severe proliferative vitreoretinopathy postoperatively (see p. 333). Therefore, specific measures to prevent the occurrence of this devastating complication are needed in such patients. Several measures can be applied, however, their clinical value remains to be fully established.

Drugs that decrease ocular inflammation and cell proliferation, such as corticosteroids and colchicine, can be administered preoperatively and postoperatively with the same protocol as in confirmed proliferative vitreoretinopathy (see p. 251). However, the value of these drugs in the prevention of proliferative vitreoretinopathy remains to be proven.

In addition, the most appropriate surgical protocol to be applied in such eyes remains to be determined. Cryotreatment may be a stimulus for epiretinal membrane formation. Therefore diathermy or argon laser photocoagulation should be used, rather than cryo, to induce the retinochoroidal scar.

HORSESHOE TEARS WITH A BRIDGING VESSEL

Management of horseshoe tears with a bridging vessel requires use of a very high scleral buckle.[21–22] The purpose of the very high buckle is to relieve vitreous traction on the bridging vessel. A high scleral buckle may be insufficient, however, to prevent recurrent vitreous hemorrhages when the bridging vessel remains under vitreous traction. An attempt should, therefore, be made to obliterate the bridging vessel at the initial operation. This attempt can consist of either cryotreatment or argon laser photocoagulation. Cryoapplications to the bridging vessel are carried out before scleral buckling. The three-thaw freeze cycle technique is applied. When argon laser photocoagulation is used rather than cryotreatment, it is carried out after scleral buckling. Both techniques may fail to permanently occlude a large bridging vessel. In addition, each technique may lead to specific complications.

Eyes with vitreous hemorrhages that recur in spite of the above treatment should be managed by vitrectomy. Vitrectomy relieves vitreous traction on the bridging vessel. In addition, permanent occlusion of the bridging vessel can be achieved by endodiathermy. Vitrectomy should also be applied as the first surgical treatment in eyes with marked vitreous hemorrhage at initial presentation.

Vitreous Body

Changes of the vitreous gel play a major role in the pathogenesis of retinal detachments with horseshoe tears. However, apart from the necessity of relieving vitreous traction on the tear flap, little

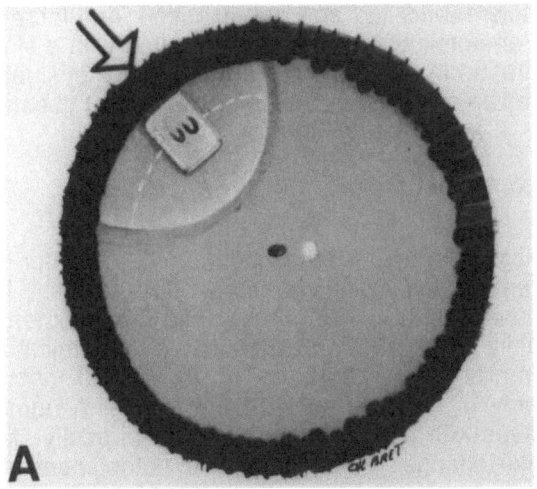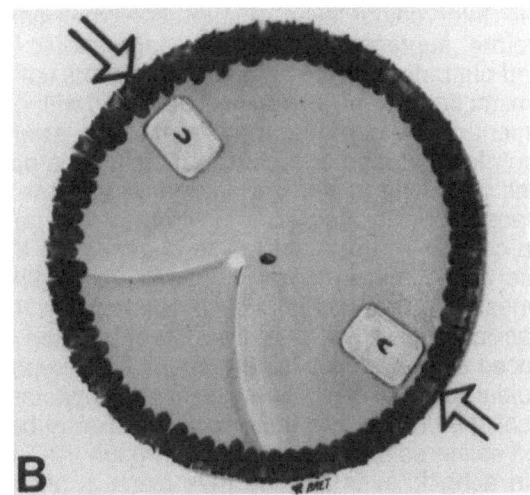

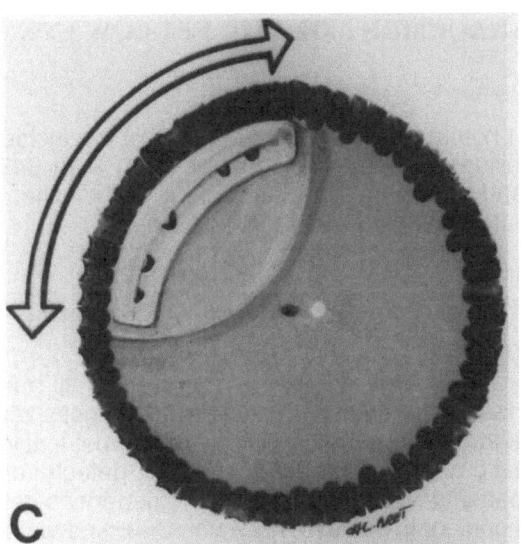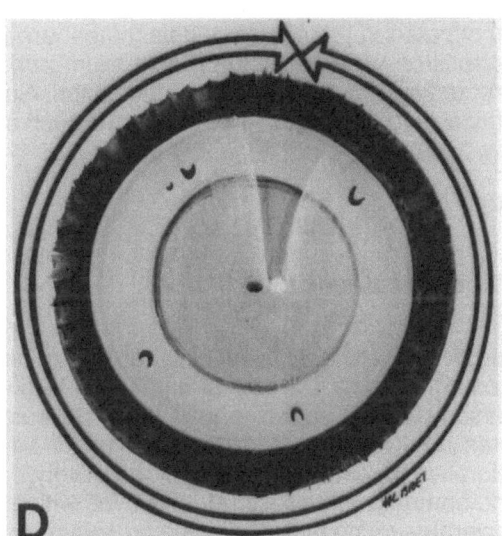

Figure 130. Guidelines for scleral buckling of horseshoe tears in mobile retinal detachments. (A) Two contiguous horseshoe tears involving less than 70° of the eye circumference are managed by a single radial buckle. (B) Two horseshoe tears more than 90° apart are managed by two separate radial buckles. (C) Multiple contiguous tears at the posterior edge of the vitreous base are managed by a segmental circumferential buckle and gas injection. (D) Retinal detachment with multiple horseshoe tears in three or more quadrants is managed by 360° circumferential buckling procedure.

is known on the choice of the most appropriate surgical protocol according to vitreous gel changes.

In particular, eyes with extensive vitreous gel liquefaction and incomplete posterior vitreous detachment are at an increased risk of recurrent retinal detachment (see p. 234). Further clinical investigations are required to determine the potential value of 360° scleral buckling or early vitrectomy in such eyes. For the surgical approach in retinal detachments with vitreous hemorrhage see p. 135.

Choroidal Detachment

Shallow and peripheral choroidal detachments do not prevent adequate cryotreatment of the retinal tears, in most eyes. Therefore the surgical protocol for retinal detachment repair is carried out in the usual way in such eyes.

In contrast, in eyes with bullous choroidal detachment, cryotreatment cannot reach the choroid owing to the intervening layer of suprachoroidal fluid. Therefore, suprachoroidal fluid drainage should be carried out before cryotreatment of the retinal tears. Choroidal detachment is always associated with detachment of the ciliary body. Therefore the scleral incision for drainage of suprachoroidal fluid is performed anteriorly to the ora serrata. It is made 4 mm posteriorly to the limbus, in front of the pars plana ciliaris. The scleral incision is parallel to the limbus and 2 mm in length. Clear or yellow fluid escapes from the suprachoroidal space when the supraciliaris space is open. Intravitreal injection of balanced saline solution is performed during suprachoroidal fluid drainage to prevent massive hypotony and collapse of the eye. Intravitreal injection of balanced saline solution is performed through the limbus in aphakic eyes and the pars plana in phakic eyes.

In a few eyes, the media remains clear in spite of the choroidal detachment. In such eyes, the retinal tears situated in the choroidal detachment area are in apposition with the pigment epithelium and can be treated by argon laser photocoagulation. Suprachoroidal fluid drainage is unnecessary in such eyes.

RESULTS

Anatomical Results

The overall anatomical success rate achieved by microsurgery in mobile retinal detachments due to horseshoe tears is approximately 95%.[20] All surgical failures are related to the development of severe proliferative vitreoretinopathy postoperatively.

The anatomical success rate achieved with a single scleral buckling or gas injection procedure shows significant variations with case selection. The anatomy of the tear posterior edge is the most significant factor in predicting the postoperative outcome after scleral buckling. In a recent series of mobile retinal detachments with horseshoe tears[20] permanent retinal reattachment was achieved with a single operation in 97.5% of eyes with tears that showed a mobile posterior edge, compared to only 63% of eyes with tears that showed a curled and fixed posterior edge. In the latter group of eyes, all recurrent retinal detachments were related to postoperative proliferative vitreoretinopathy. Permanent retinal reattachment was eventually achieved with one or several operations in 86.5% of the curled posterior edge series. Most eyes successfully reoperated on underwent vitrectomy. The poor prognosis for permanent retinal reattachment with a single scleral buckling procedure in mobile retinal detachments with horseshoe tears that show a curled and fixed posterior edge raises an important point: would vitrectomy, performed at the initial operation, be a valuable adjunct

to scleral buckling and gas injection, and increase the anatomical success rate achieved with a single operation in such eyes? Further clinical evaluation is required to answer this most important question.

Visual Results

Postoperative visual acuity of 20/40 or better can be anticipated in approximately 50% of eyes.[20] Decreased central vision after retinal reattachment is usually associated with a definable anatomical abnormality in the macula such as cystoid macular edema or macular pucker (see p. 16). A number of eyes with poor postoperative visual acuity show ocular changes unrelated to the detachment (see p. 16).

MANAGEMENT OF THE FELLOW EYE

In nontraumatic retinal detachment the incidence of bilateral involvement ranges from 9 to 34%.[35] Therefore, prophylactic treatment of the other eye should be considered in selected cases.

Indications for Prophylactic Treatment

Prophylactic treatment is indicated in all nondetached fellow eyes that show full thickness retinal breaks. Such retinal breaks may remain asymptomatic and may not lead to retinal detachment.[36] In patients who have already experienced retinal detachment in one eye, however, the disadvantages of prophylactic treatment are nearly nil compared to the potential risk of retinal breaks.

Prophylactic treatment should also be considered in nondetached fellow eyes showing lesions that may predispose to the development of horseshoe tears, in particular islands of lattice degeneration. Islands of lattice degeneration are found in approximately 22% of the nondetached fellow eyes.[37] The indications for prophylactic treatment should be based on the status of the retina and vitreous gel.

The vast majority of horseshoe tears leading to retinal detachment develop at the time of acute posterior vitreous detachment. They are due to dynamic vitreous traction on areas of vitreoretinal adhesion. Any island of lattice degeneration involves a potential risk of subsequent horseshoe tear development in eyes showing no posterior vitreous detachment, or incomplete posterior vitreous detachment without collapse of the vitreous gel.

There is an indication for prophylactic treatment in fellow eyes with lattice degeneration that show no posterior vitreous detachment or incomplete posterior vitreous detachment. In contrast prophylactic treatment is unnecessary in fellow eyes with lattice degeneration and total posterior vitreous detachment with collapse of the vitreous gel.

Methods of Prophylactic Treatment

The goal of prophylactic treatment is to induce a firm retinochoroidal adhesion in areas with open breaks or lesions that predispose to the development of retinal breaks. The induced retinochoroidal scar should seal the retinal break(s) or resist dynamic vitreous traction at the time of subsequent acute posterior vitreous detachment.

Cryotreatment and argon laser photocoagulation are the techniques most commonly used for prophylactic treatment. Both techniques have advantages and limits.

In eyes with clear media, argon laser photocoagulation is used rather than cryo. A 500 micron spot size and 0.5 second exposure time are used. No shorter exposure time should be used because the strength of the induced retinochoroidal adhesion would be insufficient. The power is determined to induce a white yellow retinal lesion. Four rows of contiguous burns are made all around the retinal break or island of lattice degeneration.

In eyes with retinal breaks the inner row of burns is placed at the very edge of the break. Great care should be taken to seal the anterior edge of the tear as well as its posterior edge. Scleral depression may be necessary to apply appropriate treatment to the tear anterior edge. In eyes with poor dilatation of the pupil or lens opacities, transconjunctival cryotreatment is used as an adjunct to argon laser photocoagulation to seal the anterior edge of the retinal break. In such eyes cryotreatment is also used rather than photocoagulation to treat retinal breaks located anteriorly to the equatorial region. Cryotreatment is performed with simultaneous biomicroscopic observation of the fundus.

In eyes with lattice degeneration the inner row of photocoagulation burns is made at the edge of the lattice island(s). All islands of lattice are treated prophylactically, even those located in the lower quadrants.

Results of Prophylactic Treatment

All patients having experienced retinal detachment due to horseshoe tear(s) in one eye and having no posterior vitreous detachment of the other eye should be followed up until complete posterior vitreous detachment has occurred in the other eye. This applies to patients who show no predisposing lesions of the fellow eye as well as patients who are prophylactically treated. In the former group of patients, retinal tears may develop at the time of acute posterior vitreous detachment, in spite of the absence of predisposing lesions detectable by clinical examination. In the latter group of patients, subsequent retinal tear(s) may develop in spite of prophylactic treatment.

The failure rate of prophylactic treatment, that is the incidence of retinal detachments occurring in spite of prophylactic treatment, is approximately 4.5%, regardless of the method used for prophylactic treatment.[37,38]

In eyes prophylactically treated for retinal tears, failures of prophylactic treatment may be related to inadequate technique, or development of subsequent retinal tears. Failures related to inadequate technique are most infrequent. The most common cause of failure is an incomplete surrounding of the retinal tear, in particular its anterior edge by the induced retinochoroidal scars. Such failures can be avoided by complete surrounding of the retinal tear with the photocoagulation or cryotreatment scars. The incidence of sequential retinal tears after prophylactic treatment of retinal breaks is approximately 7%.[39–41] The incidence is approximately the same whatever the method used for prophylactic treatment. Sequential retinal tears result in a retinal detachment in approximately 4.5% of the eyes prophylactically treated.[37,38] Sequential horseshoe tears may develop a few weeks to more than 10 years after prophylactic treatment of the initial retinal tears.[42] New retinal tears may be situated either within or adjacent to the coagulation scars or unrelated to the treated areas of the retina.[38,42]

In eyes prophylactically treated for lesions predisposing to retinal tears, failures are related to the development of horseshoe tears at the time of acute posterior vitreous detachment. After prophylactic treatment of predisposing lesions, the incidence of retinal detachment in fellow eyes is approximately 4.5% in patients followed for a few years.[43] An increased incidence may be observed in patients followed for a longer period of time. Retinal breaks that develop in spite of prophylactic treatment may be located either within or adjacent to the scars, or unrelated to the treated areas.

In most patients, the detachment, which develops in the fellow eye in spite of prophylactic treatment, is as severe as the detachment of the eye that was not prophylactically treated.[42]

Complications after prophylactic treatment with cryo or argon laser photocoagulation are infrequent. Recurrent vitreous hemorrhage have been observed in 2.2%[44] to 3.6%[45] in a large series of eyes. Vitreous hemorrhages are mainly observed after prophylactic treatment of horseshoe tears with a bridging vessel.[45] Such tears require specific treatment so as to close the patent vessel or relieve vitreous traction (see p. 168). The incidence of macular lesions in eyes that had prophylactic treatment ranges from 0.6%[46] to 3.9%.[44] It is approximately the same whatever the method used for prophylactic treatment.[44,47] Macular pucker[38,39,48] is the most common macular lesion. Cystoid macular edema is most uncommon.[38] The correlation between macular pucker and prophylactic treatment is uncertain in eyes treated with argon laser photocoagulation or cryoapplication. Eyes with horseshoe tears may show a premacular membrane before any treatment. The macular pucker may develop several years after prophylactic treatment,[39] therefore, macular pucker may be related to the vitreoretinal disease rather than prophylactic treatment.

REFERENCES

1. Ashrafzadeh MT, Schepens CL, Elzeneiny I, Moura R, Morse P, Kravshar F: Aphakic and phakic retinal detachment—I Preoperative findings. Arch Ophthalmol 89:476–483, 1973
2. Schepens CL: Retinal detachment and allied diseases. Vol 1, 47–51, 177–213 Philadelphia, W.B. Saunders, 1983
3. Schepens CL, Marden D: Data on the natural history of retinal detachment. Further characterization of certain unilateral non-traumatic cases. Am J Ophthalmol 61:213–226, 1966
4. Bonnet M: Clinical factors predisposing to severe proliferative vitreoretinopathy. Ophthalmologica, 188:148–152, 1984
5. Urrets-Zavalia J: Traitement du dècollement rhegmatogène de la rétine du sujet myope par la microchirurgie. Thèse universitaire Cordoba (to be published)
6. Haimann MH, Burton TC, Brown CK: Epidemiology of retinal detachment. Arch Ophthalmol 100:289–292, 1982
7. Schepens CL: Retinal detachment and aphakia. Arch Ophthalmol 45:1–17, 1951
8. Norton EW: Retinal detachment in aphakia. Trans Am Ophthalmol Soc 61:770–789, 1963
9. Hagler WS: Retinal detachment in the unilateral aphake, in Emery JM, Paton D (Eds): Current concepts in cataract surgery. Selected proceedings of the third biennal cataract surgical congress. St. Louis, C.V. Mosby Co, 1974, 350–352
10. Edmund J, Seedorff HH: Retinal detachment in the aphakic eye. Acta Ophthalmol, 52:323–333, 1974
11. Cox MS, Schepens CL, Freeman HM: Retinal detachment due to ocular contusion. Arch Ophthalmol 76:678–685, 1966
12. Lincoff H, Gieser R: Finding the retinal hole. Arch Ophthalmol 85:565–569, 1971
13. Chignell AH: Retinal detachment surgery. New York, Springer-Verlag, 7, 1980
14. Kirkby GR, Chignel AH: Shifting subretinal fluid in rhegmatogenous retinal detachment. Brit J Ophthalmol 69:654–655, 1985
15. Morse PH: Lattice degeneration of the retina and retinal detachment. Am J Ophthalmol 78:930–934, 1974
16. Byer NE: Lattice degeneration of the retina. Surv Ophthalmol 23:213–248, 1979
17. Boniuk M, Butler FC: An autopsy study of lattice degeneration, retinal breaks, and retinal pits, in McPherson A (ed.): new and controversial aspects of retinal detachment. New York, Harper and Row, 1968, 59–75
18. Byer NE: Cystic retinal tufts and their relationship to retinal detachment. Arch Ophthalmol 99:1788–1790, 1981
19. Straatsma BR, Zeegen PD, Foos RY, et al: Lattice degeneration of the retina. Am J Ophthalmol 77:619–649, 1974
20. Bonnet M: Grade B, a determining risk factor in the development of severe proliferative vitreoretinopathy. Graefe's Arch Clin Exp Ophthalmol. 226:201–205, 1988
21. Theodossiadis G, Velissaropoulos P, Maguritsas N, Vikas K: Behandlung und Nachuntersuchung von Netzhautrissen ohne Netzhautgefäss Klin Monatslb Augenheilkd 140:411–415, 1977
22. De Bustros S, Welch R: The avulsed retinal vessel syndrome and its variants ophthalmology 91:86–88, 1984
23. Fournier P: Décollement rétinien rhegmatogène et déchirures rétinennes avec hémorragie intravitréenne. Lyon France, Thèse université 1986
24. Bonnet M: Les indications de la vitrectomie dans le décollement de la rétine. Ophtalmologie 1:95–100, 1987
25. Seelenfreund MH, Kravshar MF, Schepens CL, Freilich DB: Choroidal detachment associated with primary retinal detachment. Arch Ophthalmol 91:254–258, 1974
26. Rachal WF, Burton TC: Changing concepts of failures after retinal detachment surgery. Arch Ophthalmol 97:480–483, 1979
27. Chawla HB, Coleiro JA: Retinal detachment treatment with intra-vitreal air: an evaluation of 241 cases. Brit J Ophthalmol 61:588–592, 1977
28. Bonnet M: Microsurgery of retinal detachment. Advantages, disadvantages, limitations, results. Developments in Ophthalmology, 2:208–213, 1981
29. Hilton GF, Grizzard WS: Pneumatic retinopexy. A two-step out patient operation without conjunctival incision. Ophthalmology 93:626–641, 1986
30. Lincoff H: The rationale for radial buckling Mod Probl Ophthalmol 12:484–491, 1974
31. Lincoff H, Kreissig I: Advantages of radial buckling Am J Ophthalmol 79:955–957, 1975
32. Goldbaum MH, Smithline M, Poole TA, and Lincoff H: Geometric analysis of radial buckling. Am J Ophthalmol 79:958–965, 1975
33. Lincoff H, Kreissig I, Lafranco F: Mechanisms of failures in the repair of large retinal tears. Am J Ophthalmol 84:501–507, 1977
34. Bonnet M, Nagao M: Microsurgery of aphakic retinal detachment. Ophthalmologica, 186:177–182, 1983
35. Schepens CL, Marden D: Data on the natural history of retinal detachment I—age and sex relationship. Arch Ophthalmol 66:631–642, 1961
36. Byer NE: The natural history of asymptomatic retinal breaks. Ophthalmology 89:1033–1039, 1982
37. McPherson A, O'Malley R, Beltangady SS: Management of the fellow eyes of patients with rhegmatogenous retinal detachment. Ophthalmology 88:922–934, 1981
38. Kanski JJ, Daniel R: Prophylaxis of retinal detachment. Am J Ophthalmol 79:197–205, 1975
39. Robertson DM, Norton EW: Long term follow-up of treated retinal breaks Am J Ophthalmol 75:395–404, 1973
40. Bec P, Ravault M, Arne JL, Trepsat C: La Périphérie du fond d'oeil. Masson, Paris 1980, 244
41. Goldberg MF: Sequential retinal breaks following a spontaneous initial retinal break. Ophthalmology 88:10–12, 1981
42. Bonnet M, Aracil P, Carneau F: Rhegmatogenous retinal detachment after prophylactic argon laser photocoagulation. Graefe's Arch Clin Exp Ophthalmol 225:5–8, 1987
43. Girard P, Goichot L, Saragoussi J, Merad I, Forest A: Le devenir de l'oeil adelphe dans le décollement de la rétine. J Fr Ophtalmol 5:681–685, 1982
44. Paupert-Ravault M, Trepsat C, Milan JJ, Nemoz C: Traitement au laser des déchirures rétiniennes non décollées. Bull Mem Soc Fr Ophtalmol 93:34–37, 1982
45. Robertson DM, Norton EW: Cause of failure in prophylactic treatment of retinal breaks. Mod Probl Ophthalmol 12:74–80, 1974
46. Zweng C, Little H: Argon laser photocoagulation P. St. Louis, C.V. Mosby, 1977
47. Boniuk I, Okun E, Johnston GP, Arribas N: Xenon photocoagulation versus cryotherapy in the prevention of retinal detachment. Mod Probl Ophthalmol 12:81–92, 1974
48. Chignell AH, Shilling J: Prophylaxis of retinal detachment. Brit J Ophthalmol 57:291–298, 1973

15

Retinal Detachment with Atrophic Round Holes in Lattice Degeneration

Retinal detachments due solely to atrophic round holes in lattice degeneration are in many respects distinct from retinal detachments associated with tractional horseshoe retinal tears. In most cases, those retinal detachments develop in eyes that have neither significant vitreous degeneration nor posterior vitreous detachment. As a consequence, the detachment has a very low progression and shares most of the clinical characteristics of retinal detachments associated with nontraumatic retinal dialysis. The risk of postoperative proliferative vitreoretinopathy is virtually nil. The surgical prognosis for retinal reattachment is excellent.

ETIOLOGY

Incidence

Phakic retinal detachments due solely to atrophic round holes in lattice degeneration are infrequent as compared to retinal detachments due to tractional horseshoe retinal tears. They account for 2.8%[1] to 6%[2,3] of all rhegmatogenous retinal detachments.

Age and Sex Distribution

Phakic retinal detachments due to atrophic round holes in lattice degeneration have been observed in patients from 9 years[4] to 80 years of age,[1] however, there is a significant prevalence in young individuals. Eighty percent of the patients are under 40 years of age[3] and 50% are less than 30 years old.[1]

Certain series[1,4] show no statistically significant sex predilection. However, in the author's own experience, those retinal detachments are more frequent in females (69%),[3] who account for 85% of patients 21–40 years of age.[3]

Refractive Errors

Approximately 75% of the patients have myopic refractive errors greater than—3 diopters spherical equivalent.[1,2,3] The distribution is almost the same in eyes with myopia under 8 diopters (41%)[3] and eyes over 8 diopters of myopia (53%).[3]

Retinal detachment due solely to round holes in lattice degeneration account for 15% of all rhegmatogenous retinal detachments in myopic eyes.[3]

Approximately 25% of retinal detachments with atrophic round holes occur in emmetropic eyes.[1,2,4]

The mean age of emmetropic patients is significantly higher than that of myopic patients (50 years versus 27 years).[2]

Bilaterality

Although lattice degeneration is present in the fellow eye in more than 60 percent of the patients,[1,3] the incidence of bilateral retinal detachment is rather low (12%).[1,3]

In most patients affected by bilateral round atrophic holes in lattice degeneration, there is mirror symmetry of the lesions in both eyes.[3]

173

Family History

A family history of retinal detachment is infrequent. However the occurrence of the same type of detachment in siblings has been observed.[3]

CLINICAL CHARACTERISTICS

Visual Symptoms

In contrast to retinal detachments due to tractional horseshoe retinal tears, retinal detachments due solely to round atrophic holes are characterized by the absence of acute visual symptoms. Light flashes, vitreous floaters, sudden visual field defect are almost never reported by the patients. The most common symptom is blurred or distorted vision of gradual onset and variable duration. Half of the patients complain of no symptoms until the macula becomes detached. Retinal detachments sparing the macula are sometimes disclosed by routine fundus examination.

There is no difference in the clinical symptoms between detachments beginning superiorly and detachments related to inferior holes.

Fundus Findings

RETINAL DETACHMENT

Retinal detachments due solely to atrophic round holes in lattice degeneration have distinct clinical features as compared to retinal detachments associated with tractional horseshoe retinal tears (Fig. 131). Actually they share most of the clinical features of retinal detachments associated with nontraumatic dialysis. Those clinical features are related to the very slow progression of the detachment in an eye that has no posterior vitreous detachment in most cases.

The retinal detachment is rather flat; it is smooth and there are no retinal folds. In spite of the common longstanding duration, the detachment is most often circumscribed. In most cases (72–78%).[1,2,3] The detachment involves less than two quadrants. Total retinal detachment is very rare (2% of all cases)[3] even in detachments of several years duration.

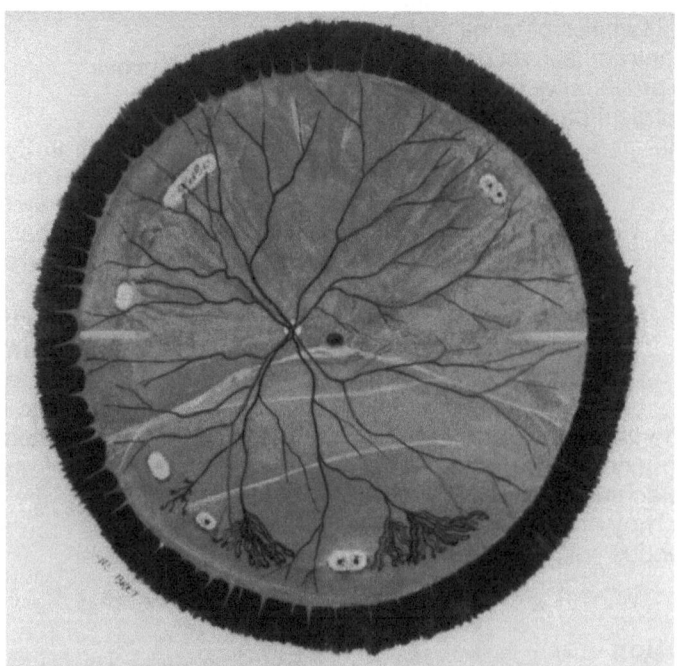

Figure 131. Longstanding retinal detachment associated with multiple atrophic holes in detached and attached retina. Retinal detachment is associated with newvessels of the equatorial region in detached retina and subretinal proliferation (Courtesy of BONNET M., Graefe's Arch Clin Exp Ophthalmol 225:59–62, 1987).

The quadrants that are most often involved by the retinal detachment are the inferior temporal quadrant (83% of the eyes) and the superior temporal quadrant (48% of the eyes).[3] The detachments beginning inferiorly are slightly more frequent than those beginning superiorly.[1]

Signs of long standing duration are common. Demarcation lines with subretinal gliosis are present in 25%[1] to more than 50%[3] of the cases. The demarcation lines are more often multiple and concentric. In a few cases there are two separate groups of concentric demarcation lines located in two quadrants (most often the supero temporal and the infero temporal quadrants). The association of two separate groups of concentric demarcation lines indicates that the detachment has gradually extended in two different directions and is, in fact, related to separate holes or group of holes located in two quadrants (Fig. 135).

The detached retina often appears rather translucent. It is actually thickened by multiple tiny confluent cystic spaces. Cystic degeneration of the retina is secondary to the long duration of the detachment. It can lead to the misdiagnosis of primary retinoschisis.

The macula is detached in approximately half of the cases.[1,3,4] Cystoid macular degeneration is present in 13% of the cases,[3] and demarcation lines run through the posterior pole in approximately 22% of the cases.[3]

In retinal detachments of several years duration, one or several groups of retinal new vessels may be present in the equatorial zone (approximately 17% of the eyes). Such new retinal vessels have the clinical characteristics of small sea fans. They are located in the detached retina and in the vicinity of the retinal holes (Figs. 131 and 132). It is assumed that they are secondary to prolonged retinal hypoxia resulting from a several year duration retinal detachment. The new vessels do not bleed. They do not require any specific treatment. They regress spontaneously after surgical retinal reattachment.[5]

In spite of the longstanding duration of most of these retinal detachments, and although subretinal proliferation is very frequent, preretinal proliferation and fixed retinal folds are never observed.[2,3,5]

The constant absence of preretinal proliferation is likely to be related to the absence of major vitreous pathology and posterior vitreous detachment.

RETINAL HOLES

The retinal detachment is associated with round atrophic retinal holes. The holes are located within one or, more commonly, several foci of lattice degeneration. Some of them are located in the detached retina and are the direct cause of the detachment.

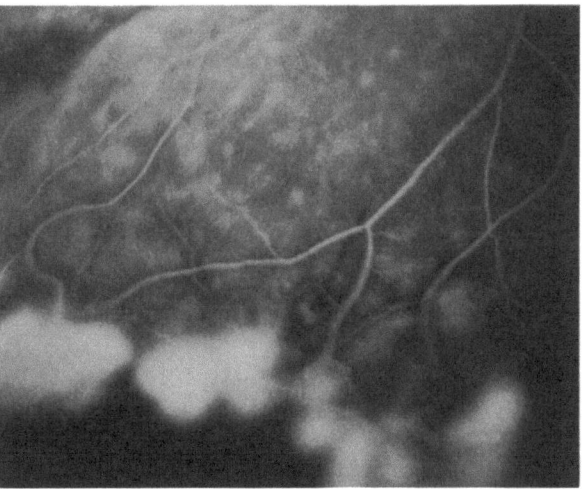

Figure 132. Fluorescein angiography of equatorial retinal new vessels in a longstanding retinal detachment associated with atrophic holes in lattice. Dye leakage from the new vessels. Capillary nonperfusion of the detached retina peripheral to the new vessels (Courtesy of BONNET M. Graefe's Arch Clin Exp Ophthalmol 225:59–62, 1987).

Others are located in attached retina and play no role in the detachment.

The number of foci of lattice degeneration varies from 1 to 25,[3] with the mean number being 3.26.[4] When they are multiple foci of lattice degeneration, only a few in number show associated full thickness retinal holes.

The number of full thickness retinal holes in lattice degeneration ranges from 1–16,[3] while the mean number of retinal holes is 4.54.[3] There is more than a single retinal hole in over 80% of the eyes.[1,3] The distribution of the full thickness retinal holes is significantly more frequent in the temporal quadrants than in the nasal quadrants. Full thickness retinal holes are found in the infero temporal quadrant in approximately 85% of the eyes,[3,4] and in the superotemporal quadrant in approximately 50% of the eyes.[3,4] Full thickness retinal holes located in the inferonasal quadrant are less frequent (approximately 20% of the eyes). Location in the superonasal quadrant is uncommon (less than 10% of the eyes). Full thickness retinal holes in the detached retina are also more often located in the temporal quadrants than on the nasal side. They are located in the inferotemporal quadrant in 45% of the eyes, in the superotemporal quadrant in 34% of the eyes, in the inferonasal quadrant in 14% of the eyes, and in the superonasal quadrant in only 7% of the eyes.[1]

The full thickness retinal holes are round and very small. Their size range from 50 μm to a 0.5 disc

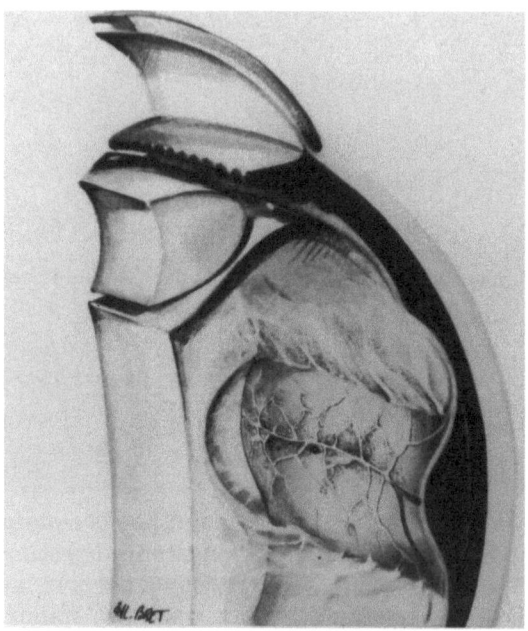

Figure 133. Vitreous gel in retinal detachment associated with atrophic hole in lattice. Vitreous gel shows a lacuna in front of the island of lattice degeneration. The posterior vitreous cortex is firmly adherent to the retina at the edge of lattice degeneration. There is no posterior vitreous detachment.

diameter. Larger holes, which span the width of the lattice lesion, are very uncommon. A cluster of two or three tiny holes in the center of a lattice lesion is frequent. The holes have no associated flap or free operculum. There is no evidence of vitreous traction. The holes are located in front of a lacuna in the vitreous cortex, which involves the area of the lattice lesion (Fig. 133).

VITREOUS GEL

Posterior vitreous detachment with collapse of the vitreous gel is very rare (6.5% of the eyes).[3]

In most eyes, associated vitreous pathology is limited to small lacunae in the cortical vitreous gel, located in front of the lattice lesions (Fig. 133). There is no clinical evidence of peripheral vitreous traction or vitreous syneresis.

Eyes with longstanding duration retinal detachments show tobacco dust pigmentation in the vitreous gel. In most cases the pigment granules are deposited in the peripheral vitreous. They are more numerous in the close vicinity of the retinal holes. Clusters of pigment granules in the equatorial region may help the identification of tiny open holes in lattice lesions.

SURGICAL MANAGEMENT

Indications for Surgical Management

Basically, any rhegmatogenous retinal detachment is an indication for surgery. This rule applies to retinal detachments due solely to round atrophic holes. However, because of the very slow progression of this particular variety of retinal detachment, the necessity of surgical treatment may appear questionable in certain instances.

The indication for surgery is beyond doubt when the patient complains of visual symptoms, and the macula is involved or threatened by the detachment.

In contrast, when a subclinical retinal detachment, confined to the peripheral fundus, is disclosed by routine examination, the necessity of surgery may be open to question. Occasionally, a subclinical peripheral detachment due to a single tiny hold spontaneously flattens after several years. The diagnosis is made retrospectively by the typical sequelae (Fig. 134). The area of the previously detached retina is limited by hyperpigmented demarcation lines, concave towards the periphery. This area shows extreme pigment epithelium atrophy with subretinal pigment migration and gliosis. The tiny atrophic retinal hole is often no longer visible in the pigmented and glial scars. There is an absolute visual field defect corresponding to the atrophic area of the fundus, of which the patient may be unaware. However, such spontaneous reattachment of a subclinical detachment is uncommon and unpredictable. In most cases the retinal hole(s) remain open and the demarcation lines do not limit the extension of the detachment for an indefinite period of time. "Walling off" the detachment with photocoagulation is contraindicated for two main reasons. First, this method is more traumatic than one or two cryoapplications applied to the retinal hole(s), and it does sacrifice the visual field corresponding to the area of detachment. Second, the new demarcation line created with photocoagulation, although much stronger than any spontaneous demarcation lines, will not limit extension of the subretinal fluid towards the posterior pole forever.[3] Therefore, subclinical retinal detachments should be surgically treated.

Very longstanding duration retinal detachments, which have been neglected by the patient for many years, are associated with subretinal white strands running through the posterior pole. This is another extreme situation in which the value of any treatment may appear questionnable. Even in such extreme cases, however, surgical sealing of the retinal holes can provide retinal reattachment, restore at least part of the visual field, and prevent further trophic complications such as cataract.[3] Therefore, indica-

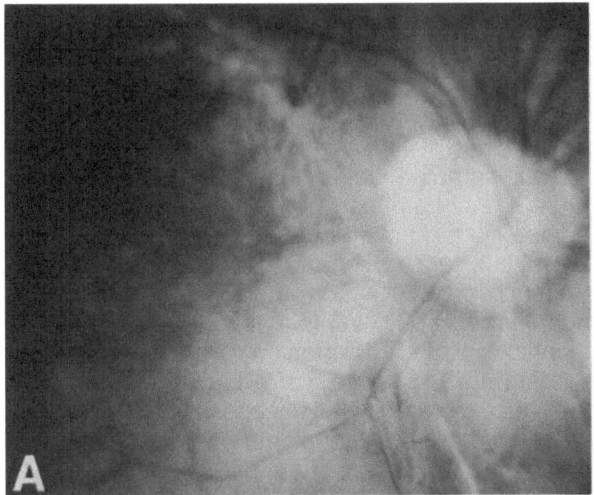

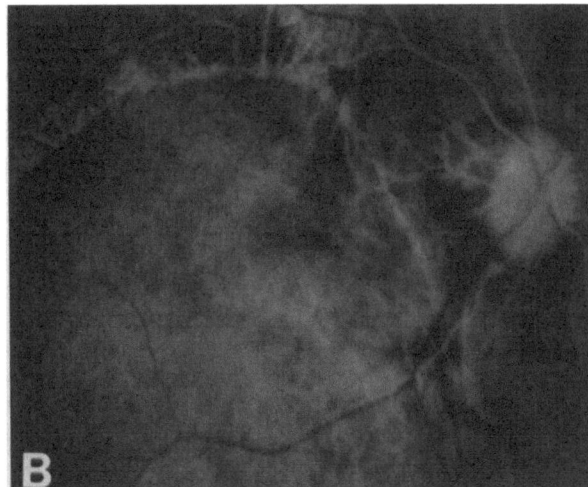

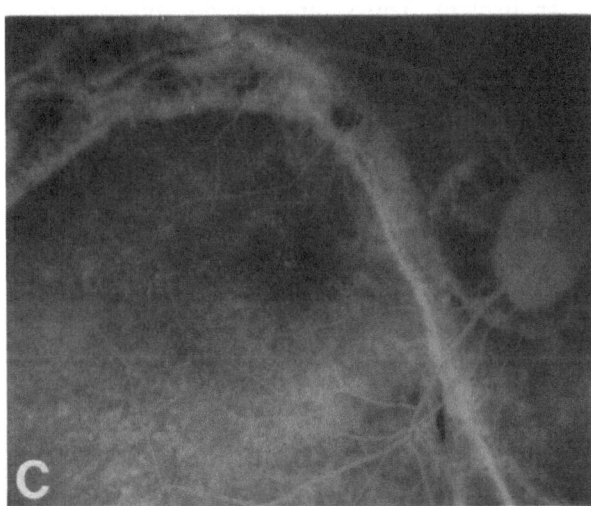

Figure 134. Sequelae after spontaneous reattachment of a retinal detachment associated with atrophic holes in a 60-year-old myopic patient. (A) Fundus photograph showing pigment epithelium atrophy and demarcation line on the posterior pole. (B) Early phase of fluorescein angiography. (C) Late phase of fluorescein angiography. Central vision is reduced to hand motion. The other eye shows subclinical retinal detachment of the inferior temporal quadrant associated with two small atrophic holes.

tion for surgical treatment should be considered as long as the light perceptions remain present.

Surgical Technique

In retinal detachments due solely to round atrophic retinal holes, surgical success depends only on adequate sealing of all open retinal holes. There is virtually no risk of surgical failures related to vitreous traction or preretinal proliferation. Subretinal strands, whatever their extension, are not an obstacle to retinal reattachment. They deserve no special attention, except for the visual prognosis when they run through the macula. All surgical failures that the author has observed in this variety of retinal detachments were due to the inability of the surgeon to identify and treat all open retinal holes. When the detachment was unsuccessfully operated on, identification of the hole(s) missed at the first operation

may be very arduous, especially when there are extensive, atrophic scars, secondary to heavy and multiple cryoapplications.

Therefore the most important step of treatment is the preoperative and operative identification of all open retinal holes. Since retinal holes are most often very tiny and multiple, the use of the surgical microscope for fundus examination under high magnification is most helpful in the treatment of those detachments.

LOCALIZATION OF THE RETINAL HOLES

Localization of the retinal holes is carried out for the holes or group of holes located in the detached retina. Accurate scleral landmarks are necessary for further adequate placement of a segmental scleral buckle.

It is not necessary to determine the scleral projection of the retinal holes located in the attached retina because their treatment does not require scleral buckling.

INDUCING A RETINOCHOROIDAL ADHESION

Holes in a Detached Retina. Holes in a detached retina are best treated with cryo. The backward shifting technique allows for a very limited and accurately centered cryotreatment. One to three cryoapplications are usually sufficient to seal a hole, or group of holes, in a lattice lesion. When cryo is carried out under high magnification, the surgeon can see dispersed pigment granules by freezing of the pigment epithelium. The pigment granules migrate through the open retinal hole from the subretinal space towards the vitreous lacuna overlying the lattice lesion. In longstanding retinal detachments associated with significant subretinal proliferation and secondary cystoid degeneration of the detached retina, migration of pigment granules through the retinal hole during cryo can help the surgeon to identify the open lesions.

Holes in the Attached Retina. Treatment is required for full thickness retinal holes in the attached retina, which may have a relationship with the retinal detachment. In particular, a retinal detachment located inferiorly may actually be superior in onset. The configuration of the detachment and the demarcation lines are the best guides for the surgeon to determine whether an atrophic hole in the attached retina plays a role in the detachment. From a theoretical standpoint, atrophic holes in the attached retina that have no relationship with the detachment could be left untreated. However, they are treated in most instances, although there is no clinical evidence that they will result in a recurrent retinal detachment years later. Any technique for inducing a retinochoroidal adhesion can be used for the treatment of atrophic holes in the attached retina. The author uses by preference argon laser photocoagulation because it allows for the most accuracy with the least trauma. Argon laser photocoagulation can indifferently be carried out the day before or a few days after surgery. If the attachment of the argon laser to the surgical microscope is available, the surgeon can also perform the treatment during the operation. The lattice lesions with full thickness holes are closely surrounded with 3–4 rows of coagulations (500 μm in size with an exposure time of 0.5 seconds) (Fig. 135).

SCLERAL BUCKLING

Treatment of retinal holes in the detached retina requires scleral buckling. The only aim of scleral buckling is to push the pigment epithelium into apposition with the retinal hole(s) allowing for the formation of an adherent retinochoroidal scar. Scleral buckling is not required to treat the retinal holes in the attached retina, since there is no associated vitreous pathology that might lead to late reopening of the retinal holes.

The scleral buckle should be segmental, a 360° scleral buckle is never necessary, even when there are multiple holes in more than two quadrants. Segmental scleral buckling is limited to the area corresponding to the lattice lesion(s) with full thickness hole(s) (Fig. 135 and Fig. 136). When there is only one lattice lesion with full thickness hole(s), and also when there are two groups of holes located in close vicinity, the necessary choroidal indentation can be achieved either with a small lamellar scleral pocket or an explant. The scleral buckle should overlap the lattice lesion(s) by 2 mm in each direction. When the condition of the sclera permits the dissection, a lamellar scleral pocket is the least traumatic and the most effective way to seal such lesions.

When there are multiple full thickness retinal holes, all lesions are treated with a single scleral buckle. It is parallel to the limbus and should overlap by 2 mm the posterior margin of the lattice lesions. An explant of lyophylized human dura mater is used. It is 3.5–4 mm in width and as long as necessary to cover all open lesions.

When a retinal fold develops and involves a retinal hole there is an indication for associated gas injection. Gas injection rather than scleral buckling can be used to seal holes in the superior quadrants.

DRAINAGE OF SUBRETINAL FLUID

In most cases drainage of subretinal fluid is not necessary to achieve surgical success[3] even in longstanding duration retinal detachments with subretinal proliferation. Subretinal fluid will spontaneously absorb within a few days when all retinal holes have been sealed. Inability to tighten the scleral sutures of an explant, insufficient intraocular space for gas injection, if required, and a very old standing retinal detachment associated with detachment of the pars plana ciliaris epithelium, are the three main indications for subretinal fluid drainage.

GAS INJECTION

Holes in the superior quadrants and circumferential or radial retinal folds induced by a circumferential buckle that involve open lesions are indications for gas injection.

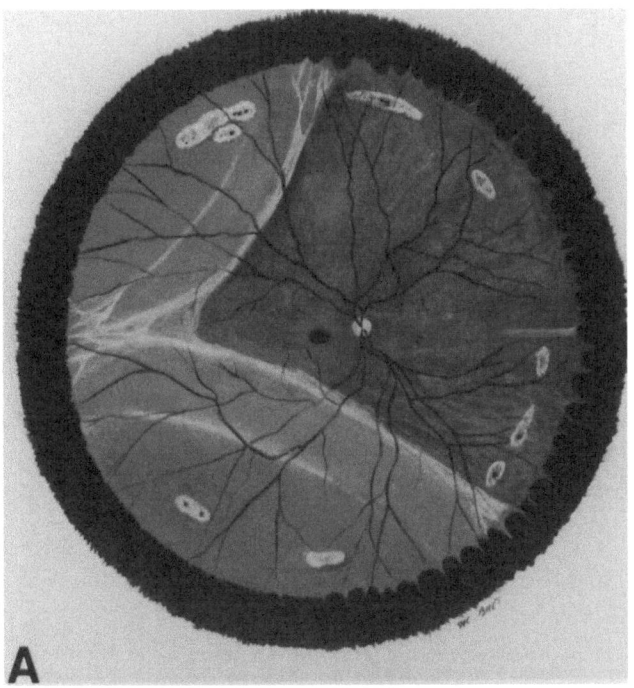

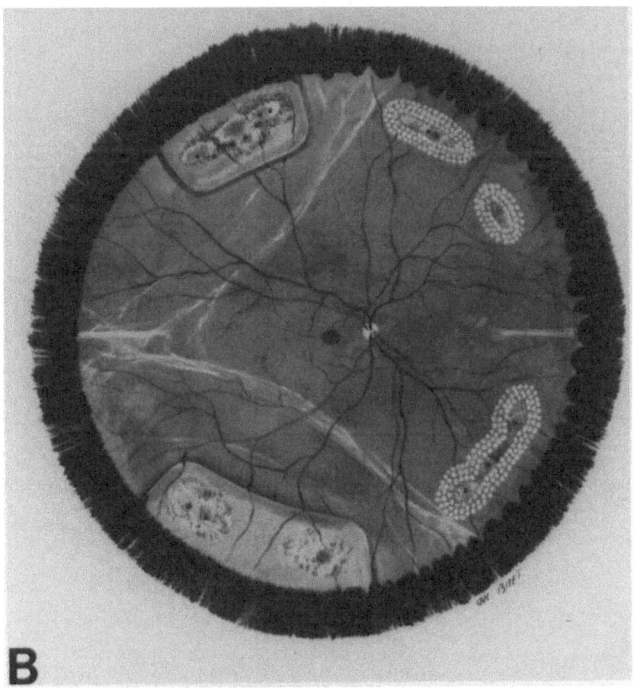

Figure 135. Longstanding retinal detachment associated with multiple atrophic holes in attached and detached retina. (A) Preoperative fundus appearance. Spread of subretinal fluid and features of subretinal proliferation indicate that detachment includes two independent components: an inferior detachment related to two tiny holes at 7 o'clock and a superior detachment related to the tiny holes at 11 o'clock (Courtesy of BONNET M. and URRETS-ZAVALIA J J Fr Ophtalmol, 9:615–624, 1986). (B) Postoperative fundus appearance. Management consisted of segmental scleral buckling of the inferotemporal holes and the superotemporal holes in detached retina, and photocoagulation treatment of the islands of lattice degeneration in attached retina. Subretinal fluid spontaneously absorbed within two weeks. White strands of subretinal proliferation remain unchanged after retinal reattachment.

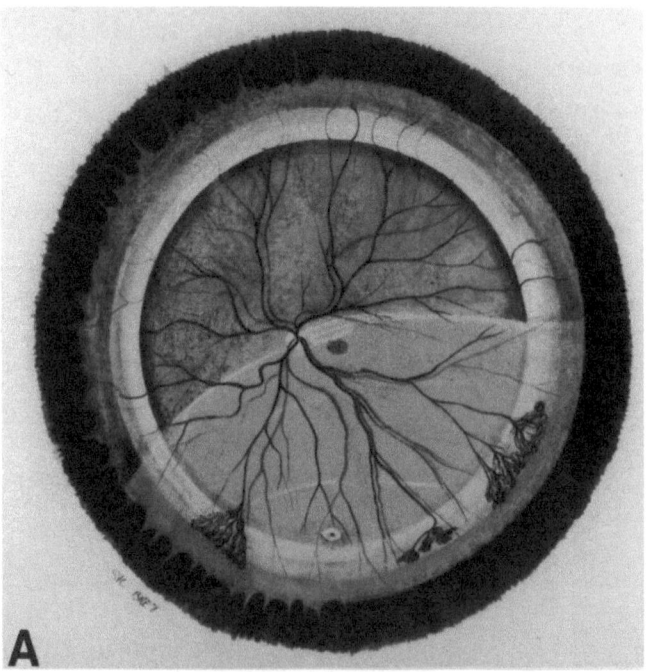

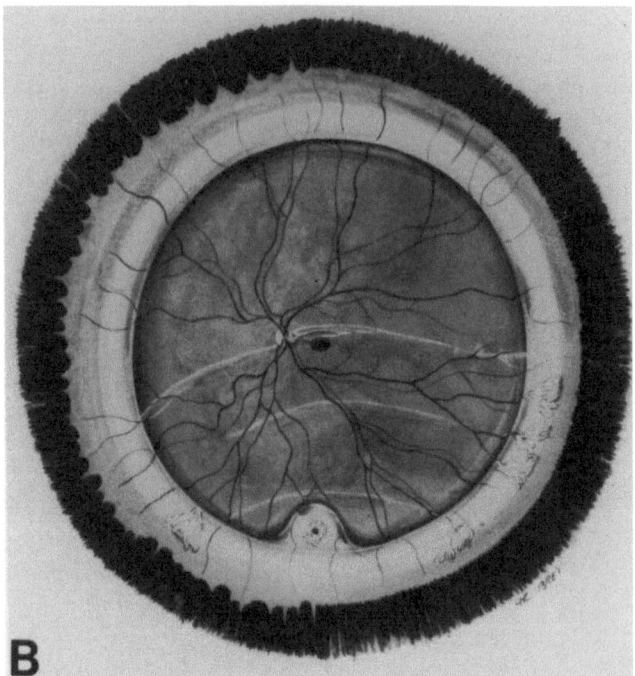

Figure 136. Longstanding duration retinal detachment associated with a single atrophic hole at 6 o'clock. (A) Fundus appearance at initial presentation. Retinal detachment of long duration is associated with new vessels in detached retina and a tiny hole at 6 o'clock. The tiny hole is posterior to the 360° buckle and the previous operation performed elsewhere had failed to reattach the retina (Courtesy of BONNET M. Graefe's Arch Clin Exp Ophthalmol 225:59–62, 1987). (B) Postoperative fundus appearance. Following two cryoapplications and segmental scleral buckling of the hole, subretinal fluid spontaneously absorbed within a week. New vessels spontaneously regressed within 6 months.

The gas to be injected is SF6, since internal tamponade is required for only a few days. 0.2 to 0.3 CC pure gas are usually sufficient provided adequate positioning of the patient's head be done during the first postoperative days.

VITRECTOMY

Vitrectomy is virtually never required in the treatment of retinal detachments solely due to atrophic holes.[2,3]

It is most infrequent that vitreous lesions, most often induced by unsuccessful previous operations, make it necessary to perform vitrectomy.

RESULTS

Anatomical Results

Provided all full thickness retinal holes have been identified and adequately sealed, the prognosis for retinal reattachment is excellent. Retinal reattachment can be achieved in nearly all cases.[1–4]

The high success rate (98–100%) is mainly related to the fact that the risk of postoperative proliferative vitreoretinopathy is virtually nil, even when there are multiple retinal holes. This is in striking contrast to the prognosis of retinal detachments associated with tractional horseshoe retinal tears.

Visual Results

In spite of the frequent long duration of the detachment and macular involvement at the time of initial presentation, the prognosis for visual improvement after surgery is fairly good. Improvement of the visual field can be expected in nearly all cases. Postoperative visual acuity of 20/40 or better can be achieved in approximately 60% of eyes.[3]

REFERENCES

1. Tillery WV, Lucier AC: Round atrophic holes in lattice degeneration. An important cause of phakic retinal detachment. Trans Am Acad Ophthalmol Otolaryngol 81:509–518, 1976
2. Malbran ES, Dodds R, Hulsbus R: Two distinct types of myopic retinal detachments. Mod Probl Ophthalmol 18:292–303, 1977
3. Bonnet M, Urrets-Zavalia J: Décollements rétiniens par petits trous de la région équatoriale. J Fr Ophtalmol 9:615–624, 1986
4. Murakami-Nagasako F, Ohba N: Phakic retinal detachment associated with atrophic hole of lattice degeneration of the retina. Graefe's Arch Clin Exp Ophthalmol 220:175–178, 1983
5. Bonnet M: Peripheral neovascularization complicating rhegmatogenous retinal detachments of long duration. Graefe's Arch Clin Exp Ophthalmol 225:59–62, 1987

16

Retinal Detachment with
Retinal Dialysis

Retinal dialyses have been observed in chronic pars planitis as a result of cyclitic membrane contraction[1] in retinal detachment following penetrating ocular wounds[2,3] and after pars plana vitrectomy. Most cases, however, occur either after ocular contusion or as a primary disease in young individuals. In this chapter we shall only consider traumatic and idiopathic dialyses.

Retinal detachment with dialysis accounts for approximately 10% of all rhegmatogenous retinal detachments.[4-8] The incidence is slightly higher in men (59%[1] to 72%[9]). Patient age ranges from 2 years[9] to 72 years.[10] However, most cases are recognized between the second and the third decade[8] and 90% of patients are under 40 years of age.[9]

NONTRAUMATIC RETINAL DIALYSIS

Etiology

Nontraumatic retinal dialysis or juvenile dialysis is a clinical entity.[11,12] The most frequent location is the lower temporal quadrant. Several etiologic theories have been proposed. The cause of nontraumatic retinal dialysis, however, is still unclear.

Refractive errors are not a significant factor. In particular, retinal dialyses are not related to myopia. Myopia, usually of small degree, is found in only 10% of patients.[8,9] This incidence is approximately the same as that of myopia in the eye clinic population, but it is significantly lower than the incidence of myopia in all nontraumatic retinal detachments.[13] Family occurence of nontraumatic retinal dialysis has been reported.[4,7,8,14] In a family survey, where siblings of affected individuals had fundus examination with scleral depression, Verdaguer et al[7] found a family incidence of 33%. The siblings of affected patients were all clinically asymptomatic. The inheritance pattern may be either autosomal recessive or autosomal dominant.[4,7] Ethnic factors may play a role and explain the differences in incidence and bilaterality observed in various series.[7,15]

A congenital weakness may predispose to nontraumatic retinal dialysis.[4,11,16]

This hypothesis is supported by the fact that the most common location is the lower temporal quadrant and some cases are bilateral. The incidence of bilateral involvement, however, shows great variations depending on the series (4%,[1] up to 54%).[17] On the other hand the anatomy of the orbit makes the inferotemporal quadrant of the eye more vulnerable to trauma.

Peripheral cystic degeneration of unknown etiology may predispose to temporal dialysis.[9,11,18]

Visual Symptoms

In contrast with most other forms of rhegmatogenous retinal detachment, retinal detachments associated with dialysis are characterized by the lack of acute visual symptoms. Light flashes, vitreous floaters, or sudden and massive visual field defects are almost never reported by patients with retinal detachment resulting from retinal dialysis.

More than half of the patients complain of no symptoms until the macula becomes detached with resulting poor central vision. Some patients complain of vague or generalized blurring vision. In children unilateral decreased central vision is often disclosed by routine examination at school. In very young children unilateral strabismus may lead to the diagnosis of retinal detachment. Although the progression of such retinal detachment is usually very slow, it is infrequent that subclinical retinal detachment is found by routine fundus examination.[9]

Fundus Findings

RETINAL DETACHMENT

Retinal detachments associated with dialysis have distinct clinical features compared to other forms of rhegmatogenous retinal detachment (Figs. 137, 138, 139). The clinical features are related to the very gradual progression of the detachment in an eye that usually has no posterior vitreous detachment. The retinal detachment is usually rather flat. The height of the detachment gradually decreases from the periphery towards the posterior pole. Hence the posterior limit of the retinal detachment is usually very slightly elevated. It is concave towards the ora serrata and the dialysis. The surface of the detached retina is smooth without retinal folds. The retinal detachment remains circumscribed in the quadrant of the dialysis for several weeks or months. This is most often (61%[9] to 64%[1]) the lower temporal quadrant. The retinal detachment gradually extends superiorly until the macula becomes involved. A total retinal detachment is very rare (10%[9]) even in retinal detachments that have lasted several years. The retinal detachment seldom flattens with bed rest.

Signs of longstanding duration are found in approximately half of the cases. Demarcation lines with subretinal gliosis, intraretinal cysts, and secondary macular changes are the typical signs of longstanding duration. However, in spite of the longstanding duration, there is no sign of preretinal membrane proliferation, in particular no star-shaped fixed retinal folds.

Demarcation Lines. Demarcation lines are present in 37%[9] to 50%[1] of the cases. They are most frequent in inferotemporal dialysis than in the other locations (55% compared with 24%).[10] They are often multiple and concentric. The multiplicity of demarcation lines indicates a successive increase in the extent of the retinal detachment. It is assumed that it takes a minimum of 3 months for a demarcation line to develop.[4] The number of concentric demarcation lines provides an indication for evaluation of the duration of the detachment.

Peripheral Retinal cysts. The detached retina is often thickened by multiple confluent cystic spaces that can mimic a retinoschisis. In very longstanding detachments, confluence of the cystic spaces can result in large retinal macrocysts (Fig. 138 and Fig.

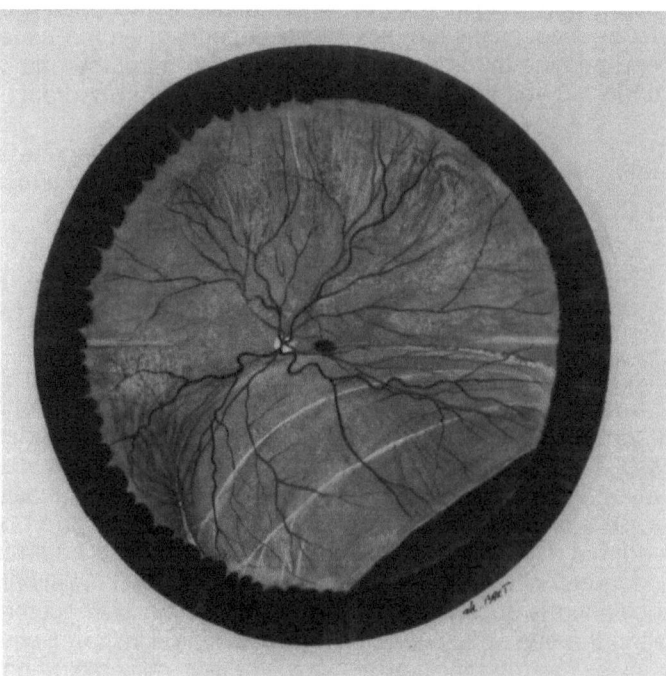

Figure 137. Retinal detachment with nontraumatic dialysis of the inferior temporal quadrant in a 22-year-old patient. Retinal detachment is associated with white lines of subretinal proliferation.

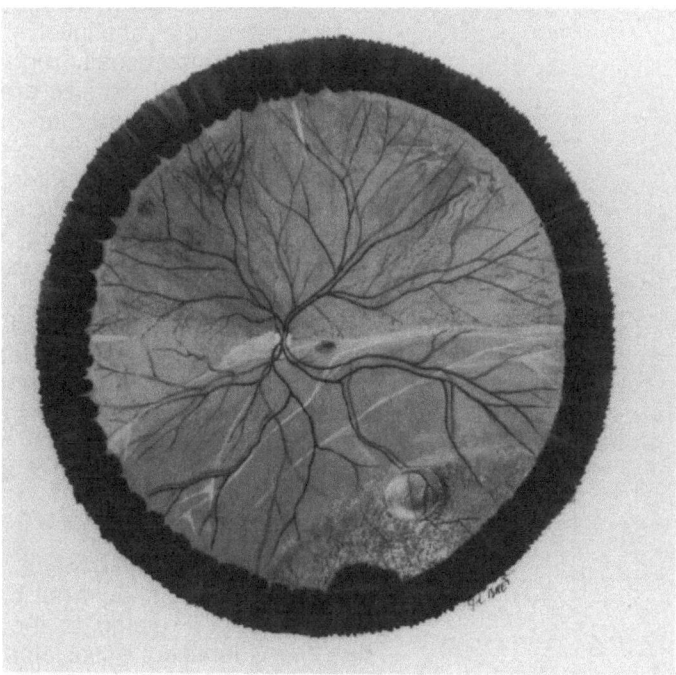

Figure 138. Longstanding duration retinal detachment associated with nontraumatic retinal dialysis. White lines of subretinal proliferation, and cystoid degeneration of the peripheral retina with a macrocyst are present.

140). Those large cysts are found in 6.5%[9] to 20%[1] of cases. The macrocysts are one to 8 disc diameters in size, round or oval in shape, and often multiple. They are usually located posteriorly to the equator. Those cysts do not require any treatment, but flatten spontaneously after surgery when the retinal dialysis is sealed.

Cystoid Macular Degeneration. Preoperative macular cysts or hole are present in 11%[10] to 43%[9] of cases. Macular lesions have the same pathogenesis as the peripheral cysts. They indicate a longstanding duration of the macular detachment. Cystic macular degeneration is the major sign for postoperative visual prognosis. Eyes with cystic macular degeneration will never recover useful central vision.[6,9]

RETINAL BREAK

Retinal dialysis related to the retinal detachment. The retinal dialysis is located in the quadrant involved by the retinal detachment. In longstanding retinal detachments that have spread to two or more quadrants, the location of the demarcation lines indicates where the dialysis should be searched for. The dialysis is situated at the basis of the arc of circle(s) delineated by the demarca-

tion line(s) (Figs. 137, and 138). Most nontraumatic dialyses are located in the inferotemporal quadrant (61%,[9] 64%,[1] 97%[7]) (Figs. 137 and 138). The superotemporal quadrant is the second most frequent location (32%[9]) (Fig. 140). The other locations account for only 7% of all cases.[9] Large dialyses are easily recognized; small dialysis are less easy to detect, especially when the retinal detachment is shallow. Their identification requires scleral depression.

Small dialyses are best seen when scleral depression is applied to the sides of the *dialyses*. In fact, when scleral depression is directly applied over a small dialysis, the posterior margin of the dialysis is brought into contact with its normal position at the ora serrata, and the dialysis may be invisible.

In contrast, when scleral depression is applied close to one extremity of the dialysis, the posterior margin of the dialysis becomes visible. The posterior margin of the dialysis is simply elevated towards the vitreous cavity. In contrast with what occurs in giant retinal tears, it does not roll back on itself, even when the dialysis is located in the upper quadrants. The posterior border is smooth or, less often, serrated with small bridges of cystic retina still attached to the ora serrata. The retina behind the dialysis often shows signs of cystic degeneration and is thicker than normal.

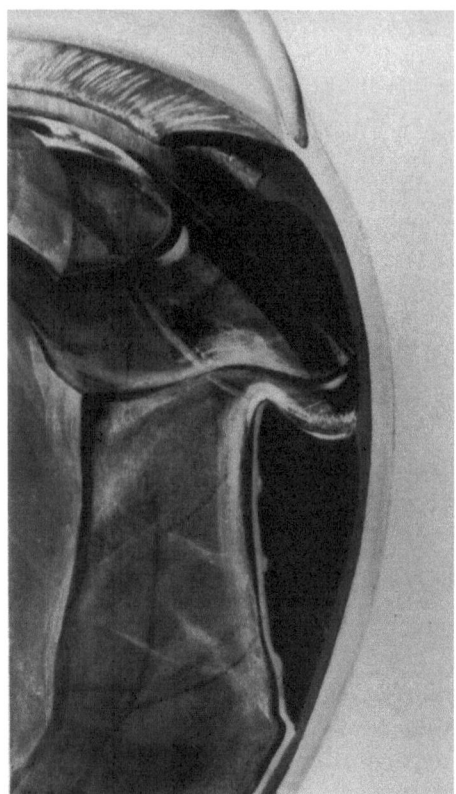

Figure 139. Vitreous gel in nontraumatic retinal dialysis. Normal vitreous gel is adherent to the posterior edge of the dialysis and the detached retina. Subretinal space is isolated from the vitreous cavity by viscous vitreous, covering the dialysis from edge to edge.

Most retinal dialyses involve less than one quadrant.[8,9] Their size usually ranges between 20° and 60°. Dialyses of 90° in size are rare (14%).[9] Large dialyses involving more than one quadrant are uncommon (8%).[8,9] Large dialyses are observed more frequently after severe blunt injury than in the nontraumatic form.[9] Large dialyses must be differenciated from giant retinal tears, since the prognosis of a large retinal tear is much more severe than that of a dialysis of the same size.

Vitreous surgery is required in the management of a number of large retinal tears. In contrast, it is virtually never required in the management of nontraumatic dialyses, regardless of their size.

The clinical signs that allow for the diagnosis between a large dialysis and a large retinal tear are summarized in Table 6.

Associated Retinal Breaks. Examination of the peripheral fundus should not be stopped when the dialysis directly related to the retinal detachment has been identified; associated retinal breaks may be present and require treatment. Association of two or more dialyses has been observed in approximately 30% of cases[7,8,9] (Fig. 140). The associated dialyses may be located in areas of detached or attached retina. Two or more retinal dialyses located in the superotemporal and the inferotemporal quadrants is the most frequent association. Full thickness retinal holes may also be associated with the dialysis, which are usually located in the intrabasal retina and situated in detached and/or attached retinas. Those holes are located in areas of primary cystic degeneration of the retina. They should be

Table 6
Summary of Clinical Signs for Diagnosis of Large Dialysis Versus Large Retinal Tear

Dialysis	Large and Giant Tear
– Anterior margin at the ora serrata	– Anterior margin posterior to the ora serrata
– No anterior flap	– Anterior retinal flap constant, although sometimes very narrow
– Anterior margin attached	– Anterior margin elevated
– Posterior margin simply elevated towards the vitreous cavity	– Posterior margin less elevated than the flap and frequently inverted
– Vitreous cortex attached to the posterior edge and the ora serrata, bridges the dialysis	– Vitreous cortex adherent to the anterior margin and detached from the posterior margin
– No vitreous detachment, no vitreous syneresis	– Vitreous detached and liquefied with large pockets of syneresis.

differenciated from pseudo holes and retinal cysts that do not require any treatment. Biomicroscopic examination with a narrow slit beam makes it possible to differenciate full thickness retinal holes from retinal cysts. In full thickness retinal holes, the pigment epithelium is directly exposed to the vitreous cortex, whereas retinal cysts correspond to an area of thickened retina. It should be stressed that horseshoe retinal tears are never seen in association with nontraumic retinal dialysis. Indentification of an associated horseshoe retinal tear should lead the surgeon to question the initial diagnosis of retinal dialysis. More thorough examination of the anterior margin of the retinal break and the vitreous cortex should be carried out. In such cases slit lamp examination with scleral depression will show that the retinal break is actually a large horseshoe tear with a very narrow flap under traction of the vitreous cortex.

VITREOUS BODY

Vitreous changes detectable by clinical examination are almost nil in nontraumatic retinal dialysis (Fig. 139). In particular there is neither a true posterior detachment nor definite vitreous liquefaction or syneresis. The vitreous base is always attached to the posterior edge of the dialysis. The pigment epithelium exposed by the dialysis is isolated from the vitreous cavity by the vitreous cortex, which covers the dialysis from edge to edge. In longstanding retinal detachments, there are often pigment clumps suspended in the vitreous base. This clinical finding is of no value with regard to the prognosis.

The absence of posterior detachment and definite vitreous syneresis may account for the specific clinical features of retinal detachments associated with dialysis, as compared with retinal detachments associated with horseshoe retinal tears. In particular the posterior edge of a retinal dialysis is adherent to the vitreous cortex and cannot role itself back on toward the vitreous cavity. The amount of vitreous fluid entering the subretinal space through the dialysis is small and the progression of the retinal detachment is very slow in spite of the large size of the retinal break. There is no available surface for the exposed pigment epithelial cells to migrate and proliferate on the inner side of the neurosensory retina. Proliferative vitreo retinopathy with fixed retinal folds cannot develop, even in a very large dialysis and longstanding retinal detachment. Pigment epithelial cells can only proliferate on the outer surface of the detached retina. Cell proliferation in the subretinal space results in demarcation lines and subretinal strands and cords, which do not prevent retinal reattachment when the dialysis is sealed.

FUNDUS EXAMINATION OF THE FELLOW EYE

The oral region of the fellow eye should be carefully examined with scleral depression since asymptomatic lesions may be present, some of them requiring treatment, and some requiring fundus examination at regular intervals.

Bilaterality of Nontraumatic Dialysis. Bilateral involvement of nontraumatic retinal dialysis may occur (Fig. 140), however the incidence of bilaterality shows great variations with the series. It is very low in certain series (2%,[8] and 7.7%[10]), as compared with other series (20%,[4]–27%,[9] and 37%).[7] Ethnic factors may also play a role in the incidence of bilateral involvement.[7] The dialysis in the fellow eye, when present, is associated with a retinal detachment, which is subclinical in 40%[7] to 60%[9] of patients. Most dialyses found in the fellow eye are also inferotemporal; however, they are not always symmetrical with regard to location and size.[7,9]

Peripheral Cystic Degeneration. Predetachment changes in the ora region of the fellow eye may be present[9,18,19] (Fig. 140). They consist of peripheral cystic degeneration, which is most often located in the temporal quadrants. Cystic degeneration may already be associated with small holes.

DIALYSIS AFTER BLUNT TRAUMA

Contusion injuries can cause retinal dialysis. Trauma accounts for approximately 35% of retinal detachments with dialysis.[9]

Pathogenesis

The pathogenesis of retinal dialysis resulting from ocular contusion was demonstrated by Weindenthal and Schepens.[20] Experiments on enucleated pig eyes produced traumatic changes of the peripheral fundus similar to those seen clinically in human eyes. Those changes included detachment of the nasal ora serrata, nasal retinal dialysis, festoon formation, peripheral pigmentary changes, and tears in the epithelium of the pars plana. Experimentally, damage to the superonasal ora serrata was most common when the projectile struck the center of the cornea.

Temporal dialysis was produced when the projectile struck the temporal limbus.

It is assumed from experimental data[20,21] that superonasal dialysis results from rapid expansion of the sclera in the equatorial region following the impact. A high-speed projectile that strikes the center of the cornea initiates a shock wave, which results in rapid distension of the sclera in the equatorial region. As a result, the vitreous base and ciliary epithelium pull away from the pigment epithelium of the pars plana.

Experimentally, temporal dialyses were produced when the projectile struck the temporal limbus.[2] Temporal dialyses are probably caused by the violent indentation of the coats of the eye near the temporal ora serrata and pars plana. Experimentally, temporal dialyses were usually associated with tears in the nonpigmented epithelium of the pars plana.[20]

Specific Clinical Features

Retinal dialyses following blunt trauma have specific clinical features compared to nontraumatic dialyses. In addition to their clinical significance, these clinical features may be of value in medico–legal cases.

LATENT INTERVAL

Retinal dialysis develops at the time of the contusion, hence, it should be diagnosed immediately after trauma. However, few retinal dialyses are discovered early after the trauma.[9] There is usually a latent interval between the injury and the time of diagnosis. The latent interval may be very long. In Zion's series,[10] only 15.8% of the cases were recognized within one month of injury, 41% of the cases were diagnosed more than 1 year after injury, and the latent interval was 5 years or more in 14% of patients. The latent interval is significantly longer in inferotemporal dialysis than in dialyses located in other quadrants.[10]

FUNDUS FINDINGS

Retinal detachments secondary to traumatic retinal dialysis share the main clinical characteristics of retinal detachments associated with nontraumatic dialysis. Therefore, the aspect of the detached retina does not in itself reveal the traumatic origin of the detachment. The diagnosis of traumatic origin is based on the specific features of peripheral fundus lesions and the associated sequelae of ocular contusion; all lesions are unilateral. It is mandatorily re-

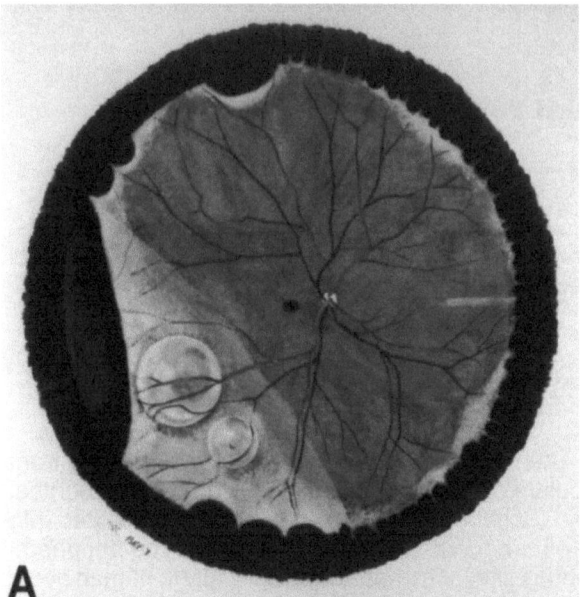
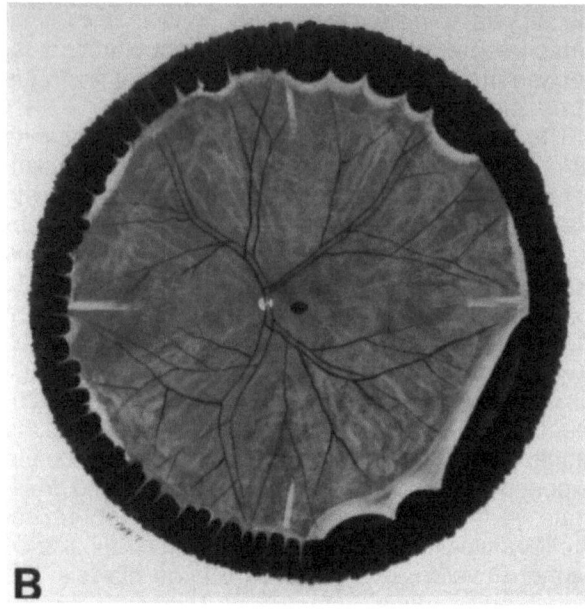

A   **B**

Figure 140. Bilateral nontraumatic dialysis in a 28-year-old patient. (A) Right eye shows retinal detachment with two retinal cysts. A large retinal dialysis in the temporal quadrants is associated with multiple smaller dialyses in detached and attached retina; cystic degeneration of the oral region is visible in the nasal quadrants. (B) Left eye shows multiple dialyses, in attached retina, in both temporal quadrants. Retinal dialyses are associated with cystic degeneration of the oral region.

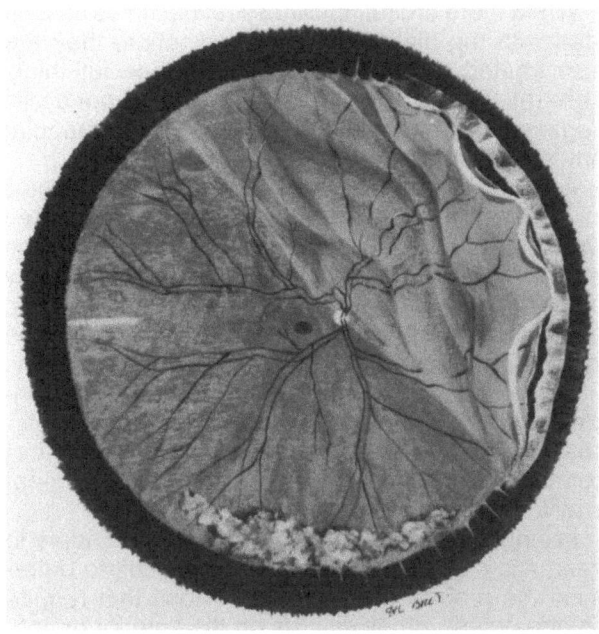

Figure 141. Retinal detachment with multiple oral dialyses in the nasal quadrants, following blunt trauma by a ball in a 30-year-old patient. Dialyses are associated with a festoon of avulsed nonpigmented epithelium of the pars plana. Blood is present in the lower part of the vitreous cavity.

quired that fundus examination be performed with scleral depression of the pars plana and ora serrata region. Traumatic retinal dialyses may be located in any quadrant, however, they are significantly more frequent in the upper nasal quadrant[8,9,20] (Fig. 141), and (78.3%) at the posterior border of the vitreous base than at the anterior border (11.2%).[22] Simultaneous anterior and posterior border dialyses result in avulsion of the vitreous base, which is pathognomonic of retinal detachment due to contusion injury. The nonpigmented epithelium of the pars plana is avulsed with the vitreous base. In some cases it can be seen suspended in the vitreous cavity like a festoon (Fig. 141). The dialysis is frequently associated with chorioretinal atrophy and pigmentation. The lesions are located in the ora serrata region and the pars plana, and they are found more frequently in superonasal dialysis than in inferotemporal dialysis. The lesions of the pars plana epithelium have no specific implication in terms of the treatment. They should, however, be carefully examined for their value in medico–legal cases.

ASSOCIATED SEQUELAE OF BLUNT TRAUMA

A contusion injury severe enough to cause a retinal dialysis usually results in associated traumatic lesions of the eye such as sphincter tears, iridodialysis, angle recession, lens subluxation, or choroidal ruptures. Angle recession, which may be associated with secondary glaucoma, is often located in the same quadrant as the retinal dialysis. At least one

sequela of ocular contusion is required to establish the traumatic origin of a retinal detachment.[22]

Surgical Management

INDICATIONS FOR SURGICAL TREATMENT

Affected Eye. Any retinal detachment associated with retinal dialysis is an indication for surgical treatment. Even very longstanding duration retinal detachments should be treated provided light perceptions are still present, since surgical retinal reattachment will restore at least part of the visual field. Retinal dialysis associated with asymptomatic peripheral retinal detachment with demarcation lines should also be operated on because the demarcation lines will not limit the extension of the detachment for an indefinite period of time. "Walling off" the detachment with cryoapplication or photocoagulation should be restricted to dialysis with subclinical retinal detachment extending no more than one disc diameter beyond the dialysis.

Fellow Eye. When fundus examination has disclosed bilateral dialysis, the indications for surgical treatment are identical for the fellow eye. Peripheral cystic degeneration of the fellow eye, which is not associated with retinal breaks, should not be prophilactically treated, since one cannot predict where a retinal dialysis or full thickness retinal hole might develop. Although the occurence of a retinal dialysis several years later is rare,[9] such patients should be examined once a year for a virtually indefinite period of time.

SURGICAL TECHNIQUE

Surgical treatment of retinal detachments associated with dialysis is easy in most cases. Treatment does not present any special difficulty excepting for some cases of giant dialyses. Giant dialyses are infrequent, however, and the surgical difficulties that may occur can be overcome with adequate technique.

The simplicity of the surgical treatment and the excellent prognosis for retinal reattachment (even in most cases of giant dialyses) are related to the fact that there is no significant vitreous pathology associated with retinal dialysis.

Care in sealing, not only the posterior edge, but also both extremities of the dialysis, is the single most important key for surgical success.

Localization. localization of the scleral projection of the dialysis is done on both extremities and the median part of the posterior edge. These scleral landmarks are then used for adequate placement of the scleral buckle.

Inducing a Retinochoroidal Adhesion. Cryoapplication for inducing retinochoroidal adhesion has only advantages in the treatment of retinal dialysis. There is no contraindication for the use of cryotreatment even in a very large dialysis, since the risk of proliferative vitreoretinopathy is virtually nil. The virtually nonexistent risk of proliferative vitreoretinopathy in retinal dialysis is the striking difference between retinal detachment associated with dialysis and detachment associated with large or giant retinal tears.

Cryoapplication is carried out under simultaneous biomicroscopic observation of the fundus with the three-mirror contact lens. The first cryoapplication is done on one of the extremities of the dialysis. Cryoapplications are then methodically performed on the posterior border of the dialysis up to the other extremity. A single row of cryoapplications performed along the posterior margin of the dialysis is sufficient in most cases, as there is virtually no risk of secondary slipping of the posterior edge of the dialysis on the choroidal indentation. Most failures in the treatment of retinal dialysis result from the inability to seal one or both extremities of the dialysis.[9] To avoid such failures, the surgeon has to make sure that the first and last cryoapplications on both extremities of the dialysis reach the ora serrata.

When there are full-thickness retinal holes associated with the dialysis in detached retina, they are also treated with cryoapplication. Those full-thickness retinal holes must be differentiated from cystic degeneration and macrocysts that do not require any specific treatment.

Associated dialysis or full thickness retinal holes in attached retina, when present, can be treated with cryoapplications. Argon laser photocoagulation is, however, more accurate. Photocoagulation may be performed before, during, or after surgery. The author usually performs photocoagulation of the lesions in attached retina the day before surgery. Photocoagulation during surgery unnecessarily increases the duration of general anesthesia. Photocoagulation treatment soon after surgery is less comfortable for the patient as compared to preoperative photocoagulation treatment.

In longstanding retinal detachments secondary to traumatic dialysis, it is sometimes difficult to determine the precise extent of the lesions that require cryotreatment. Small dialysis on the anterior or posterior border of the vitreous base may be associated with the main dialysis. One or both extremities of the dialysis may be partially hidden by the avulsed epithelium of the pars plana. Associated breaks may be difficult to identify in the pigmented and atrophic scars resulting from the contusion, which may extend far beyond the extremities of the main dialysis. In such cases observation of the lesions under very high magnification makes it easier to identify all lesions that require cryotreatment.

Scleral Buckling. Scleral buckling is necessary when the dialysis is associated with a retinal detachment extending more than two disc diameters beyond the posterior edge of the dialysis.

The scleral buckle should be segmental and parallel to the limbus. A 360° scleral buckle is never required to achieve surgical success, even in very large dialysis.[9]

Choroidal indentation can be achieved by means of either an explant or a lamellar scleral pocket. Scleral buckling with an explant is performed when the dialysis is more than 75° in size or when its scleral projection is behind a rectus muscle. The indications for a lamellar scleral pocket are usually restricted to dialysis less than 75° in size. Small dialysis located in the inferotemporal quadrant are the most suitable indication for a lamellar scleral pocket.

The choroidal indentation obtained by scleral buckling must involve the posterior edge of the dialysis up to the ora serrata (Fig. 142). The dialysis must not be simply "walled off" by placement of a buckle posterior to the dialysis. This type of buckle leaves the extremities of the dialysis untreated;

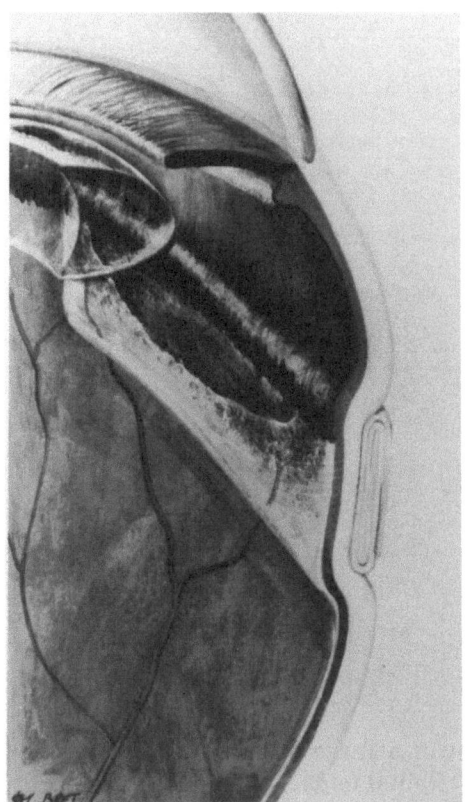

Figure 142. Scleral buckling of a retinal dialysis. The buckle should involve the ora serrata and extend 2 mm beyond the posterior edge of the dialysis. Both extremities of the dialysis should be supported by the buckle.

subretinal fluid accumulates anteriorly to the buckle and will subsequently extend posteriorly.

In order to achieve a choroidal indentation that involves the ora serrata, the anterior incision of a lamellar scleral pocket, or the anterior bites of the sutures for an explant are placed on the scleral projection of the ora serrata. Laterally, the buckle should extend 2 mm beyond both extremities of the dialysis. Posteriorly, the buckle should extend beyond the median part of the dialysis for 2 mm when an explant is used, and 4 mm when a lamellar scleral pocket is performed.

When the dialysis is more than 75° in size, the buckle should not be too high in order to avoid or minimize the risk of inducing radial folds and a fishmouth phenomenon.

Drainage of Subretinal Fluid. Drainage of subretinal fluid is unnecessary in most cases.

Subretinal fluid spontaneously absorbs within a few days after sealing of the dialysis, even in longstanding duration retinal detachments. The only indication for release of the subretinal fluid is the inability to tighten the scleral sutures of an explant when paracentesis of the anterior chamber and intravenous administration of acetazolamide have failed to provide intraocular space (see p. 63).

Gas Injection. Intravitreal gas injection is rarely required in the treatment of retinal dialysis, however, indication for gas injection may occur in large dialysis more than 75° in size, associated with a highly detached retina. In such cases gas injection is indicated when close approximation of the entire dialysis and pigment epithelium is not achieved by scleral buckling or when the scleral buckle induces radial retinal folds and a fishmouth phenomenon (Fig. 143).

The gas to be used is SF6, since internal tamponade is required for a short period of time. A small amount of pure gas is injected. The amount of gas is calculated by taking into account only the usually limited area of the dialysis that requires internal tamponade. A small gas bubble is sufficient for flattening a radial fold, provided the patient's head is adequately positioned for two or three days after surgery.

Vitrectomy. Vitrectomy is virtually never required in the treatment of idiopathic dialysis or dialysis after blunt trauma. In contrast with large and giant retinal tears, even very large and giant retinal dialysis after blunt trauma can successfully be treated without vitreous surgery.[9] Giant dialyses, 180° or more in size, after blunt trauma, which are very uncommon, can be successfully managed with a combination of posterior sclerotomy, gas injection, and early postoperative manipulation of the retina with the gas bubble.[9] Those simple maneuvers can be successful in the management of giant dialysis after blunt trauma because there is no static vitreous traction on the dialysis. The vitreous base was avulsed at the time of injury, but the vitreous body remains otherwise healthy. The vitreous body status is very different from the vitreous changes associated with giant retinal tears (see p. 187).

Vitreous surgery is not only unnecessary in the treatment of retinal dialysis, but it may also have deleterious effects on the course of the retinal detachment. Most retinal dialyses occur in eyes having no posterior vitreous detachment. Vitrectomy may be followed by the development of massive proliferative vitreoretinopathy, which never develops spontaneously in retinal detachments associated with dialyses.[9]

Indications for vitreous surgery in retinal dialyses are restricted to dialyses associated with traction retinal detachment. Traction retinal detachments, which may be associated with retinal dialysis, develop after penetrating injury of the eye (see p. 289) and in the late stages of severe pars planitis.

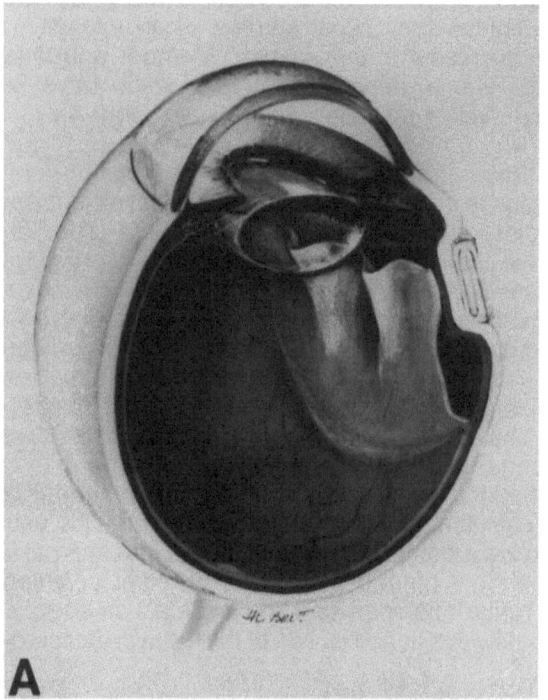
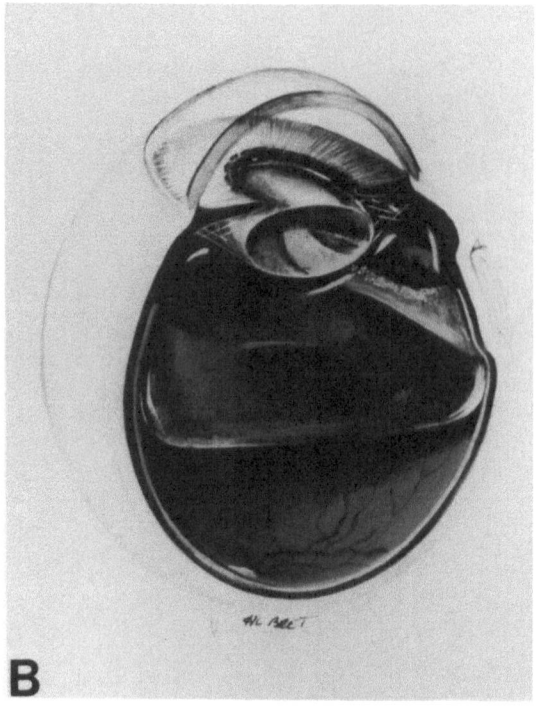

Figure 143. Intravitreal gas injection in the management of a large retinal dialysis. (A) Radial retinal folds have been induced by scleral buckling. (B) Radial folds have been flattened by the gas bubble.

Results

ANATOMICAL RESULTS

Anatomical results of the treatment are excellent. Permanent retinal reattachment can be achieved in 100% of eyes.[1,8,9,23]

Retinal reattachment can be achieved with a single operation in 91% of all cases regardless of the size of the dialysis, and 100% of dialysis 90° or less in size.[9] In the author's experience, the few cases that required two operations for retinal reattachment were retinal detachments associated with dialysis of 100° to 130° in size, which developed radial folds after scleral buckling and were not immediately managed by intravitreal gas injection.

The excellent anatomical results are related to two main parameters. The first parameter is related to the disease itself: the risk of proliferative vitreoretinopathy is virtually nonexistent in retinal detachments associated with dialyses. The second parameter is related to the care given by the surgeon in sealing the entire posterior edge of the dialysis up to the ora serrata.

FUNCTIONAL RESULTS

In spite of the severely impaired vision at the time of initial examination and the frequent longstanding duration of the retinal detachment in most cases, the majority of patients can expect visual improvement after retinal reattachment. Even in retinal detachments of several years duration, significant improvement of the visual field almost invariably occurs.

Functional results in terms of central visual acuity depend on the status of the macula before surgery. As expected, functional results are usually excellent when the macula is not involved by the detachment. The visual results are still good with vision of 20/40 or better in 58% of eyes when the macula was preoperatively detached but with no signs of cystic degeneration.[9] In contrast, the visual results in terms of central visual acuity are poor when preoperative examination reveals cystic macular degeneration of the detached macula.[6,9]

Angiographic cystoid macular edema after retinal reattachment is uncommon (approximately 10% of eyes).[9] The low incidence of cystoid macular edema is likely related to the young age of the patients.[24]

REFERENCES

1. Hagler WS, North AW: Retinal dialysis and retinal detachment. Arch Ophthalmol 79:376–388, 1968
2. Cox MS, Freeman HM: Retinal detachment due to ocular penetration. I—Clinical characteristics and surgical results Arch Ophthalmol 96:1354–1361, 1978
3. Bonnet M: Treatment of retinal detachment after penetrating eye injury: heavy cryotreatment of the fibrous ingrowth as an adjunct to vitreoretinal microsurgery. Ophthalmologica 194:164–168, 1987
4. Lefferstra LJ: Disinsertions at the ora serrata. Ophthalmologica 119:1–16, 1950
5. Tullock CG: Distribution of holes and tears in primary retinal detachment. Brit J Ophthalmol 49:413–431, 1965
6. Chignell AH: Retinal dialysis Brit J Ophthalmol 57:572–577, 1973
7. Verdaguer J: Juvenile retinal detachment. Am J Ophthalmol 93:145–156, 1982
8. Hagler S: Retinal dialysis: a statistical and genetic study to determine pathogenic factors. Trans Am Ophthalmol Soc 78:686–732, 1980
9. Bonnet M, Moyenin P, Pecold C, Grange JD: Décollements de la rétine par desinsertion À l'ora serrata. J Fr Ophthalmol 9:231–242, 1986
10. Zion VM, Burton TC: Retinal dialysis. Arch Ophthalmol 98:1971–1974, 1980
11. Shapland CD: Diseases of the retina. 1—Retinal detachment and gonin' operation Trans Ophthalmol Soc UK 52:170–202, 1932
12. Gonin J: Le décollement de la rétine Pathogénie—Traitement. Lausanne, Payot, Switzerland, 1934, 70–73
13. Ashrafzadeh MT, Schepens CL, Elzeneiny I, Moura R, et al: Aphakic and phakic retinal detachment. I—Preoperative findings. Arch Ophthalmol 89:476–483, 1973
14. Levy J: Inherited retinal detachment. Brit J Ophthalmol 35:626–636, 1952
15. Rodriguez ZA: Retinal pigmentation in cases of detachments with spontaneous dialysis, in Pruett RC, Regan CD (eds). Retina congress, Twenty-fifth meeting New York, Appleton-Century-Crofts 1972, 479–487
16. Tornquist R: Bilateral retinal detachment. Acta Ophthalmol. 41:126–133, 1963
17. Verdaguer TJ, Rojas B, Lechuga M: Genetical studies in nontraumatic retinal dialysis. Mod Probl Ophthalmol 15:34–39, 1975
18. Schepens CL: Retinal detachment and allied diseases. Philadelphia, W.B. Saunders 1983, Vol. 1 pp. 42
19. Scott JD: Retinal dialysis. Trans Ophthalmol Soc UK 97:33–35, 1977
20. Weidenthal DT, Schepens CL: Peripheral fundus changes associated with ocular contusion. Am J Ophthalmol 62:465–477, 1966
21. Delori F, Pomerantzeff O, Cox MS: Deformation of the globe under high-speed impact: its relation to contusion injuries. Invest Ophthalmol 8:290–301, 1969
22. Cox MS, Schepens CL, Freeman HM: Retinal detachment due to ocular contusion. Arch Ophthalmol 76:678–685, 1966
23. Saito T, Koda N, Kikuchi H: Juvenile bilateral disinsertion at the ora serrata II—statistic survey. Folia Ophthal Jap 25:1225, 1974
24. Bonnet M, Fernandez Pastor D: Rupture de la barrière hematorétinienne après microchirurgie du décollement de la rétine. Ophtalmologie 1:29–31, 1988

17

Retinal Detachment with Giant Retinal Tear

Giant retinal tears extend 90 degrees or more around the circumference of the eye. Those associated with giant retinal tears are the most severe rhegmatogenous retinal detachments. In most cases retinal detachment is associated with severe vitreous change. There is a close correlation between the severity of the vitreous changes and the retinal tear size.

At present, microsurgical techniques make it possible to achieve mechanical repositioning of the detached, and often inverted, retina in most cases. However the prognosis for permanent retinal reattachment remains poor. Poor prognosis is related to the high incidence of severe proliferative vitreo retinopathy that develops or recurs after surgery.

ETIOLOGY

Incidence

Retinal detachments associated with giant retinal tears are infrequent. The actual incidence cannot be evaluated from the series emanating from retinal referral centers because most patients with giant retinal tears are operated on in retinal referral centers where most patients with easy retinal detachments are not referred. In the author's experience, retinal detachments with giant retinal tears account for 4.6% of rhegmatogenous retinal detachments.

Age and Sex Distribution

Retinal detachments with giant retinal tears have been observed in patients from 5 years[1] to 82 years of age.[2] There is a prevalence in young patients,

however. Fifty-three per cent[3] to 56%[1] of the patients are under age 40. Twenty percent of the patients are children.[3] The average age of the patients is approximately 35 years.[1,3,4] This is younger than the average age of the patients in series of nonselected retinal detachments.[5] There is also a prevalence in males who account for 69%[4] to 88%[1] of all patients with giant retinal tears.

Trauma Cases

The incidence of trauma cases is approximately 20% in most series.[2–4,6] There is a significant male prevalence in trauma cases. Giant retinal tears have been observed after penetrating ocular injury as well as blunt truma. Blunt trauma may be only a precipitating factor in highly myopic or aphakic eyes with preexisting vitreoretinal changes. Giant retinal tears after blunt trauma must be differenciated from giant dialysis (see p. 186).

Nontrauma Cases

Retinal detachments with nontraumatic giant retinal tears have been observed in phakic as well as aphakic and pseudophakic eyes.

Aphakic eyes account for approximately 10%[2–4] to 35%[1] of retinal detachments with giant retinal tears. Aphakia is less common in nontrauma cases than in trauma cases. Thirty-three percent[4] to 60%[3] of nontraumatic cases in aphakic eyes have been observed in eyes that underwent repeated surgery for congenital cataract. Giant retinal tears after lensectomy through the pars plana have also been observed.[7] There is a high prevalence of myopic eyes in nontraumatic giant tears. The incidence of myopia is approximately 70%.[3,4] The incidence of bilateral retinal detachment is very high. It is approximately 40%[4,8] at the time of initial presentation. This incidence does increase with time.[8] The retinal detachment in the fellow eye may be associated with horseshoe retinal tears less than 90° in size or a giant retinal tear. The incidence of bilateral giant tears is estimated to be approximately 13%[8] in patients followed during an average period of 4 years. The actual incidence of bilateral giant tear is probably underestimated since a secondary cataract often prevents ophthalmoscopic examination of the fellow eye at the time of initial presentation. In addition giant retinal tears may develop in the fellow eye after periods of time that range from 1 year to 26 years.[3]

Family history of retinal detachment and giant retinal tears is found in 10%[4] to 18% of the patients.[3] Some cases develop in patients affected by Wagner's hereditary vitreoretinal degeneration.

CLINICAL CHARACTERISTICS

Visual Symptoms

As in most retinal detachments associated with horseshoe retinal tears visual symptoms are acute.

Light flashes and vitreous floaters are associated with sudden and massive visual field defect in most patients. Therefore, the retinal detachment is recognized at an early stage in most patients. In very young children, however, the retinal detachment is often not recognized until a secondary cataract develops.

On the other hand economic and geographical reasons result in late examination of the patient.[3]

Fundus Findings

RETINAL TEAR

Most giant retinal tears develop at the posterior border of the vitreous base. Only a few cases develop along the posterior edge of lattice degeneration. In most cases there is no detectable evidence of retinal degeneration in the area of the giant retinal tear. The vast majority of giant retinal tears are located anteriorly to the equator. However, the ends of the retinal tear may curve posteriorly towards the optic disc, making the prognosis more severe[6,9] (Fig 144). The anterior flap is most often very narrow. When the slit in the retina is very close to the ora serrata, the anterior flap is so narrow that the retinal tear may be misdiagnosed as a retinal dialysis. However, a more careful slit lamp examination will reveal the nature of the retinal break. An anterior flap is

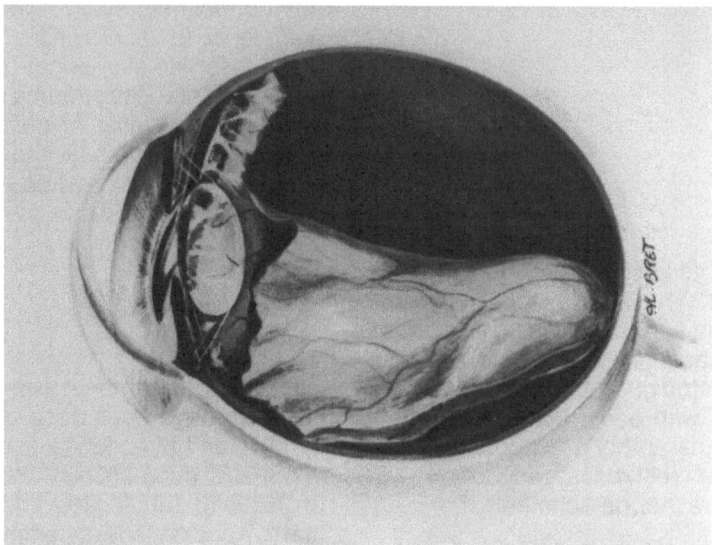

Figure 144. Cross section of a myopic eye with a 210° tear involving both superior quadrants. Owing to the site and size of the tear and severe vitreous gel liquefaction, the superior retina is inverted. Condensed anterior vitreous gel pulls on the narrow anterior flap of the tear. (Cross section corresponds to the eye shown in Fig. 152.)

always present in giant retinal tears. It is dragged anteriorly toward the vitreous cavity by contraction of the vitreous base. The epithelium of the pars plana, which is also under traction of the vitreous base is detached with the anterior edge of the retinal tear in more than 90% of eyes.

The posterior edge of a giant retinal tear shows a significant tendency to become inverted. Folding of the posterior edge relates to two distinct groups of parameters that can be recognized by clinical examination. It is most important for surgical management and prognosis to differenciate mobile from fixed folding. Mobile folding of the posterior edge of a giant retinal tear is related to the inward movements of the vitreous gel and gravity. The degree of mobile folding depends on 4 parameters: (1) the degree and extent of vitreous gel liquefaction and posterior vitreous detachment, (2) the circumferential extent of the retinal tear, (3) the posterior extension of the extremities of the retinal tear, and (4) the quadrantic location of the retinal tear.

The tendency of mobile folding to the posterior edge most often parallels the circumferential extent of the retinal tear and the degree of vitreous gel liquefaction and posterior vitreous detachment. In retinal tears less than 180° in size, mobile inversion of the posterior edge increases with the posterior extension of the retinal tear extremities. Nearly all giant retinal tears located in the superior quadrants show an inverted posterior edge (Fig. 144).

Mobility of the inverted flap can and should be recognized by preoperative fundus examination. It is evaluated by slit lamp examination in the seated and supine positions and ophthalmoscopic examination in the prone position. Head exercises for unfolding mobile retinal flaps have been described by Freeman.[10] A mobile inverted flap will unfold with a fast head movement in the direction the flap is folded, followed by a short pause and slow return movement to the opposite direction.

In contrast to mobile folding, fixed folding of the posterior edge of a giant retinal tear is related to the development of proliferative vitreoretinopathy. It is a sign of poor prognosis. Fixed folding of the posterior edge is not dependent on the size, posterior extent, or quadrantic location of the retinal tear. It is related to cell proliferation and contraction of the layer of vitreous cortex that remains adherent to the posterior retina. The posterior edge of the retinal tear is rolled over and fixed. The position of the retinal flap does not respond to head positioning and exercises. Giant retinal tears extend circumferentialy from 90° up to 360°. Giant retinal tears involving less than 180° are twice as frequent as those of 180° and over.[3] Giant retinal tears extending on more than 270° are infrequent (13% of giant retinal tears.[1,3]

Horseshoe retinal tears are often associated with giant retinal tears. They are present in approximately 35% of eyes.[3,9] They are invariably situated at the same circumferential level of the retina as the giant tear. The size of the associated horseshoe retinal tears may range from 2° to 90° and over.[3,9] Giant retinal tears may involve any of the retinal quadrants. Involvement of the temporal quadrants is the most frequent; location limited to the inferior quadrants is the least frequent.[3]

RETINAL DETACHMENT

Extent of the retinal detachment is directly related to the size of the retinal tear, degree of vitreous gel liquefaction, and posterior vitreous detachment. The ciliary epithelium is also detached in the area of the giant retinal tear in more than 90% of eyes (Fig. 145). In some eyes detachment of the ciliary epithelium involves 360° of the eye circumference. It is of primary importance to carefully evaluate the detached posterior retina with regard to signs of proliferative vitreoretinopathy. In the author's experience proliferative vitreoretinopathy is already present preoperatively in 95% of nontraumatic giant retinal tears.

VITREOUS GEL

Changes of the vitreous body are a constant finding in giant retinal tears. The vitreous findings are dependent on the etiology of the giant retinal tear. Two distinct groups of vitreous findings should be differenciated. They are of major importance with regard to the surgical prognosis.

Severe Vitreous Gel Liquefaction without Posterior Vitreous Detachment. Slit lamp examination reveals three major findings: (1) extensive liquefaction of the vitreous gel posteriorly to the equator, (2) condensation of the anterior vitreous gel, and (3) a thin layer of vitreous cortex that remains adherent to the inner surface of the posterior retina. (Fig. 145)

Vitreous gel liquefaction involves the entire vitreous gel except for the anterior vitreous gel and the posterior vitreous cortex. In spite of extensive liquefaction of the posterior vitreous gel, there is no posterior vitreous detachment. Liquid vitreous gel overlies the giant retinal tear, but a thin layer of vitreous cortex covers the posterior retina. Intravitreal membranes and bands, originating from the vitreous base, are often visible within the liquefied posterior vitreous gel and condensed anterior vitreous gel. Freeman[8] demonstrated that such modifications of the vitreous gel precede the giant retinal tear

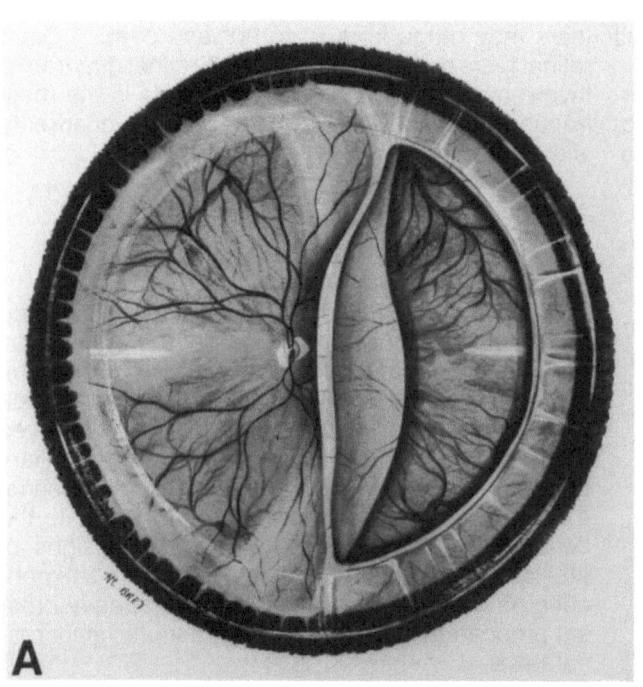 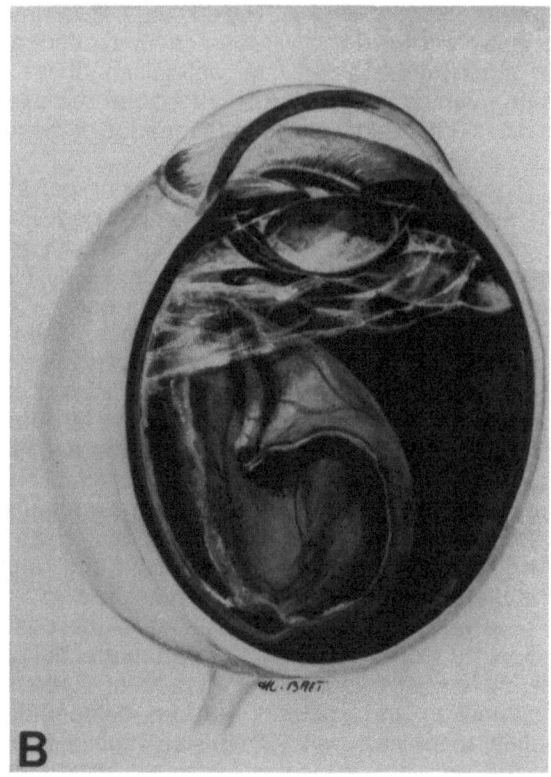

Figure 145.   Giant tear in a 20-diopter myopic eye. (A) Fundus appearance. The nonpigmented ciliary epithelium is detached in the retinal tear area. The posterior edge of the tear is inverted. (B) Cross-section of the eye. The anterior vitreous gel is condensed and pulls on the anterior flap of the tear. The central vitreous gel shows nearly complete liquefaction. A thin layer of vitreous cortex remains adherent to the retina. Intravitreal bands extending from the optic disc to the anterior vitreous gel are visible.

formation, and they can help to predict the development of a giant retinal tear in the fellow eye.

Intravitreal membranes and bands originating from the region of the vitreous base are often visible within the liquefied posterior vitreous and condensed anterior vitreous gel. Such major changes of the vitreous gel are a constant finding in giant retinal tears that develop in young myopic patients. They are associated with a poor surgical prognosis. Such eyes show a very high incidence of severe proliferative vitreoretinopathy.

Posterior Vitreous Detachment with or without Vitreous Gel Liquefaction.   Posterior vitreous detachment is the major finding. In this group the vitreous gel changes that may be associated with posterior vitreous detachment depends mainly on the etiology of the giant retinal tear. In nontraumatic cases occurring in emmetropic eyes, usually in patients over 45, posterior vitreous detachment may be complete or incomplete. It is associated with some

degree of vitreous gel liquefaction. However, vitreous liquefaction remains limited to part of the vitreous gel. Formed vitreous gel remains visible in the lower part of the vitreous cavity. When the giant retinal tear is located inferiorly, viscous vitreous overlies the tear and may seep into the subretinal space.

In trauma cases in nonpredisposed eyes, posterior vitreous detachment is limited to the region of the giant retinal tear in most cases (Fig. 146). There is no vitreous gel liquefaction. Vitreous hemorrhage is a common finding. In young patients it is the only significant vitreous change associated with posterior vitreous detachment. The surgical prognosis is excellent in most cases, whatever the size of the giant retinal tear. In trauma cases in predisposed eyes the vitreous changes associated with posterior vitreous detachment depend on preexisting vitreous lesions. As a whole the surgical prognosis appears to be better in the group of eyes with posterior vitreous detachment than in the group of eyes with extensive vitreous liquefaction and no posterior vitreous detachment.

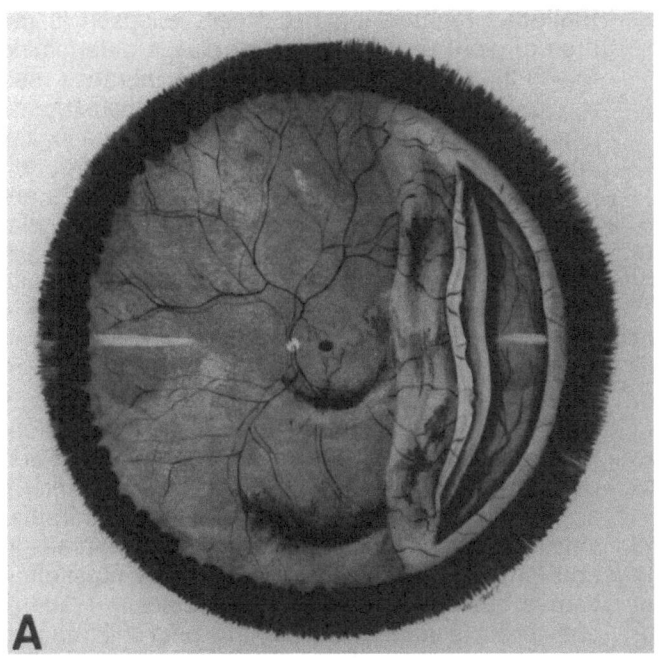
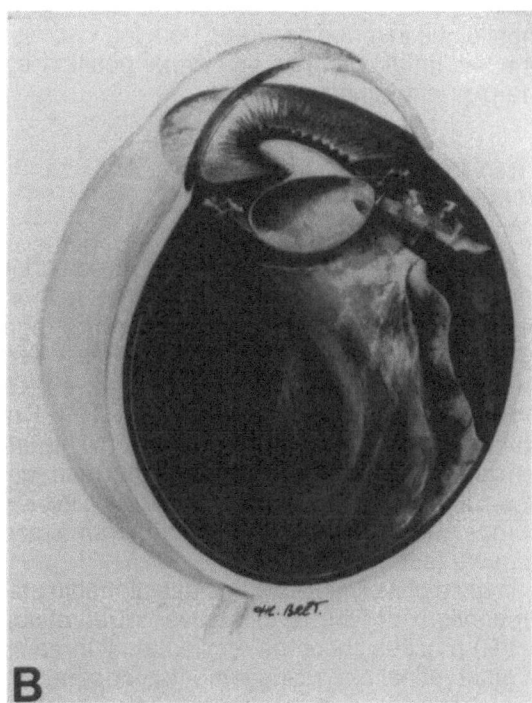

Figure 146. Giant tear after blunt trauma in an emmetropic eye of a 35-year-old patient. (A) Fundus appearance. In spite of the tear size the tear posterior edge is slightly inverted. Retinal detachment does not extend to the posterior pole. Hemorrhages are present in the retrovitreal space. (B) Cross-section of the eye. Posterior vitreous detachment is limited and vitreous gel is normally viscous. The narrow anterior flap of the tear is not pulled anteriorly and the nonpigmented ciliary epithelium is attached.

TREATMENT

Preoperative Management

Two specific measures should be considered in preoperative management of a patient with a giant retinal tear: (1) preoperative head positioning and exercises, and (2) prophylaxis of proliferative vitreoretinopathy.

PREOPERATIVE HEAD POSITIONING AND EXERCISES

Development of improved surgical techniques for repositioning an inverted retina has decreased the indications for preoperative head positioning and exercises in giant retinal tears. At present preoperative positioning for a period of one to two or three days is limited to giant retinal tears that can be surgically managed without vitrectomy. In contrast, preoperative head positioning for more than 24 hours is useless when vitrectomy is required. Preoperative head positioning is indicated in the following circum-

stances: (1) giant retinal tears of any size, after blunt trauma in eyes with no previous predisposing vitreous changes and (2) giant retinal tears less than 180° in size in emmetropic eyes with posterior vitreous detachment and no extensive liquefaction of the vitreous gel. In both circumstances preoperative head positioning is indicated when the posterior flap is inverted and mobile.

In contrast, preoperative head positioning is of little value, excepting for diagnosis of flap mobility, in myopic eyes with extensive vitreous liquefaction, giant retinal tears over 180° in size, and retinal detachments already associated with fixed retinal folds. When indicated, head positioning is limited to a short period of time that shoud not exceed two or three days.

The head maneuvers and positioning for unfolding an inverted retinal flap have been described in details by Freeman[10] and Schepens.[6] First, the patient's head should be placed in the prone position. Displacement of viscous vitreous downward, towards the anterior part of the vitreous cavity in order to free the inverted retinal flap, is the goal of the prone position. The patient's head kept prone, is then rotated so that the inverted flap is dependent. When mobile, the inverted flap freed from the viscous vitreous will unfold towards its normal position against the pigment epithelium.

PREVENTION OF PROLIFERATIVE VITREORETINOPATHY

At present severe proliferative vitreoretinopathy remains the major complication of giant retinal tears and the most frequent cause of failure to permanently reattach the retina (see p. 209). In most series[1,3] the incidence of failures related to severe proliferative vitreoretinopathy is approximately 45%. Prevention of the proliferative process should, therefore, be one of the main objectives in the management of giant retinal tears. Unfortunately, the clinical value of most means currently used today remains questionable (see p. 251).

In spite of its limitations and questionable efficacy, prevention of the proliferative vitreoretinopathy (PVR) process shoud be applied at all three stages of giant retinal tear management: preoperatively, intraoperatively, and postoperatively. Preoperative prevention of PVR includes three means: (1) early surgery, (2) systemic treatment, and (3) destruction of the exposed pigment epithelium by argon laser photocoagulation.

Early Surgery. Ocular and systemic examination are performed without delay so that surgery can be performed very rapidly. Development of proliferative vitreoretinopathy is a very early process in giant retinal tears. In the author's own experience, 60% of patients referred shortly after the onset of visual symptoms already show PVR, grade B. Most patients referred 2 weeks or more after the onset of visual symptoms show proliferative vitreoretinopathy, grade C or D. Treatment of giant retinal tears is an emergency. Early surgery can deal with giant retinal tears that are not yet associated with full thickness fixed retinal folds. Therefore, surgical management at an early stage is easier. It remains most uncertain, however, that early surgery effectively decreases the rate of severe postoperative PVR. In spite of early and proper surgical management, the incidence of severe postoperative PVR remains very high in giant retinal tears associated with extensive vitreous gel liquefaction and no posterior vitreous detachment.

Systemic Treatment for Inhibition of the Proliferative Process. Systemic treatment for inhibition of the proliferative process is started two days before surgery. At present intravenous synacthene and oral colchicine are the drugs most commonly used (see p. 251). Other drugs and Roentgentherapy may be used in the future (see p. 252).

Early Destruction of the Exposed Pigment Epithelium. Pigment epithelial cells exposed in the area of giant retinal tears may play a determining role in the formation of preretinal membranes (see p. 233). Therefore, early destruction of the exposed pigment epithelium appears to be one of the logical approaches for preventing proliferative vitreoretinopathy. The exposed pigment epithelial cells are destroyed by means of argon laser photocoagulation. Laser treatment is carried out as soon as possible. It is performed before any attempt to unfold the inverted retina. It is followed by head maneuvers and adequate positioning for one or two days. Surgical management will be carried out within 24 or 48 hours after argon laser photocoagulation. Argon laser photocoagulation of the exposed pigment epithelium is usually performed in the supine position using the argon laser attached to the surgical microscope. In giant retinal tears, treatment is rather lengthy owing to the large area to be treated. In addition, it may be painful. It is therefore, most often carried out under retrobulbar anesthesia. General anesthesia is usually required in young children and nervous patients. A 350 or 500 μm size spot and an exposure time of 0.5 seconds are used. The power should be sufficient to obtain mild whitening of the pigment epithelial cells. The burns should be confluent. When the hinge of the folded retina is located very posterior to the equator, such as it is often the case in retinal tears of 180° and over located superiorly, argon laser photocoagulation is performed on approximately half of the midperiphery.

Anteriorly, photocoagulation should reach the edge of the anterior retinal flap. When photocoagulation of the exposed pigment epithelium is completed, photocoagulation of the anterior flap and lateral edges of the giant tear are performed under scleral depression, which temporarily places the detached retina into apposition with the underlying pigment epithelium. White burns on the retina shoud be obtained. Head maneuvering and positioning are carried out immediately after photocoagulation treatment.

Surgical Management

Because of the complexity and length of the surgical procedure in most cases, surgery is usually performed under general anesthesia.

Choice of the surgical procedure is dictated by four main parameters: (1) the etiology of the giant retinal tear, (2) the size of the giant tear, (3) the location of the posterior retinal fold hinge, and (4) the absence or presence, and degree, or proliferative vitreoretinopathy.

With regard to their surgical management, giant

retinal tears can be classified into two distinct groups: (1) giant retinal tears that can and should be managed without vitreous surgery and (2) giant retinal tears in which vitreous surgery is required.

SURGICAL MANAGEMENT WITHOUT VITRECTOMY

Giant retinal tears that can, and should preferably be managed without vitrectomy are those that fulfil the following criteria: (1) giant retinal tears after blunt trauma in emmetropic and healthy eyes, (2) those under 180° in size, (3) those with a hinge of the posterior fold located anteriorly to the equatorial region, and (4) those having a mobile retina without any clinical evidence of incipient proliferative vitreoretinopathy (grade 0) and absence of viscous vitreous gel in the subretinal space (Fig. 146).

Giant retinal tears that fulfill all these criteria are by far the least common.

Satisfactory surgical management of such easy cases can be achieved by the combination of scleral buckling and gas injection (Fig. 147). The surgical procedure includes six consecutive steps.

Exposure of the Surgical Field. Temporary disinsertion of a rectus muscle is carried out in most cases in order that scleral surgery can be performed with the greatest accuracy and the least tissue trauma.

Localization of the retinal Tear. Localization of the scleral projection of the retinal tear is made for the posterior extremities of both lateral edges and the hinge of the posterior flap when the retina is slightly inverted or the margin of the posterior edge when the retina is not folded.

Choroidal Irritation. Cryotreatment is limited to the margins of the retinal tear. When the retinal tear is over 120° in size, argon laser photocoagulation rather than cryotreatment is used. When the posterior retinal flap is not inverted or the inversion is less than 1.5 mm in width, argon laser photocoagulation is performed intraoperatively. It is done before scleral buckling. Temporary apposition of the retina and the pigment epithelium is obtained by scleral depression. When the posterior flap is not inverted, 4–5 rows of photocoagulation burns are made on the posterior edge of the retinal tear. The lateral edges and the anterior flap were submitted to photocoagulation before surgery. When the posterior flap is slightly inverted, one row of photocoagulation burns is placed on the hinge of the posterior flap. Four additional rows are made on the retina behind the posterior border of the flap. When the inverted flap is more than 1.5 mm in width, argon laser photo-

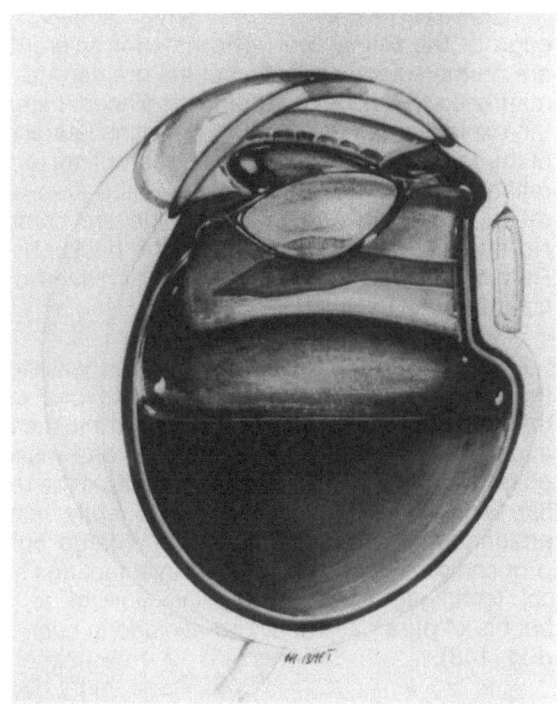

Figure 147. Surgical management of a giant tear after blunt trauma in an emmetropic eye (case shown in Figure 146). Surgical management consisted of segmental scleral buckling of the tear and intravitreal gas injection without vitrectomy. Permanent retinal reattachment was achieved with 20/20 central vision.

coagulation cannot be performed before unfolding the retina. In such cases argon laser photocoagulation is performed postoperatively in aphakic eyes. In phakic eyes, postoperative argon laser treatment through the gas bubble is most often difficult to perform, especially when the retinal tear is located in the lower quadrants. In such cases cryotreatment is applied during surgery. Cryo is performed before scleral buckling and unfolding of the flap. One row of cryoapplications is performed on the hinge of the folded retina. An additional row of cryoapplications is made more posteriorly.

Scleral Buckling. Scleral buckling is limited to the retinal tear (Fig. 147). Choroidal indentation should be broad and moderately high to buckle the retinal tear and induce the least radial retinal folds. A rather broad explant is used. The width of the explant is equal to the radial size of the tear. Explants of 5–8 mm in width are commonly used in giant retinal tears. The posterior scleral bites of the mattress sutures are placed 3–4 mm as a maximum posteriorly to the scleral projection of the posterior edge of the retinal tear. The anterior scleral bites are on the scleral projection of the ora serrata. Two mattress sutures per quadrant are placed. Laterally, the explant extends 4 mm beyond each lateral edge of the tear. In most cases the buckle will not provide retinochoroidal apposition on the entire area of the retinal tear, and radial retinal folds are common. No attempt is made to increase the buckle height. Retinochoroidal apposition will be achieved by intravitreal gas injection.

Gas Injection. Gas injection is the last step of the procedure. Pure perfluoropropane gas rather than sulfur-hexafluoride gas is used in most cases. Injection of a small volume of pure gas makes it possible, with a single injection, to unfold the retinal flap with a small bubble and subsequently, achieve prolonged retinal tamponade with a large bubble. (For choice of gas, volume to be injected, and surgical technique see p. 122.) Injection of a large bubble of pure gas should be avoided in such eyes (Fig. 148).

Head Maneuvers for Unfolding the Retinal Flap. Head maneuvering is done as early as the patient is returned to his bed. Maneuvering includes three consecutive steps (Fig. 149): (1) the patient is positioned so that the gas bubble is opposite the retinal tear; (2) the patient is rotated prone and maintained in this position for 30 seconds to one minute so that the small gas bubble moves towards the posterior pole while the retinal flap unfolds towards the eye wall; and (3) the patient is slowly rotated so that the gas bubble passes beneath the retinal flap and pushes it against the pigment epithelium (Fig. 149). For unfolding a giant retinal tear located in the superior quadrants, the patient is first placed in the supine position (the gas bubble moves towards the anterior part of the vitreous cavity); then the head is flexed and the patient is rotated to the prone position, the apex of his head oriented towards the floor (the gas bubble moves towards the lower part of the vitreous cavity, while the retinal flap moves under gravity towards the upper quadrants of the eye). Then the patient is positioned in the seated position, his head resting on pillows.

A rotating table facilitates manipulation of an inverted flap with a small gas bubble. When a rotating table is not available, however, three strong staff members can do the job with the same efficacy and safety. Soon after general anesthesia, when manipulation must be done, one cannot rely on patient coop-

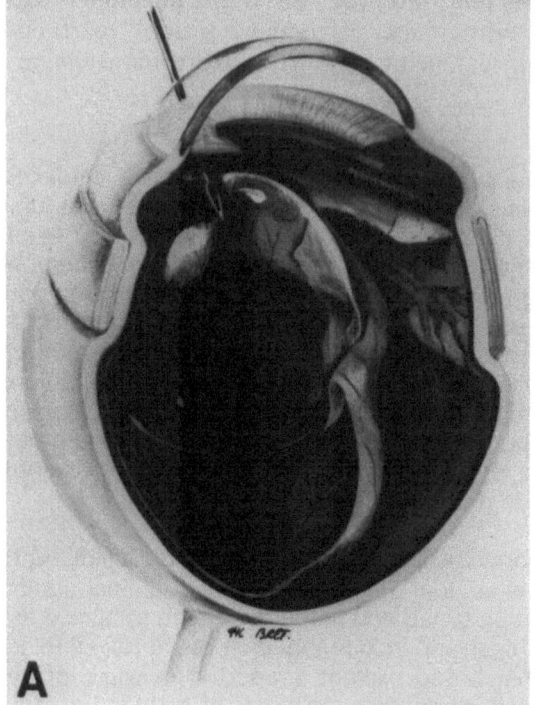

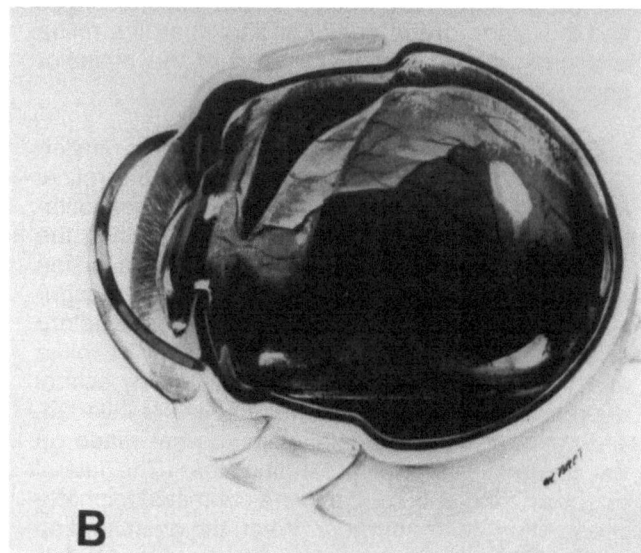

Figure 148. Error to avoid in the management of a giant tear with intravitreal gas injection. (A) The bubble of pure gas injected intraoperatively is too large. The gas bubble compresses the inverted posterior flap of the tear. (B) Postoperative appearance after gas bubble expansion. Early head maneuvering failed to unfold the inverted retina.

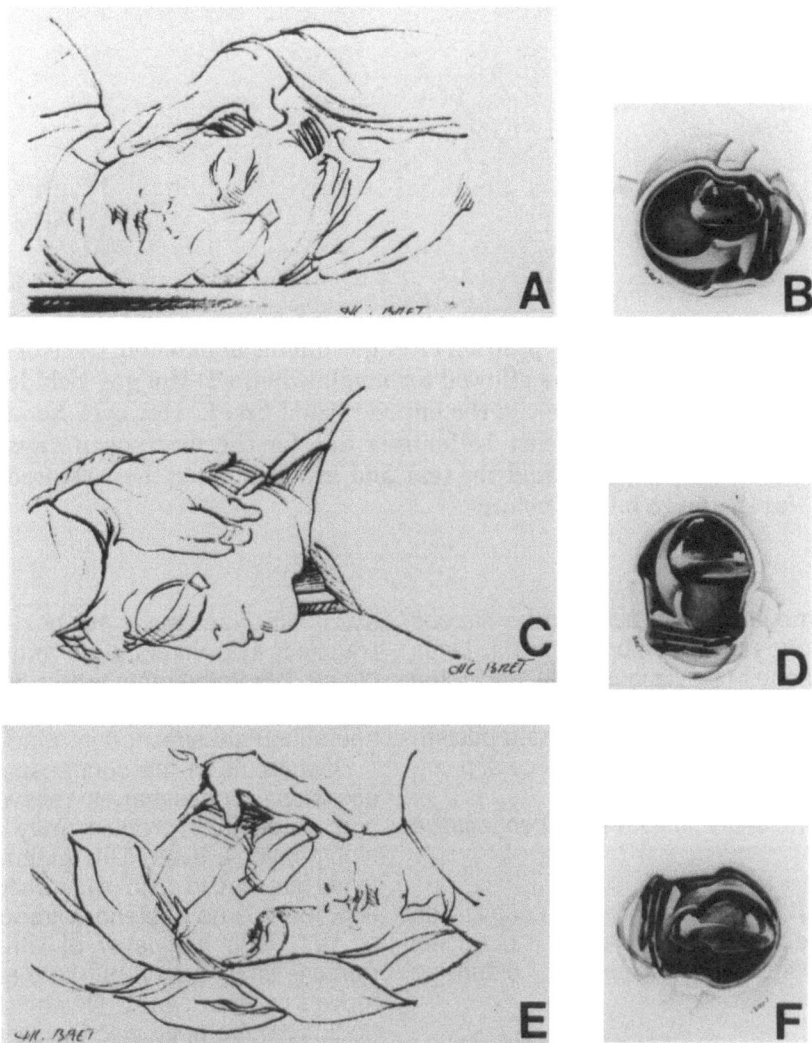

Figure 149. Head maneuvers to unfold the posterior flap of a giant tear of the temporal quadrants in the left eye (case shown in Figures 146 and 147). (A) The patient is placed on the left side. (B) The gas bubble is on the nasal side, distant from the tear posterior flap. (C) The patient is rotated to the prone position. (D) The gas bubble moves toward the posterior pole. (E) The patient is gently rotated to his right side. (F) The gas bubble moves beneath the retinal flap and unfolds the inverted retina.

eration. The patient should, therefore, be maneuvered like a heavy bag. One staff member takes care of the lower part of the body, the second staff member takes care of the shoulders and the third one holds the patient's head. Performing these maneuvers takes 2–3 minutes. The patient will be allowed to move normally after complete expansion of the gas bubble (Fig. 150).

SURGICAL MANAGEMENT WITH VITREOUS SURGERY

Vitreous surgery is required in surgical management of giant retinal tears associated with the following characteristics: (1) major vitreous changes such as extensive vitreous gel liquefaction, condensation

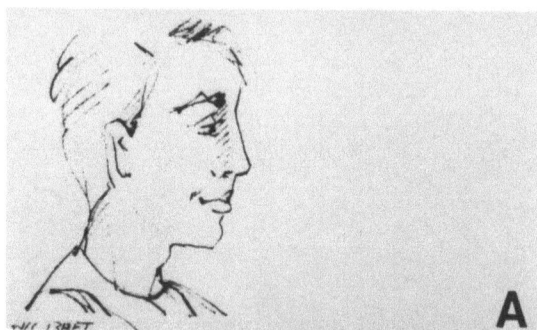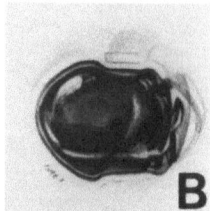

Figure 150.　Head position after gas bubble expansion. (A) Normal head position is allowed for meals when (B) the gas bubble has expanded and seals the entire retinal break. However head positioning for at least 15 hours a day for the first seven days is recommended to seal the tear and avoid complications related to the large bubble volume.

of the anterior vitreous and contraction of the vitreous base, vitreous bands and membranes, and dense vitreous hemorrhage, (2) viscous vitreous in the subretinal space, (3) retinal tears 180° and over in size, (4) hinge of the inverted retina located posteriorly to the equator, and (5) clinical evidence of proliferative vitreoretinopathy.

The surgical procedure includes six consecutive steps.

Localization of the Retinal Tear.　Localization of the scleral projection of the retinal tear is restricted to each lateral edge and their posterior extension when present.

Vitreous Surgery.　Endosurgery is performed with the 3-entry technique.

The infusion cannula is placed, whenever possible, in an area where the ciliary epithelium is not detached.

Vitreous surgery for giant retinal tears includes four consecutive steps: (1) lensectomy, (2) vitreous gel removal, (3) epiretinal membrane segmentation, and (4) unfolding and securing the inverted retina.

Lensectomy.　Lensectomy is required in most retinal tears of 180° and over in size and in giant tears associated with severe proliferative vitreoretinopathy. In such eyes an inferior peripheral iridectomy is performed to avoid pupillary block by the gas bubble.

Vitreous Gel Removal.　Relief of vitreous traction is the goal of vitreous gel removal. Vitreous gel removal is performed with very low suction force. Great care is taken to remove all condensed anterior vitreous gel up to the vitreous base. In most myopic

eyes with giant tears the posterior vitreous gel is liquefied, thus vitreous gel removal is rapidly completed. When the giant tear is located inferiorly, viscous vitreous gel may be present in the retinal tear and subretinal space; it is removed.

Radial cuts in the condensed vitreous base are occasionally necessary to relieve anterior loop traction. One major problem may be encountered in highly myopic eyes. This major problem is related to the fact that, in spite of extensive vitreous liquefaction, there is no posterior vitreous detachment (see p. 197). The thin layer of vitreous cortex, which remains firmly adherent to the retina, cannot be removed in most cases. Delamination with the blunt hook from the optic disc towards the periphery can be attempted. However, satisfactory delamination can rarely be achieved.

Epiretinal Membrane Segmentation.　When the giant tear is already associated with fixed retinal folds, delamination and segmentation of epiretinal membranes is performed (see p. 245). When the posterior edge of the inverted flap is stiff and shrunken by periretinal proliferation, radial cuts are made to relax circumferential shortening. Radial cuts are made using automated scissors (Fig. 151).

Unfolding and Securing the Inverted Retina.　Several techniques have been developed to unfold the inverted retina and secure the flap until the adjunctive choroidal irritation develops a firm adhesion.[2,9,11–27,30–34] All techniques have their own advantages, limits, and complications. A rotating operating table is used by many surgeons[1,15,20,21,26] for unfolding the retina by gravity. When vitrectomy is completed, the patient is rotated from the supine into the prone position. In this position the retina

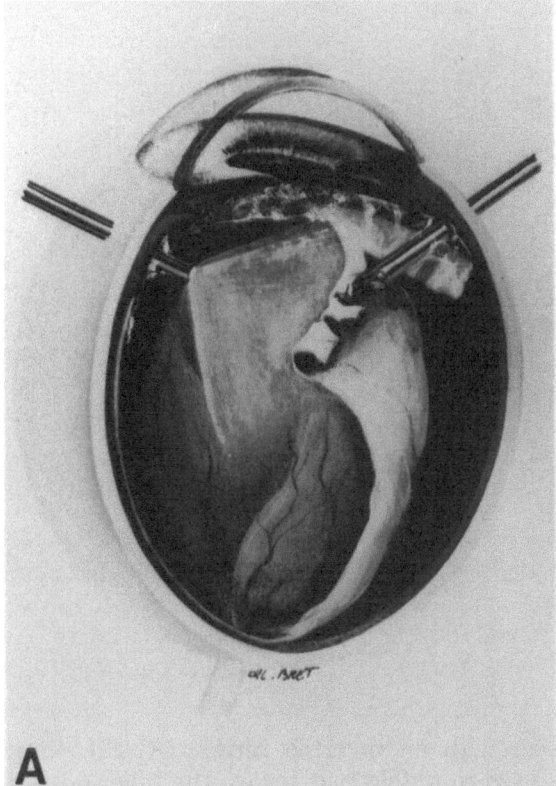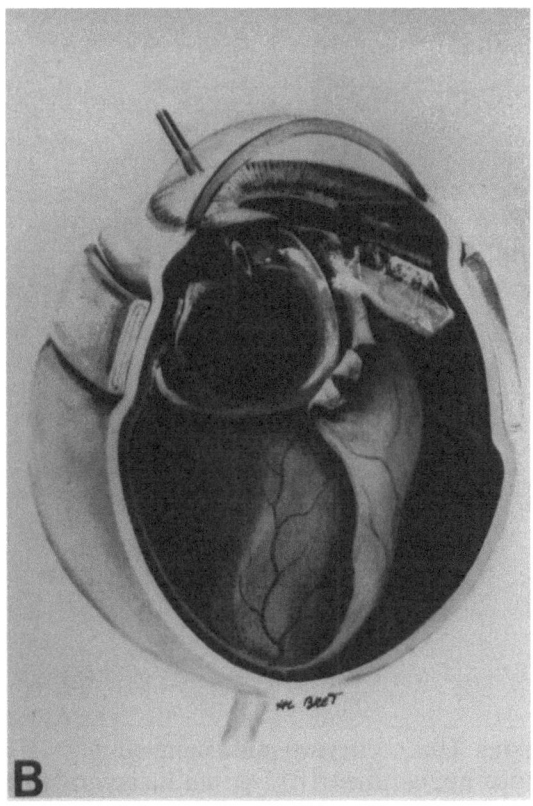

Figure 151. Surgical management of a nontraumatic giant tear in a myopic eye. (A) Following lensectomy and vitrectomy, radial cuts are made in the shrunken posterior edge of the tear to relax circumferential shortening. (B) Following a 360° scleral buckling, a small bubble of pure perfluoropropane is injected into the vitreous cavity. (Preoperative fundus appearance of the same case is shown in Figure 145)

hangs down. Complete fluid gas exchange is carried out in the prone position under ophthalmoscopic control. The surgeon position during fluid gas exchange is a disadvantage of the technique. In addition, in spite of total fluid gas exchange, slipping of the retina may occur when the patient is rotated into the supine position.

Sodium hyaluronate has been used with success for unfolding the retina with the patient in the normal supine position.[3,27] Because of its high viscosity and density sodium hyaluronate acts as a soft instrument. Slowly injected beneath the inverted retina, it will gently unfold the flap. Unfortunately, in the author's experience, all eyes developed severe proliferative vitreoretinopathy and failed to reattach,[3] and therefore, this technique is no longer used. Trans-scleral magnetic fixation of the retina was developed experimentally by Lobel et al.[16] The first clinical applications of this technique are encouraging.[17]

Securing the retinal flap to the eye wall to prevent slippage or recurrent folding before development of a firm retinochoroidal adhesion is required in most

giant retinal tears over 180° or giant tears associated with severe proliferative vitreoretinopathy.

Three main techniques can be used for securing the retinal flap: retinal sutures, retinal incarceration, and retinal tacks.

Choice of the technique depends mainly on the degree of retinal shortening that is always present in giant retinal tears with an inverted flap.

Retinal suturing and retinal incarceration are used when retinal shortening is moderate. In such cases the posterior edge of the giant tear can be repositioned anteriorly to the equator.

The first use of retinal sutures was reported by Galezowski in 1889. In recent years sophisticated techniques for retinal suturing have been developed.[18,19,25,29,30] Choroidal bleeding, retinal tearing, and necrosis are potential complications of the procedure that can be avoided by proper technique.[19,25,30] The best technique for retinal sutures is that with which the surgeon is most familiar. In our own experience retinal sutures combined with retinal incarceration has been the best surgical ap-

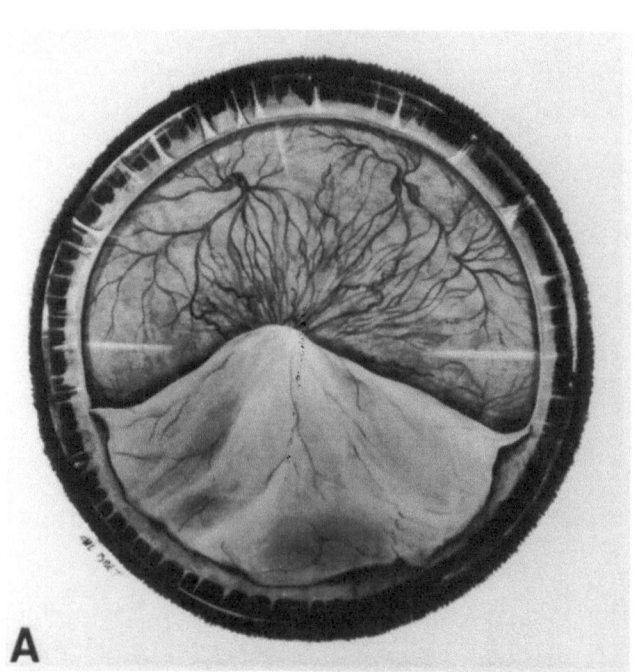
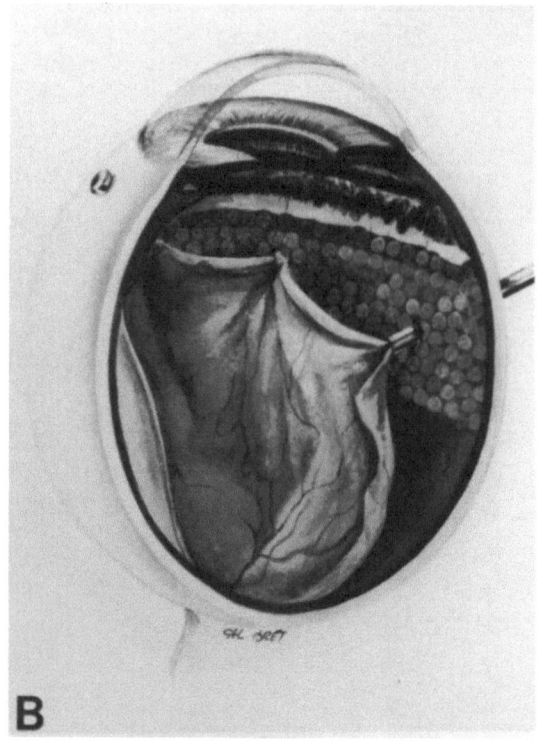

A   **B**

Figure 152. Surgical management of a giant tear with an inverted retina. (A) Preoperative fundus appearance. (B) Retinal incarcerations are used to unfold and secure the inverted retina. Argon laser photocoagulation of the exposed pigment epithelium in the peripheral fundus was performed preoperatively.

proach for immediate anterior fixation of the inverted retina (Figs. 152 and 153). The surgical technique is close to the technique described by Heiman.[31]

The surgical technique has two main advantages: (1) it is rapid to perform and (2) repositioning and securing the inverted flap are achieved with a single surgical maneuver.

In most cases one retinal incarceration and suture is made every 60°. For a retinal tear of 180°, three retinal incarcerations and sutures are made (Fig. 152). The sclerotomies are prepared in advance. They are made 1 mm posterior to the point where the posterior edge of the retinal tear is expected to flatten. In most cases sclerotomies are performed just anterior to the equator. The sclerotomies are oriented radially. They are 1 mm in length. The choroid is cauterized with diathermy to avoid choroidal bleeding and to induce further retinochoroidal adhesion. The fiberoptic probe combined with a needle connected to linear suction is used for retinal incarceration. Retinal incarcerations are performed under simultaneous observation of the fundus using the three-mirror contact lens. The two-function probe, used as a smooth forceps, is inserted into the sclerotomy prepared for retinal incarceration. The tip is

placed into contact with the posterior edge of the inverted retina at approximately 60° of the lateral edge of the tear. Then gentle suction is applied to lift the retina with the probe. The probe is gently moved towards the equator and the sclerotomy site. Suction is released as early as the probe tip and retina are in the sclerotomy. Suture of the incarcerated retina is performed under high magnification. An 8–0 nylon suture and a round-bodied needle are used. The needle is inserted into one of the sclerotomy edges, the incarcerated retina, and the opposite sclerotomy edge. The suture is tied so that it places both sclerotomy edges in apposition without traction. The same maneuvers are repeated for each retinal incarceration. When the sutures are completed, the infusion cannula is removed from the vitreous cavity and the pars plana incisions are secured.

Retinal incarceration combined with transscleral suture may be associated with complications. Choroidal bleeding may occur, but it is uncommon. The sclerotomy sites should be distant from the vortex veins and the long posterior ciliary arteries.

Inability to achieve retinal incarceration into the sclerotomy may occur. Shortening of the retina has

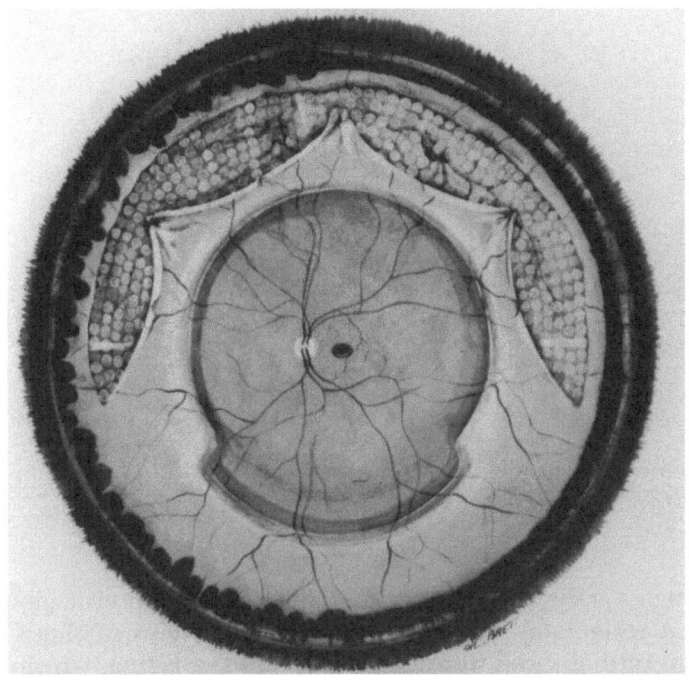

Figure 153. Early postoperative appearance of the fundus following retinal incarceration (Preoperative and intraoperative appearance of the same case shown in Figures 144 and 152).

been underestimated when the sclerotomy is too anterior. In this case, the sclerotomy is secured and a new sclerectomy is performed more posteriorly.

If the surgeon releases the suction too late excessive retinal incarceration with retinal prolapse can occur. This can be avoided through proper technique by releasing the suction as soon as the probe tip and retina are in the sclerotomy.

Tearing of the retina during suturing can be avoided by placing the suture with a single and gentle rotating motion. Sharp spatuled needles should not be used. Round bodied needles are used. Each needle should be used for only one suture.

Retinal incarceration and suturing should not be attempted when the posterior retina is shrunken by the proliferative process to such a degree that the edge of the posterior flap cannot be mobilized anteriorly to the equator after completion of the vitrectomy. In such cases retinal tacks are used for immediate fixation of the retina.

Retinal tacks were introduced in the treatment of giant retinal tears by Ando and Kondo in 1983.[24] At present, various models for permanent or temporary fixation are commercially available.[24,32,33] The basic idea is to nail the retina against the eye wall with small tacks pierced through the retina into the choroid and sclera (Fig. 154). Special instrumentation has been developed to guide the tack into the eye and remove it once it is no longer needed.[32] After vitrectomy and membrane peeling a small area of the retina is flattened and held into place using the flute needle connected to linear suction while the tack is being placed. Tack displacement, choroidal hemorrhage, postoperative tack dislocation, and late proliferation at the site of tack insertion are podal hemorrhage, postoperative tack dislocation, and late proliferation at the site of tack insertion are potential complications of the technique. The technique is used in the most severe cases that otherwise would not be considered operable. Owing to the extreme severity of such cases, surgical results are poor. The indications for surgical management of giant retinal tears over 270° in size associated with severe proliferative vitreoretinopathy are considered only for patients with no useful vision of the fellow eye.

Choroidal Irritation. Choroidal irritation achieved by preoperative argon laser photocoagulation of the exposed pigment epithelium and anterior flap is completed after repositioning of the inverted retina. Cryotreatment associated with an increased risk of choroidal bleeding and release of viable pigment cells[35] is not used in such eyes. Argon laser photocoagulation in the supine position is performed through the gas bubble postoperatively (see p. 81).

Scleral Buckling. Scleral buckling is performed after vitrectomy and repositioning of the inverted flap. A 360° buckling procedure is performed. The main purpose of scleral buckling is to counteract ring contraction of the vitreous base. An explant of lyophylized dura mater is used. It is 4–5 mm in width

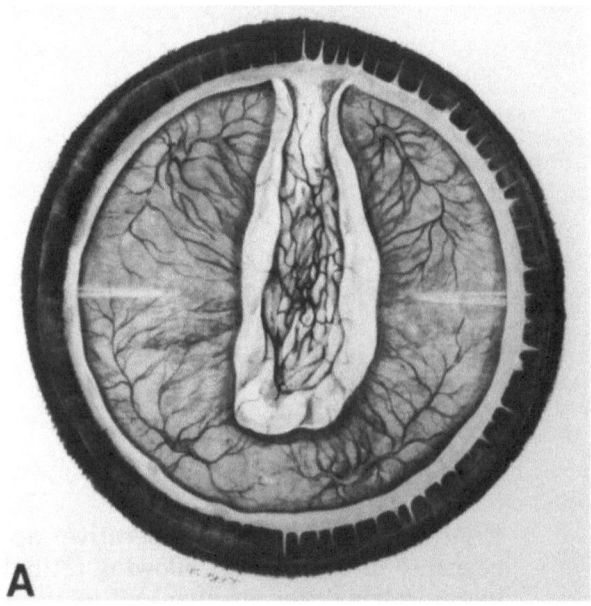
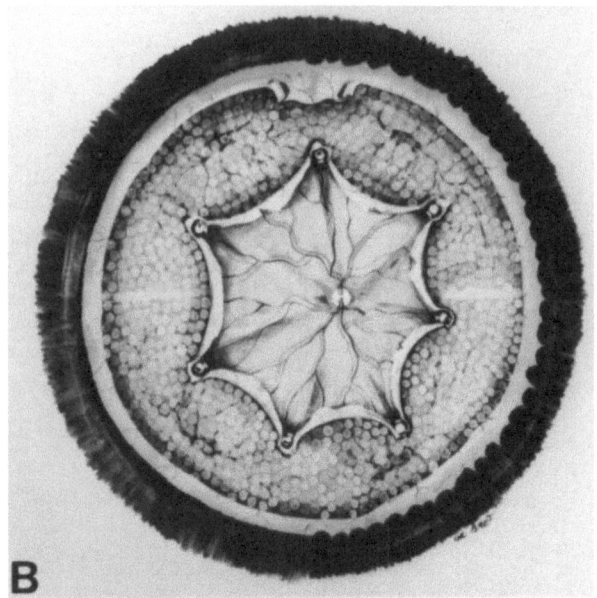

Figure 154. Surgical management of a giant tear associated with severe proliferative vitreoretinopathy. (A) Preoperative fundus appearance. (B) A retinotomy was performed to relieve vitreous base traction on the superior part of the tear. Seven retinal tacks were used to secure the retina, which remained greatly shortened after periretinal membrane peeling. Recurrent proliferative vitreoretinopathy and intractable retinal detachment developed after gas absorption.

in the quadrants where the retina is not torn and broader in the quadrants corresponding to the retinal tear. A circumferential explant 8 mm in width is used. A 0.2 ml of intraocular fluid is removed using a 30-gauge blunt needle, inserted through the limbus for tightening of each suture. The total amount of intraocular fluid removed from the eye for tightening all sutures is recorded for calculation of intraocular space available for gas expansion.

Gas Injection. Gas injection is performed through the pars plana in phakic eyes and the limbus in aphakic eyes. Pure perfluoropropane is used rather than sulfur-hexafluoride because of its longevity and expansion properties. Total or subtotal retinal tamponade by the expanded gas bubble is required in most cases. The optimum volume of pure gas to be injected is calculated by taking into account three parameters: (1) the vitreous cavity volume (see p. 122), (2) intraocular fluid displacement resulting from scleral buckling (see p. 23), and (3) expansion properties of the gas (see p. 117).

Patient Head Maneuvering and Positioning. Patient head maneuvering is performed when the patient is returned to bed. Maneuvers to ensure proper positioning of the retinal flap are required only in eyes managed without retinal incarceration and suture. In all cases the patient is positioned in

the prone position, the head rotated so that the gas bubble seals the retinal tear.

Postoperative Management

Postoperative management of any giant retinal tear includes: (1) early and careful monitoring of intraocular pressure (see p. 130), (2) continuation of systemic treatment to inhibit, or at least reduce, the proliferative process associated with most non-traumatic giant tears, and (3) early photocoagulation of the posterior edge of the giant tear.

The patient is examined using the slit lamp on the first postoperative day. Fundus examination is performed in the seated position. No corneal contact lens is required when the eye is aphakic. The position of the posterior edge of the retinal tear, patency of the central retinal artery, and absence of major intraocular inflammation are verified.

Three to four days after surgery, the gas bubble expansion has reached its maximum and subretinal fluid has been absorbed in most cases. Argon laser photocoagulation of the posterior edge of the retinal tear is performed. In most cases the argon laser attached to the operating microscope is used. Four rows of burns are placed on the posterior edge of the tear. A 350 μm spot size and a 0.5 second exposure time are used. The power is gradually increased to obtain white burns. Special care is taken to avoid overtreatment, which is more likely to occur in the gas filled eye than in the fluid filled eye (see p. 81).

When argon laser photocoagulation is completed, the patient is returned to his or her room and instructed about appropriate head positioning. When the retinal tear is superior and retinal incarcerations have been made, the patient can move around normally. When no retinal incarcerations have been made, the patient is instructed to keep the face tilted toward the floor for three days. When the retinal tear is inferior the patient's head must be completely prone. This can be easily done in a seated position with the forehead resting on a table. When the retinal tear is temporal or nasal, the patient should lie on the side opposite to the tear, the face rotated toward the bed. The same position can be done in the seated position, the head kept rotated and prone on a table. Head positioning should be done 18 hours a day for three days after surgery and photocoagulation treatment. Normal head position is allowed for meals and using the bath room. After three days a greater latitude of movements is allowed, however, head positioning remains recommended for at least 15 hours a day during the first seven days. The patient is instructed never to lie in the supine position as long as the gas bubble remains of effective size to avoid pupillary block in the aphakic eye and cataract formation in the phakic eye.

RESULTS

At present microsurgical techniques make it possible to achieve retinal reattachment in the early postoperative period in approximately 94% of eyes.[3] The long term results remain disappointing, however, owing to the high incidence of severe proliferative vitreoretinopathy and recurrent retinal detachment two weeks to 2 months postoperatively. Repeated gas injections for prolonged retinal tamponade do not reduce the incidence of recurrent detachment related to proliferative vitreoretinopathy.[3]

The rate of permanent retinal reattachment is greatly dependent on case selection.

In the author's experience, the overall success rate with at least 6 month follow-up is 50%.[3] It is 80% in giant tears after blunt trauma in emmetropic

Permanent retinal reattachment with useful vision can be achieved in 80% of retinal tears 90° to less than 180° in size versus only 40% of retinal tears 180° to 340° in size. The success rate is greatly dependent on the presence and degree of proliferative vitreoretinopathy before surgery. In the author's experience, permanent retinal reattachment with useful vision can be achieved in 85% of giant tears without clinical evidence of preoperative proliferative vitreoretinopathy, and in approximately 50% of eyes with preoperative proliferative vitreoretinopathy (Fig. 155).

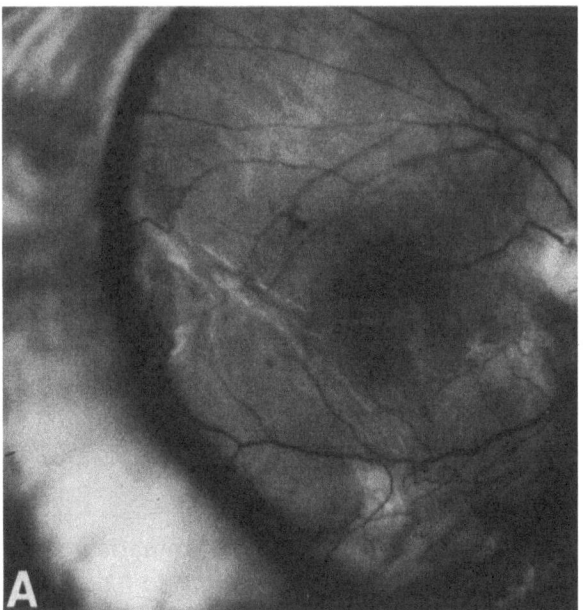 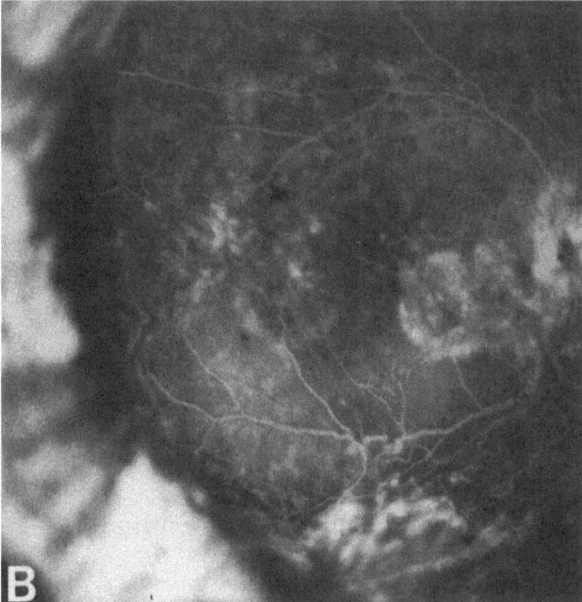

Figure 155. Postoperative fundus appearance of a 320° tear associated with severe proliferative vitreoretinopathy, managed with vitrectomy, retinal incarceration, scleral buckling and C3F8 gas injection. (A) Fundus photograph 12 months postoperatively. (B) Fluorescein angiography shows cystoid macular edema. Central vision is 20/400.

Far visual acuity of 20/40 or better can be expected in 33% of successful eyes. Near reading visual acuity is a more reliable criteria to assess the visual results in highly myopic eyes. Normal near reading visual acuity can be expected in 62% of successful eyes.[3]

Prolonged follow-up after retinal reattachment shows that 50% of phakic eyes develop cataract 2–10 years postoperatively.[3]

The author's results are roughly similar to those achieved by other surgeons[1,15,26,34] who use microsurgical techniques, which are different in their details but quite similar in their basic principles. Anatomical result achieved at 6 months by fluid silicone oil exchange[2] are better than those achieved by gas tamponade. However, the long term outcome of eyes operated with silicone oil remains unknown, and visual results after silicone oil tamponade are somewhat disappointing.[2]

The disappointing long term anatomical results of microsurgery in nontraumatic giant tears of 180° and more in size are related to the severity of the vitreoretinal disease, which results in a giant retinal tear rather than surgical problems related to the tear size. In nontraumatic cases the size of the retinal tear reflects the severity of the underlying vitreoretinal disease. In such eyes most surgical failures are related to the severity of the underlying vitreoretinal disease rather than mechanical problems encountered during surgical management. This assessment is supported by the fact that in all series the anatomical success rate is significantly higher (approximately 80%) in giant tears, after blunt trauma in healthy eyes.

MANAGEMENT OF THE FELLOW EYE

Prophylactic treatment of the fellow eye should be considered in nontraumatic giant tears, especially in highly myopic patients, for two main reasons: (1) in spite of sophisticated microsurgical techniques, a high percentage of retinal detachment with giant retinal tears fail to reattach and (2) the incidence of retinal detachment and retinal breaks in the fellow eye is very high (see p. 196).

Indications for Prophylactic Treatment

The indications for prophylactic treatment of the fellow eye in nontraumatic giant tears are as follows:

1. Retinal tears, even asymptomatic,
2. Lattice degeneration,

3. Severe vitreous gel liquefaction, condensation of the vitreous base and white with, or without, pressure.

Most nontraumatic giant tears develop in eyes without detectable degenerative lesion of the peripheral retina. In such eyes, vitreous changes and white with or without pressure are the most important clinical findings with regard to the indications for prophylactic treatment (Fig. 156).

Methods of Prophylactic Treatment

Production of a firm retinochoroidal adhesion in the peripheral fundus and relief of vitreous traction are the two techniques currently used for prophylactic treatment.

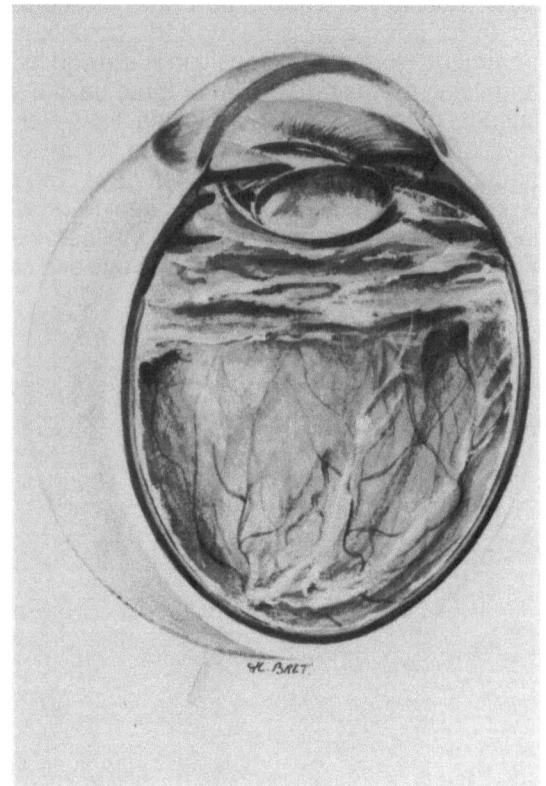

Figure 156. Vitreous gel changes preceding the development of nontraumatic giant tears: Condensation of the vitreous base and anterior vitreous gel, severe syneresis of the central vitreous gel, vitreous bands, and absence of posterior vitreous detachment. Such findings are an indication for prophylactic treatment.

INDUCED RETINOCHOROIDAL ADHESION

Retinochoroidal adhesion can be induced using either cryo or photocoagulation. Cryotreatment has been advocated and used with success.[8] However, accurate monitoring of induced lesions is easier to achieve by photocoagulation.

Argon laser photocoagulation is carried out under topical anesthesia in adults and general anesthesia in children. A 500 μm spot size and a 0.5 second exposure time are used. Power is determined to induce a white retinal lesion. A broad retinochoroidal scar involving 360° of the peripheral fundus, which must resist the increasing vitreous base traction should be obtained (Fig. 157).

Photocoagulation scars should extend from the ora serrata to the equatorial region. Some eyes show a small circumferential retinal ridge on the posterior limit of white with or without pressure. This ridge corresponds to the posterior border of the vitreous base. Four to five rows of photocoagulation burns are made posteriorly to the retinal ridge. When the posterior border of the vitreous base is not visible the most posterior row of photocoagulation burns is placed just behind the vortex veins ampulae. Then photocoagulation is completed up to the ora serrata on 360°. Treatment requires 4–5 consecutive sessions to be completed. The sessions are performed at 1–3 week intervals.

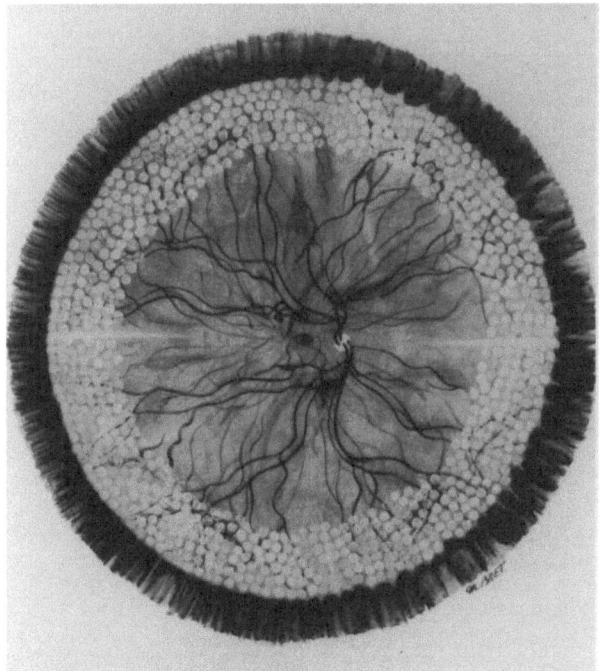

Figure 157. Extent of laser burns for prophylactic treatment of the fellow eye in a myopic patient with nontraumatic giant tear.

VITREOUS TRACTION RELIEF

Relief of vitreous traction on the peripheral retina is considered in myopic eyes with major vitreous changes,[8] especially in children with a family history. In such eyes photocoagulation treatment is associated with scleral buckling. The circumferential scleral buckle should involve approximately 180–220 degrees of the eye circumference. When both eyes are affected by giant retinal tears, it is commonly with mirror symmetry. Therefore, the buckle is placed in the symmetric quadrants of the quadrants affected by the giant tear in the other eye. The explant is 3.5–4 mm in width. Two mattress sutures per quadrant are placed. The posterior and anterior bites of the mattress sutures are placed 6–7 mm apart. Intraocular pressure monitoring is achieved by carbonic anhydrase inhibitors and osmotic agents administered intravenously, and repeated paracentesis of the anterior chamber. Patency of the central retinal artery is carefully monitored at the end of the procedure.

The patients should be followed up at 6 month or 1 year intervals for extended periods of time, regardless of the method used for prophylactic treatment. Retinal tears and retinal detachment may develop, in spite of proper prophylactic treatment, after periods of time that range from a few months to several years.[3,36] Most retinal tears and retinal detachments in eyes that underwent prophylactic treatment are less severe than in eyes that underwent no prophylactic treatment.[3,36]

REFERENCES

1. Freeman HM: Current management of giant retinal breaks: results with vitrectomy and total air fluid exchange in 95 cases Tr Am Ophthalmol Soc 79:89–101, 1981
2. Leaver PK, Cooling RJ, Feretis EB, et al: Vitrectomy and fluid/ silicone—oil exchange for giant retinal tears: results at six months Brit J Ophthalmol 68:432–438, 1984
3. Fleury J: Décollements de la rétine par déchirures de grande taille et déchirures géantes. Thèse Doctorat Lyon 10 Octobre 1986
4. Kanski JJ: Giant retinal tears. Amer J Ophthalmol 79:846–852, 1975
5. Haimann HM, Burton TC, Brown CK: Epidemiology of retinal detachment. Arch Ophthalmol 100:289–292, 1982
6. Schepens CL: Retinal detachment and allied diseases Philadelphia W. B. Saunders Company, 1983, Vol. 2, 520–542
7. McLeod D: Giant retinal tears after central vitrectomy. Brit J Ophthalmol 69:96–98, 1985
8. Freeman HM: Fellow eyes of giant retinal breaks. Mod Probl Ophthal 1979, Vol. 20 pp. 267–274
9. Holland PM, Smith TR: Broad scleral buckle in the management of retinal detachments with giant tears. Amer J Ophthalmol 83:518–525, 1977
10. Freeman HM: The treatment of giant retinal tears, in Mc Pherson

A. (Ed). New and controversial aspects of retinal detachment. New-York, Harper and Row, 1968, 391–399

11. Schepens CL, Freeman HM: Current management of giant retinal breaks. Trans Am Acad Ophthalmol Otolaryngol 71:474–487, 1967

12. Freeman HM, Couvillion GC, Schepens CL: Vitreous surgery, IV intraocular balloon: clinical application. Arch Ophthalmol 83:715–721, 1970

13. Wessing A, Spitznas M, Palomar A: The surgical treatment of retinal detachment due to equatorial giant tears. Mod Probl Ophthalmol 15:328–331, 1975

14. Norton EW, Aaberg T, Fung W, Curtin VT: Giant retinal tears. Clinical management with intravitreal air. Am J Ophthalmol. 68:1011–1021, 1969

15. Machemer R, Allen AW: Retinal tears 180 degrees and greater. Management with vitrectomy and intravitreal gas. Arch Ophthalmol 94:1340–1346, 1976

16. Lobel D, Hale JR, Montgomery DB: A new magnetic technique for the treatment of giant retinal tears. Am J Ophthalmol 85:699–703, 1978

17. Eckardt C, Henning G: Transsklerale Magnet Fixierung der Netzhaut bei Komplizierter Amotio. Klinische Monatsblätter für Augenheilkunde 4:235–314, 1984

18. Usui M, Hamazaki S, Takano S, Matsuo H: A new surgical technique for the treatment of giant tear: Transvitreoretinal fixation. Jpn J Ophthalmol 23:206–215, 1979

19. Federman JL, Shakin JL, Lanning RG: The microsurgical management of giant retinal tears with transscleral retinal sutures. Ophthalmology 89:832–838, 1982

20. Peyman GA: A new operative table for the management of giant retinal breaks. Arch Ophthalmol 99:498–499, 1981

21. Schepens CL, Freeman HHM, Thompson RF: A power driven multipositional operating table. Arch Ophthalmol 73:671–673, 1965

22. De Juan E, McCuen BW, Machemer R: The use of retinal tacks in the repair of complicated retinal detachments. Am J Ophthalmol 102:20–24, 1986

23. Heiman K: Zur Behandlung Komplizierter Riesenrisse der Nethaut. Klin Monatsbl Augenheilkd 176:491–492, 1980

24. Ando F, Kondo J: A plastic tack for the treatment of retinal detachment with giant tear. Am J Ophthalmol 95:260–261, 1983

25. Hirose T, Schepens CL, Lopansri C: Subtotal open-sky vitrectomy for severe retinal detachment occurring as a late complication of ocular trauma. Ophthalmology 88:1–9, 1981

26. Charles S: Vitreous microsurgery. Baltimore, Williams and Wilkins, 1981, 135–141

27. Fitzgerald CR: The use of healon in a case of rolled-over retina. Retina 1:227–231, 1981

28. Galezowski X: Du décollement de la rétine et de son traitement. Bull Mem Soc Fr Ophtalmol 8:200–202, 1889

29. Scott JD: A new approach to the vitreous base. Mod Probl Ophthalmol 12:407–410, 1974

30. Michels RG, Rice TA, Blankenship GR: Surgical techniques for selected giant retinal tears. Retina 3:139–153, 1983

31. Heiman K: Zur Behandlung Komplizierter Riesenrisse der Netzhaut. Klin Monatsbl Augenheilk 176:491–492, 1980

32. De Juan E, Hickingbotham D, Machemer R: Retinal tacks. Am J Ophthalmol 99:272–274, 1985

33. Abrams GW, Williams GA, Neuwirth J, McDonald HR: Clinical results of titanium retinal tacks with pneumatic insertion. Am J Ophthalmol 102:13–19, 1986

34. Vidaurri-Leal J, De Bustros S, Michels RG: Surgical treatment of giant retinal tears with inverted posterior retinal flap. Am J Ophthalmol 98:463–466, 1984

35. Campochiaro A, Kaden IH, Vidaurri-Leal J, Glaser BM: Cryotherapy enhances intravitreal dispersion of viable retinal pigment epithelial cells Arch Ophthalmol 103:434–436, 1985

36. Loyer JP, Lemer Y, Ganen C, Heligon GT: Devenir de l'oeil adelphe chez 50 sujets ayant presenté une inversion rétinienne non traumatique Bull et Mem SFO 97:351–354, 1986

18

Retinal Detachment with Posterior Paravascular Retinal Tears

Posterior paravascular retinal breaks include 3 distinct clinical entities: (1) posterior paravascular retinal breaks secondary to proliferative retinopathies (see p. 271), (2) linear paravascular retinal breaks secondary to severe proliferative vitreoretinopathy (see p. 239), and (3) primary linear paravascular retinal tears.

ETIOLOGY

Retinal detachments with primary posterior paravascular tears are observed only in highly myopic eyes.[1] They are very rare.[1-2] In a retina referral center, they accounted for only 1.5% of all rhegmatogenous retinal detachments operated on during the same time period.[1] In the same series[1] they were approximately 4 times less frequent than retinal detachments due to macular holes in highly myopic eyes.

There is no sex prevalence; patient age may range from 20 to 70 years.

CLINICAL FINDINGS

Retinal Detachment

In most patients the onset of retinal detachment is an acute with sudden loss of central vision and rapid visual field defect.

The retinal detachment may be confined to a small area around the retinal tear(s). More commonly, however, the retinal detachment extends far beyond the area of the retinal tear(s). It may involve two or three quadrants. The macula is detached in most eyes. The retinal detachment may be extensive and high with large mobile retinal folds (Fig. 158). Maximum height of the detachment is on the posterior pole or the midperiphery. The retina anterior to the equator may show a shallow detachment or no detachment (Figs. 158 and 159).

At an early stage there is no clinical evidence of proliferative vitreoretinopathy. However proliferative vitreoretinopathy may develop later on. In particular, it is common in eyes in which the posterior tears were not identified and a peripheral scleral buckling procedure was performed although no peripheral retinal tears were present.

Retinal Tears

Paravascular retinal tears should be carefully looked for in any highly myopic eye with acute retinal detachment and no detectable retinal tear of the peripheral retina. They may be difficult to identify owing to the atrophic choroidal background. They may be located in the close vicinity of an atrophic staphyloma. However, the retinal tear(s) will be found, when methodical slit lamp examination is performed along all retinal vessels from the optic disc to the equator.

The retinal tear shows a linear shape with a narrow flap (Fig. 158). The flap is on the tear side opposite the retinal vessel. There may be a single retinal tear. However approximately 62% of eyes[1] show 2

213

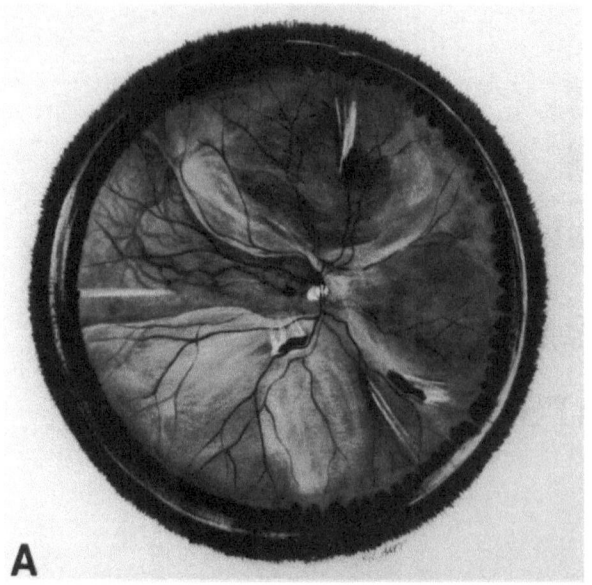

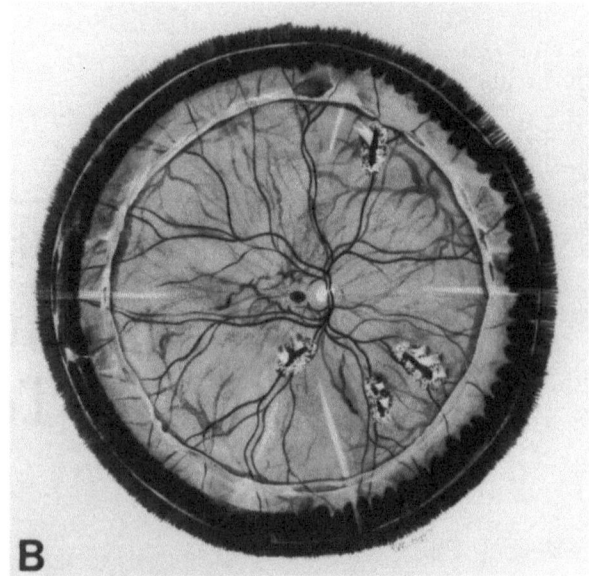

Figure 158. Retinal detachment with multiple posterior paravascular tears in a twelve-diopter myopic eye. (A) Preoperative fundus appearance. (B) Postoperative fundus appearance. Treatment consisted of vitrectomy, cryotreatment of the retinal tears and intravitreal injection of 1.5 cc of pure SF6.

or more retinal tears (Figs. 158 and 159). All retinal tears may be located along the same retinal vessel, and close to each others. They may also be located in different retinal quadrants (Fig. 158).

Location along the temporal arcades and/or major branches of the temporal vessels is the most common. However the tears may also be located in the nasal midperiphery of the fundus.

Vitreous Body

Significant vitreous gel liquefaction and posterior vitreous detachment are common in myopic eyes with posterior paravascular retinal tears. However, biomicroscopic examination shows that posterior vitreous detachment is incomplete. In most cases vitreous strands still adherent to the small tear flap can be identified by slit lamp examination using high magnification. All vitreoretinal adhesions should be carefully recorded on the preoperative fundus chart to accomplish the main objective of the surgical procedure: relief of vitreoretinal traction.

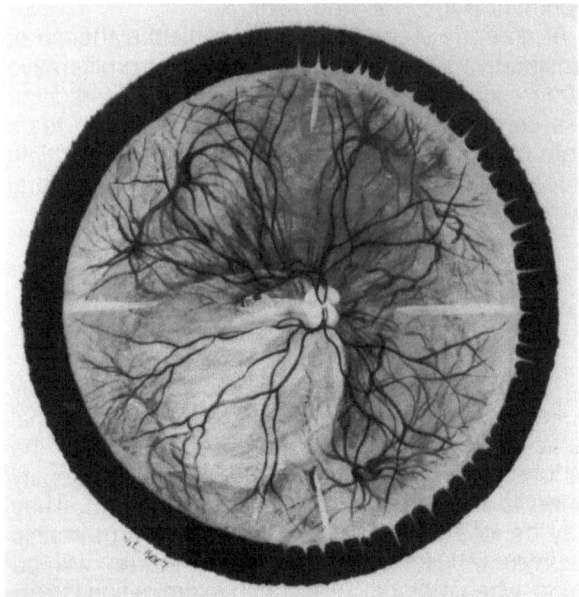

Figure 159. Retinal detachment with two tiny paravascular tears in a twenty-diopter myopic eye. The tears are situated along a tributary of the superior temporal artery in the paramacular region.

SURGICAL MANAGEMENT

Before the development of vitrectomy, retinal detachments with posterior paravascular retinal tears were among the most difficult detachments to manage. Surgical difficulties were related to the anatomy of the posterior sclera in highly myopic eyes and the hazards of posterior scleral buckling procedures in such eyes. Intraoperative complications, frequent inability to achieve a buckle height sufficient to counteract vitreous traction, and severe postoperative proliferative vitreoretinopathy accounted for the rather disappointing surgical results.

At present, the most appropriate surgical approach in the management of these detachments includes three steps: (1) vitrectomy, (2) choroidal irritation in the area of the retinal tear(s), and (3) retinal tamponade with gas.

Vitrectomy

Vitrectomy has two objectives: (1) to relieve vitreoretinal traction and (2) to create space for gas injection. Relief of vitreoretinal traction is the main objective of vitrectomy. This can be achieved by complete removal of the posterior vitreous face up to the posterior edge of the vitreous base. In most cases posterior vitreous detachment is incomplete. Complete separation of the posterior vitreous face can usually be achieved using the hooked fiber optic. All vitreous strands still adherent to the retinal flap(s) should be cut (Fig. 158). this is accomplished with automated scissors. Removal of the anterior vitreous gel is unnecessary.

Inducement of a Retinochoroidal Adhesion

A retinochoroidal adhesion must be induced in the area of the retinal tear(s). This procedure has no disadvantage since the retinal tears do not involve the macula. Permanent sealing of the retinal tear(s) is necessary, even in eyes with a very small paravascular tear, in order to avoid recurrent retinal detachment after gas absorption or at a later date.

In phakic eyes, inducement of the retinochoroidal adhesion is performed before, rather than after, vitrectomy and gas injection because visualization of small retinal tear(s) through a gas bubble is difficult in highly myopic and phakic eyes. Cryotreatment or argon laser photocoagulation are used. Cryotreatment is performed with a very thin and long cryoprobe. It is performed with simultaneous biomicroscopic observation of the fundus. Cryotreatment is strictly limited to retinal tear(s). Placing of the cryoprobe tip exactly in front of the retinal tear(s) requires preliminary opening of Tenon's space with microscissors beyond the scleral projection(s) of the retinal tear(s). Argon laser photocoagulation is used, rather

than cryotreatment, in eyes with retinal tear(s) close to the macula or the optic disc (Fig. 159 and Fig. 160). In most highly myopic eyes, the sclera on the posterior pole is very thin. Therefore, tissue freezing may spread very rapidly and result in macular or optic nerve damage. Argon laser photocoagulation is performed as the first step of the procedure. Temporary apposition of the retina onto the pigment epithelium is necessary to obtain visible burns. It is achieved by simultaneous scleral depression. The thin and long cryoprobe originally designed for treatment of macular holes is used as a scleral depressor (Fig. 160). Since the sclera may be very thin in the area of a staphyloma, scleral depression should be performed with great care. Decreased intraocular pressure obtained by paracentesis of the anterior chamber may be helpful to obtain retinochoroidal apposition at the cryoprobe tip and eliminate the risk of scleral laceration. If the maneuver is not sufficient for temporary retinochoroidal apposition at the cryoprobe tip, subretinal fluid is drained off. Two to three rows of photocoagulation burns are placed around the retinal tear with a 250 μm micron spot size and a 0.5 second exposure time.

In aphakic eyes, argon laser photocoagulation is

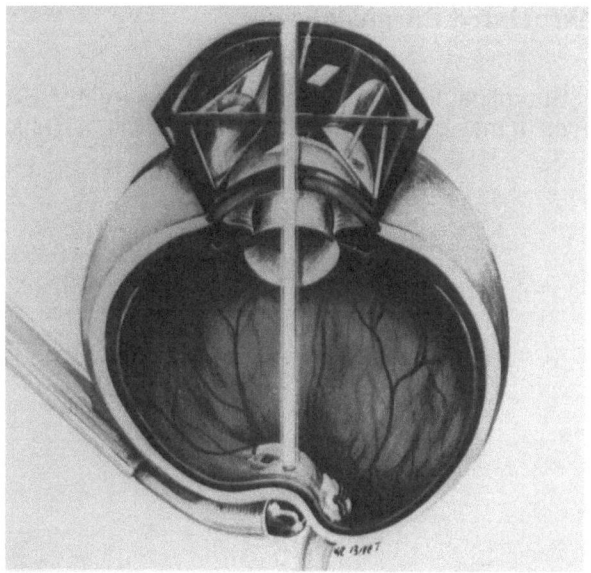

Figure 160. Surgical management of paravascular tears close to the macula (see case shown in Figure 159). Argon laser photocoagulation of both tears is performed intraoperatively using simultaneous scleral depression of the posterior pole. Retinal detachment is rather shallow on the posterior pole and temporary apposition of the pigment epithelium to the detached retina is easily achieved by scleral depression.

usually performed 3–4 days postoperatively, when maximal gas expansion has occurred. At that time the subretinal fluid has absorbed. Argon laser photocoagulation is performed through the gas bubble. No contact lens is needed (see p. 81).

Gas Injection

Fluid-gas exchange is performed as the last step of the surgical procedure (see p. 123). Pure SF6 is used in most cases, since internal sealing of the retinal tear(s) by the gas bubble is required for a short period of time. The optimal volume of pure gas to be injected is determined according to two parameters: (1) the volume of the vitreous cavity and (2) the location of the retinal tear(s).

The volume of the vitreous cavity is determined with preoperative ultrasonography (see p. 122).

When the retinal tears are located in the lower midperiphery, a rather large volume of gas is injected to give the patient more liberty of movement in the early postoperative days. Appropriate head positioning will be required for the first five postoperative days.

Associated Surgical Steps

Subretinal fluid drainage is unnecessary in most eyes. It may be required in phakic eyes with a highly detached retina that could prevent accurate intraoperative cryotreatment or argon laser photocoagulation. Subretinal fluid can be drained off internally or externally (see p. 66). Scleral buckling of the retinal tear(s) is unnecessary because vitreoretinal traction is relieved by vitrectomy. Scleral buckling of the vitreous base is also unnecessary in eyes with a mobile retina; however, it may be necessary in eyes with clinical evidence of proliferative vitreoretinopathy (see p. 250).

RESULTS

Permanent retinal reattachment with a single operation was achieved in all eyes of a small series of patients operated by the above procedure[1] (Fig. 158)

REFERENCES

1. Normand-Guyonnet F: Décollements de la rétine par trou maculaire ou déchirure du pôle postérieur chez le myope fort. Thèse Doctorat—Université Lyon, 1986
2. Schepens CL: Retinal detachment and allied diseases. Philadelphia W.B. Saunders, 1983, Vol. 2, 553

19

Retinal Detachments with Macular Holes in Myopic Eyes

Retinal detachments associated with macular holes in myopic eyes are a specific clinical entity. In fact, the vast majority of retinal detachments in emmetropic eyes associated with macular lesions resembling macular holes are actually due to peripheral retinal breaks.

"Macular holes" have been observed in a large variety of retinal detachments, including retinal detachments after penetrating eye injury, retinal detachments after blunt trauma, and rhegmatogenous detachments in nonmyopic eyes.[1] From a theoretical point of view, a full thickness macular hole may occur after penetrating injury of the eye and result in a rhegmatogenous retinal detachment. Direct damage to the macula may be due to a penetrating object or a foreign body. However, retinal detachments due to direct traumatic macular tearing is most uncommon, since spontaneous healing of posterior retinal wounds generally occurs within a few days after trauma. Most retinal detachments after penetrating eye injury are traction detachments associated with intravitreal fibrous ingrowth (see p. 286). An iatrogenic macular break may also occur during vitrectomy, particularly during epiretinal membrane removal. However, iatrogenic breaks of the macula have not yet been reported in the literature to the author's knowledge. Macular lesions that mimic macular holes are common in retinal detachments associated with peripheral retinal breaks of any etiology. Cystoid macular degeneration with secondary macular hole is the most common in longstanding duration retinal detachments associated with round atrophic holes in the equatorial region or retinal dialysis (see p. 185). In such eyes the macular hole does not play any role in the development of retinal detachment. Retinal reattachment will be achieved by sealing of the peripheral retinal break(s). Treatment of the macular lesion is not required to achieve permanent retinal reattachment.

Retinal detachments associated with macular holes in myopic eyes are of a specific clinical entity. In recent years, their surgical management has been significantly improved by vitrectomy and intravitreal gas injection. It has been demonstrated that neither scleral buckling of the posterior pole nor choroidal irritation in the macular area were required to achieve permanent retinal reattachment in most eyes. However, a small percentage of retinal detachments with macular holes in a myopic eye still fail to reattach after vitrectomy or gas tamponade. The small number of eyes that fail to respond to vitrectomy and internal tamponade are still managed with scleral buckling of the posterior pole or choroidal irritation.

This chapter illustrates the continuing evolution of surgical techniques and pathogenesis concepts in retinal detachment.[1]

ETIOLOGY

Incidence

Retinal detachments with macular holes are most infrequent, accounting for approximately 0.5% of all rhegmatogenous retinal detachments.[2–4] The high incidence in certain series[5–8] reflects the specific activity of referral retina centers rather than a geographical prevalence.

Age and Sex Distribution

Retinal detachments due to macular holes have been observed in patients from 25 to 84 years of age.[8] However there is a high prevalence in adults between 45 and 65 years of age.[8] There is also a significant prevalence in female patients (78%).[8]

Refractive Errors

All patients have myopic refractive errors over minus 3 diopters. Most retinal detachments with macular holes are observed in highly myopic patients. In our series,[8] approximately 74% of 59 patients had myopia over minus 10 diopters. The axial length of the eye was measured by A-scan ultrasonography in 42 eyes. It ranged from 27 to 29 mm in approximately 47% of the patients, and 30–36 mm in approximately 45%.

Retinal detachments associated with macular holes accounted for 6% of all retinal detachments in myopic eyes operated on in the author's clinic during the last decade.[8]

Bilaterality

Bilateral retinal detachment associated with a macular hole in both eyes is observed in approximately 10% of patients.[8,9]

CLINICAL FINDINGS

Visual Symptoms

Most patients are referred because of blurred vision with central scotoma. The onset of visual symptoms is gradual in most cases. The onset of the retinal detachment may be uncertain in patients with significant degenerative lesions of the posterior pole related to myopia. The visual acuity is under 0.05 in most patients. However, a few patients (approximately 10%) retain useful near reading visual acuity. These patients generally have a shallow detachment localized at the posterior pole. The detachment may be disclosed by routine fundus examination.

Fundus Examination

RETINAL DETACHMENT

The retinal detachment begins at the posterior pole in the macular area. In most cases it extends very gradually, over weeks or months, towards the midperiphery and the lower quadrants.

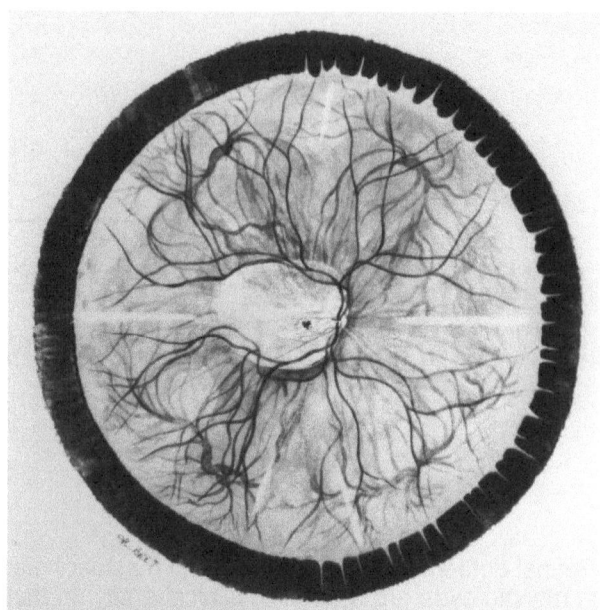

Figure 161. Retinal detachment associated with a tiny macular hole in a 18-diopter myopic eye. The detachment is confined to the posterior pole.

Depending on the extent of the retinal detachment at initial presentation, two distinct stages can be differentiated: (1) the retinal detachment is confined to the posterior pole and (2) the retinal detachment extends to the equator.

Retinal Detachment Confined the Posterior Pole. The retinal detachment is localized within the temporal arcades (Fig. 161 and Fig. 162). It is shallow. The detachment height measured by A-scan ultrasonography ranges from 1 to 4 mm.[8] The detached retina shows no retinal folds. The detachment cannot be modified by eye movements and bed rest.

In most patients, the progression will be very gradual.[3] It may remain unchanged for months or several years (Fig. 162). A shallow detachment confined to the posterior pole may regress spontaneously.

Retinal Detachment Extending to the Equator When the retinal detachment involves the posterior pole and extends to the lower quadrants, mainly the inferotemporal quadrant, the detachment extends to the equatorial region. It does not, however, reach the ora serrata (Fig. 163). A retinal detachment extending to the ora serrata is likely to be associated with peripheral retinal breaks rather than a macular break. Therefore, in such eyes, a thorough miomicroscopic examination of the periph-

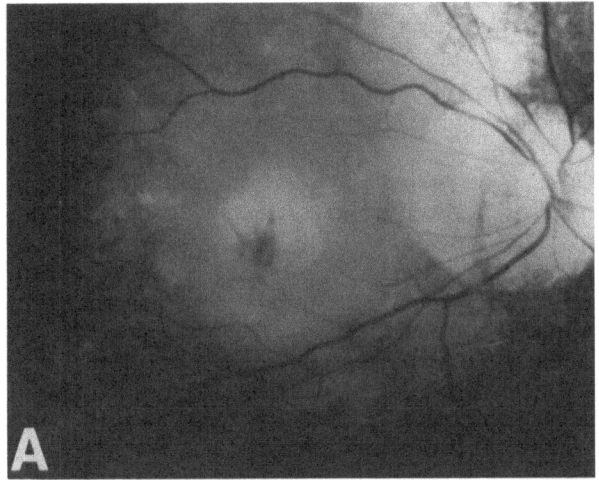

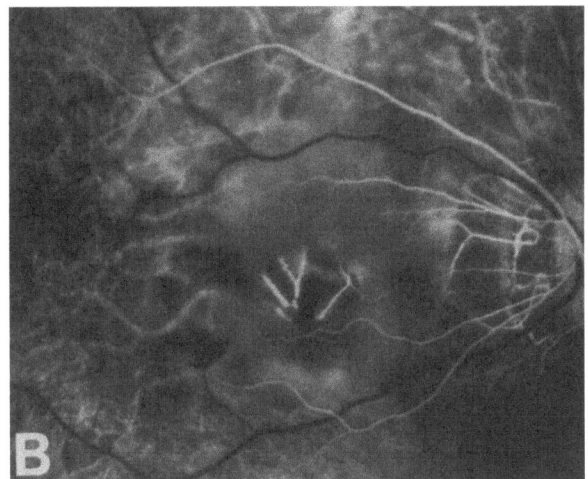

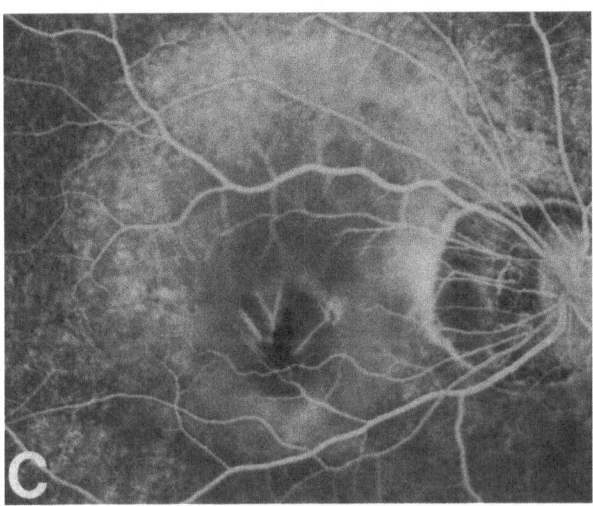

Figure 162. Retinal detachment associated with a macular hole in a 12-diopter myopic eye. The detachment has remained unchanged for a 3-year period. Near-reading visual acuity is nearly normal. The detachment height measured by A-scan ultrasonography is 1 mm. (A) Fundus photograph before dye injection. (B) Early stage of fluorescein angiography. (C) Late stage of fluorescein angiography.

eral fundus with scleral depression should be performed to find the peripheral retinal break(s).

In most eyes, the height of a retinal detachment due solely to a macular hole gradually increases from the posterior pole towards the midperiphery and decreases from the midperiphery to the equatorial region. The detachment height is maximal in the postequatorial region of the lower temporal quadrant (Fig. 163). The detached retina may show numerous tiny radial folds. There is no clinical evidence of proliferative vitreoretinopathy even in eyes with longstanding duration detachments.

The typical clinical features of retinal detachments due to macular holes may be significantly modified after unsuccessful surgery. The detachment may be very high with large retinal folds, particularly in eyes that failed to reattach after vitrectomy. In such eyes, the detachment may extend to the ora serrata in the lower quadrants and involve the midperiphery of the superior temporal quadrant.

MACULAR BREAK

The only retinal break associated with retinal detachment involves the macula. It is best recognized using a narrow slit beam, high magnification, and bright illumination. Retroillumination with the slit beam may be helpful to differentiate a full thickness macular break from a retinal cyst.

In most eyes with a retinal detachment confined to the posterior pole, the macular break is tiny. It may be less than 200 microns in size. In most cases, it involves the center of the macula. In most eyes the surrounding retina within the macular area shows cystic spaces. It may be difficult to differentiate the tiny full thickness break in the foveola from cystic cavities in the surrounding macula. At present there are no clinical means that allow the surgeon to determine with certainty whether the lesion that looks like a tiny full thickness hole actually is a full thickness retinal break or a hole in the inner wall of a macular

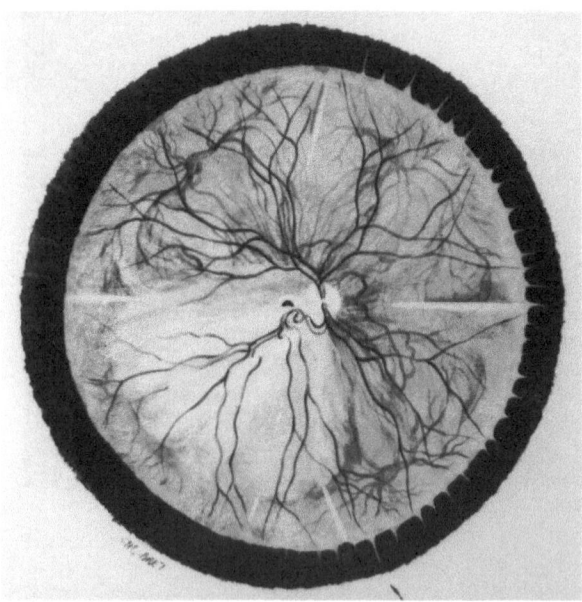

Figure 163. Retinal detachment associated with a macular hole in a 19-diopter myopic eye. The retina is highly detached in the inferior temporal quadrant. It is, however, attached in the preequatorial region.

cyst. Therefore, clinically, it may be impossible to determine whether the associated retinal detachment within the temporal arcades is a traction retinal detachment or a rhegmatogenous detachment, or both.

In most eyes with retinal detachment that extends beyond the lower temporal arcade, the diagnosis of macular break involves no difficulty. The macular break is clearly visible, although it rarely exceeds 500 μm in size. It shows a coarse, round shape. The choroidal pattern is clearly visible through the break. It shows a grey-white or red color, depending on the presence or absence of an atrophic staphyloma. A small retinal operculum, adherent to the posterior vitreous cortex may be present.

VITREOUS BODY

Vitreous liquefaction and posterior vitreous detachment are constant findings in retinal detachments associated with macular holes in myopic eyes. However the extent of posterior vitreous detachment shows important variations. There is a clinical correlation between the extent of posterior vitreous detachment and the extent of retinal detachment.

Eyes with shallow detachments confined within the temporal arcades generally exhibit a limited detachment of the posterior vitreous cortex on the posterior pole. In most eyes vitreous strands adherent

to the retina are visible by slit lamp examination, particularly on the temporal margin of the disc and along the superotemporal arcade. However, the precise extent of all vitreoretinal adhesions on the posterior pole cannot be determined by clinical examination.

Most eyes with retinal detachments extending beyond the temporal arcades show extensive posterior detachments. However, vitreous strands that are still adherent to the temporal arcades may be visible. The precise extent of the posterior vitreous detachment is difficult to determine clinically.

TREATMENT

Indications for Surgical Management

Immediate surgical management is not indicated in eyes with a shallow detachment confined to the perimacular area for two reasons: (1) the retinal detachment may remain unchanged for a prolonged period of time with conservation of useful reading visual acuity; and (2) the retinal detachment may spontaneously regress. Such patients should be followed up every 3 months. Surgery is indicated when repeated eye examinations reveal extension of the retinal detachment and increased visual defects.

Surgical management is indicated in all retinal detachments that extend beyond the inferior temporal arcade. These eyes have no useful visual acuity and show a deep visual field defect corresponding to the retinal detachment.

Surgical Technique

Clinical experience gained in recent years with vitrectomy and intravitreal gas injection has demonstrated that neither scleral buckling of the posterior pole, nor choroidal irritation in the macular area were required to reattach the retina in most eyes.[10–13] However a few eyes fail to reattach with gas injection only, or gas injection associated with vitrectomy.[8–11] The criteria for predicting which retinal detachments will not respond favorably to endosurgery have not yet been established. Consequently, in any given clinical case, the surgeon should apply the simplest surgical technique. More sophisticated technique(s) will be performed in the small number of eyes that fail to reattach after simple surgery.

At present, the surgical techniques currently used in the management of retinal detachments associated with macular holes can be classified from the simplest to the most sophisticated and are as follows:

(1) intravitreal gas injection, (2) vitrectomy associated with intravitreal gas injection, (3) choroidal irritation and gas injection in a previously vitrectomized eye, and (4) scleral buckling and gas injection in eyes that failed to reattach with the former procedures.

INTRAVITREAL GAS INJECTION

Intravitreal gas injection without vitrectomy or any direct surgical action on the macular break was introduced by Miyake.[11]

It is the most simple technique in the management of macular holes and has two main advantages: (1) it is rapidly performed and (2) the remaining central vision is preserved. The technique should be applied as the first and, most often, single surgical procedure in most eyes.

Pure sulfur hexafluoride is used. The volume of pure gas to be injected is determined so that internal tamponade of the macular break is achieved and also to give the patient some latitude of movement postoperatively (Fig. 164). The maximal volume of gas to be injected with minimal risk of inducing severely increased intraocular pressure depends on three main parameters: (1) the volume of the vitreous cavity, (2) the degree and extent of vitreous liquefaction, and (3) the amount of subretinal fluid.

The vitreous cavity volume is determined by preoperative measurement of the axial and transverse diameters of the vitreous cavity with A-scan ultrasonography (see p. 122). It is significantly increased in highly myopic eyes. The degree and extent of vitreous liquefaction is evaluated with biomicroscopic examination, however, clinical evaluation is approximate.

The technique for providing sufficient intraocular space for the gas bubble and for avoiding induced increased intraocular pressure depends on the amount of subretinal fluid.

In eyes with retinal detachment extending to the equatorial region, subretinal fluid is drained off (Fig. 165). The incision for subretinal fluid drainage is performed in the inferotemporal quadrant. The scleral projection of the peripheral limit of the detachment should be determined intraoperatively to make sure that the drainage site is in an area of detached retina. A syringe containing pure SF6 is prepared in advance. The choroidal incision is performed. When subretinal fluid escapes from the eye, gas is injected into the vitreous cavity through the pars plana in the inferotemporal quadrant. Gas is injected during subretinal fluid escape to avoid collapse of the eye (Fig. 165). Intraocular pressure is roughly estimated during gas injection using a spatula held with the left hand. Gas injection is discontinued at the first evidence of increasing intraocular pressure. In most eyes a volume of 1 ml to 1.5 ml of pure SF6 is injected. If the intraocular pressure is increased, paracentesis of the anterior chamber is performed as an adjunct to subretinal fluid drainage. The retinal circulation on the optic disc is monitored (see p. 123).

In eyes with flat detachment that does not reach the equatorial region, subretinal fluid is not drained

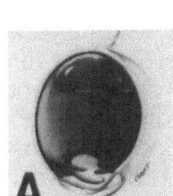
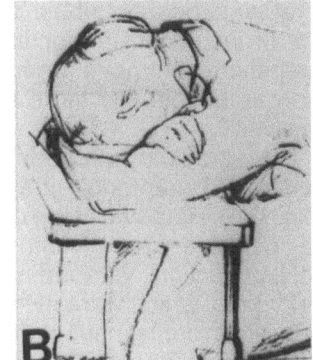
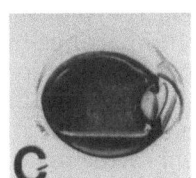
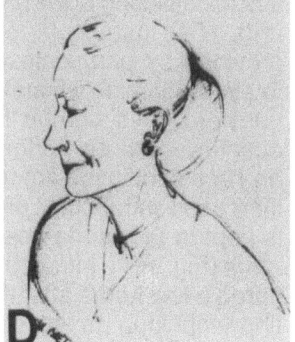

Figure 164. Head positioning after gas injection in management of retinal detachment with macular hole in a highly myopic patient. (A) Intravitreal space available for gas injection was limited. A small gas bubble was used so as to avoid increased intraocular pressure. (B) The patient must keep her head in the prone position to ensure macular tamponade by the small gas bubble. (C) Following repeated paracentesis of the anterior chamber and subretinal fluid drainage, intraocular space was sufficient to inject 1.5 ml of pure SF6. After bubble expansion, the macular hole is sealed by the large gas bubble, regardless of the patient head position. (D) The patient can move around normally.

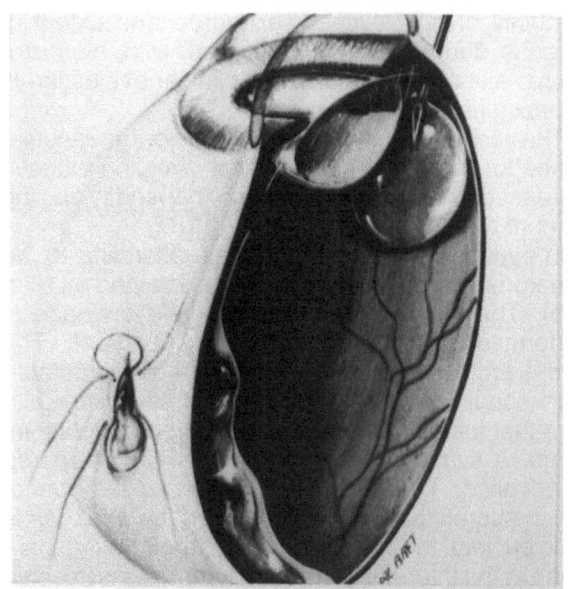

Figure 165. Surgical management of retinal detachment with a macular hole by gas injection with simultaneous release of subretinal fluid. The drainage site is rather posterior because subretinal fluid does not spread beyond the equator. The goal of subretinal fluid drainage is to create intraocular space for gas injection so as to avoid increased intraocular pressure.

off because drainage would be hazardous. The volume of pure SF6 to be injected should not exceed 0.6 to 0.7 ml. This small volume of gas will require strict positioning of the patient's head postoperatively (Fig. 164). Intraocular space for the gas bubble is provided by paracentesis of the anterior chamber. In eyes with highly liquefied vitreous gel, liquid vitreous percolates through the zonula and repeated paracentesis can be performed. Intravenous mannitol and acetazolamide are useful adjuncts in preventing increased intraocular pressure. The patient's head is kept in the prone position following return to the room (Fig. 164). Intraocular pressure should be monitored a few hours after the operation. The gas injection technique provides permanent retinal reattachment in approximately 80% of eyes.[12]

Failures may be related to inadequate patient's head positioning in the first postoperative days, an insufficient volume of the gas bubble, or unknown reasons. In failed eyes, gas injection may be performed a second time and succeed.

Although the procedure is successful in a high percentage of eyes, the actual cause(s) for success remain speculative. The gas bubble may peel away weak vitreoretinal adhesions on the posterior pole.[12,13] The technique has been developed re-

cently and the long-term outcome remains unknown. The technique has a major potential risk in eyes with a small amount of subretinal fluid that cannot be drained off: gas injection may result in severely increased intraocular pressure. The complication is more likely to occur in eyes with slight, vitreous liquefaction or impaired aqueous humor outflow. Highly myopic eyes are the most vulnerable to increased intraocular pressure. A high, although transient increase in intraocular pressure may result in acute optic disc or retinal ischemia with permanent visual field defect. Therefore, gas injection with vitrectomy should be performed rather than just gas injection alone in eyes with a limited retinal detachment, slight vitreous liquefaction, or impaired aqueous outflow.

VITRECTOMY AND GAS INJECTION

Vitrectomy and gas injection was introduced for the management of retinal detachment with macular hole by Gonvers and Machemer.[10] The value of this technique has been confirmed by several publications.[8,14–18] This surgical approach should be used (1) as the first surgical procedure in eyes at high risk of increased intraocular pressure after gas injection alone and (2) as the third surgical procedure in eyes that fail to reattach after two consecutive gas injections.

The procedure shares the same major advantage as gas injection: the remaining central vision is preserved. It is more invasive and less rapid a procedure than gas injection. However, it has the major advantage of providing a large space for the gas bubble. A rather large gas bubble can be used with minimal risk of increased intraocular pressure. In addition, the patient can move around almost normally when the gas bubble fills more than half of the vitreous cavity.

The vitrectomy procedure is easy and rapid to perform. The anterior vitreous gel is left untouched (Fig. 166). Removal of the central and posterior vitreous gel is very rapid in most eyes owing to vitreous gel liquefaction. Vitreoretinal adhesions on the posterior pole, which were invisible preoperatively, may be visible during vitrectomy (Fig. 166). However, weak vitreoretinal adhesions may be missed by the surgeon because they are relieved by fluid currents induced by vitrectomy. The diagnosis of a full thickness macular break is confirmed during vitrectomy by the observation of subretinal fluid passing into the vitreous cavity (Schlieren phenomenon)[19] (Fig. 167). As in the former procedure, no choroidal irritation is carried out, and subretinal fluid drainage is unnecessary.

The pars plana incisions are secured on a rather soft eye and 1.5 ml to 2.5 ml of pure SF6, depending

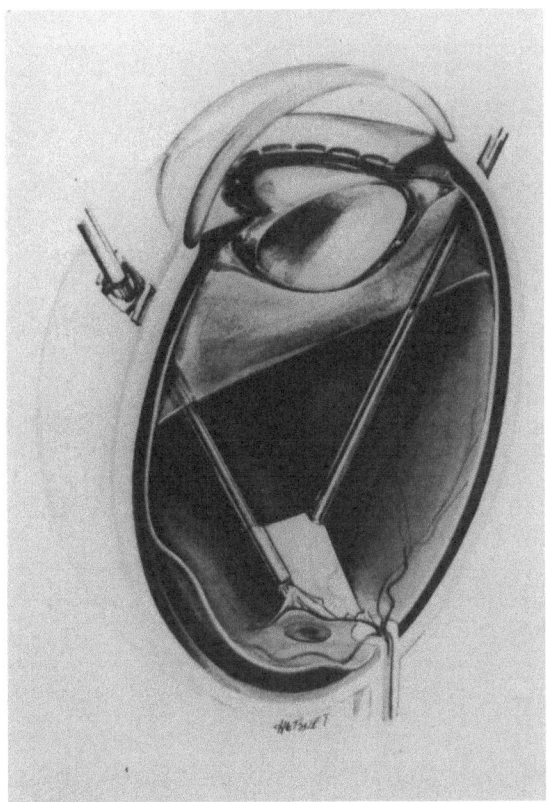

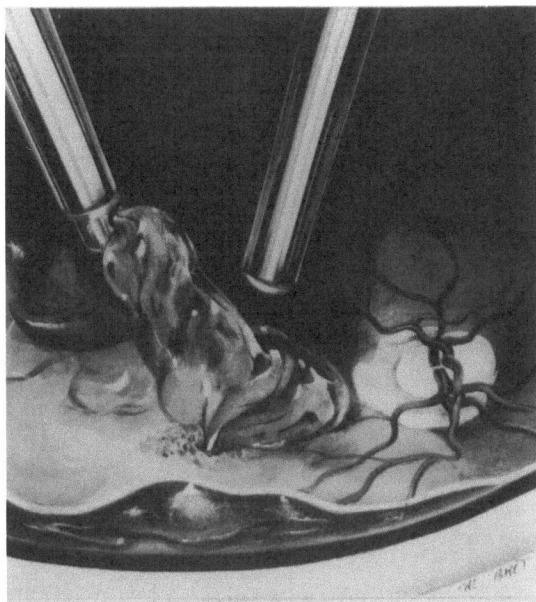

Figure 167. Schlieren phenomenon: During vitrectomy subretinal fluid migrates toward the vitreous cavity through a full-thickness macular hole.

Figure 166. Vitrectomy in the management of retinal detachment with macular hole in highly myopic eyes: The anterior vitreous gel is left in place. In this case attachment of the posterior vitreous face to the superior temporal arcade was clearly visible intraoperatively.

on eye biometry, are injected into the vitreous cavity.

The procedure provides retinal reattachment in approximately 85% of the eyes[8,10,15,18] (Fig. 168). In eyes that fail to reattach, the retinal detachment generally increases in height and extent; however, an additional gas injection may successfully permanently reattach the retina. Late recurrences of the detachment may occur a year to 18 months postoperatively. They are successfully managed with gas injection and no choroidal irritation.

The vitrectomy-gas technique developed by Gonvers and Machemer was based on the concept that vitreous traction plays a major role in most retinal detachments associated with macular holes. Observations during vitrectomy and early postoperative results correlate well with this hypothesis. However the actual cause of the beneficial effect of repeated gas injection in failed eyes, remains speculative. The causes of late recurrences are also unclear.

GAS INJECTION AND CHOROIDAL IRRITATION IN THE MACULAR AREA

Gas injection and choroidal irritation in the macular area has a major disadvantage: it introduces iatrogenic loss of the remaining central vision. However, the technique should be used in eyes that failed to reattach after the former procedures. Internal tamponade with silicone oil has been advocated to preserve central vision.[20–23] The value of this technique remains questionable because of the short and long-term complications of intraocular silicone oil.

Inducement of an efficacious and limited retinochoroidal adhesion in the close vicinity of the macular break is best achieved by argon laser photocoagulation. In aphakic eyes it is carried out a few days postoperatively after complete gas expansion. In phakic myopic eyes argon laser photocoagulation of a macular hole through a gas bubble is difficult to perform. Therefore, intraoperative photocoagulation treatment with simultaneous scleral depression of the posterior pole, rather than postoperative photocoagulation, is used. Scleral depression is performed with the tip of the long and thin cryoprobe, especially designed for management of macular holes. The conjunctiva is disinserted 2 mm from the limbus in the lower temporal quadrant. Bridle sutures are placed in the lateral and inferior recti muscles. An additional bridle suture is placed transconjunctivally in the superior rectus muscle inser-

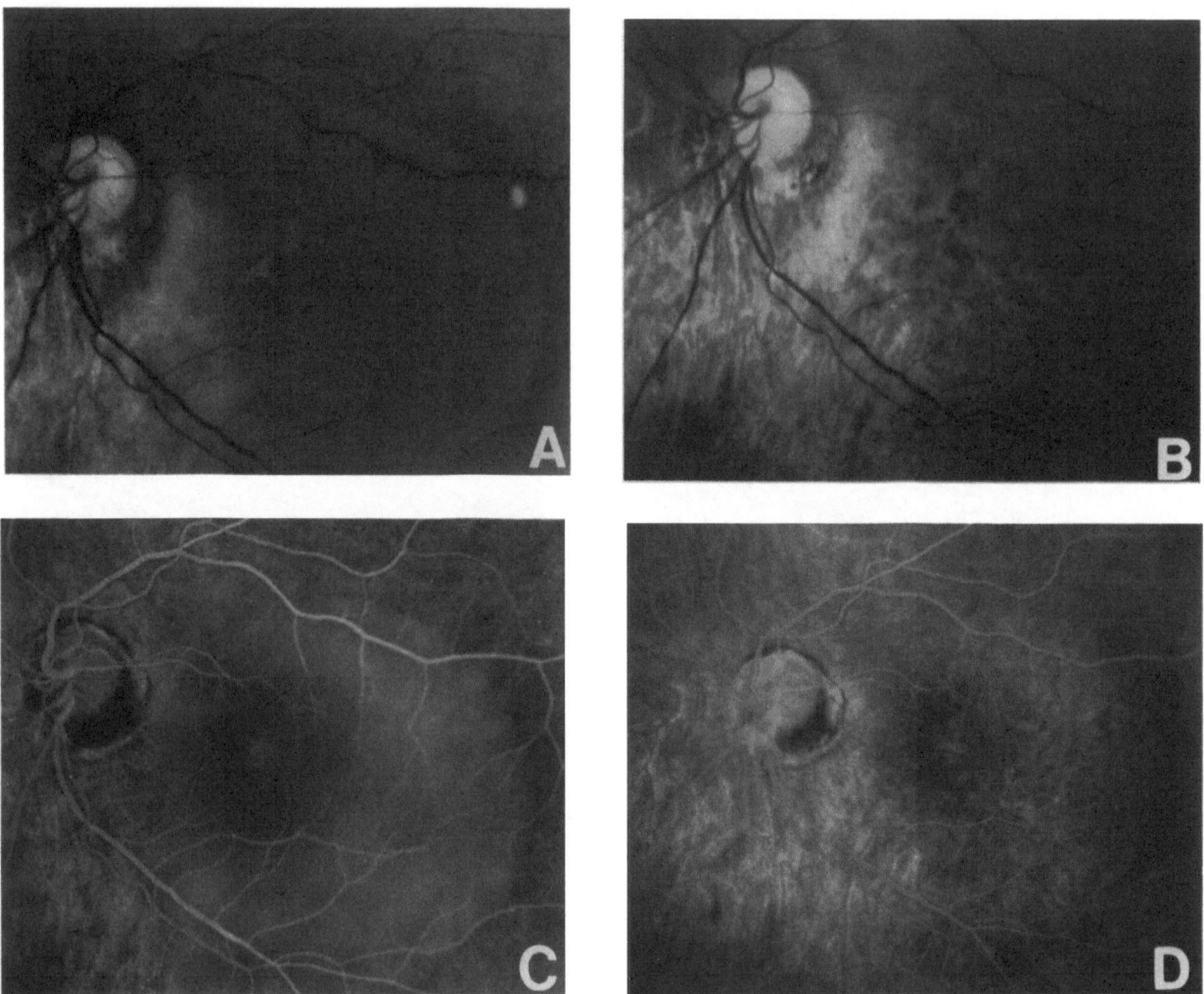

Figure 168. Retinal detachment with a macular hole and decreased visual acuity in a 9-diopter myopic eye, managed by vitrectomy and gas injection. (A) Preoperative fundus photograph. (B) Postoperative fundus photograph. (C) Preoperative fluorescein angiography. (D) Postoperative fluorescein angiography.

tion. Tenon's space is opened with scissor blades under visual control up to the posterior pole. Then, the bridle sutures are fixed to the surgical drapes with forceps to place and maintain the eye in the straight ahead position during argon laser photocoagulation. The cryoprobe tip is inserted into Tenon's space under visual control. Then the contact lens is placed on the cornea. The cryoprobe tip is moved towards the macular hole with simultaneous biomicroscopic observation of the fundus. Scleral depression on the posterior pole should be very gentle. The posterior sclera of highly myopic eyes is often very thin, and excessive scleral depression on the posterior pole may result in scleral perforation. Apposition of the pigment epithelium and retina in the area of the macular break is generally easy to achieve with gentle scleral depression, since the

retinal detachment is rather shallow on the posterior pole in most eyes. Two rows of burns are placed all around the macula. Burns should not be made on the macula itself which must be preserved as much as possible for the remaining central vision. A 250 μm-size spot and 0.5 second exposure time are used. Laser photocoagulation is begun with a low power. The power is gradually increased until a yellow-white burn of the retina is obtained.

A retinochoroidal burn cannot be achieved by photocoagulation in eyes with total atrophy of the pigment epithelium and choroid in the macular area. Cryotreatment, although much more destructive than argon laser photocoagulation, is used in such eyes. It is performed with simultaneous biomicroscopic observation of the fundus. A single cryoapplication is performed. Before freezing, the surgeon should verify that scleral depression in front of the macular break is achieved by the very tip of the cryoprobe (see pp. 77). This is most important since misplacement of the cryoprobe tip and scleral depression in front of the macular break by the cryoprobe shaft would result in freezing of the surrounding retina, or even the optic nerve.

Gas injection is performed after argon laser photocoagulation or cryotreatment, using the technique described above.

In the author's experience,[8] choroidal irritation associated with gas injection provides permanent retinal reattachment in approximately 90% of eyes that failed to reattach with gas injection and vitrectomy. Most patients will recover peripheral visual field, but no useful central vision.[8]

SCLERAL BUCKLING OF THE POSTERIOR POLE

Indications for scleral buckling of the posterior pole are restricted to the very small percentage of eyes (approximately 10%) that fail to reattach with the procedures described above.

Difficulty and surgical hazards of the procedure, as well as permanent loss of central vision in most patients, are the main disadvantages of scleral buckling. The numerous techniques that were developed in the past for scleral buckling of macular holes[2,5,6,24-48] reflect the difficulty of scleral surgery on the posterior pole, as well as the fertile imaginations of retina surgeons.

In the author's experience, the patch pocket technique has been the most efficient, the least hazardous, and the easiest procedure to perform for direct scleral buckling of the macular break.[8, 45] The author, therefore, still uses the patch pocket technique as the last surgical procedure in the small number of eyes that fail to reattach after vitrectomy and two gas injections with choroidal irritation.

Instrumentation. Three specific instruments are required to perform the procedure. They include forceps, scissors, and a hook. The forceps and scissors are used for tissue dissection on the posterior pole in the close vicinity of the posterior ciliary arteries and optic nerve. The forceps with atraumatic teeth and the blades of the blunt scissors are similar respectively, to those of Bonn forceps and corneal blunt scissors. However, the instrument shaft is twice the length of the equivalent instruments used in anterior segment microsurgery (Fig. 169).

A special hook has been developed to shift the nasal straps of the patch pocket behind the eye and alongside the optic nerve (Fig. 170). The hook makes a 25° angle with the handle. Hook orientation allows for easier rotation behind the eye. A hole at

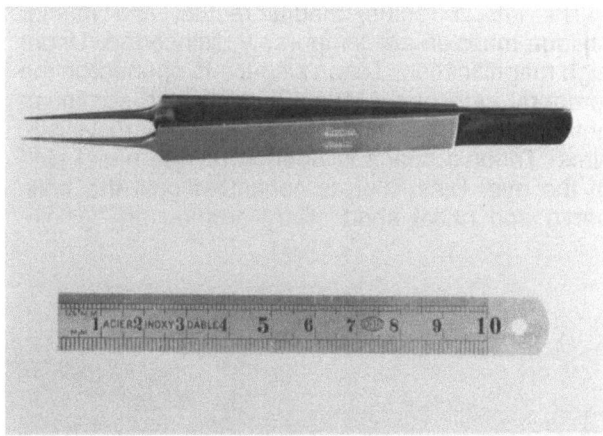

Figure 169. Forceps for tissue dissection on the posterior pole [Moria (Paris)].

the hook tip is used to insert the threads used as leaders of the nasal straps of the patch pocket.

Surgical Technique. Placement of scleral sutures on the posterior pole is the most difficult and hazardous step of scleral buckling of macular holes because of the surgical field depth, and the usually thin sclera on the posterior staphyloma. Therefore the shape of the patch pocket has been developed to make scleral sutures on the posterior pole unnecessary.

The patch pocket is made up with lyophylized human dura mater. It is composed of a medial part, 7 mm by 15 mm in size, and four straps 1.5 mm in width and 14 mm in length. A double-armed 5–0 nonabsorbable suture is preplaced at the extremity of each strap. The sutures will be used as leaders for the placing of the patch pocket and fixation of the straps to the anterior sclera. An explant made of six thicknesses of dura mater is stuck onto the medial part of the pocket with histoacryl glue.

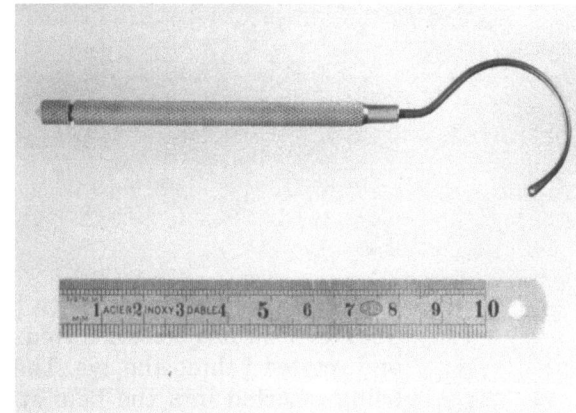

Figure 170. Hook for placing the nasal straps of the patch pocket.

The lateral rectus, medial rectus, and inferior oblique muscles are temporarily disinserted. Under high magnification, Tenon's space is opened on the temporal side of the eye. Dissection is continued until the short posterior ciliary arteries are visible. Next, Tenon's space is opened on the nasal side of the eye. Dissection is continued until the optic nerve and nasal short ciliary arteries are visible.

Then, two funnels are created below and above the optic nerve. The upper funnel is made between the medial short posterior ciliary arteries and the superior nasal vortex vein. The lower funnel is made between the posterior ciliary arteries and the inferior nasal vortex vein. Accurate dissection of the funnel is most important because it will determine the position of the nasal pocket straps. The straps must not jeopard-

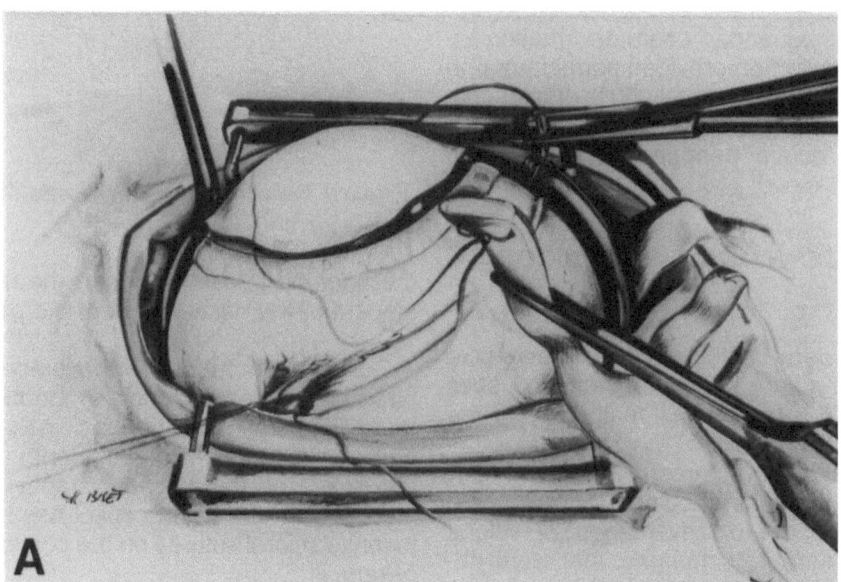

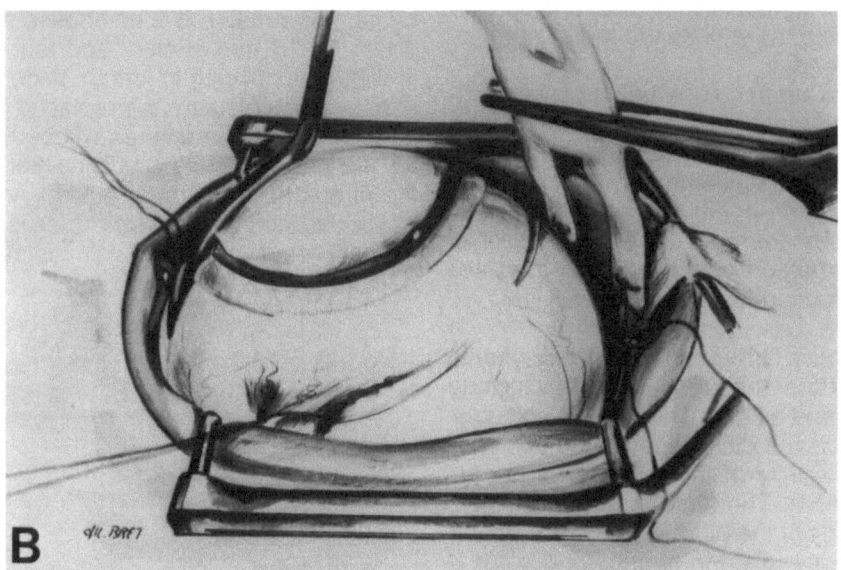

Figure 171. Patch pocket on the posterior pole: surgical technique. (A) The hook has been inserted into the funnel above the optic nerve, and rotated behind the eye. The suture of the superior nasal strap is being inserted into the hole at the hook tip. (B) The suture of the superior nasal strap has been placed on the nasal side of the eye. The suture of the inferior nasal strap is being pulled by the hook toward the nasal side of the eye.

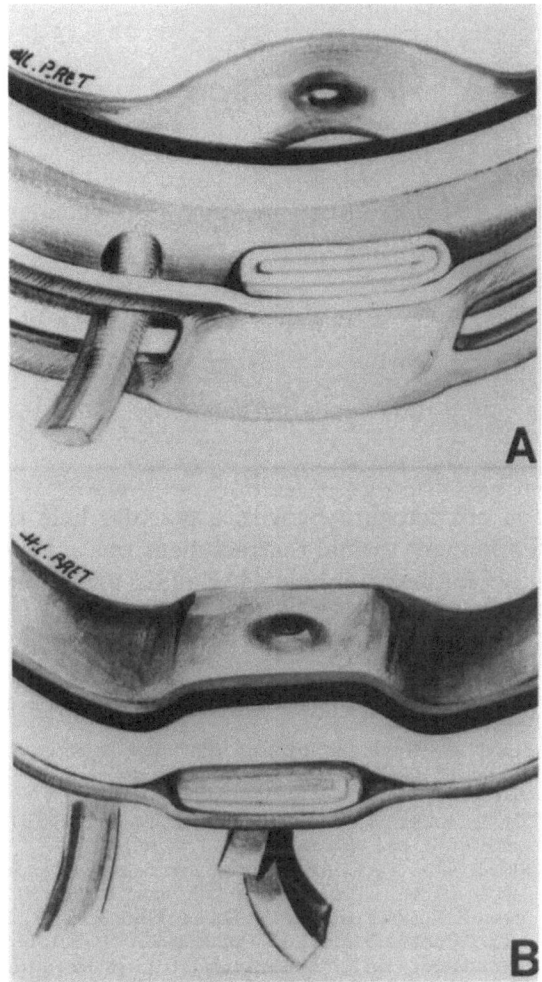

Figure 172. Scleral buckling of the posterior pole with the patch pocket technique: (A) Buckle positioning in front of the macular hole. (B) Approximation of the pigment epithelium and the detached retina is achieved by securing the straps of the patch pocket to the sclera anterior to the equator.

nasally while placement of the medial part of the patch pocket in Tenon's space on the posterior pole is monitored by the assistant.

Proper positioning of the patch pocket in front of the macular break (Fig. 172) is verified by fundus examination before suturing the straps to the sclera. The nasal straps are sutured first. The preplaced sutures are used to fix the straps to the sclera. The scleral sutures are placed anteriorly to the equator (Fig. 173). Then, fundus examination is performed. If the buckle height appears insufficient, subretinal fluid is drained off and the straps are shortened. Completion of the procedure takes approximately 90 minutes. Proper opening of Tenon's space and dissection of both funnels above and below the optic nerve are the keys for a successful and uneventful operation. In contrast, intraoperative and postoperative complications may occur when these surgical steps are not properly carried out. Insufficient opening of Tenon's space up to the short posterior ciliary arteries will result in major difficulties in proper placement of the buckle. Inadequate dissection of the funnels above and below the optic nerve may result in the inability to carry out the hook maneuver behind the eye, scleral perforation, and compression of the nasal vortex veins by the straps.

In most vitrectomized eyes, retinal folds remain on the posterior pole after scleral buckling and may involve the macular break. Therefore, intravitreal gas

ize the blood circulation in the vortex veins and posterior ciliary arteries.

The special hook is then inserted in the superior funnel and passed behind the eye from the nasal side to the temporal side. The preplaced suture of the superior nasal strap is inserted in the hole at the hook tip (Fig. 171). Then the hook tip is gently moved backward with a rotating motion towards the nasal side of the eye. When the strap is visible along the optic nerve, the suture is freed from the hook.

The same maneuver is carried out for placement of the inferior nasal strap of the patch pocket (Fig. 171).

Both sutures of the nasal straps are gently pulled

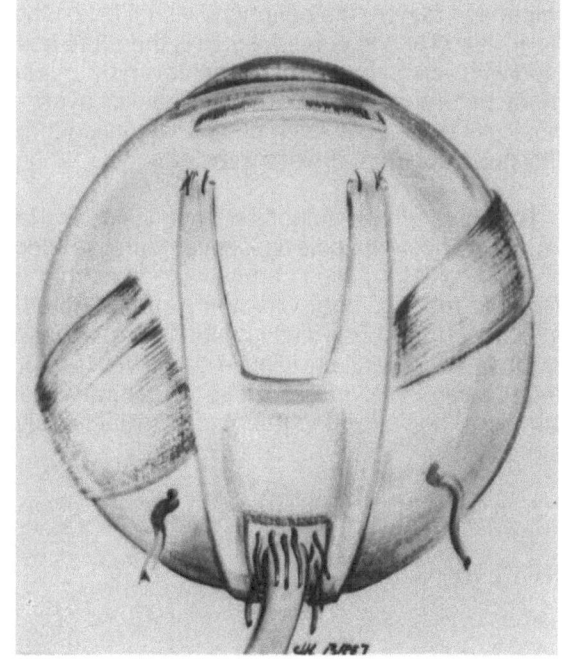

Figure 173. Posterior view of the eye after completion of the patch pocket. Each nasal strap of the buckle runs between the short posterior ciliary arteries and the vortex vein.

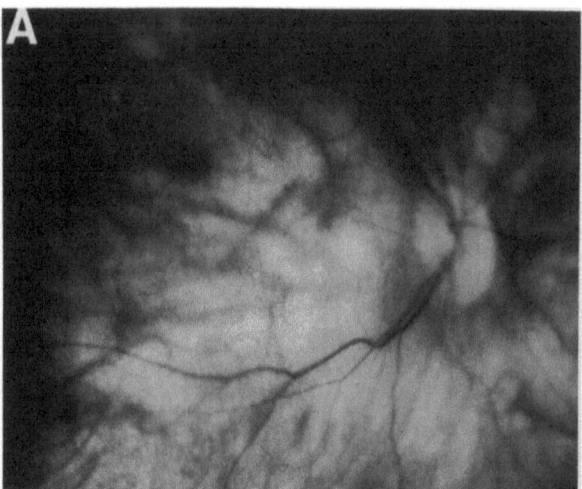 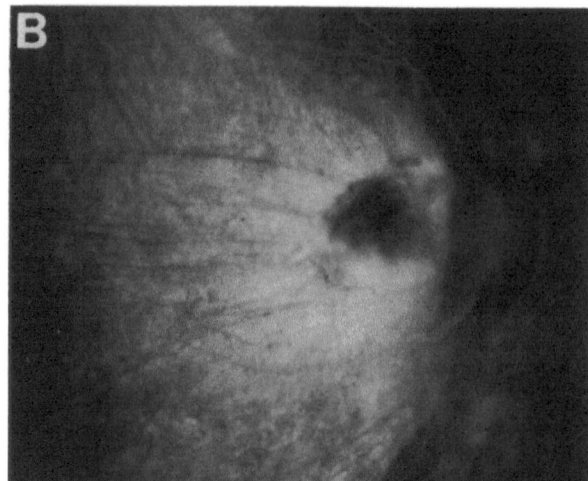

Figure 174. Postoperative fundus photographs of a retinal detachment with a macular hole that failed to reattach after vitrectomy and gas tamponade. Permanent retinal reattachment was achieved by scleral buckling of the posterior pole and cryotreatment of the macular hole. (A) Fundus photograph. (B) Fluorescein angiography.

injection is performed as an adjunct to scleral buckling.

Permanent retinal reattachment may be achieved by scleral buckling of the posterior pole without choroidal irritation.[49] However, in eyes that have failed to reattach after several operations, scleral buckling is performed as the ultimate attempt to reattach the retina and restore the peripheral visual field. Choroidal irritation on the posterior pole is therefore associated with scleral buckling. It is achieved by cryotreatment before scleral buckling in phakic eyes, and postoperative argon laser photocoagulation through the gas bubble in aphakic eyes.

Results. In the author's experience scleral buckling of the posterior pole associated with gas injection and choroidal irritation can salvage eyes that have failed to reattach after vitrectomy and repeated gas injection (Fig. 174). The anatomical success rate achieved by scleral buckling in such eyes is approximately 87%.[8] Permanent loss of central vision is constant, however, the peripheral visual field is restored.

REFERENCES

1. Machemer R: The importance of fluid absorption, traction, intraocular currents, and chorioretinal scars in the therapy of rhegmatogenous retinal detachment. Am J Ophthalmol 98:681–693, 1984
2. Margherio RB, Schepens CL: Macular breaks. I—Diagnosis, etiology and observations. Am J Ophthalmol 74:219–232, 1972
3. Urrets-Zavalia A: Le décollement de la rétine. Paris, Masson, 1968, 135–144
4. Feman SS, Hepler RS, Straatsma BR: Rhegmatogenous retinal detachment due to macular hole. Arch Ophthalmol 91:371–372, 1974
5. Theodossiadis G: Treatment of retinal detachment arising from macular hole. Mod Probl Ophthalmol 12:322–329, 1974
6. Klöti R: Silver clip for central retinal detachments with macular hole. Mod Probl Ophthalmol (Karger Edit., Basel) 12:330–336, 1974
7. Muños A, Mateus F, Heredia CD: Retinal detachments with holes in the posterior pole. Mod Probl Ophthalmol 12:315–321, 1974
8. Normand-Guyonnet F: Décollements de la rétine par trou maculaire ou déchirure du pole postérieur chez le myope fort. Thèse doctorat, Université Lyon, 1986
9. Schepens CL: Retinal detachment and allied diseases, Philadelphia, W. B. Saunders, 1983, Volume 2, 542–553
10. Gonvers M, Machemer R: A new approach to treating retinal detachment with macular hole. Am J Ophthalmol 94:468–472, 1982
11. Miyake Y: A simplified method for treating retinal detachment with macular hole. Am J Ophthalmol 97:243–245, 1984
12. Mikaye Y: A simplified method of treating retinal detachment with macular hole. Arch Ophthalmol 104:1234–1236, 1986
13. Blodi CF, Folk JC: Treatment of macular hole retinal detachments with intravitreal gas. Am J Ophthalmol 98:811, 1984
14. Clarkson JG: Traitement du décollement rétinien par trou maculaire. J Fr Ophthalmol 6:436, 1983
15. Vallat M, Van Coppenolle F, Detre J, Moze M, et al: Traitement chirurgical des décollements de la rétine avec trou maculaire par vitrectomie suivie d'échange air-serum. Bull Soc Ophtalmol Fr 84: 421–423, 1984
16. De Molfeta V, Arpa P, Decasa N, et al: La vitrectomia via pars plana nel trattamento del distacco della retina da foro maculare. Ann Ottalmol Clin Ocul 110:311–315, 1984
17. Laqua H: Die behandlung der Ablatio mit Makulaforamen nach der methode von Gonvers und Machemer. Klin Monatsbl Augenheilk 186:13–17, 1985
18. Girard P, Navarro F, Boscher C, Mercier P: Le traitement des décollements rétiniens par déhiscence du pole postérieur. J Fr Ophtalmol 8:613–618, 1985
19. Friberg TR, Tano Y, Machemer R: Schlieren (streaks) as a sign of rhegmatogenous detachment in vitreous surgery. Am J Ophthalmol 88:943, 1979

20. Cockerman W, Schepens CL, Freeman HM: Silicone injection in retinal detachment. Mod Probl Ophthalmol 8:525–540, 1969

21. Haut J, Van Effentere G, Ullern M, Chermet M: Traitement chirurgical des décollements de la rétine avec trou maculaire par la technique de la vitrectomie associée à l'injection de silicone liquide. J Fr Ophtalmol 3, 2:115–118, 1980

22. Haut J, Van Effentere G, Flamand M: Treatment of macular hole retinal detachment with silicone oil, with or without argon laser photocoagulation. Ophthalmologica 187:25–28, 1983

23. Larricart P, Faure IF, Monin C, Sfeir T: Indications respectives des différentes techniques opératoires du traitement d'un décollement rétinien par trou maculaire. Bull Mem Soc Fr Ophtalmol 97:363–366, 1986

24. Schepens CL, Okamura ID, Brockhurst RJ: The scleral buckling procedures: I—surgical techniques and management. Arch Ophthalmol 58:797–811, 1957

25. Bangerter A: Zür therapie beim Maculaloch. Klin Monatsbl Augenheilk 136:593–598, 1960

26. Adams ST: Retinal detachment due to macular and small posterior holes. Arch Ophthalmol 66:528–533, 1961

27. Pannarale MR: Techniques de traitement du décollement avec déchirures très postérieures. Mod Probl Ophthalmol 4:239–245 1, 1966

28. Rosengren B: The silver plombs method in macular holes. Trans Ophthalmol Soc U.K. 86:49–53, 1966

29. Hager G: Die T: Plomben plastik line Neuablatioperation. Klin Monatsbl. Augenheilk. 153, 624, 1968

30. Paufique L, Bonnet M: Traitement du décollement de la rétine avec déchirure vraie de la macula par la technique de la poche sclérale. Ann Oculist (Paris) 201:290–302, 1968

31. Bouchat J, Marsol C: Trou maculaire, décollement de la rétine et marsupialisation sclérale. Bull Soc Ophtalmol Fr 68:550–556, 1968

32. Long RS, Mittl R, Chuanico R: Experimental scleral buckling of the posterior pole using tissue adhesive. Amer J Ophthalmol 69: 419–422, 1970

33. Ravault PM, Maugery J, Franck JP, Demilliere B: Traitement du décollement rétinien maculaire par une méthode de sanglage maculaire. Bull Soc Ophtalmol Fr 71:230–232, 1971

34. Haut J, Lecoq PJ, Clay C, Limon S, Moschos M: Traitement par éponge en élastique localisée et cryothérapie des décollements de la rétine par trou maculaire. Arch Ophtalmol (Paris) 32:541–548, 1972

35. Kapuscinski WJ: Cerclage postero-antérieur dans les décollements rétiniens avec trou maculaire. Ann Oculist (Paris) 205:1115–1121, 1972

36. Bagolini B, Ravalico G: Traitement chirurgical du décollement de la rétine avec trou maculaire. Arch Ophtalmol (Paris) 33:553–559, 1973

37. Linnen HJ, Gareis-Helferich E: Erfahrungen mit der plombenoperation bei Netzhaut foramina im hinterem Bulbusberlich. Klin Monatsbl Augenheilk 162:729–735, 1973

38. Feman SS, Hepler RS, Straatsma BR: Rhegmatogenous retinal detachment due to macular hole. Arch Ophthalmol 91:371–372, 1974

39. Mortada A: Retinal detachment surgery for giant tear or macular hole. The oblique silastic band without evacuation of subretinal fluid. Jap J Ophthalmol 18:245–252, 1974

40. Harris GS: Treatment of retinal detachments due to macular holes. Mod Probl Ophthalmol, 12:337–341, 1974

41. Gloor BP: Operation der Netzhautablösung bei Löchern im Bereich des hinteren Poles mit einfacher, lang verträglicher sieberspange und cerclage. Klin Monatsbl Augenheilk 171:271–277, 1977

42. Tolentino F, Schepens CL, Freeman HM: Vitreoretinal disorders. Diagnosis and management. Philadelphia, W. B. Saunders, 1976, 406

43. Bagolini B, Peduzzi M: Implant de silicone armé dans le traitement chirurgical du décollement de la rétine avec trou maculaire. Bull Mem Soc Fr Ophtalmol 91:161–163, 1980

44. Siam AL: Décollement de la rétine causé par un trou maculaire. Bull Mem Soc Fr Ophtalmol 91:151–160, 1980

45. Bonnet M, Nagao M: Poche sclérale sur le pole postérieur dans le traitement des décollements de la rétine par trou maculaire. J Fr Ophtalmol 5:505–513, 1982

46. Bagolini B, Peduzzi M: Permanent buckling for retinal detachment due to macular hole. Ophthalmologica 2:77–80, 1983

47. Wollensak J, Engels T: Traitement des trous rétiniens au pole postérieur par les techniques de buckling. J Fr Ophtalmol 6:435–437, 1983

48. Meyer Schwickerath G, Gerke E: Décollement de rétine par trou maculaire. J Fr Ophtalmol 6:434–436, 1983

49. Theodossiadis GP: Traitement du décollement de la rétine consécutif à un trou maculaire sans application d'aucune forme d'énergie. J Fr Ophtalmol 5:427–431, 1982

20

Rhegmatogenous Retinal Detachment with Proliferative Vitreoretinopathy

In 1983[1] the Retina Society suggested the name of Proliferative Vitreoretinopathy for the clinical entity previously known as massive vitreous retraction, massive preretinal retraction, or massive preretinal proliferation. This clinical condition is the major complication of rhegmatogenous retinal detachment. At present severe proliferative vitreoretinopathy remains the most common cause of surgical failure in the management of rhegmatogenous retinal detachment.[2] Proliferative vitreoretinopathy is characterized by the proliferation of cellular membranes on both surfaces of the detached retina and on the posterior surface of the vitreous gel. These membranes contract and result in further elevation and extension of the retinal detachment and fixed retinal folds. The retinal detachment that was initially purely rhegmatogenous has become a tractional retinal detachment. In severe cases the traction forces are so strong that previously sealed retinal breaks reopen and new breaks occur.

Experimental studies[3–11] and histologic examinations of epiretinal and retroretinal membranes removed during vitrectomy[10–15] have led to improved understanding of the pathogenesis of proliferative vitreoretinopathy.

Development of sophisticated vitreous microsurgery has brought about significant improvement in the surgical management of severe proliferative vitreoretinopathy. At present, permanent retinal reattachment can be achieved in approximately 70% of eyes treated without silicone oil.[16–20] The overall anatomical success rate achieved with silicone oil is higher.[21–22] However, the long-term outcome of eyes treated with silicone oil remains unknown.

Treatment of retinal detachments associated with severe proliferative vitreoretinopathy is time-con-suming for the retina surgeon and may be a strain for the patient. Visual results, although priceless for the patient who has already lost vision of the fellow eye, are often disappointing. Most patients with severe proliferative vitreoretinopathy recover only ambulatory vision after successful surgery.

Therefore, prevention of severe proliferative vitreoretinopathy should be one of the main objectives of retinal detachment surgeons. Identification of the clinical factors that predispose to the development of severe proliferative vitreoretinopathy is the first step in the prevention of this devastating complication of rhegmatogenous retinal detachment.

ETIOLOGY—PREDISPOSING FACTORS

Severe proliferative vitreoretinopathy occurs in approximately 5–10% of all rhegmatogenous retinal detachments.[1] The actual incidence greatly depends on case selection. In most instances, severe proliferative vitreoretinopathy develops after surgery for retinal reattachment. Therefore, for the clinician, it is of primary importance to recognize preoperatively, those eyes that are at risk of developing severe proliferative vitreoretinopathy postoperatively.

Ametropia

Retrospective studies[23–24] have shown that there is a tendency toward an increased incidence of severe proliferative vitreoretinopathy in aphakic retinal detachments. In the author's own experience,[25] the incidence of severe proliferative vitreoretinopathy after microsurgery was 11% in aphakic retinal detachments, as compared to 10% in myopic retinal detachments, and 5.4% in senile retinal detachments. However, statistical analysis showed that the differences in the incidence of severe proliferative vitreoretinopathy between the three groups was not significant.

It has also been reported that severe proliferative vitreoretinopathy was more frequent at initial examination in pseudophakic retinal detachment.[26] However, in the author's knowledge no statistical analysis as yet demonstrated that surgical failures due to severe proliferative vitreoretinopathy were more frequent in pseudophakic retinal detachment.

Clinical Characteristics of the Retinal Detachment and Associated Lesions

The clinical characteristics of retinal detachment and associated lesions at initial examination can be used to identify most eyes at risk of developing severe proliferative vitreoretinopathy postoperatively.

FAILURES OF PREVIOUS SURGERY

Retinal detachments that have already failed to reattach after one or several operation(s) are at a high risk for developing severe proliferative vitreoretinopathy after additional surgery for retinal reattachment.[2] In the author's own experience,[25] the incidence of failed surgery due to severe proliferative vitreoretinopathy after microsurgical management without vitrectomy was 19.5% in retinal detachments, which had already undergone unsuccessful surgery for retinal reattachment, as compared to 7.8% for retinal detachments managed by conventional microsurgery at the first operation. The difference between the two groups is statistically, highly significant.

In spite of their statistical value, those figures bring about no useful information of the actual causes for the higher incidence of severe proliferative vitreoretinopathy in retinal detachments that failed to reattach after a first operation. Indeed, two different causes may account for failure of the first operation(s): (1) inadequate surgical technique or intraoperative complications and (2) specific clinical characteristics of the retinal detachment at initial presentation.

RETINAL DETACHMENTS BEFORE ANY SURGICAL ATTEMPT TO REATTACH THE RETINA

The overall incidence of severe proliferative vitreoretinopathy in retinal detachments treated with conventional microsurgery at the first operation is approximately 8%.[25] However, the rate of severe proliferative vitreoretinopathy after microsurgery shows significant variations, depending on the clinical characteristics of the retinal detachment and associated lesions at initial presentation.

CLINICAL CHARACTERISTICS OF THE RETINAL DETACHMENT

Location and Extent of the Detachment. The location and extent of the retinal detachment at initial presentation do not determine the risk of severe proliferative vitreoretinopathy after surgery. This complication may develop in eyes with total retinal detachments as well as in eyes with limited and shallow detachments. Severe proliferative vitreoretinopathy has been observed after surgery for retinal detachments of the lower quadrants as well as detachments of the superior retina.

Demarcation Lines and Subretinal Proliferation. Demarcation lines and subretinal white strands at initial presentation are associated with a very low incidence of severe proliferative vitreoretinopathy after appropriate surgery for retinal reattachment. Indeed, the incidence of surgical failures related to severe proliferative vitreoretinopathy is significantly lower in retinal detachments with demarcation lines and subretinal strands (1.5%)[27] as compared to retinal detachments with no demarcation lines and cell proliferation in the subretinal space (6.9%).

Subretinal strands do not prevent the retina from settling on the pigment epithelium. Although subretinal white strands are secondary to pigment epithelium cell proliferation in the subretinal space,[4, 15] the process will no longer progress after retinal reattachment.

Demarcation lines and subretinal white strands indicate slow progression of the retinal detachment. Thus, retinal detachments that progress slowly are associated with a very low risk of severe proliferative vitreoretinopathy aftrer surgery for retinal reattachment. Therefore, the length of time a retina is detached before surgery is not, by itself, a determining factor in the development of severe proliferative vitreoretinopathy.

Preretinal Proliferation. Preoperative fixed retinal folds involving 1–3 quadrants of the retinal surface (grade C) at initial examination are a significant risk factor in the development of severe proliferative vitreoretinopathy postoperatively. In the author's experience,[25] the incidence of severe proliferative vitreoretinopathy after scleral buckling was 32.5% in retinal detachments with preoperative fixed retinal folds involving 1–3 quadrants, compared to 6% in retinal detachments without any full-thickness fixed folds. This clinical finding is not surprising. One would expect an increased incidence of severe proliferative vitreoretinopathy after scleral buckling when the process of preretinal membrane formation and contraction has already started before surgery. In this group of eyes, however, the surgeon should distinguish retinal detachments of recent onset from detachments of over 1 month's duration. When the retinal detachment is associated with full thickness retinal folds in less than two quadrants preoperatively, the risk of severe proliferative vitreoretinopathy after scleral buckling is significantly increased in eyes with retinal detachments of recent onset, compared to eyes with retinal detachments of over 1 month's duration. In the former group, early development of fixed retinal folds reflects a very active cellular process. In contrast, full thickness retinal folds that remain confined to less than two quadrants in retinal detachments of over 1 month's duration, indicate a rather slow and mild proliferative process, which may spontaneously subside after scleral buckling of retinal tear(s).

CLINICAL CHARACTERISTICS OF THE RETINAL BREAKS

Preretinal membrane formation and severe proliferative vitreoretinopathy is a complication specific of retinal detachments associated with horseshoe retinal tears.[25] In eyes operated on with microsurgical techniques, the incidence of preretinal membrane formation and severe proliferative vitreoretinopathy after scleral buckling is virtually nil in retinal detachments associated with oral dialysis, regardless of their sizes,[28] round atrophic holes in lattice[29] regardless of their number,[30] and macular holes in highly myopic eyes.[31] In contrast, the overall incidence of proliferative vitreoretinopathy after scleral buckling is nearly 11% in retinal detachments associated with horseshoe retinal tears.[25] The actual incidence of severe proliferative vitreoretinopathy after scleral buckling shows large variations depending on clinical characteristics of the horseshoe tears. The size, and the morphology of the posterior edge of the horseshoe tear are the two most important parameters to predicting the risk of severe proliferative vitreoretinopathy postoperatively.

Size of Horseshoe Retinal Tears. Severe proliferative vitreoretinopathy and failure to surgically reattach the retina are significantly more frequent in retinal detachments associated with large or giant retinal tears (see p. 209). The incidence of severe proliferative vitreoretinopathy increases with the size of the horseshoe retinal tears.[32] The incidence of severe proliferative vitreoretinopathy in eyes treated with cryo is 23% in retinal tears 70° to less than 90° in size, and 50% in retinal tears 90° to 180° and over.[32] There is a correlation, which is statistically, highly significant, between the surface of pigment epithelium cells exposed by horseshoe retinal tears and the incidence of severe proliferative vitreoretinopathy after surgery.[25] The incidence of severe proliferative vitreoretinopathy is 24% in retinal detachments associated with horseshoe retinal tears that expose a total surface of pigment epithelium cell of 3 disc diameters or more in size, compared to only 2.4% in retinal detachments with horseshoe retinal tears that expose a total surface of pigment epithelium cells less than 3 disc diameters in size.[33]

Posterior Edge of Horseshoe Retinal Tears. With regard to the morphology of their posterior edges, horseshoe retinal tears should be subdivided into two categories: (1) horseshoe retinal tears with mobile posterior edges and (2) horseshoe retinal tears with curled and fixed posterior edges (see p. 163).

Horseshoe retinal tears with curled and fixed posterior edges are observed in retinal detachments associated with proliferative vitreoretinopathy of any grade. They are a most conspicuous sign of proliferative vitreoretinopathy, grade B and may also be present in an eye with a retina that is still attached. Curled and fixed posterior edged retinal tears are a major predicting factor of impending proliferative vitreoretinopathy. In fact, they are the first clinical evidence of proliferative vitreoretinopathy. The rolled over posterior edge of the retinal tear is stuck to the underlying retina by a preretinal membrane, which may not yet be visible in any other part of the fundus. However, the proliferative process has already started.

The incidence of recurrent retinal detachment and active proliferative vitreoretinopathy after a single scleral buckling procedure is approximately 36% in eyes with curled and fixed posterior edged retinal tears, compared to only 2.5% in eyes with mobile posterior edged retinal tears.[34] The incidence of severe proliferative vitreoretinopathy after one or several scleral buckling procedure(s) is 20% in retinal detachments with curled and fixed posterior edged retinal tears. In contrast, the risk of severe proliferative vitreoretinopathy is virtually nil in retinal detachments with mobile posterior edged retinal tears.[34]

STATUS OF THE VITREOUS BODY

Vitreous Gel Liquefaction and Posterior Vitreous Detachment. The role of the degree and extent of vitreous gel liquefaction and posterior vitreous detachment in the development of severe proliferative vitreoretinopathy has not yet been fully studied. However, clinical experience suggests that vitreous changes associated with retinal detachment play a major role in the development of severe proliferative vitreoretinopathy. With regard to the associated vitreous changes, rhegmatogenous retinal detachments should be subdivided into two distinct groups: (1) retinal detachments assocated with normal or nearly normal vitreous gel and (2) retinal detachments associated with posterior vitreous detachment and/or extensive vitreous liquefaction.

Retinal detachments in eyes with no posterior vitreous detachment and no significant vitreous liquefaction include detachments associated with oral dialyses and detachments associated with round atrophic holes in lattice degeneration (see pp. 183 and 173). The risk of severe proliferative vitreoretinopathy after scleral buckling is virtually nil in such eyes. The absence of significant vitreous changes may account for the absence of severe proliferative vitreoretinopathy. In particular, severe proliferative vitreoretinopathy never develops after microsurgical management of large and giant dialyses at the ora serrata, although the dialyses most commonly, expose a very large surface of pigment epithelium cells. This is in striking contrast with what occurs in giant horseshoe retinal tears. Pigment epithelial cells exposed by giant dialysis at the ora serrata remain isolated from the vitreous cavity by the vitreous gel, which is adherent to the anterior and posterior edges of the dialysis. They cannot migrate towards the inner surface of the retina and vitreous cavity, thus, preretinal membranes cannot develop. In contrast, pigment epithelium cells can migrate into the subretinal space. Subretinal proliferation is a common finding in retinal detachments associated with oral dialysis. However, subretinal proliferation does not prevent the retina from being surgically reattached. Subretinal proliferation will subside after retinal reattachment.

Retinal detachments in eyes with significant vitreous gel liquefaction and posterior vitreous detachment include the vast majority of retinal detachments associated with horseshoe retinal tears. Severe proliferative vitreoretinopathy that develops in rhegmatogenous retinal detachment is a specific complication of detachments associated with horseshoe retinal tears. It can, therefore, be postulated that vitreous changes associated with horseshoe retinal tears should either induce the proliferative process, or at least create the requisite conditions for preretinal membrane formation. Findings of careful biomi-croscopic examination of the vitreous gel and posterior vitreous face suggest that incomplete posterior vitreous detachment with no collapse of the vitreous gel in eyes with horseshoe tears may be a determining risk factor in the development of severe proliferative vitreoretinopathy.[34]

Vitreous Hemorrhage. Experimental studies[9, 11] have shown that blood in the vitreous cavity can induce the formation of thick epiretinal membranes originating from glial retinal cells. Clinically, vitreous hemorrhage is associated with an increased incidence of severe proliferative vitreoretinopathy in retinal detachments associated with horseshoe retinal tears. The incidence of active proliferative vitreoretinopathy and failure to reattach the retina with a single scleral buckling procedure is 30% in retinal detachments associated with horseshoe retinal tears and preoperative vitreous hemorrhage.[34]

Surgical Trauma

Severe proliferative vitreretinopathy occurs most commonly after surgery for retinal detachment repair. It is particularly common when an initial retinal reattachment procedure fails and additional surgery is required.[2, 25]

Surgical trauma is likely a precipitating factor for the proliferative process in eyes with predisposing factors. The surgical trauma may also be a determining factor in eyes that show no predisposing factor preoperatively.

It would be of major importance for the retinal detachment surgeon to know which steps of the detachment surgeon to know which steps of the surgical procedures for retinal reattachment are the most likely to induce or precipitate the proliferative process. This knowledge would permit the surgeon to avoid use of certain surgical procedures in high risk eyes.

Any factors that may induce intraocular inflammation and breakdown of the blood ocular barrier may be a stimulus for cell proliferation and periretinal membrane formation.[35]

Cryotreatment may play a determining role in the development of proliferative vitreoretinopathy under specific conditions. Cryotreatment may induce breakdown of the blood ocular barrier with release of stimuli of cell proliferation and migration. In addition, cryotherapy enhances dispersion of viable pigment epithelium cells into the vitreous cavity.[36] Retinal pigment epithelial cells are a major component of the cellular membranes in proliferative vitreoretinopathy.[4,8,10,37]

Any surgical trauma that induces choroidal detachment may play a role in the development of proliferative vitreoretinopathy. Indeed, choroidal detachment is associated with a breakdown of the blood ocular barrier and release of stimuli of cell proliferation.[35]

Surgical trauma of the vitreous gel may also play a role in the development of postoperative proliferative vitreoretinopathy. Vitreous hemorrhage can induce glial cell migration onto the retina.[9, 11] The role of intravitreal gas injection in proliferative vitreoretinopathy has been questioned,[38] but it remains uncertain. Cell proliferation induced by intravitreal gas has not been demonstrated. Vitrectomy performed in eyes with retinal detachments associated with normal viscous vitreous gel and no posterior vitreous detachment may result in severe proliferative vitreoretinopathy.[28]

Intraoperative complications, such as choroidal hemorrhage, retinal incarceration, and vitreous gel incarceration may play a role in the development of severe proliferative vitreoretinopathy. They are often observed in retinal detachments that failed to reattach after initial operation, and which developed proliferative vitreoretinopathy. However, the role of these complications in the proliferative process has not been demonstrated.

CLINICAL FINDINGS

Four clinical classifications of proliferative vitreoretinopathy have been reported.[1,39–41] At present, the classification established by the retina society terminology committee is the most widely accepted by retina and vitreous surgeons. This classification distinguishes four grades of increasing severity: grade A or minimal, grade B or moderate, grade C or marked, and grade D or massive.

The retina society classification has the advantage of being schematic and easily applicable to clinical practice. It permits uniform evaluation of similar cases and facilitates proper comparison of results achieved with various treatment approaches. However, some additional features should be taken into account in clinical evaluation of any retinal detachment with proliferative vitreoretinopathy.

Grade A

Grade A, or minimal proliferative vitreoretinopathy was not clearly defined by the retina society terminology committee. Pigment clumps in the vitreous gel and vitreous haze were the two clinical features given by the retina society to define this stage. The findings, however, are not specific of proliferative vitreo-

retinopathy. In particular, they are most common in longstanding retinal detachments. Clusters of pigment cells on the retinal surface, rather than pigment clumps in the vitreous gel are the major clinical feature of impending proliferative vitreoretinopathy. They indicate that pigment epithelium cells have already migrated onto the inner surface of the retina and begin to form epiretinal membranes.[4] Clusters of pigment cells are most commonly found in the lower midperiphery of the fundus. Numerous clusters of pigment cells are often present in the same area. They are commonly located in the close vicinity of retinal vessels. Clusters of pigment cells may also be located in front of the optic disc.

Marked vitreous liquefaction with condensation and haziness of the anterior vitreous gel and vitreous base, as well as incomplete posterior vitreous detachment with no collapse of the vitreous gel are common biomicroscopic features in such eyes.

Grade B

Grade B, or moderate proliferative vitreoretinopathy, is defined by the presence of wrinkling of the inner retinal surface or the curled posterior edge of the retinal breaks. At this stage, preretinal membranes are already present. However, they are often not visible as such clinically. Their presence is indicated by secondary changes. The retina shows a pale gray color with irregular reflexes and wrinkling of the internal limiting membrane. The retina appears to be stiff in the involved area. It does not undulate after quick eye movements, although there are no full thickness fixed retinal folds. In the wrinkled retina the vessels exhibit marked tortuosity. Those changes usually begin in the retina posterior to the retinal tears. They may be very subtle and be missed by the surgeon.

The curled posterior edges of horseshoe retinal tears is the major clinical feature of proliferative vitreoretinopathy, grade B. In the author's clinical experience, this finding is always present at this stage.

Retinal tears with curled and fixed posterior edges most often expose areas of pigment epithelium significantly larger in size than the anterior retinal flaps. The discrepancy between the large surface of bare pigment epithelium and the small size of the anterior flap is indicative of incipient retraction of the preretinal membrane which sticks the curled tear edge and the underlying retina.

Grade C

Grade C, or marked proliferative vitreoretinopathy, is defined by the presence of full-thickness fixed

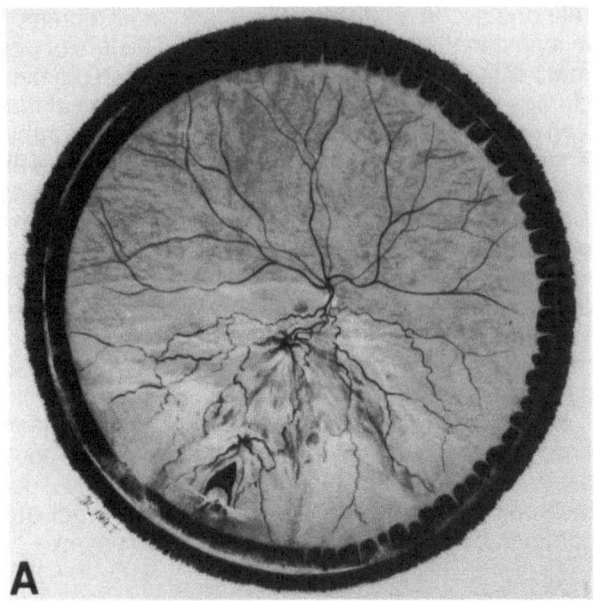
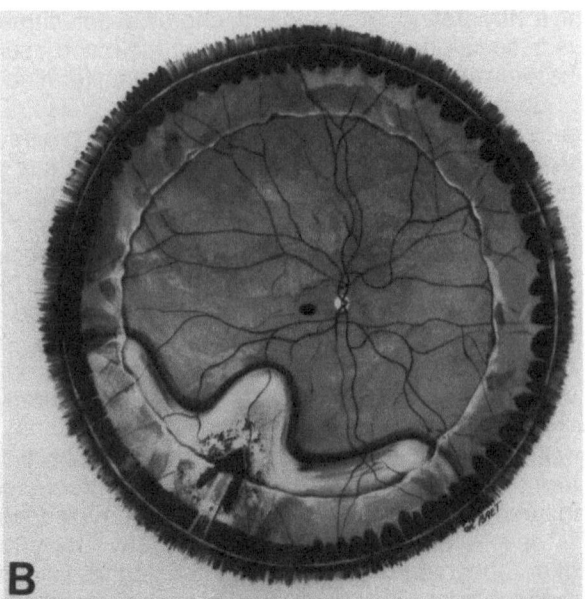

Figure 175. Retinal detachment complicated by proliferative vitreoretinopathy grade C1. (A) Fundus appearance at initial examination, four weeks after onset of visual symptoms. Two groups of star-shaped retinal folds are present on the meridian of the tear. Fixed retinal folds involve the posterior pole. (B) Fundus appearance six months postoperatively. Surgical management included pars plana vitrectomy, epiretinal membrane peeling on the posterior pole, epiretinal membrane segmentation in the midperiphery of the inferior fundus, high radial scleral buckling of the horse-shoe tear and segmental scleral buckling of the vitreous base.

retinal folds that involve up to nine clock hours of the retinal circumference. This grade is subdivided into 3 stages, Stage C1 is characterized by fixed folds involving up to three clock hours of the retinal circumference (Fig. 175). The clock hours may not be contiguous. Stage C2 includes retinal detachments with full thickness fixed folds involving up to six clock hours. Stage C3 is defined by full thickness fixed folds involving up to nine clock hours (Fig. 176).

In most cases, full thickness fixed retinal folds begin in the lower quadrants. They often remain more conspicuous in the inferior retina when the proliferative process involves three quadrants (Fig. 176).

Full thickness fixed retinal folds exhibit three major clinical aspects: (1) star-shaped folds, (2) irregular folds, and (3) circumferential folds.

Star-shaped folds are most often located in the midperiphery of the fundus. They converge towards a depressed center and are due to contraction of a preretinal membrane that covers the depressed center. The preretinal membrane is most often visible at biomicroscopic examination.

Irregular folds are most often located in the vicinity of the optic disc and the macular region. They usually are smaller in size than star-shaped folds. In most

cases they are numerous and pulled tightly together (Fig. 176). The retina looks crumpled up, thickened, and shows a pale gray color.

Circumferential full thickness folds are most conspicuous in grade D. However they may be already present in grade C. At this stage, there is a single circumferential fold involving only part of the eye circumference (Fig. 176). The circumferential fold is typically located at the posterior edge of the vitreous base. It is parallel to the ora serrata. The retina posterior to the circumferential fold exhibits star-shaped and irregular fixed folds. In contrast, the retina anterior to the circumferential fold shows a smooth, regular, surface. The circumferential fold is due to contraction of the vitreous base. Horseshoe retinal tears are often located at the posterior border of the circumferential fold (Fig. 176).

Full-thickness fixed retinal folds are associated with increased condensation and haziness of the vitreous gel and vitreous base.

Grade D

Grade D, or massive proliferative vitreoretinopathy, is defined by the presence of full thickness fixed

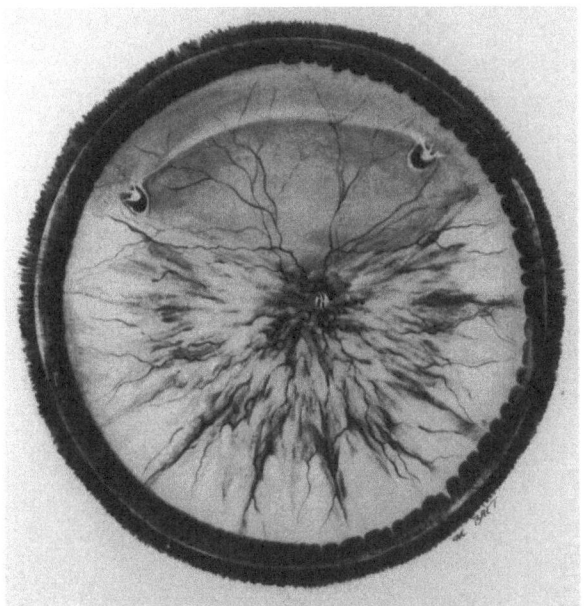

Figure 176. Rhegmatogenous retinal detachment complicated by proliferative vitreoretinopathy grade C2-C3 in a 60 year old emmetropic patient. Visual symptoms related to the detachment were neglected by the patient for two months. The retinal detachment is associated with two horse-shoe tears with a curled posterior edge, at the posterior border of the vitreous base. In spite of the superior site of the tears full thickness fixed retinal folds are more conspicuous in the inferior fundus. A circumferential fold is present in the superior fundus.

retinal folds in all four quadrants (Fig. 177). This results in a funnel-like configuration of the detached retina (Figs. 178,179). Grade D is subdivided into three stages according to the width of the funnel. Stage D1 is defined as a wide funnel, stage D2 as a narrow funnel, and stage D3 as a funnel that is so narrow, or closed, that the optic disc cannot be seen. Increasing contraction of preretinal membranes and vitreous body accounts for the decreasing width of the funnel.

Circumferential fixed folds are a common clinical feature in massive proliferative vitreoretinopathy. The most conspicuous circumferential fold is located at the posterior edge of the vitreous base. The retina peripheral to this fold is adherent to the vitreous base and remains flat, although it is detached (Fig. 177). With increasing contraction of the vitreous base, the peripheral circumferential fold gradually shrinks to form a smaller circle and moves toward the optical axis of the eye. The retina peripheral to the circumferential fold gradually moves anteriorly. In grade D3 the peripheral retina is in a frontal plane

(Fig. 179). The ciliary epithelium of the pars plana is also detached and pulled anteriorly. The detached ora serrata is identifed by a scalloped outline between the ciliary epithelium and the peripheral retina. Detachment of the ciliary epithelium results from ring contraction of the vitreous base. One or two additional circumferential fixed folds may be present in grade D1 and D2 which are posterior to the circumferential fold located at the posterior border of the vitreous base. Most often circumferential fixed folds are located in the midperiphery or in the vicinity of the temporal arcades, and they are superimposed onto radial folds. Although less conspicuous than the circumferential fold located at the posterior edge of the vitreous base, they are easily visible by biomicroscopic examination. The posterior concentric folds indicate that posterior vitreous detachment is incomplete. Circumferential adhesions remain between the radially folded retina and the posterior vitreous face (Fig. 177,179).

Associated Clinical Findings

Certain clinical features associated with proliferative vitreoretinopathy are of major importance for surgical management and evaluation of the prognosis. They include: (1) the life-cycle of the proliferative process, (2) the clinical characteristics of the retinal tears, (3) iatrogenic lesions induced by previous surgery, and (4) clinical findings indicative of a highly compromised eye trophicity.

LIFE-CYCLE OF THE PROLIFERATIVE PROCESS

The proliferative process may be gradual over months (Fig. 176) or it may be explosive, creating the full picture of a massive retinal retraction within a few days (Fig. 179). The full picture of massive proliferative vitreoretinopathy may even develop within hours, a few days or weeks after an uneventful, and apparently, successful operation for retinal detachment repair.

The prognosis for permanent retinal reattachment with a single operation is usually good when the proliferative process is very gradual. In contrast, the prognosis is more uncertain when the disease appears to be very active at initial examination. For example, the prognosis for permanent retinal reattachment with a single operation is most often good in proliferative vitreoretinopathy grade C1 associated with a retinal detachment of over one month duration. The slow natural course of the process probably accounts for the good surgical prognosis. In contrast, the prognosis for permanent retinal reattachment

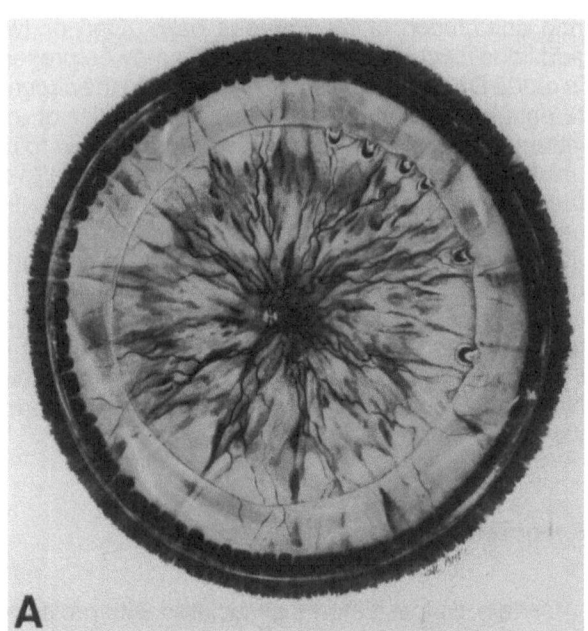

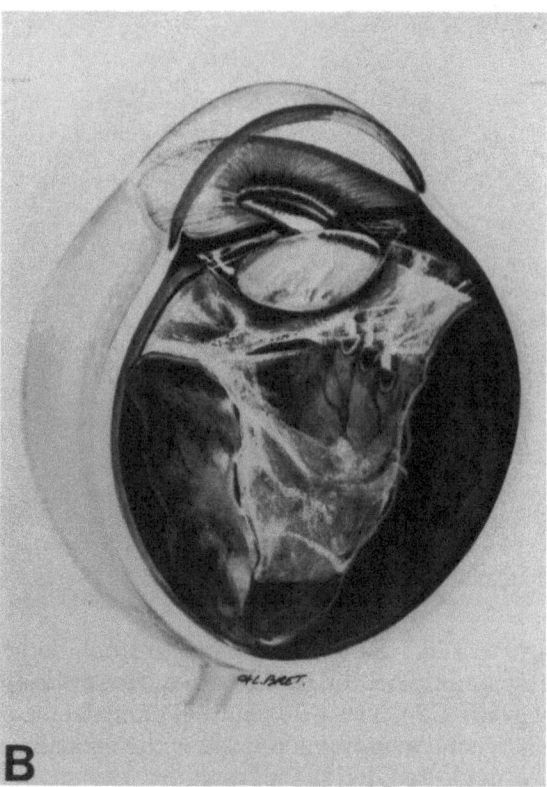

Figure 177. Rhegmatogenous retinal detachment complicated by proliferative vitreoretinopathy grade D1. (A) fundus appearance at initial presentation: Full thickness fixed retinal folds involve all four quadrants. A circumferential fold at the posterior border of the vitreous base runs on 360° of the eye circumference. The detachment is associated with 6 small horse-shoe tears at the posterior border of the vitreous base in the superior temporal quadrant. Tears show a curled posterior edge and their small anterior flap is dragged anteriorly by contraction of the vitreous base. (B) Cross-section of the same eye. The detached retina shows a funnel-like configuration. The funnel is wide. Vitreous changes include a large lacuna in the superior temporal quadrant, incomplete posterior vitreous detachment, condensation and contraction of the vitreous base.

with a single operation is usually more uncertain in retinal detachments of recent onset which are already associated with full thickness fixed folds or even merely retinal tears with curled posterior edges. Clinical evidence of proliferative vitreoretinopathy in recent rhegmatogenous retinal detachment is indicative of active disease. In such eyes there is a high risk that the surgical trauma stimulates the proliferative process and results in the full picture of early massive proliferative vitreoretinopathy after scleral buckling, or recurrent preretinal membranes after vitrectomy.

CLINICAL CHARACTERISTICS OF THE RETINAL TEARS

The absence of open retinal tears in eyes previously operated on with scleral buckling indicates a

rather good prognosis.[18] However such cases are infrequent. In most cases proliferative vitreoretinopathy is associated with open retinal tears. In severe proliferative vitreoretinopathy, mainly in grades D2 and D3, the retinal tears may be hidden by fixed retinal folds and contraction of the retina (Fig. 179). However the retinal tears will be found during vitrectomy. The prognosis is more severe when the proliferative disease is associated with giant tears.

In eyes that developed proliferative vitreoretinopathy after surgery for retinal reattachment, two groups of retinal tears may be observed: (1) primary retinal tears and (2) secondary retinal tears.

Primary retinal tears are those that were present, and usually treated, at the initial operation and most commonly located in the peripheral retina and equatorial region. After appropriate treatment at the initial operation, they may remain sealed in spite of the proliferative process (Fig. 180). Primary retinal tears

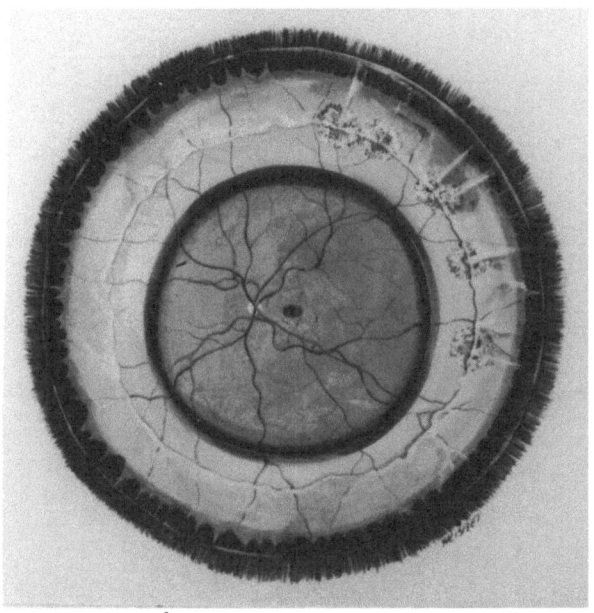

Figure 178. Retinal detachment complicated by proliferative vitreoretinopathy grade D1 6 months after surgical repair. Surgical management included vitrectomy, epiretinal membrane dissection, cryotreatment of the retinal tears, broad and high scleral buckling of the tears and the vitreous base, and retinal tamponade with C3F8.

may also reopen under tangential traction exerted by preretinal membrane contraction and anterior traction of the vitreous gel. Reopening of retinal tears, which were adequately sealed, is indicative of severe proliferative disease. Reopening of the retinal tears may be associated with enlargement of the retinal tear size. It results from severe contraction of the preretinal membranes. It is a sign of rather poor prognosis. In extreme conditions small horseshoe retinal tears may transform into very large tears extending very posteriorly.

Secondary retinal tears are those that were not present when the retinal detachment was operated on the first time. Sequential retinal tears are likely related to the proliferative process itself. With regard to their location and shape, secondary retinal tears should be subdivided into two distinct categories: (1) horseshoe retinal tears at the posterior edge of the vitreous base and (2) retinal tears posterior to the equator.

Secondary horseshoe retinal tears that develop at the posterior edge of the vitreous base are the most common type (Fig. 180). They occur in areas where the retina was usually normal and flat before the first operation. In most cases they are rather small and multiple, contiguous in the same retinal quadrant, or may involve two or more quadrants. The anterior flap is small and under traction of the

vitreous base, and the posterior edge is curled and fixed.

Secondary retinal tears that develop posteriorly to the equator also occur in areas where the retina was preoperatively normal. They exhibit two different aspects: (1) tiny horseshoe tears located in the midperiphery and (2) slit-like paravascular retinal tears. Secondary retinal tears located posteriorly to the equator are much more common in the lower quadrants than in the upper retina.

The presence of secondary retinal tears does not seem to modify the surgical prognosis, provided all retinal tears are identified and adequately treated.

IATROGENIC LESIONS DUE TO PREVIOUS SURGERY

Iatrogenic lesions secondary to previous surgery are most common in retinal detachments associated with proliferative vitreoretinopathy. They include extensive chorioretinal atrophy secondary to cryo or laser treatment, scleral erosion, buckle intrusion into the subretinal space, vitreous or retinal incarceration at the sites of subretinal fluid drainage or the entry sites of pars plana vitrectomy, choroidal and vitreous hemorrhages, silicone oil in the subretinal space, iatrogenic retinal tears, and open retinotomies.

Most iatrogenic lesions secondary to scleral buckling procedures do not interfere directly with the prognosis. However, their presence, which may be recognized only at surgery, will make the surgical procedure much more complex and lengthy.

In contrast, certain iatrogenic lesions resulting from previous vitreous surgery are a contraindication to further surgery because they leave no hope of restoring any vision. Such is the case, in particular, of the presence of silicone oil in the subretinal space and large iatrogenic retinal tears involving the posterior pole, large retinotomies, or retinectomies with the entire retina retracted in a small area of the fundus.

CLINICAL FINDINGS INDICATIVE OF HIGHLY COMPROMISED EYE TROPHICITY

Specific clinical findings are indicative of highly compromised eye trophicity and very poor surgical prognosis. They are common in eyes that have already undergone several failed operations, including vitrectomy, for retinal reattachment. Most often such eyes exhibit proliferative vitreoretinopathy, grade D2 or D3. Certain clinical findings indicate that there is virtually no hope to reattach the retina or restore any useful vision.

No light perception is an absolute contraindication

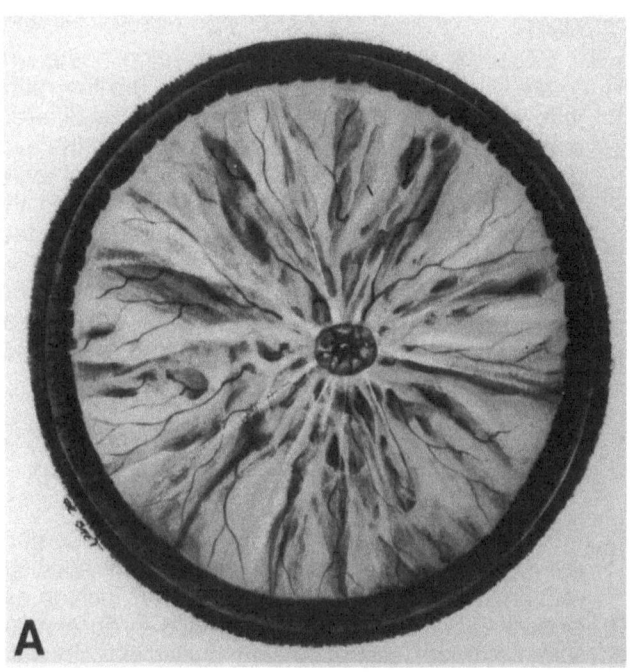
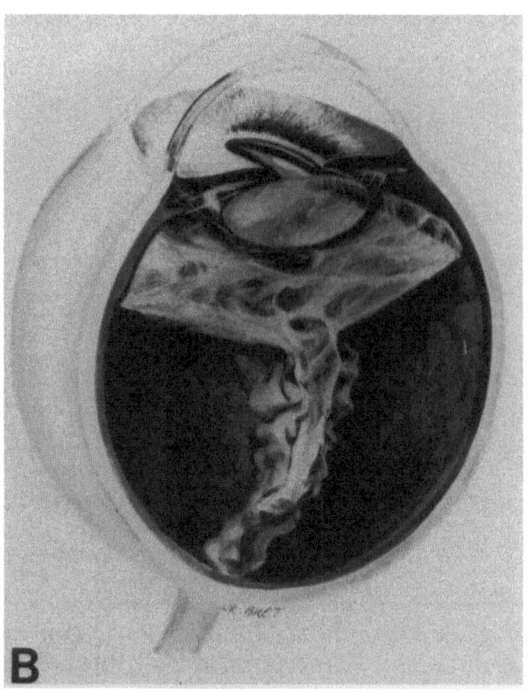

Figure 179. Rhegmatogenous retinal detachment complicated by proliferative vitreoretinopathy grade D3 in a 20-year-old myopic patient. (A) Fundus appearance at initial examination, two weeks after onset of visual symptoms. The funnel is so narrow that the optic disc is hardly visible. The retinal detachment was associated with a single retinal tear in the superior nasal quadrant. The tear was hidden by fixed retinal folds. It was found during vitrectomy. (B) Cross-section of the same eye. The funnel is nearly closed. Posterior vitreous detachment is incomplete. The peripheral retina is in a frontal plane.

to surgery. In contrast, poor light localization is not by itself a contraindication to surgery in specific cases. Electroretinography is of no value in predicting visual outcome after surgery. The electroretinogram is most often nonrecordable in eyes with total retinal detachment. Therefore, a nonrecordable electroretinogram is not, per se, a contraindication to surgery. Careful clinical evaluation of light perception and localization remains the most relevant test of visual function in eyes with total retinal detachment and proliferative vitreoretinopathy.

Iris neovascularization and ectropion uvea may be associated with severe proliferative vitreoretinopathy, most often associated with fibrous proliferation on the vitreous base and ciliary body. These symptoms indicate the end-stage of the disease. They are a contraindication to surgery, regardless of associated clinical findings.

Extensive choroidal detachment is not a contraindication to surgery, however, the surgical prognosis is poor in most cases. Measurement of the choroidal thickness on the posterior pole with A-scan ultrasonography provides useful information on the postoperative anatomic outcome. Increase in the

choroidal thickness over 3 mm is indicative of a poor surgical prognosis.

TREATMENT

Indications for Surgery

Unless there are associated systemic or a local contraindication to surgery, all eyes with proliferative vitreoretinopathy, grade C or D1 should be operated on since permanent retinal reattachment with recovery of useful vision can be expected in approximately 75% of patients.[19,20]

In contrast, indications for surgery may be more questionnable in grades D2 and D3; the anatomical success rate remains low in spite of improved microsurgical techniques, and the visual results are uniformly poor. There is an indication for surgical treatment in all patients with no useful vision of the fellow eye, provided light perception is present. In patients

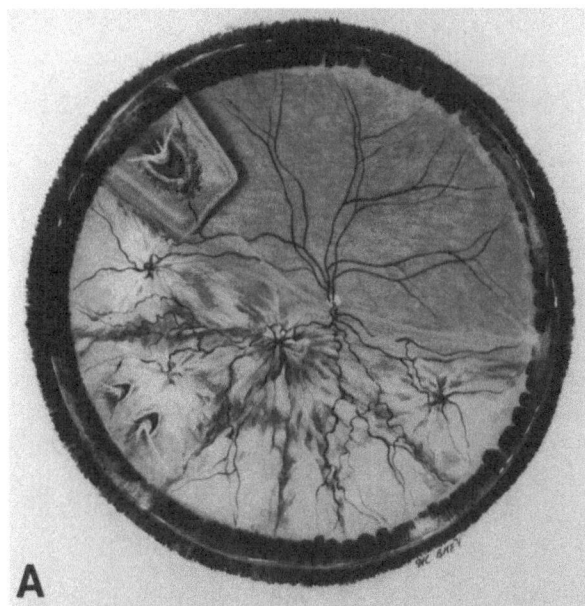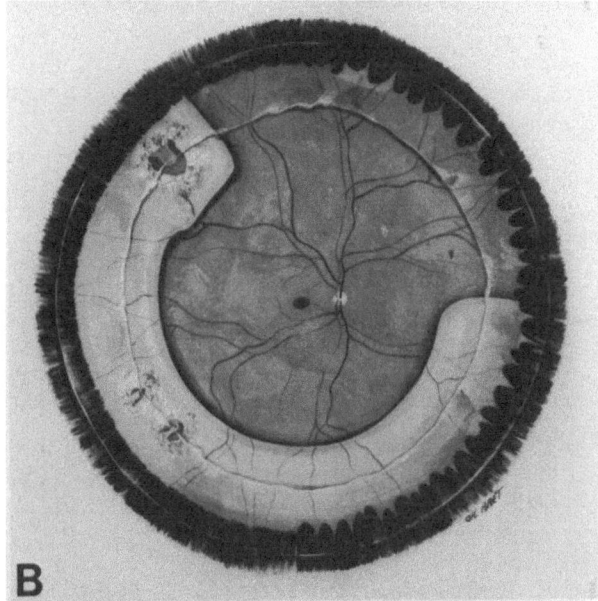

Figure 180. Recurrent retinal detachment complicated by proliferative vitreoretinopathy grade C2 in a 62 year old emmetropic patient. (A) The initial retinal tear in the superior temporal quadrant has been sealed by a segmental radial buckling procedure. Its posterior edge was curled and fixed at initial presentation. Recurrent detachment occurred five weeks postoperatively. It is associated with two sequential tears with a curled posterior edge in the inferior temporal quadrant. (B) Fundus appearance six months after reoperation. Surgical management included vitrectomy, epiretinal membrane dissection, cryotreatment of the sequential tears, segmental scleral buckling of the retinal tears, and the vitreous base in the inferior quadrants, and retinal tamponade with C3F8.

with useful vision of the fellow eye indications for surgery should be limited to the young or highly motivated patients.

Surgical Management

The surgical procedure includes four steps in most cases: (1) vitrectomy, (2) treatment of the retinal break(s), (3) scleral buckling of the vitreous base and (4) intravitreal gas injection (Figs. 181 and 182). Subretinal fluid drainage is carried out in a few eyes.

VITREOUS SURGERY

The goal of vitreous surgery in proliferative vitreoretinopathy is to relieve most of the anteroposterior and tangential tractions exerted on the retina by the altered vitreous body and epiretinal membranes. Closed vitrectomy was first introduced in the management of proliferative vitreoretinopathy by Machemer in 1973.[42] However, the initial results were disappointing. Then, the development of microsurgical techniques to dissect epiretinal membranes brought about significant improvement in the surgical results.[43–45] The goal of vitreous surgery is purely mechanical. Vitreoretinal tractions are relieved to allow retinal apposition on the pigment epithelium. Surgical relief of traction should be achieved with minimal trauma to minimize stimuli for reproliferation.

Indications for Vitreous Surgery. Several years ago the indications for vitreous surgery in proliferative vitreoretinopathy were tied to the most severe cases in eyes that could not be salvaged with scleral buckling. Most of those eyes were unsuccessfully managed with conventional techniques before an indication for vitrectomy could be considered. Today vitreous surgery is no longer reserved as a last resort. There is general agreement among retinal detachment surgeons that vitrectomy must be used as a primary procedure in retinal detachments associated with severe proliferative vitreoretinopathy. A question, however, still remains debated: should vitreous surgery be used as a primary procedure in the initial and less severe stages of proliferative vitreoretinopathy? In grade C1, high success rates have been achieved with scleral buckling,[46,47] but

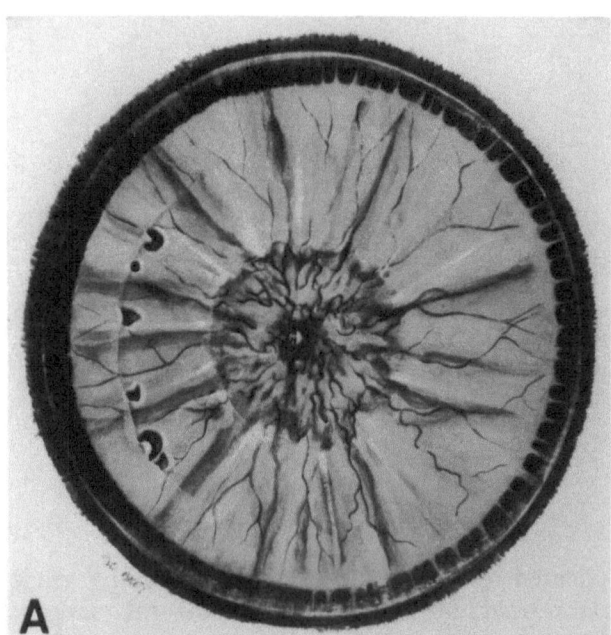 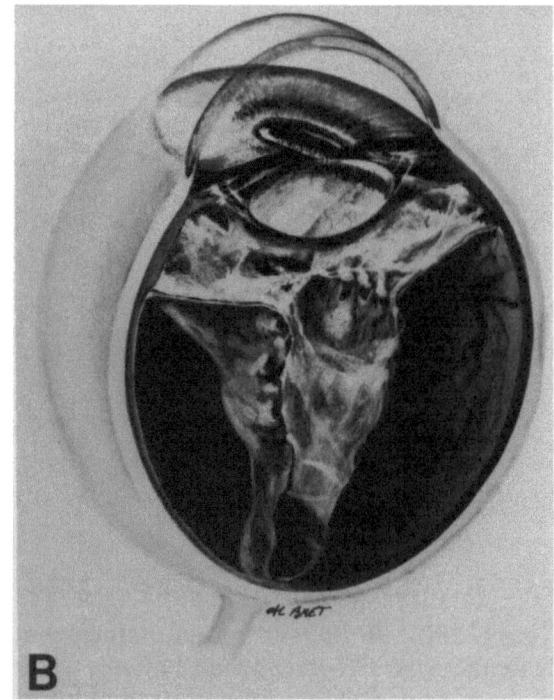

Figure 181. Rhegmatogenous retinal detachment complicated by severe proliferative vitreoretinopathy—grade D2—Preoperative findings (left eye). (A) Fundus appearance at initial examination. (B) Cross-section of the vitreous cavity.

poor results after vitrectomy have been published.[24] Indeed, the indications for vitrectomy or scleral buckling alone in grade C1 should be based on three parameters: (1) the life cycle of the proliferative process, (2) the extent of posterior vitreous detachment, and (3) the presence or absence of epiretinal membrane on the posterior pole.

Full thickness fixed retinal folds involving only one quadrant of the peripheral retina in eyes with retinal detachments of over 1 month's duration are associated with a slightly active proliferative process, which should spontaneously subside after sealing of the retinal break. Scleral buckling alone is probably the procedure of choice for the treatment of such eyes, when there is a complete posterior vitreous detachment and no epiretinal membrane on the posterior pole. In contrast, vitreous surgery should be used as a primary procedure in eyes with recent onset retinal detachments that are already associated with full thickness fixed folds in one quadrant. This clinical picture is indicative of active proliferative disease that will continue to evolve after scleral buckling. There is a high risk that a full picture of explosive severe proliferative vitreoretinopathy may develop in the early postoperative course after scleral buckling alone, especially when posterior vitreous detachment is incomplete. Vitrectomy is also indicated when the macula is involved by epiretinal mem-

branes, regardless of the life-cycle of the proliferative process. Indeed, the visual results obtained with scleral buckling alone are very poor in such cases. Removal of epiretinal membranes on the posterior pole is necessary to obtain visual improvement. Epiretinal membrane peeling can be done as a second operation after retinal reattachment with scleral buckling alone. However, the success rate is not improved by the two-step surgical management. Therefore, the author performs the scleral buckling operation and epiretinal membrane removal in a single step procedure. This is more advantageous in terms of a patient's comfort and health cost.

The high incidence of failed surgery and active proliferative vitreoretinopathy after scleral buckling in retinal detachments with curled and fixed posterior edged retinal tears, grade B, (see p. 233) raises the question of the potential value of vitrectomy at the initial operation in such eyes. Prospective clinical studies are still required to evaluate the advantages and hazards of early vitreous surgery in this indication.

Timing of Surgery. It has been postulated that delayed surgery might be advantageous in proliferative vitreoretinopathy. If the cellular process has run its course, the recurrences after surgery might be less frequent, however, this hypothesis has not been

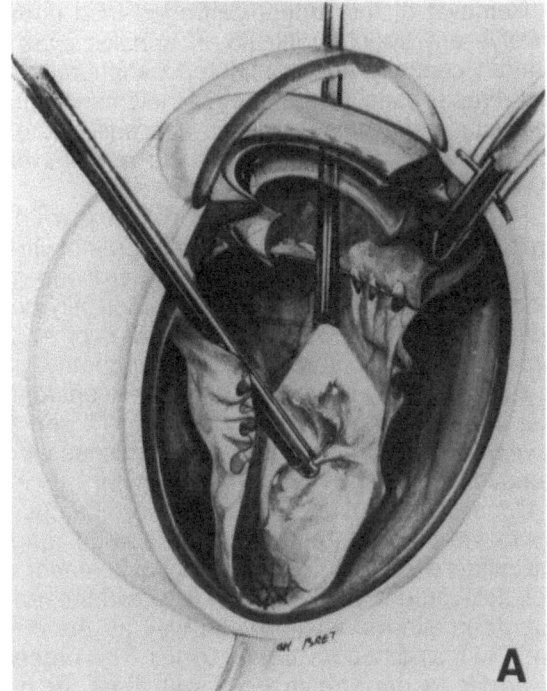

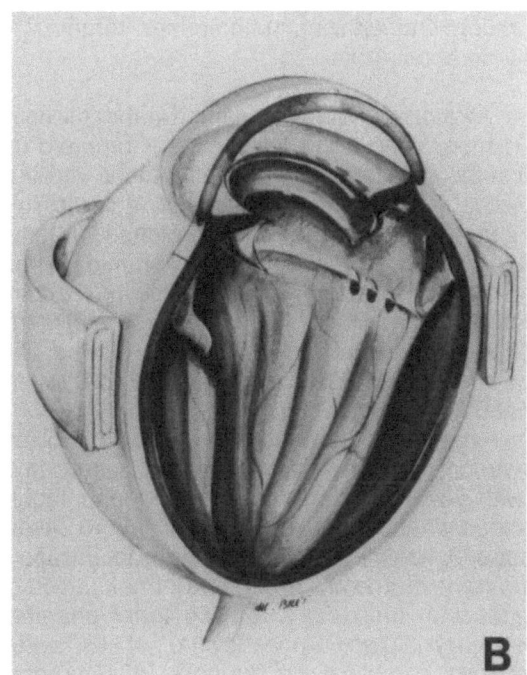

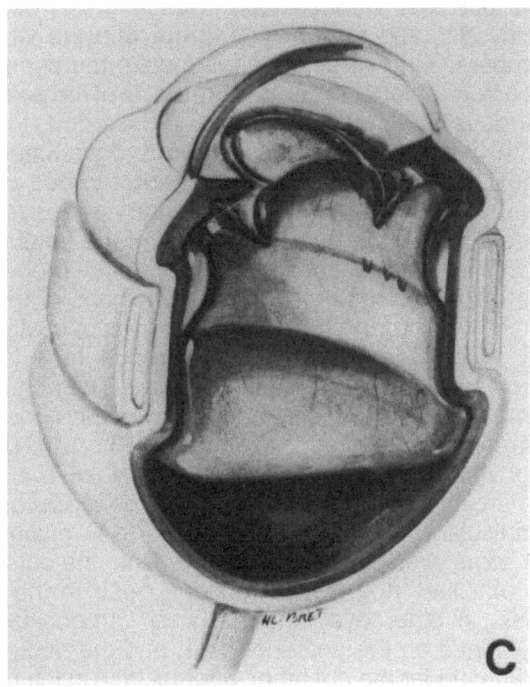

Figure 182. Surgical management of case shown in Figure 181. The surgical procedure included: (A) Lens removal, vitreous gel removal and epiretinal membrane dissection. (B) Broad and high scleral buckling of peripheral retinal tears and the vitreous base. (C) Retinal tamponade with a long-lasting gas.

confirmed.[18] Whenever possible, the author operates early, because delay may make the case worse. In addition, the longer a retina has been detached, the worse the visual results. A short period of time is used, however, for medical preparation to minimize postoperative inflammation and cell proliferation (see p. 251).

Surgical Technique. The two instrument technique is used. Remote control of linear aspiration is particularly helpful in such eyes.

The vitrectomy procedure includes two consecutive steps in all cases: (1) vitreous body removal and (2) epiretinal membrane dissection. Lens removal should also be considered in selected cases.

The clinical value of a surgical approach to subretinal proliferation and relaxing retinotomies remains to be fully demonstrated.

Lens Removal. Surgical work at the vitreous base is more difficult in phakic eyes. Complete removal of the anterior vitreous face up to the vitreous base without damaging the posterior lens capsule may be most difficult in eyes with condensed anterior vitreous gel. Therefore, lens removal should be performed before vitrectomy in the following circumstances: (1) when there is marked contraction of the vitreous base and radial cuts are planed and (2) when the anterior vitreous gel is highly condensed with bands in a frontal plane.

Lens removal is performed in all eyes with proliferative vitreoretinopathy grade D2 and D3 and most eyes with grade D1. Removal of a clear lens should be avoided whenever possible in less severe cases.

In pseudophakic eyes, the indications for intraocular lens removal mainly depends on the location of the intraocular lens. As a rule posterior chamber lenses are left in place, since they are not associated with specific complications during or after surgery for proliferative vitreoretinopathy management. In contrast, anterior chamber lenses are removed when a large bubble of expanded gas is planed for retinal tamponade. Retinal tamponade with a large bubble of gas involves a high risk of pupillary block and lens-corneal endothelium touch, when the patient is not in a strictly prone position. The indications for removal of pupillary supported lenses depend more on associated lesions than the intraocular lens itself, although the lens creates specific difficulties in posterior segment observation and participates to stimulate intraocular inflammation. The intraocular lens is removed in eyes with too poor a pupillary dilatation so as to obtain a clear view of the entire posterior segment. The intraocular lens is also removed in eyes with a dense cyclitic membrane or heavy precipitates on the lens.

Vitreous Body Removal. Vitreous body removal in proliferative vitreoretinopathy must include three consecutive steps: (1) removal of the anterior vitreous face, (2) removal of the vitreous gel, and (3) removal or segmentation of the posterior vitreous face. The technical ease or complexity of the procedure depends on the specific vitreoretinal anatomy of any given case. It can be predicted preoperatively by thorough biomicroscopic examination of the vitreous body and vitreoretinal relationship rather than the extent of star-shaped folds. There is a wide range of variation in the vitreous body status and relationship of the posterior vitreous face with the retina in eyes showing the same extent of fixed retinal folds. These variations are observed in all grades of proliferative vitreoretinopathy.

Removal of the anterior vitreous face does not involve any special difficulty in aphakic eyes. It is started centrally and completed peripherally up to the vitreous base. In phakic eyes the anterior vitreous face can be removed with no damage to the lens capsule when the anterior hyaloid remains elastic (see p. 141).

Removal of the vitreous gel will take a varying amount of time depending on the degree of vitreous gel liquefaction. In some eyes the vitreous gel is extensively liquefied and there is practically no viscous vitreous to be removed, whereas in other eyes, with the same proliferative vitreoretinopathy grade, the vitreous body is densely viscous except for lacunae in front of the retinal tears (Fig. 177 and 181). A very low suction force is used for viscous vitreous removal to prevent vitreoretinal traction.

Complete removal of the posterior vitreous face up to the vitreous base involves a wide range of difficulties depending on the extent of posterior vitreous detachment, strength, and extent of the remaining vitreoretinal adhesions, as well as the consistency of the posterior vitreous cortex. This procedure is easier to perform in eyes with total, or nearly total, posterior vitreous detachment. In such eyes the posterior vitreous face is usually well defined, fairly stiff, and rather easy to cut with the vitreous probe. During vitrectomy it is most often orientated in a frontal plane. In contrast, removal of the posterior vitreous face may be difficult and hazardous in eyes with incomplete posterior vitreous detachment. In most of these eyes, the posterior vitreous cortex remains viscous, and the posterior vitreous face is poorly defined in numerous parts of the fundus. Direct suction and section with the vitreous probe may be quite hazardous, owing to adhesions of the detached retina and to the posterior viscous vitreous. In such eyes the posterior vitreous face is approached with the hooked fiber optic. The angulated portion of the pipe is inserted between the posterior vitreous face and retina at any place where the posterior vitreous face is detached and visible. The place where the hook can be inserted depends on the particular vitreoretinal anatomy of any given eye. In some eyes the hook is inserted into the detached prepapillary ring, which remains close to the optic disc. In other eyes the posterior vitreous face is detached on the posterior pole, and the hook is inserted under the posterior vitreous face in the region of the temporal arcades. Then, the posterior vitreous face is gently lifted and separated from the underlying retina with a side-to-side motion of the instrument tip. Dissection is carried out from the posterior pole towards the periphery. In less complex cases, the adhesions between the posterior vitreous face and retina are weak, and the thin translucid layer of posterior vitreous is lifted in almost one piece up to the posterior edge of the vitreous base. In the more

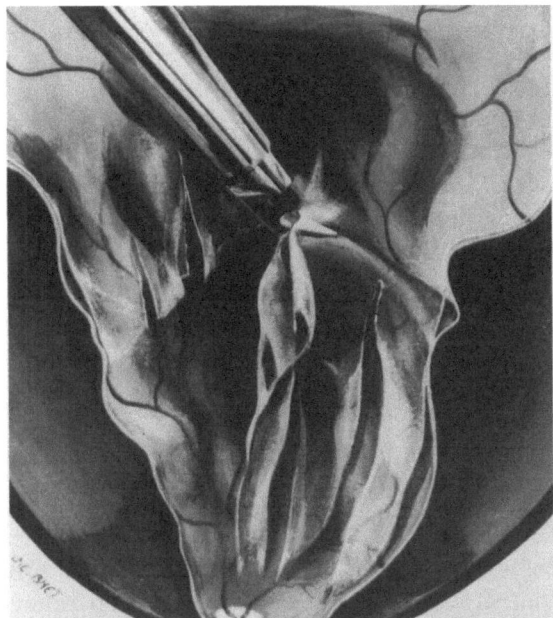

Figure 183. Segmentation of the posterior vitreous face in eyes with incomplete posterior vitreous detachment and firm vitreoretinal adhesions.

difficult cases, there are numerous bridges of strong retinochoroidal adhesions. The adhesions are most often found along large retinal vessels, posterior circumferential folds, and tops of radial retinal folds. The adhesions may be so strong that attempts to free them would result in serious damage to the inner layers of the retina or even iatrogenic full thickness retinal breaks. In such eyes the posterior vitreous face is not removed. It is only cut wherever this can safely be done. Automated scissors are used for this purpose. Radial cuts are done in front of deep valleys between radial retinal folds, and at the posterior edge of circumferential folds (Fig. 183), dissection is carried out from the posterior pole towards the periphery. It is done in each retinal quadrant. Cutting of the posterior vitreous face with scissors may be difficult when a thick layer of viscous vitreous cortex remains in place. The posterior edge of the vitreous base marks the anterior limit of posterior vitreous face dissection. Its location shows variations depending mainly on the patient's age.[48]

In severe proliferative vitreoretinopathy, ring contraction of the condensed vitreous base is common. Whenever possible, radial cuts using automated scissors are made to relax the ring contraction.

Epiretinal Membrane Dissection. Membrane peeling and membrane segmentation are the two techniques used for epiretinal membrane dissection.

Membrane peeling may involve a higher risk of damage to the inner layers of the retina and recurrent cell proliferation than membrane segmentation. Therefore, membrane peeling is used mainly on the posterior pole where complete removal of epiretinal membranes is necessary for improved visual results. Scissors-segmentation is used for epiretinal membranes located outside the temporal arcades. It is sufficient to allow retinal reattachment.

Various instruments have been developed to dissect epiretinal membranes including hooked fiber optic pipes, hooked needles, vitreoretinal pics,[45] spatulas,[49] forceps,[21] and pic-forceps.[50] All instruments have advantages and limitations. Instrument choice varies with the surgeon. Any instrument designed for this purpose can be used except for a bent 20-gauge sharp needle. A sharp needle must not be used for epiretinal membrane peeling owing to the risk of puncturing the retina with the sharp tip, or lacerating the retina with the sharp edge of the needle.

The author uses three instruments for epiretinal membrane dissection: (1) a hooked fiber optic probe, (2) right angulated automated scissors, and (3) a suction fiber optic probe connected to linear aspiration.

The tip of the hooked fiber optic probe is blunt and thin. Its upper surface is flat. It is easily inserted under epiretinal membranes with low risk of retinal damage. The fiber optic provides retroillumination of the engaged membrane. The hooked fiber optic is used for membrane peeling and to create tunnels between fixed folds. The scissors are used to cut membranes after peeling or delamination. The suction fiber optic probe is used to lift and hold the free edge of a membrane during delamination and scissors-segmentation.

Membrane peeling on the posterior pole is performed with the hooked fiber optic probe (Figs. 184 and 185). The tip of the probe is inserted under the membrane at a point where an edge is visible. The membrane is gently elevated and peeled from the retina with side-to-side motions. Peeling is carried out in a centrifugal direction. When membrane peeling on the posterior pole is completed, the free edge of the membrane is held with the suction fiber otpic probe while the membrane is cut with the scissors along its remaining adhesions to the retina. No attempt is made to peel off peripheral extensions of the epiretinal membrane. In particular, epiretinal membranes located in the temporal midperiphery are not peeled off. In most eyes adhesion to the underlying retina is quite strong, and membrane peeling would involve a high risk of damaging the internal limiting membrane or creating a iatrogenic retinal break.

Membrane segmentation is performed wherever there are full thickness fixed retinal folds, from the temporal arcades to the posterior edge of the vitre-

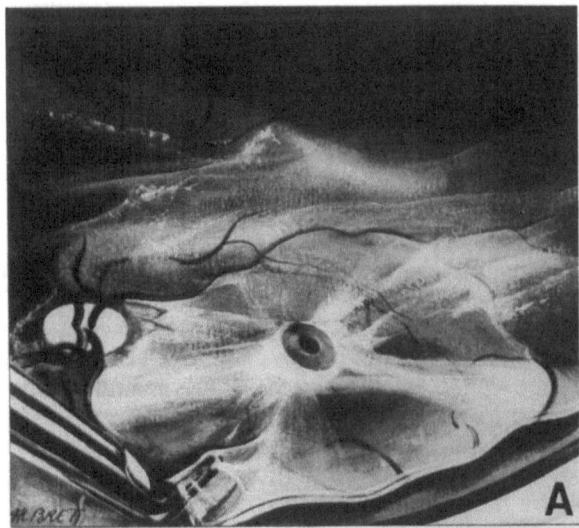
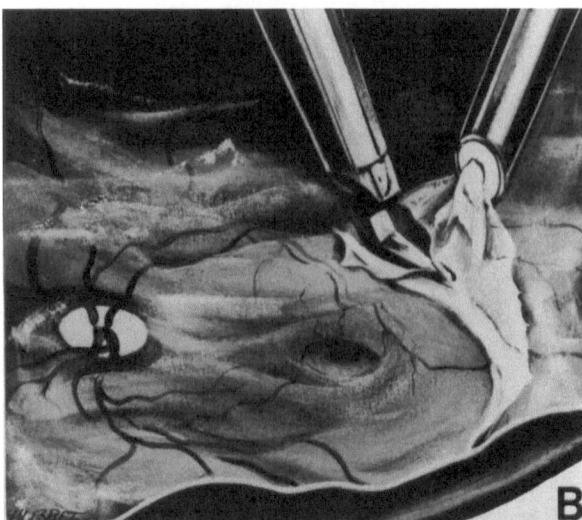

Figure 184. Epiretinal membrane removal on the posterior pole. (A) The hooked fiberoptic probe is used to peel the membrane from the retina. (B) When traction on the macula has been relieved by membrane peeling, the membrane is cut along firm vitreoretinal adhesion using automatic scissors. The cut edge of the membrane is held using the suction fiberoptic probe.

ous base. Membrane segmentation is performed between large radial retinal folds and star-shaped folds (Figs. 186 and 187). Visibility of epiretinal membranes greatly varies, depending on the duration of the proliferative process. Recent onset membranes are most often thin and transparent. Clumps of pigmented cells may help to identify them. They are most easily identified between large radial retinal folds. The bent tip of the fiberoptic probe is inserted posteriorly into the valley between two radial folds. Retroillumination provided by the fiberoptic increases visibility of the membrane bridging the retinal folds. The hooked probe is gently elevated and moved towards the periphery. Because the membrane is thin, it is most often torn off by the gentle centrifugal motion of the probe. Use of scissors to cut the membrane is unnecessary. In contrast, long duration membranes are most often thick and opaque and are of a white grey color, and are easily identified. Long duration membranes are delaminated and cut with automated scissors between radial and star-shaped folds. Marked space can develop between the cut edges of the membrane as a result of the released elasticity of the membrane.

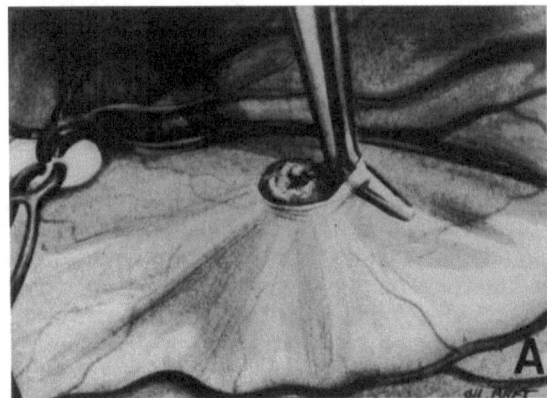
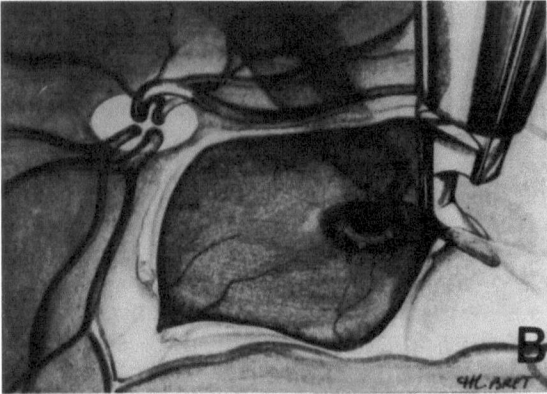

Figure 185. Epiretinal membrane dissection on the posterior pole. (A) In a few cases a thick membrane firmly adherent to the temporal arcades shows an edge around the macula. The perimacular edge is used to lift the membrane. (B) Scissors are used to make radial cuts in the membrane which retracts toward the sites of firm attachment along the temporal vessels.

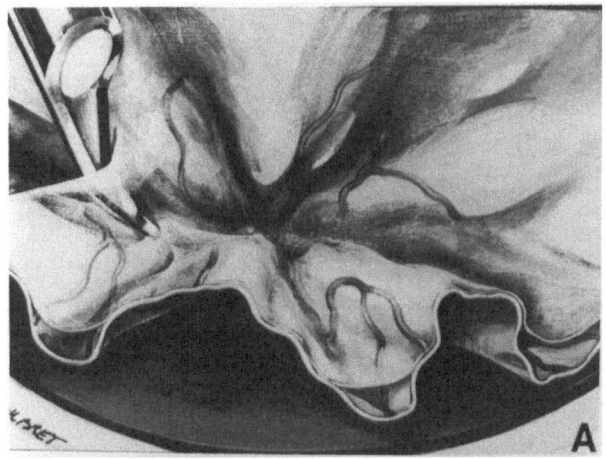
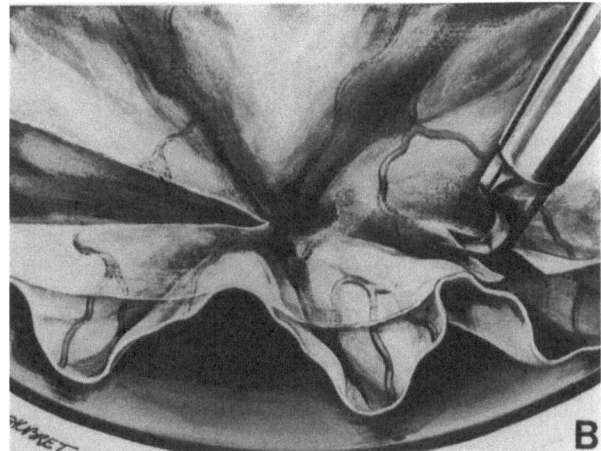
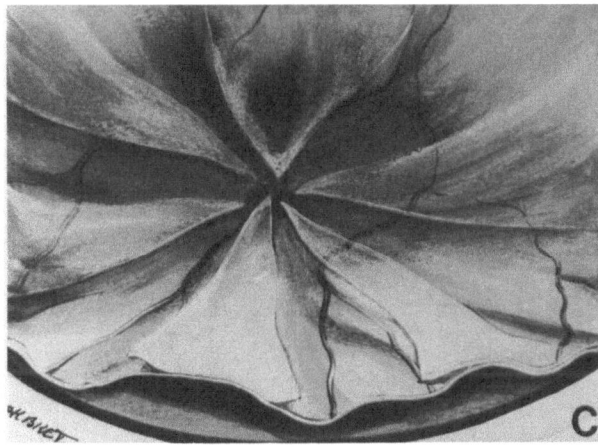

Figure 186. Epiretinal membrane segmentation at the site of star-shaped retinal folds. (A) The hooked fiberoptic probe is used to free the membrane between two retinal folds. (B) Then automatic scissors are used to cut the membrane. (C) Traction on the retina is relieved when epiretinal membrane segmentation is completed. Space has developed between the cut edges of the membrane and the retina is less prominent.

After epiretinal membrane segmentation, retinal mobility is verified by gently opening the retinal folds using the instrument back. If the retinal folds cannot be fully opened remaining bridges of epiretinal membrane are looked for and segmented.

In the future, enzyme assisted delamination of the posterior vitreous face and epiretinal membranes may be a useful adjunct to current techniques in difficult cases.

Excessive traction on the retina should be avoided during epiretinal membrane dissection. Motions of the surrounding retina are the best indicator of how much traction is exerted on the retina, which should be minimal.

Three main complications may occur during epiretinal membrane dissection: (1) inability to identify the membranes and open the fixed folds, (2) bleeding from small retinal vessels, and (3) full thickness iatrogenic retinal breaks (Figs. 188 and 189). Inability to identify the membranes and open the fixed folds will result in surgical failure. Bleeding from small retinal vessels may result from excessive traction on the retina or damage to the inner layers of the retina by the instrument. This may result in recurrent proliferation. Full-thickness iatrogenic retinal breaks result from excessive traction on the retina or improper orientation of the microscissors. Retinal breaks must be identified and treated (see p. 150). Iatrogenic retinal breaks that are not identified and treated will often enlarge postoperatively. They may result in an inoperable recurrent detachment after gas absorption.

Subretinal Membrane Discussion. Subretinal proliferation is a frequent component of proliferative vitreoretinopathy.[3,15] Segmentation and removal of subretinal membranes and cords have been advocated by several vitreous surgeons. However, significant subretinal proliferation with membranes and cords is most common in longstanding retinal detachments associated with round atrophic holes in lattice, or disinsertion at the ora serrata, and virtually never prevent surgical reattachment of the retina in those eyes. For this reason the author believes that a surgical approach of subretinal proliferation in proliferative vitreoretinopathy is unnecessary in most cases. Inability to relieve traction from the posterior vitreous face and epiretinal membranes, in-

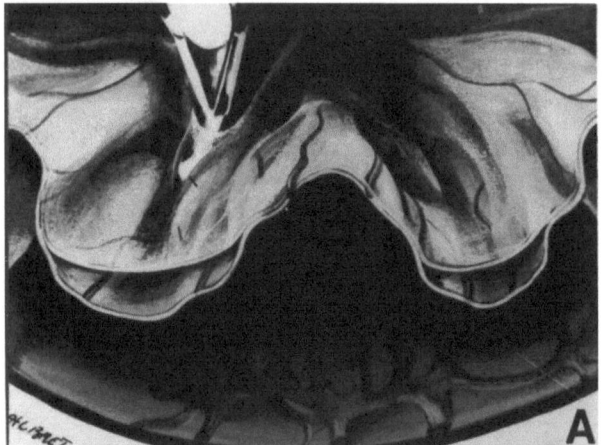
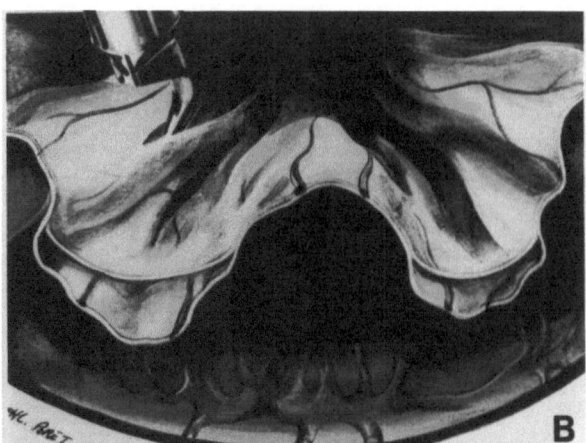
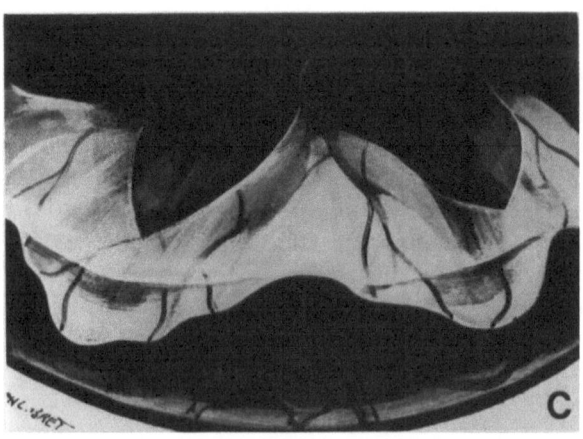
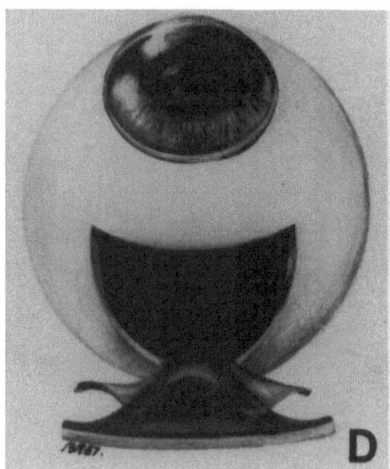

Figure 187. Epiretinal membrane segmentation at the site of radial retinal folds. (A) The hooked fiberoptic probe is used to delaminate the membrane between two retinal folds. Delamination is carried out from the posterior pole toward the peripheral fundus. (B) The membrane is firmly adherent to the retinal ridges. Bridges of epiretinal membrane are cut using automatic scissors. (C) Segmentation of epiretinal membrane bridges has relieved traction on the retina. (D) Whole-eye view.

traoperative complications, and recurrent epiretinal membranes, rather than subretinal proliferation, are the major causes for failed surgery in proliferative vitreoretinopathy.

Relaxing Retinotomies. When, in spite of membrane peeling, the detached retina remains too short to be reattached, relaxing retinotomies and retinectomies have been advocated.[22, 51] However, the value of these techniques has not yet been fully demonstrated.

RETINAL TEAR MANAGEMENT

As in any rhegmatogenous retinal detachment, treatment of all retinal tears is a requisite for perma-

nent retinal reattachment. Retinal tears may be primary or secondary to the proliferative process (see p. 239) or iatrogenic process (see p. 247). All retinal tears must be identified by thorough examination of the fundus performed preoperatively and during vitrectomy.

The basic principles of retinal tear management are the same in retinal detachments associated with proliferative vitreoretinopathy as in any retinal detachment. The treatment must include two components: (1) inducement of a firm retinochoroidal adhesion in the area of the retinal tear and (2) relief of vitreoretinal traction. Specific rules should be followed in applying these basic principles, however, because of the specific anatomical and biological conditions associated with proliferative vitreoretinopathy and the modifications of the inner anatomy of the eye after vitrectomy.

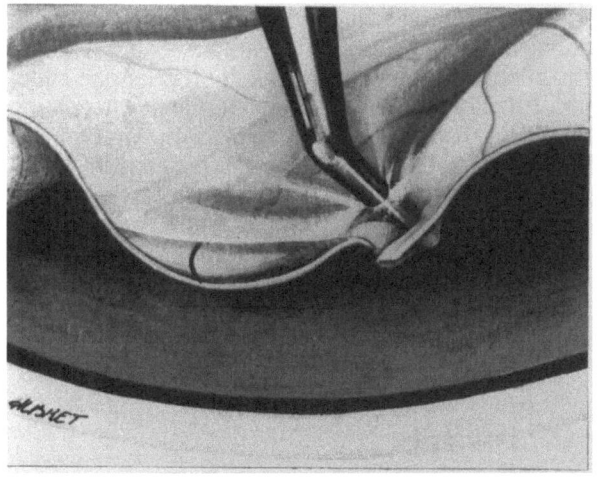

Figure 188. Error to avoid in epiretinal membrane dissection: The hooked fiberoptic probe has not been inserted beneath the membrane in a valley between two retinal folds. It is not orientated in the proper direction. Attempts to free the membrane, and/or use of a sharp needle, will result in a iatrogenic retinal tear.

Inducing a Firm Retinochoroidal Adhesion.

It is thought that the retinochoroidal adhesion required to permanently seal a retinal break in proliferative vitreoretinopathy should be stronger than those in the usual retinal detachments. This belief is based on the fact that the induced retinochoroidal adhesion should resist traction forces related to the proliferative process, which will persist as long as the proliferative process remains active. The period of time that the proliferative process will remain active postoperatively is unknown. Variations depending on unknown factors are likely. As a rule the author tries to create a retinochoroidal scar in the area of the retinal tear(s) twice as large as that routinely obtained in usual retinal detachments (see p. 74).

Cryotherapy or argon laser photocoagulation are used to induce the retinochoroidal adhesion. A choice between the two techniques mainly depends on the size and number of retinal breaks.

Cryotreatment may play a determining role in the development or recurrence of proliferative vitreoretinopathy under specific conditions (see p. 234). Therefore, use of cryotreatment is minimized as much as possible in retinal detachments associated with proliferative vitreoretinopathy. The indications for cryotreatment are limted as follows: (1) it can be anticipated from preoperative examination that less than 20 cryoapplications will be necessary to seal the retinal breaks and (2) full thickness fixed retinal folds involve less than four retinal quadrants (grade C).

Argon laser photocoagulation is used rather than cryo in the following circumstances: (1) when there are multiple, large, or giant retinal tears, (2) when the fixed retina is highly detached, or (3) when full thickness fixed retinal folds involve all four quadrants (grade D).

When cryotreatment is used, it is performed through the sclera and under simultaneous biomicroscopic observation of the retinal tear. It is routinely performed at the beginning of the surgical procedure before vitrectomy. However, retinal breaks that are identified at the time of vitreous surgery can obviously be treated only after completion of vitrectomy. Performing cryotreatment of the retinal tears before, rather than after, vitrectomy has three main advantages:

1. Viable pigment epithelium cells released into the vitreous cavity by cryo will likely be washed out during vitrectomy.[52]
2. Choroidal thickness is commonly increased after completion of the vitrectomy. Therefore, if retinal tear treatment is performed after vitrectomy, cryoapplications of increased duration are often necessary to freeze the outer layers of the neurosensory retina. This may result in an increased inflammatory response postoperatively.
3. Height of the retinal detachment is frequently increased after completion of the vitrectomy. This makes cryo and retinal tear localization less accurate than at the beginning of the operation.

When argon laser photocoagulation is used to seal retinal tears, it is performed 3–4 days postoperatively. At that time, maximal expansion of the gas bubble is achieved and subretinal fluid has absorbed.

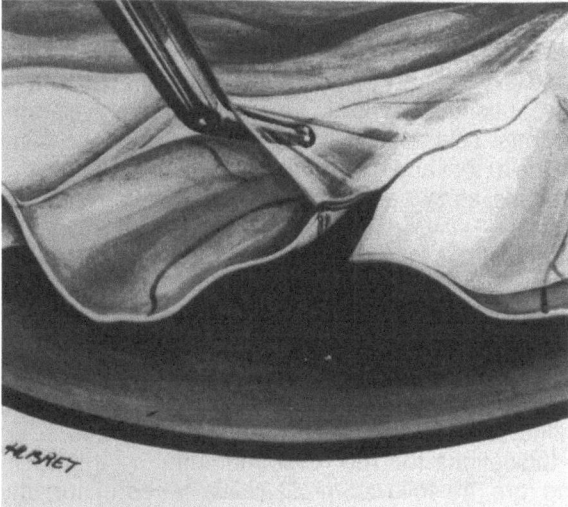

Figure 189. Error to avoid in epiretinal membrane dissection: Excessive traction on the retina results in a iatrogenic retinal tear at the site of firm epiretinal attachment along a retinal vessel.

(For the technique of argon laser photocoagulation through a gas bubble see p. 000.) Four rows of burns are made all around each retinal break. Small retinal tears are often difficult to identify through a gas bubble. This difficulty is overcome by making a retinal landmark with endodiathermy during vitrectomy. The white retinal burn made by endodiathermy will remain clearly visible through the gas bubble for a week.

Relief of Vitreoretinal Traction. Relief of vitreoretinal traction can be achieved by vitrectomy or scleral buckling. On a theoretical basis, when vitrectomy is performed, all vitreoretinal tractions are relieved and scleral buckling of the retinal breaks is unnecessary. However, in practical terms, this applies only to retinal breaks located posteriorly to the equator.

In vitrectomized eyes, scleral buckling is unnecessary in the management of retinal breaks located posteriorly to the equator. Induced choroidal irritation and gas tamponade provide permanent sealing of such breaks, since they are no longer under vitreous traction.

In contrast, scleral buckling remains a requisite for permanent sealing of most peripheral retinal tears in proliferative vitreoretinopathy, because most peripheral tears are submitted to the ring contraction of the vitreous base. Broad and high scleral buckles are performed either circumferentially or radially.

Radial buckles are used for large retinal tears that overlap the posterior edge of the vitreous base or when fixed retinal folds remain in the vicinity of the tears.

SCLERAL BUCKLING OF THE VITREOUS BASE

Circumferential scleral buckling of the vitreous base is necessary in most eyes. Its goal is to counteract concentric traction of the vitreous base. A circumferential scleral buckle is 360° or less, depending on the extent and biological course of the proliferative process, as well as the number and location of retinal tears.

Indications for 360° scleral buckling are as follows: (1) all eyes with proliferative vitreoretinopathy grade C3 and over, (2) most eyes with lesser extent of full thickness fixed folds when there is clinical evidence of a very active proliferative process associated with recent onset retinal detachment, and (3) retinal tears involving more than 2 quadrants.

Indications for 180° circumferential scleral buckling are as follows: proliferative vitreoretinopathy grade C1 or C2 associated with longstanding retinal detachments and small retinal tears involving two quadrants or less of the peripheral retina.

High and broad scleral buckles used in the man-

agement of proliferative vitreoretinopathy result in significant reduction of the vitreous cavity volume and intraocular space available for further gas injection. Precise reduction of the vitreous cavity volume should be known for evaluation of the optimal volume of pure gas to be injected. For this purpose intraocular fluid removed from the eye to tighten the scleral sutures and maintain normal intraocular pressure is collected in a syringe. The total amount of fluid removed from the eye indicates the precise reduction of the vitreous cavity volume induced by scleral buckling.

GAS INJECTION

Intravitreal injection of pure gas is the last step of the procedure. At present, perfluoropropane gas is used, preferably because of its expansion properties and longevity (see p. 120). The optimal volume to be injected is calculated according to four parameters: (1) the location and size of the retinal breaks (see p. 121), (2) the severity and extent of the proliferative process, (3) the biometry of the eye (see p. 122), and (4) the volume of intraocular fluid removed for scleral buckling.

Large bubbles, which fill approximately 80% of the vitreous cavity after maximal expansion, are used in proliferative vitreoretinopathy, grade C3 and over, in large, multiple or giant retinal tears, and in retinal tears located inferiorly. Smaller bubbles, which fill approximately 50% of the vitreous cavity after maximal expansion, are used in proliferative vitreoretinopathy, grades C1 and C2, associated with small retinal tear(s) located in the upper quadrants.

Gas injection is performed via the limbus in aphakic eyes and through the pars plana in phakic eyes. The same amount of fluid as the volume of pure gas to be injected is removed from the vitreous cavity just before gas injection. Drainage of subretinal fluid to give space for intravitreal gas injection in unnecessary in most cases.

SUBRETINAL FLUID DRAINAGE

Subretinal fluid drainage is unnecessary to achieve retinal reattachment in proliferative vitreoretinopathy, as in any retinal detachment. Subretinal fluid will spontaneously absorb within a few days, provided all retinal breaks are sealed, and vitreoretinal tractions are relieved.[20] Therefore subretinal fluid drainage is not carried out unless it might be helpful for completion of other surgical steps.

There are two main indications for subretinal fluid drainage in proliferative vitreoretinopathy: (1) to make the vitrectomy procedure easier, and (2) to create intraocular space available for intravitreal gas injection.

Adjuncts to Surgical Treatment

In retinal detachments associated with proliferative vitreoretinopathy, most failures to permanently reattach the retina are related to recurrence of the proliferative process postoperatively, rather than from the surgeon's inability to satisfactorily complete the operation. Recurrent proliferative vitreoretinopathy after surgery most commonly results in an anatomical situation of the eye that is more severe than preoperatively. A significant number of detachments with recurrent proliferative vitreoretinopathy are inoperable. The anatomical success rate in eyes that appear to be still operable is very low.[20]

Surgical trauma is likely a stimulus for the cellular events that result in preretinal membrane formation (see p. 234). Therefore, any therapeutic measure that could prevent epiretinal membrane formation would be a valuable adjunct to surgery.

In recent years, most efforts have been centered on finding a pharmacologic solution to the problem. A varity of drugs have been tested for their ability to inhibit the biological process of membrane formation. The cellular process that leads to proliferative vitreoretinopathy includes three distinct stages: (1) migration of retinal pigment epithelial cells,[10] glial cells,[53] and fibroblasts[8] into the vitreous cavity and both surfaces of the retina, (2) proliferation of these cells, and (3) contraction.

In vitro and in vivo experimental studies have been conducted to determine the ability of various drugs to inhibit the proliferative process. Those studies have provided most useful information. However, animal models of proliferative vitreoretinopathy do not reproduce the human disease. Therefore, extrapolation from experimental data to human disease requires great care. Randomized clinical studies are required to determine which drug(s) or what other means, is the most effective in the prevention of the human disease.

PHARMACOLOGIC AGENTS

Pharmacologic agents that have been extensively studied both experimentally and clinically include corticosteroids and 5-Fluorouracil. Other drugs such as Daunomycin, Collagen cross linking inhibitors, and Colchicine are still under evaluation.

Corticosteroids. Corticosteroids have a high level of antiinflammatory action, antimitotic activity, and an inhibitory effect on the growth of fibroblasts.

Experimental studies have shown that intravitreal injection of 1 mg dexamethosone alcohol,[54] or 1 mg triamcinolone acetonide[55] inhibits the growth of fibroblasts transplanted into the rabbit vitreous cavity. However, the effects were not as pronounced in a refined model of proliferative vitreoretinopathy, which resembles more the human disease, as in the previous studies.[56] The lack of toxicity of intravitreally administered triamcinolone acetonide was demonstrated in the rabbit eye.[57] However, the beneficial effects of intravitreal injection of corticosteroids in the human disease remain to be fully demonstrated.

The effects of systemic corticosteroids in the prevention of the human disease seem to be weaker than that of intravitreal injection in the rabbit eye.[58] However, systemic corticosteroids significantly decrease the incidence of autoimmunity against the retina associated with the development of proliferative vitreoretinopathy.[59–60] The inhibitory effect of corticosteroids on the development of autoimmunity against the retina, and probably proliferative vitreoretinopathy, requires that the treatment be started preoperatively.[60] Synacthene administered intravenously is used to start treatment. After eight days, it is replaced by oral prednisone. Treatment is begun three days before surgery and continued for a 2-month period. 0.5 to 1 mg prednisone per kilo are given daily for 10 days, and then the daily dosage is gradually decreased. Treatment is administered for 2 months because this time period is thought to be that of maximal biological activity of the proliferative process. Systemic side effects and systemic contraindications are two major disadvantages of the treatment. Efficacy in preventing recurrent proliferative vitreoretinopathy remains to be fully demonstrated by randomized clinical studies.

5-Fluorouracil. 5-Fluorouracil has extensively been studied as a promising pharmacological adjunct in the treatment of proliferative vitreoretinopathy.[61–67] It is a synthetic pyrimidine analog with cytostatic activity. Its mode of action in proliferative vitreoretinopathy is through inhibition of fibroblast, glial, and pigment epithelial cells proliferation. Intravitreal and periocular administration of the drug has proven to be effective to decrease proliferative vitreoretinopathy both experimentally,[62–64] and clinically.[61] However the neurotoxicity of the drug[65–66] limits its use to low dosages. Experimentally, the inhibitory effect on cell proliferation is approximately the same for 1 mg 5-fluorouracil and 1 mg dexamethosone alcohol.[64]

Daunomycin. Daunomycin has been shown to decrease the incidence of recurrent proliferative vitreoretinopathy and improve the anatomical results in the most severe grades of proliferative vitreoretinopathy.[68]

Colchicine. Experimental studies[69-70] suggest that oral therapy with colchicine may prove to be of value in the treatment of proliferative vitreoretinopathy. In vitro, low dose colchicine is an effective inhibitor of retinal pigment epithelium, astrocyte, and fibroblast migration and proliferation.[69-70] The possibility of oral administration and maintainence of a constant drug level during the active stage of the disease are potential advantages, however, digestive side effects may limit its use. Moreover, the intraocular penetration and optimal dosage are unknown.

EYE ROENTGENTHERAPY

Experimentally, roentgentherapy has been proven to inhibit growth of fibroblasts transplanted into the vitreous cavity.[71] A randomized clinical trial is being conducted to determine whether this mode of treatment is of any value in the prevention of recurrent proliferative vitreoretinopathy.

RESULTS

In the author's experience, total retinal reattachment can be achieved in approximately 80% of eyes with proliferative vitreoretinopathy, grade C, and in 40% of eyes with grade D.[19-20] These results are achieved with a single operation in approximately 90% of successful eyes. There is a close correlation between the anatomical success rate and the severity of the proliferative process. The anatomical success rate is approximately 85% in grade C1 and C2, 70% in grade C3, 60% in Grade D1, but only 33% in grades D2 and D3.

Visual results are dependent on the severity of the proliferative process and duration of macular detachment. Rather good visual recovery, with visual acuities ranging from 0.1 to 0.7 can be expected in grade C. In contrast, the vast majority of patients with proliferative vitreoretinopathy, grade D recover only ambulatory vision.

The author's results are comparable with those achieved by other surgeons[16-17,24,72] who use microsurgical techniques, which are different in their detailed performance but basically similar in their principles. These results are not as good as those reported with the use of silicone oil,[21,22] however, the visual

results after retinal tamponade with silicone oil are often disappointing and the long-term anatomical outcome of the eyes remain most uncertain. In contrast, retinal reattachment achieved 6 months after gas absorption, will remain permanent. The patients will not require reoperation for retinal reattachment later on. In eyes that have been left phakic, cataract may develop several months or years postoperatively. However, this complication which is benign as compared to the retinal disease, is infrequent.[20]

REFERENCES

1. The retina Society terminology committee: The classification of retinal detachment with proliferative vitreoretinopathy. Ophthalmology 90:121–125, 1983
2. Rachal WS, Burton TC: Changing concepts of failures after retinal detachment surgery. Arch Ophthalmol 97:480–483, 1979
3. Laqua H, Machemer R: Glial proliferation in retinal detachment (massive periretinal proliferation). Am J Ophthalmol 80:602–618, 1975
4. Machemer R, Laqua H: Pigment epithelium proliferation in retinal detachment (massive periretinal proliferation). Amer J Ophthalmol 80:1–23, 1975
5. Mandelcorn MS, Machemer R, Fineberg E: Proliferation and metaplasia of intravitreal retinal pigment epithelium cell auto transplants. Am J Ophthalmol 80:227–237, 1975
6. Mueller-Jensen K, Machemer R, Azarnia R: Auto transplantation of retinal pigment epithelium in intravitreal diffusion chambers. Am J Ophthalmol 80:530–537, 1975
7. Newsome DA, Kenyon KR: Collagen production in vitro by retinal pigmented epithelium of the chick embryo. Dev Biol 387–400, 1973
8. Newsome DA, Rodrigues MM, Machemer R: Human massive periretinal proliferation. In vitro characteristics of cellular components. Arch Ophthalmol 99:873–880, 1981
9. Miller B, Miller H, Ryan SJ: Experimental epiretinal proliferation induced by intravitreal red blood cells. Am J Ophthalmol 102:188–195, 1986
10. Machemer R, Van Horn D, Aaberg T: Pigment epithelial proliferation in human retinal detachment with massive peripheral proliferation. Am J Ophthalmol 85:181–191, 1978
11. Ehrenberg M, Thresher RJ, Machemer R: Vitreous hemorrhage nontoxic to retina as a stimulator of glial and fibrous proliferation. Am J Ophthalmol 97:611–626, 1984
12. Harada T: An electron microscopic study of the epiretinal membrane in human eyes. Acta Soc Ophthalmol Jap 85:631–645, 1981
13. Kampik A, Kenyon K, Michels R, Green W, De la Cruz Z: Epiretinal and vitreous membranes. Comparative study of 56 cases. Arch Ophthalmol 99:1445–1454, 1981
14. Ohira A, Oshima K: Histological study of proliferating membrane of human massive periretinal proliferation (MPP). Acta Soc Ophthalmol Jap 85:622–630, 1981
15. Sternberg P, Machemer R: Subretinal proliferation. Amer J Ophthalmol 98:456–462, 1984
16. Chang S, Coleman D, Lincoff H, Wilcox L, et al: Perfluoropropane gas in the management of proliferative vitreoretinopathy. Amer J Ophthalmol 98:180–188, 1984
17. De Bustros S, Michels RG: Treatment of retinal detachments complicated by proliferative vitreoretinopathy. Am J Ophthalmol 98:694–699, 1984

18. Sternberg P, Machemer R: Results of conventional vitreous surgery for proliferative vitreoretinopathy. Am J Ophthalmol 100:141–146, 1985

19. Bonnet M: Les gaz expansifs de longue durée dans le traitement des décollements rétiniens associés à une rétraction rétinovitréenne. J Fr Ophtalmol 8:607–611, 1985

20. Bonnet M, Santamaria E, Mouche J: Intraoperative use of pure perfluoropropane gas in the management of proliferative vitreoretinopathy. Graefe's Arch Clin Exp Ophthalmol 225:299–302, 1987

21. Gonvers M: Temporary silicone oil tamponade in the management of retinal detachment with proliferative vitreoretinopathy. Am J Ophthalmol 100:239–245, 1985

22. Haut J, Coulombel P, Larricart P, Ullern M, Van Effenterre G: L'intervention vitrectomie-silicone. A propos de 1000 cas. Paris, Masson, 1984

23. Ashrafzaden MT, Schepens CH, Elzeneiny I, et al: Aphakic and phakic retinal detachment, I-preoperative findings. Arch Ophthalmol 89:476–483, 1973

24. Jalkh AE, Avila MP, Schepens CH, Azzolini C, Duncan JE, Trempe CL: Surgical treatments of proliferative vitreoretinopathy. Arch Ophthalmol 102:1135–1139, 1984

25. Bonnet M: Clinical factors predisposing to massive proliferative vitreoretinopathy in rhegmatogenous retinal detachment. Ophthalmologica (Basel) 188:148–152, 1984

26. Wilkinson CP: Retinal detachment following intraocular lens implantation. Ophthalmology 88:410–413, 1987

27. Benson WE, Nantawan P, Morse PH: Characteristics and prognosis of retinal detachments with demarcation lines. Amer J Ophthalmol 84:641–644, 1977

28. Bonnet M, Moyenin P, Pecold K, Grange JD: Décollements rétiniens par désinsertion à l'ora serrata. J Fr Ophtalmol 9:231–242, 1986

29. Tillery WV, Lucier AC: Round atrophic holes in lattice degeneration. An important cause of phakic retinal detachment. Trans Amer Acad Ophthalmol Otolaryngol 81:509–518, 1970

30. Bonnet M, Urrets-Zavalia J: Décollements rétiniens par petits trous de la région equatoriale. J Fr Ophtalmol 9:615–624, 1986

31. Normand F: Décollements de la rétine par trou maculaire ou déchirure du trou postérieur du myope fort—Analyse de 60 cas successifs. Thèse Université, Lyon, 1986

32. Fleury J: Microchirurgie des décollements de la rétine par déchirures grandes ou géantes. Thèse Université, Lyon, 1986

33. Bonnet M: Epithélium pigmenté exposé par les déchirures rétiniennes et rétraction rétinovitréenne massive. Bull Mem SFO 97:271–273, 1986

34. Bonnet M: Grade B a determining factor in the development of proliferative vitreoretinopathy. Graefe's Arch Clin Exp Ophthalmol 226:201–205, 1988

35. Ryan SJ: The pathophysiology of proliferative vitreoretinopathy in its management. Am J Ophthalmol 100:188–193, 1985

36. Campochiaro PA, Kaden IH, Vidaurri-Leal J, et al: Cryotherapy enhances intravitreal dispersion of viable retinal pigment epithelial cells. Arch Ophthalmol 103:434–436, 1985

37. Radtke ND, Tamo Y, Chandler D, et al: Simulation of massive periretinal proliferation by autotransplantation of retinal pigment epithelial cells in rabbits. Am J Ophthalmol 91:76–87, 1981

38. Lincoff H, Kreissig I, Fuchs W, Jakobiec F, Iwamoto T: Vollstandiger Ersatz des Glaskorpers durch ein intraokular expandierendes Gas. Fortschr Ophthalmol 81:1, 95–98, 1984

39. Havener WH: Massive vitreous retraction. Ophthalmic Surg 4:22–67, 1973

40. Scott JD: The treatment of massive vitreous retraction by the separation of preretinal membranes using liquid silicone. Mod Probl Ophthalmol 15:285–290, 1975

41. Machemer R: Pathogenesis and classification of massive periretinal proliferation. Brit J Ophthalmol 62:737–747, 1978

42. Machemer R: Subtotal vitrectomy through the pars plana. Ophthalmology 77:198–201, 1973

43. Machemer R, Laqua H: A logical approach to the treatment of massive periretinal proliferation. Ophthalmology 85:584–593, 1978

44. Charles ST: Vitreous Microsurgery. Baltimore, Williams and Wilkins, 1981

45. Michels R: Vitreous Surgery. St. Louis, C. L. Mosby Co, 1981

46. Bonnet M: Scleral shortening for the surgical repair of retinal detachments with peripheral retinal retraction. International symposium and first training course on retinal detachment. Rome, September 29–October 1, 1981.

47. Grizzard WS, Hilton GF: Scleral buckling for retinal detachments complicated by periretinal proliferation. Arch Ophthalmol 100:419–422, 1982

48. Eisner G: Biomicroscopy of the peripheral fundus. New York, Springer-Verlag, 1973, 48

49. Olk RJ, Escoffery RF: Modified vitreoretinal pics and spatulas. Am J Ophthalmol 99:610–611, 1985

50. De Juan E, Hickingbotham D, Mc Cuen BW, Machemer R: The pic-forceps for removal of epiretinal membranes. Am J Ophthalmol 98:519, 1984

51. Machemer R, Mc Cuen BW, De Juan E: Relaxing retinotomies and rectinectomies. Am J Ophthalmol 102:7–12, 1986

52. Vidauri-Leal J, De Bustros S, Michels RG: Surgical treatment of giant retinal tears with inverted posterior retinal flap. Am J Ophthalmol 98:-463–466, 1984

53. Van Horn DL, Aaberg TM, Machemer R, et al: Glial cell proliferation in human retinal detachment with massive periretinal proliferation. Am J Ophthalmol 84:383–393, 1977

54. Trano Y, Chandler DB, Mc Cuen B, Machemer R: Glucocorticosteroid inhibition of intraocular proliferation after injury. Am J Ophthalmol 91, 184–189, 1981

55. Tano Y, Chandler D, Machemer R: Treatment of intraocular proliferation with intravitreal injection of triamcinolone acetonide. Am J Ophthalmol 90:810–816, 1980

56. Chandler DB, Rozakis G, De Juan E, Machemer R: The effect of triamcinolone acetonide on a refined experimental model of proliferative vitreoretinopathy. Am J Ophthalmol 99:686–690, 1985

57. Mc Cuen B, Bessler M, Tano Y, Chandler D, Machemer R: The lack of toxicity of intravitreally administered triamcinolone acetonide. Am J Ophthalmol 91:785–788, 1981

58. Koerner F, Merz A, Gloor B, Wagner E: Postoperative retinal fibrosis. A controlled clinical study of systemic steroid therapy. Graefe's Arch Clin Exp Ophthalmol 119:268–271, 1982

59. Remy Ch: Recherche de l'auto immunité contre la rétine dans les décollements rétiniens idiopathiques (étude de 50 cas). J Fr Ophtalmol 4:213–217, 1981

60. Remy Ch: Décollement de la rétine et rétraction rétinienne. Effet des anti inflammatoires stéroidiens et non stéroidiens sur la réaction auto immune contre la rétine dans les décollements de la rétine avec rétraction. J Fr Ophtalmol 5:621–632, 1982

61. Blumenkranz M, Hernandez E, Ophir A, Norton EW: 5-fluorouracil: new applications in complicated retinal detachment for an established antimetabolite. Ophthalmology 91:122–130, 1984

62. Blumenkranz M, Ophir A, Claflin AJ, Hajek A: Fluorouracil for the treatment of massive periretinal proliferation. Am J Ophthalmol 94:458–467, 1982

63. Stern WH, Lewis GP, Erickson PA, Guerin CJ, et al: Fluorouracil therapy for proliferative vitreoretinopathy after vitrectomy. Am J Ophthalmol 96:33–42, 1983

64. Binder S, Riss B, Skoppik Ch, Kulnig W: Inhibition of experimental intraocular proliferation with intravitreal 5-fluorouracil. Graefe's Arch Clin Exp Ophthalmol 221:126–129, 1983

65. Nao IN, Honda Y: Toxic effect of fluorouracil on the rabbit retina. Amer J Ophthalmol 96:641–643, 1983

66. Kulnig W, Binder S, Riss B, Skoppik Ch: Inhibition of experimental intraocular proliferation with intravitreous 5-fluorouracil. Basel, Ophthalmologica 188:248–258, 1984

67. Rootman J, Tisdall J, Gudauskas G, Ostry A: Intraocular penetration of subconjunctivally administered 14 C Fluorouracil in rabbits. Arch Ophthalmol 97:2375–2378, 1979

68. Wiedemann P, Lemmen K, Schmiedl R, Heimann K: Intraocular daunorubicin for the treatment and prophylaxis of traumatic prolif-

erative vitreoretinopathy. Am J Ophthalmol 104:1, 10–14, 1987

69. Lemor M, De Bustros S, Glaser BM: Low-dose colchicine inhibits astrocyte, fibroblast, and retinal pigment epithelial cell migration and proliferation. Arch Ophthalmol 104:1223–1225, 1986

70. Lemor M, Yeo JH, Glaser BM: Oral colchicine for the treatment of experimental traction retinal detachment. Arch Ophthalmol 104:1226–1229, 1986

71. Binder S, Skoppik C, Paroussis P, Kulnig W, Menapace R, Prokesch E: High-energy electrons used to inhibit experimental intraocular proliferation and detachment. Ophthalmologica 195, 3:128–134, 1987

72. Blumenkranz M, Gardner T, Blankenship G: Fluid-gas exchange and photocoagulation after vitrectomy indications, technique and results. Arch Ophthalmol 104:291–296, 1986

21

Aphakic and Pseudophakic Retinal Detachment

RETINAL DETACHMENT FOLLOWING SENILE CATARACT SURGERY

Etiology

INCIDENCE

Aphakia is associated with an increased incidence of retinal detachment. Before the development of modern cataract surgery with intraocular lens implantation, aphakic retinal detachments accounted for approximately 25% of all retinal detachments treated in referral retinal centers.[1–3] Owing to the increasing popularity of intraocular lens implantation, the incidence of aphakic retinal detachment has shown a steady decrease over the last years, whereas pseudophakic retinal detachment has become more common. Variations in the incidence of retinal detachment in aphakic and pseudophakic eyes are probably related to the surgical technique used for lens removal rather than the absence or presence and type of intraocular lens.

After an uneventful intracapsular cataract extraction, the incidence of rhegmatogenous retinal detachment is 3.3%.[4] There is an increased risk of retinal detachment in patients with lattice degeneration, a history of retinal detachment in the other eye, and severe myopia.[5,6] The incidence of retinal detachment after intracapsular cataract extraction in eyes with myopia of 6 diopters or more is approximately 6.5%.[5] Intracapsular cataract extraction complicated by vitreous loss and vitreous gel incarceration in the corneal wound significantly increases the risk of subsequent retinal detachment.[4,7,8]

It is generally believed that modern extracapsular cataract surgery has reduced the incidence of subsequent rhegmatogenous retinal detachment, as compared to intracapsular cataract surgery.[9–11] The incidence of retinal detachment is less than 1% in eyes with an intact posterior capsule.[4,10,12] There is however ample evidence in the literature that secondary opening of the posterior capsule increases the incidence of subsequent retinal detachment, regardless of the technique used for posterior capsulotomy.[12–17] The incidence of retinal detachment is 3.1% following a primary knife-needle discision and 6.1% following a secondary knife-needle discision.[12]

BILATERAL INVOLVEMENT

The incidence of bilateral retinal detachment in bilateral aphakic patients varies from 20%[1,2] to 48%.[19]

PATIENT AGE

Aphakic retinal detachment shows a peak incidence in patients between 60 and 70 years old.[18,19] The peak age incidence is related to the peak age for development of posterior vitreous detachment.

TIME INTERVAL BETWEEN CATARACT SURGERY AND RETINAL DETACHMENT

The time interval between cataract surgery and occurrence of retinal detachment varies depending on the surgical technique used for cataract extraction.

After uneventful intracapsular cataract extraction, approximately 50% of retinal detachments develop within the first postoperative year.[1,3,20] Sixty percent of retinal detachments develop within 2 years following cataract surgery, and 72% within five years.[19] Most aphakic retinal detachments develop at the time of posterior vitreous detachment or shortly thereafter. The time interval between uneventful intracapsular cataract surgery and occurrence of posterior vitreous detachment is correlated with patient-age. It is longer in patients under 60 compared with patients over 60 years.

The risk of early retinal detachment within 3 months following cataract surgery is increased in patients who had vitreous loss at cataract extraction.[8]

Time interval between cataract surgery and occurrence of retinal detachment is longer after extracapsular cataract extraction compared to intracapsular surgery. Most retinal detachments develop more than a year after extracapsular cataract surgery. In most patients, retinal detachment develops after capsulotomy.

In pseudophakic eyes, the time interval between lens implantation and occurrence of retinal detachment varies depending on the technique used for cataract extraction rather than the type of intraocular lens. In eyes that have undergone extracapsular cataract extraction, most retinal detachments occur after capsulotomy. The time interval between capsulotomy and retinal detachment approximates that of aphakic retinal detachment after intracapsular extraction.[12,13,18]

Clinical Findings

Some clinical features are more common in aphakic and pseudophakic retinal detachment following senile cataract surgery, as compared to phakic retinal detachment.

RETINAL DETACHMENT

Retinal detachment is generally more extensive at initial presentation in aphakic and pseudophakic eyes compared to phakic eyes.[1,3,20–23] Total retinal detachment is present in 22%[3] to 37.9% of eyes.[1] Macular detachment is observed in 62.5%[3] to 83% of eyes.[1] The greater extent of retinal detachment in aphakic and pseudophakic eyes suggests that subretinal fluid spreads more rapidly in aphakic eyes. This may be related to the increased mobility of the vitreous gel and the decreased concentration of hyaluronic acid[24] in aphakic eyes.

The incidence of longstanding retinal detachment with demarcation lines and subretinal proliferation, is nearly the same as that of phakic retinal detachment. It is approximately 10%.[1,22]

Aphakic and pseudophakic retinal detachments show a trend for a higher incidence of proliferative vitreoretinopathy as compared to phakic retinal detachment. Full thickness fixed retinal folds were observed preoperatively in 34%[3] to 54.7%[1] of aphakic retinal detachments, and 49% of pseudophakic retinal detachments.[23] The trend for a higher incidence of proliferative vitreoretinopathy in aphakic and pseudophakic eyes compared to phakic eyes may be related to three main causes: (1) the high incidence of horseshoe tears and the low incidence of atrophic holes and oral dialysis in aphakic and pseudophakic retinal detachments, (2) modifications of the vitreous gel related to aphakic, in particular in eyes with vitreous gel incarceration in the cataract wound, and (3) low grade intraocular inflammation and breakdown of the blood ocular barrier associated with pseudophakia.

Preoperative choroidal detachment is more common—3%—in aphakic retinal detachment compared to phakic retinal detachment (1%).[1,25]

RETINAL BREAKS

In a significant number of aphakic and pseudophakic retinal detachments, identification of all retinal breaks is more difficult than in phakic eyes. This is related to two main parameters: (1) the small size and anterior location of retinal tears in most aphakic and pseudophakic retinal detachments and (2) modifications of anterior segment anatomy associated with aphakia and pseudophakia. Poor pupillary dilation, posterior iris synechiae, lens remnants, secondary opacification of the lens capsule, and intraocular lenses are the most common causes of difficult examination of the peripheral fundus. When indirect ophthalmoscopy was used as the only method for fundus examination, no retinal break could be identified in 7%[1] to over 15%[26] of aphakic retinal detachments, and 5%[27] to approximately 18%[28–29] of pseudophakic retinal detachments. When slit lamp biomicroscopy combined with scleral depression is used for fundus examination, retinal breaks can be identified in virtually all eyes.[3,19] However, repeated and prolonged fundus examination using the surgical microscope is required in a number of patients, particularly in pseudophakic patients.

The clinical characteristics of retinal breaks are similar in aphakic and pseudophakic retinal detachments.

Characteristically the retinal break location is very anterior in most cases. Retinal breaks are oral or postoral in approximately 73% of eyes, equatorial in 24% and postequatorial in 3%.[3,20]

Most aphakic and pseudophakic retinal detachments following senile cataract surgery are associated with horseshoe tears.[3] In most eyes with an axial length within the normal range, the retinal detachment is associated with small horseshoe tears at the posterior edge of the vitreous base. Owing to their anterior location and very small size, these tiny flap tears may be undetected or misdiagnosed as small retinal holes when the fundus is observed with the indirect ophthalmoscope. In a number of eyes, the tiny flap is visible only when using the surgical microscope under high magnification. The small magnification provided by indirect ophthalmoscopy may account for the high incidence of retinal holes reported in a series of aphakic retinal detachments examined by indirect ophthalmoscopy.[1,20] In the author's clinical experience, aphakic and pseudophakic retinal detachments associated with atrophic retinal holes are uncommon. They account for less than 5% of eyes.

As in phakic retinal detachment, the incidence of temporal retinal tears is greater than that of nasal breaks. However, nasal retinal breaks are more frequent in aphakic retinal detachment as compared to phakic retinal detachment.[1]

The average number of retinal breaks is similar to that of phakic retinal detachment.[20] Multiple retinal breaks are found in approximately 72% of eyes.[3] Multiple retinal tears may be located in the same quadrant or in different quadrants (approximately 56% of eyes).[3]

VITREOUS GEL

Posterior vitreous detachment is a constant finding. Retinal tears develop at the time of posterior vitreous detachment. Posterior vitreous detachment may be complete with collapse of the vitreous gel, or incomplete.

The incidence of associated vitreous hemorrhage sufficient to obscure details in some portion of the fundus is similar to that of phakic retinal detachment and is found in approximately 20% of the eyes.[1]

In eyes with vitreous gel incarcerated in the cataract wound, condensed vitreous sheets and bands may be present. In most cases they show a fan configuration from the cataract wound to the lower part of the vitreous (Fig. 190). Light and electron microscopy of autopsied aphakic eyes with vitreous gel incarceration in the cataract wound demonstrated that fibrous ingrowth was present in 84% of eyes.[30] Contraction of fibrous ingrowth from the cataract wound may contribute to the development of retinal detachment. Characteristically, the retinal tear(s) are located in the inferior quadrants, and the nonpigmented epithelium of the pars plana is detached in eyes with combined traction and rhegmatogenous aphakic retinal detachments (Fig. 190).

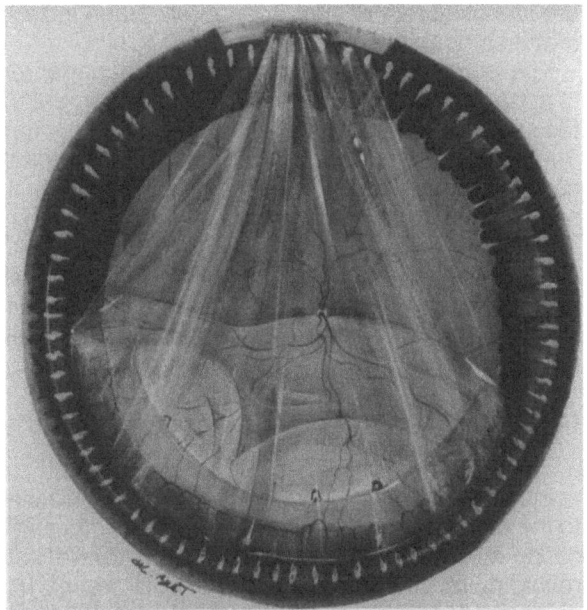

Figure 190. Retinal detachment after cataract surgery complicated by vitreous gel incarceration in the cataract wound in a myopic eye. Condensed vitreous strands fan from the cataract wound to the inferior part of the vitreous cavity. Retinal detachment is associated with three small horseshoe tears at the posterior edge of the vitreous base. The nonpigmented epithelium of the pars plana is detached in the inferior quadrants. Permanent retinal reattachment was achieved by scleral buckling of the retinal tears and the vitreous base in the inferior quadrants associated with vitrectomy.

Surgical Management

The basic principles of surgical management of aphakic and pseudophakic retinal detachment are the same as those of phakic retinal detachment. Permanent sealing of all retinal breaks and relief of static traction on the retina are the goals of surgery. Surgical objectives should be achieved with the least trauma. Aphakic and pseudophakic eyes with retinal detachment are more susceptible to surgical trauma. The increased susceptibility of aphakic eyes to surgical trauma is demonstrated by the higher incidence of postoperative choroidal detachment and cystoid macular edema in aphakic retinal detachment as compared to phakic retinal detachment.[3] Therefore, every effort should be made to minimize surgical trauma and to achieve permanent retinal reattachment with a single operation. In most cases this goal can be achieved, provided all retinal breaks are identified by thorough preoperative and intraoperative fundus examination.

The surgical methods used in the management of aphakic and pseudophakic retinal detachment are the same as those used in phakic retinal detachment. Their indications are also the same. In any given case, choice of the most appropriate surgical technique is dictated by the vitreous and retinal findings. The choice is not modified by the association of aphakia or pseudophakia. Only a few surgical details are modified in aphakic and pseudophakic eyes to make performance of the surgical procedure feasible and less hazardous.

INDUCING A RETINOCHOROIDAL SCAR

Inducing a retinochoroidal scar is strictly restricted to the retinal break area(s). In a few cases cryoapplication is used as a diagnostic tool to differentiate retinal cysts from tiny retinal breaks. However, use of cryoapplication for diagnostic purposes should be limited to a minimum.

SCLERAL BUCKLING

Many surgeons tend to perform a 360° scleral buckling procedure in the management of most aphakic and pseudophakic retinal detachments. Routine use of encircling bands has been advocated because of the erroneous belief that aphakic retinal detachment was associated with multiple small holes scattered throughout the postoral region, which could not be disclosed by indirect ophthalmoscopy. Use of an encircling band was advocated to wall off tiny holes that could not be identified[21] and to prevent recurrent retinal detachment.[31]

Routine use of the slit lamp under high magnification and with scleral depression has demonstrated that all retinal breaks can be disclosed in most aphakic and pseudophakic retinal detachments. This method of fundus examination has also demonstrated that small atrophic holes of the oral region are uncommon in aphakic detachments. The incidence of subsequent recurrent retinal detachment is not any higher in aphakic and pseudophakic eyes managed by a segmental scleral buckling procedure than in those eyes managed by an encircling band.[19,32] The indications for segmental scleral buckles and for 360° scleral buckles in aphakic and pseudophakic eyes are the same as those in phakic retinal detachment (see p. 168).

INTRAVITREAL GAS INJECTION

The indications for intravitreal gas injection in the management of aphakic and pseudophakic retinal

detachment are the same as those in phakic retinal detachment (see p. 117).

In pseudophakic eyes with an anterior chamber lens, or an iris-supported lens, intravitreal injection of a large gas bubble may push the intraocular lens against the cornea and damage the endothelium. In such eyes a small air bubble or hyaluronic acid is injected into the anterior chamber through the limbus before intravitreal gas injection to avoid endothelial damage by the intraocular lens.

Postoperatively, proper head-positioning is mandatory to avoid pupillary block by the gas bubble (see p. 130).

A peripheral inferior iridectomy is performed in vitrectomized eyes when a large volume of longlasting gas is used. Iridectomy is performed to avoid pupillary block by the gas bubble when the patient is in the upright position (see p. 146).

SUBRETINAL FLUID RELEASE

Subretinal fluid release is unnecessary to achieve retinal reattachment in aphakic and pseudophakic retinal detachment, as in any retinal detachment. However, subretinal fluid release is more often carried out in aphakic and pseudophakic eyes than in phakic eyes. In a number of aphakic and pseudophakic eyes, releasing subretinal fluid is the only surgical technique that can be used to create intraocular space for scleral buckling or gas injection and to avoid increased intraocular pressure. Aspiration of fluid from the retrovitreal space is more hazardous a procedure than external release of subretinal fluid. Paracentesis of the anterior chamber is contraindicated in pseudophakic eyes and in most nonvitrectomized aphakic eyes (see p. 64).

VITRECTOMY

Indications for vitrectomy in aphakic and pseudophakic retinal detachments after uncomplicated cataract surgery are the same as those in phakic retinal detachment (see p. 133). Severe proliferative vitreoretinopathy, and vitreous hemorrhage preventing visualization of the retinal tears, are the most common indications for vitrectomy. Although the vitreous gel plays a major role in the development of aphakic retinal detachment, the surgical prognosis for retinal reattachment is not improved by routine vitrectomy.[33] Therefore, an indication for vitrectomy, merely because the eye is aphakic, should not be considered in retinal detachments after uncomplicated cataract surgery.

In contrast, an indication for vitrectomy should be considered in most aphakic retinal detachments after cataract surgery complicated by vitreous loss and vitreous gel incarceration in the cataract wound.[34] Such retinal detachments are usually associated with static vitreous traction caused by condensed vitreous sheets and fibrous ingrowth from the cataract wound (Fig. 190). Pathogenesis of the retinal detachment is close to that of retinal detachment after penetrating injury of the eye. Relief of static vitreous traction on the detached retina is the goal of vitrectomy. Removal of the condensed anterior vitreous face with section of any vitreous strand adherent to the corneal wound is the first and most important step of vitrectomy in such eyes.

Indications for vitrectomy are more frequent in pseudophakic retinal detachment as compared with phakic and aphakic retinal detachment after uncomplicated cataract surgery. Specific indications for vitrectomy in pseudophakic retinal detachment are mainly dictated by modifications of the anterior segment, secondary to complicated cataract surgery and lens implantation or opacification of the posterior lens capsule preventing visualization of the retinal tears. Reconstruction of the pupil, removal of dense retropseudophakic membranes, and removal of an opaque posterior lens capsule to make detailed fundus examination possible, are the goals of vitrectomy in such eyes. Collapse of the anterior chamber during vitrectomy may result in permanent damage to the corneal endothelium in eyes with anterior chamber and iris-supported intraocular lenses. A low-suction force is used to avoid this complication. In addition, the anterior face of the intraocular lens is coated with hyaluronic acid before starting the vitrectomy procedure. Owing to light reflections from the surfaces of the intraocular lens and the posterior lens capsule, and the ring scotoma induced by the intraocular lens, visualization of the vitreous gel and vitreoretinal relationship during vitrectomy is often more difficult in pseudophakic eyes than in phakic and aphakic eyes. However, difficulties related to the intraocular lens can be overcome in most cases when associated lesions of the anterior segment do not prevent dilation of the pupil. The ring scotoma induced by the intraocular lens can be eliminated by increasing the microscope magnification to observe the fundus only through the optic of the intraocular lens.

INTRAOCULAR LENS REMOVAL

Indications for intraocular lens removal as a preliminary step of pseudophakic retinal detachment management are infrequent. The indications are restricted as follows: (1) iris-supported lens associated with a small pupil that prevents fundus examination and (2) retinal detachment associated with proliferative vitreoretinopathy, grade D in eyes with an anterior chamber lens or an iris-supported lens.

Iris-supported lenses associated with an absence of pupillary dilation are removed to make identification of the retinal tears possible. Intraocular lens removal is combined with a sectorial superior iridectomy.

Anterior chamber lenses and iris-supported lenses are removed in most pseudophakic retinal detachments associated with severe proliferative vitreoretinopathy. Improved visualization during epiretinal membrane segmentation, prevention of postoperative pupillary block and endothelial damage from the intraocular lens (induced by a large intravitreal gas bubble), and removal of a stimulus of intraocular inflammation are the main objectives of intraocular lens removal in such eyes. In most cases, the intraocular lens is removed as a preliminary surgical procedure. Surgery for retinal detachment management is carried out 1 or 2 weeks after lens removal, depending on the clarity of the cornea.

Results

ANATOMICAL RESULTS

The overall anatomical success rate achieved in aphakic retinal detachment is lower than that achieved in phakic retinal detachment. It is approximately 85%. The overall anatomical success rate achieved in pseudophakic retinal detachment is slightly lower than that achieved in aphakic retinal detachment. The trend for a more guarded surgical prognosis in aphakic and pseudophakic retinal detachments has been observed after conventional management[8,23,27–29,31,35–37] and after microsurgical management.[19] After microsurgical management, failures related to the inability to identify all retinal breaks or development of subsequent retinal tears and retinal detachment are uncommon.[3,19] Most failures are related to the development of postoperative proliferative vitreoretinopathy.

The main risk factors associated with a lower anatomical success rate in pseudophakic retinal detachment include: (1) preoperative uveitis, (2) early signs of proliferative vitreoretinopathy, (3) inadequate visualization of the peripheral fundus, (4) vitreous hemorrhage, and (5) vitreous gel incarceration in the cataract wound.[27,29] In a large series published in the United States,[27,29] the prognosis for retinal reattachment is significantly worse in eyes with anterior chamber lenses compared to eyes with posterior chamber lenses. The poor results achieved in eyes with anterior chamber lenses are possibly related to complications of cataract surgery, which dictated the choice of the intraocular lens type, rather than the type of intraocular lens.

VISUAL RESULTS

The visual results achieved by microsurgery in aphakic retinal detachment are the same as those achieved in phakic retinal detachment. Visual acuity of 0.5 or better can be achieved in approximately 50% of successful eyes.[19] Approximately 70% of successful eyes recover the visual acuity preexistent to the occurrence of retinal detachment.[19] However, recovery of the best postoperative visual acuity is delayed by cystoid macular edema in a number of eyes. Angiographic cystoid macular edema is significantly more frequent after retinal detachment repair in aphakic eyes compared to phakic eyes.[38-40] The incidence of angiographic cystoid macular edema after microsurgical repair is 30% in aphakic retinal detachments compared to 7% in phakic retinal detachments.[40] In spite of aphakia, the prognosis of postoperative cystoid macular edema is good in most cases. Spontaneous clearing of cystoid macular edema with improvement of the visual acuity occurs in 75% of eyes.[41] Complete absorption of cystoid macular edema and restoration of nearly normal visual acuity may occur more than a year after retinal detachment repair.[41]

The visual results achieved in pseudophakic retinal detachment are less satisfactory than those achieved in aphakic retinal detachment. An increased incidence of macular pucker, permanent cystoid macular edema, and low grade uveitis account for the poor visual results in a significant number of eyes.

RETINAL DETACHMENT AFTER CONGENITAL CATARACT SURGERY

Etiology

Retinal detachment is a common complication in patients who have undergone congenital cataract surgery using traditional surgical techniques, in particular repeated needling. However, retinal detachments after congenital cataract surgery account for only 0.5% of all rhegmatogenous retinal detachments.[42] The low incidence of congenital cataract accounts for the small number of retinal detachments after congenital cataract surgery.

Characteristically, the time interval between conventional surgery for congenital cataract and the occurrence of retinal detachment is prolonged. The average time interval varies between 23 years[42] and 33 years.[43] Seventy-two percent of retinal detachments develop more than 10 years after congenital cataract surgery. Less than 10% develop within the first postoperative year.[42]

Prolonged follow-up is required to determine whether modern congenital cataract microsurgery, in particular lens removal through the pars plana, will reduce the incidence and severity of subsequent retinal detachment. Central vitrectomy associated with lens aspiration through the pars plana may predispose to the development of giant tears.[44]

The incidence of axial myopia (43.6%) is higher than that found in senile aphakic retinal detachment (30%). It is comparable to that found in phakic retinal detachment.[42]

Fundus Findings

Difficulties are encountered in fundus examination of most patients with retinal detachment after congenital cataract surgery. Difficulty in fundus examination is related to: (1) sequelae of cataract surgery, in particular poor pupillary dilation, posterior synechiae, and lens remnants, and (2) other defects frequently associated with congenital cataract, such as nystagmus and strabismus. In a number of patients detailed fundus examination with scleral depression can be satisfactorily performed only under general anesthesia.

RETINAL DETACHMENT

The incidence of total retinal detachment (39%) is higher than in phakic retinal detachment.[42] The incidence of macular detachment is high (81.5%).[42] Clinical evidence of proliferative vitreoretinopathy with full thickness retinal folds is present in 26% of eyes.[42] Detachment of the pars plana epithelium is found in approximately 23% of eyes.[42] This clinical finding is likely indicative of vitreoretinal traction in the anterior part of the vitreous cavity.[42] Signs of longstanding retinal detachment, such as demarcation lines, subretinal proliferation, and cystoid degeneration of the detached retina are infrequent.

RETINAL BREAKS

Owing to difficulty encountered in fundus examination, the inability to disclose the retinal breaks was common in series of eyes examined by indirect ophthalmoscopy 24%,[42] 73.5%.[43] In contrast, retinal breaks can be identified in approximately 95% of eyes when fundus examination is performed using the operating microscope and when reconstruction of the anterior segment is performed as the first step of the surgical procedure for retinal detachment management in eyes with a small pupil or lens remnants, which prevent visualization of the peripheral fundus.

Retinal detachment after congenital cataract surgery may be associated with any category of retinal break, such as small horseshoe tears, atrophic round holes in lattice, oral desinsertion, or giant tears. Atrophic round holes in lattice and oral desinsertion are uncommon. Most retinal detachments are associated with tractional horseshoe tears. Horseshoe tears are related to islands of lattice degeneration or situated at the posterior edge of the vitreous base. The incidence of giant tears (13.5%[42] to 24%[45]) is significantly higher than in unselected retinal detachments. Giant tears are usually observed in eyes with an increased axial length.

VITREOUS GEL

Posterior vitreous detachment is present in the majority of eyes. Condensation of the anterior vitreous gel is a common finding in eyes that have undergone conventional congenital cataract surgery. Most eyes show organized anterior vitreous gel that is adherent to lens remnants. A few eyes show incarceration of vitreous gel in the corneal wound. Histologically, a cyclitic membrane is found in 37% of eyes.[46]

Surgical Management

The basic surgical procedures for retinal detachment management are the same as those used in any retinal detachment. However, vitreous surgery as an adjunct to scleral buckling is required in an increased number of eyes compared with unselected retinal detachments. The indications for vitrectomy are the same as those in any retinal detachment, particularly in the association of severe proliferative vitreoretinopathy and a giant tears. In addition, vitreous surgery is required to improve visualization of the peripheral fundus and to relieve anterior vitreous traction in a number of eyes. When changes in the anterior segment secondary to congenital cataract surgery prevent visualization of the retinal break(s), reconstruction of the anterior segment combined with vitrectomy should be performed as the first step of the surgical procedure for retinal detachment management. This surgical approach makes identification of retinal breaks possible in most cases. It improves the prognosis for retinal reattachment. Therefore, reconstruction of the anterior segment anatomy, and vitrectomy as an adjunct to retinal detachment surgery should be performed rather than an uncontrolled encircling operation in eyes with lens remnants or iris and anterior vitreous gel changes, which prevent visualization of retinal breaks. Choice of the surgical approach for reconstruction of the anterior segment anatomy depends on the extent and severity of congenital cataract surgery sequelae. Thin lens remnants can easily be removed through the pars plana approach using the vitrectomy probe, however, the equatorial remnants of the opaque lens capsule cannot be removed in most cases. Radial cuts are made with scissors to improve visualization of the peripheral fundus. Thick secondary cataracts are best managed through a limbal incision. In such eyes, lens remnants are removed in one piece using alphachymotrypsine. Iris synechiae are freed using a blunt spatula before removal of lens remnants. A sectorial superior iridectomy is performed in all eyes to improve fundus visualization. Then, vitrectomy is performed. Great care is taken to remove the condensed anterior vitreous gel as completely as possible. Any vitreous strand adherent to the cataract wound is cut. After completion of the anterior segment surgery and vitrectomy procedure, thorough examination of the peripheral fundus using the microscope slit lamp and the three-mirror contact lens is carried out with scleral depression to identify the retinal breaks. Choice of the scleral buckling procedure and associated procedure(s) for retinal detachment management is based upon fundus changes revealed by intraoperative fundus examination.

Results

The anatomical success rate achieved by conventional surgery in retinal detachments after congenital cataract surgery was rather poor (50%).[43] Difficulty in visualization of the retinal breaks and vitreous changes related to cataract surgery were the main causes of the unfavorable surgical prognosis. The prognosis for retinal reattachment has been significantly improved by anterior segment reconstruction surgery and vitrectomy combined with retinal detachment surgery.[45] Visual results are modest, however, in a number of patients, owing to ocular defects, such as nystagmus and amblyopia, which are commonly associated with congenital cataract.

REFERENCES

1. Ashrafzadeth MT, Schepens CL, Elzeneiny II, et al: Aphakic and phakic retinal detachment. Arch Ophthalmol 89:476–483, 1973
2. Benson WE, Grand MG, Okun E: Aphakic retinal detachment. Arch Ophthalmol 93:245–249, 1975
3. Bonnet M: Microchirurgie du décollement de la rétine de l'aphake. An Inst Barraquer 16:381–396, 1982–1983
4. Percival SP, Anand V, Das SK: Prevalence of aphakic retinal detachment. Brit J Ophthalmol 67:43–45, 1983
5. Hyams SW, Bialik M, Neumann E: Myopia—aphakia. I prevalence of retinal detachment. Br J Ophthalmol 59:480–482, 1975

6. Clayman HM, Jaffe NS, Light DS, et al: Intraocular lenses, axial length, and retinal detachment. Am J Ophthalmol 92:778–780, 1981

7. Urrets-Zavalia A: Le décollement de la rétine. Paris, Masson 238, 1968

8. Le Mesurier R, Vickers S, Booth-Mason S, Chignell AH: Aphakic retinal detachment. Brit J Ophthalmol 69:737–741, 1985

9. Bronner A, Baikoff G, Charleux J, Flament J, et al: La correction de l'aphakie. Paris, Masson 413–417, 1983

10. Jaffe NS, Clayman HM, Jaffe MS: Retinal detachment in myopic eyes after intracapsular and extracapsular cataract extraction. Am J Ophthalmol 97:48–52, 1984

11. Coonan P, Fung WE, Webster JR, et al: The incidence of retinal detachment following extracapsular cataract extraction. A ten-year study. Ophthalmology 92:1096–1101, 1985

12. Fung WE, Coonan P, Ho BT: Incidence of retinal detachment following extracapsular cataract extraction. A prospective study. Retina 1:232–237, 1981

13. Winslow RL, Taylor BC: Retinal complications following yag laser capsulotomy. Ophthalmology 92:785–789, 1985

14. Ober RR, Wilkinson Ch P, Fiore JV, et al: Rhegmatogenous retinal detachment after neodymium-yag laser capsulotomy in phakic and pseudophakic eyes. Am J Ophthalmol 101:81–89, 1986

15. Aron-Rosa DS, Aron JJ, Cohn HC: Use of a pulsed picosecond Nd-yag laster in 6,664 cases. Am Intraocul Implant Soc J 10:35, 1984

16. Keates RH, Steinert RF, Puliafito CA, Maxwell SK: Long-term follow-up of Nd-yag laser posterior capsulotomy. Am Intraocul Implant Soc J 10:164, 1984

17. Stark WJ, Worthen D, Holladay JT, Murray G: Neodymium-yag lasers. An FDA report. Ophthalmology 92:209–212, 1985

18. Fastenberg DM, Schwartz PL, Lin HZ: Retinal detachment following neodymium-yag laser capsulotomy. Am J Ophthalmol 97:288–291, 1984

19. Bonnet M, Nagao M: Microsurgery of aphakic retinal detachment. Ophthalmologica (Basel) 186:177–182, 1983

20. Menezo JL, Frances J, Suarez Reynolds R: Number and shape of tears in aphakic retinal detachment. Its relationship with different surgical techniques of cataract extraction. Mod Probl Ophthal (Basel) 18:457–463, 1977

21. Norton EW: Retinal detachment in aphakia. Am J Ophthalmol 58:111–124, 1964

22. Benson WE: Aphakic retinal detachment. in Emery JM (Ed) Current concepts in cataract surgery. St. Louis C.V. Mosby 385–405, 1978

23. Wilkinson CP: Retinal detachment following intraocular lens implantation. Ophthalmology 88:410–413, 1981

24. Österlin S: Preludes to retinal detachment in the aphakic eye. Mod Probl Ophthalmol 18:464–467, 1977

25. Gottlieb F: Combined choroidal and retinal detachment. Arch Ophthalmol 88:481–486, 1972

26. Edmund J, Seedorf HM: Retinal detachment in aphakic eyes. Acta Ophthalmol 52:323–333, 1974

27. Cousins S, Boniuk I, Okun E, et al: Pseudophakic retinal detachments in the presence of various IOL types. Ophthalmology 93:1198–1207, 1986

28. Freeman HM, Dobbie JG, Friedman MN: Pseudophakic retinal detachment. Mod Probl Ophthalmol 20:345–353, 1979

29. Ho PC, Tolentino FI: Pseudophakic retinal detachment. Ophthalmology 91:847–852, 1984

30. McDonnell PJ, De La Cruz Z, Green WR: Vitreous incarceration complicating cataract surgery. A light and electron microscopic study. Ophthalmology 93:247–253, 1986

31. Urrets-Zavalia A: Recurent retinal detachment in the aphakic myopic eye. Mod Probl Ophthalmol 12:109–122, 1974

32. Lincoff H, Kreissig I, Farber M: Results of 100 aphakic detachments treated with a temporary balloon buckle. A case against routine encircling operations. Brit J Ophthalmol 69:798–804, 1985

33. Verbraeken H: Pars plana vitrectomy in aphakic retinal detachment. XIV the meeting of the Gonin club Lausanne Sept. 24–28, 1984

34. Norton EW, Machemer R: New approach to the treatment of selected retinal detachments secondary to vitreous loss at cataract surgery. Am J Ophthalmol 72:705–707, 1971

35. Saracco JB, Cornand A, Estachy G, Bense M: Résultats comparatifs du traitement du décollement de l'aphake par sanglage avec et sans ponction (À propos de 120 cas). Bull Soc Ophtalmol Fr 78:497–501, 1978

36. Francois P, Constantinides G: Encircling silicon rod in retinal detachment in aphakia. Mod Probl Ophthalmol 12:109–122, 1974

37. Marion J: Le décollement rétinien de l'aphake. Thèse université Lyon, 1977

38. Lobes L, Grand D: Incidence of cystoid macular edema following scleral buckling procedure. Arch Ophthalmol 98:1230–1232, 1980

39. Meredith TA, Reeser F, Toppino T, Aaberg T: Cystoid macular edema after retinal detachment surgery. Ophthalmology 87:1090–1095, 1980

40. Bonnet M, Bievelez B, Noel A, Bensoussan B, Pingault C: Fluorescein angiography after retinal detachment microsurgery. Graefe's Arch Clin Exp Ophthalmol 221:35–40, 1983

41. Bonnet M: Prognosis of cystoid macular edema after retinal detachment repair. Graefe's Arch Clin Exp Ophthalmol 224:13–17, 1986

42. Toyofuku H, Hirose T, Schepens CL: Retinal detachment following congenital cataract surgery. I preoperative findings in 114 eyes. Arch Ophthalmol 98:669–675, 1980

43. Kanski JJ, Elington AR, Daniel R: Retinal detachment after congenital cataract surgery Br J Ophthalmol 58:92–95, 1974

44. McLeod D: Giant retinal tears after central vitrectomy Brit J Ophthalmol 69:96–98, 1985

45. Bonnet M: unpublished data

46. Cordes FC: Retinal detachment following congenital cataract surgery. A study of 112 enucleated eyes. Am J Ophthalmol 50:716–729, 1960

22
Retinal Detachment Associated with Retinoschisis

Retinoschisis includes two distinct fundus lesions: (1) X-chromosome-linked retinoschisis and (2) senile retinoschisis.

X-CHROMOSOME-LINKED RETINOSCHISIS

X-chromosome-linked retinoschisis, or juvenile retinoschisis, is characterized by a splitting of the retina at the level of the nerve fiber layer.[1] In most cases the disease is recognized because of poor central visual acuity disclosed by routine school examination, or by possibly, routine fundus examination of the brother(s) of the young boy affected by the disease. In a few cases, the disease is recognized in boys under 3 years of age with early complications, particularly vitreous hemorrhage.

Fundus disease is bilateral. Fundus lesions consist mainly of macular retinoschisis, peripheral retinoschisis, and vitreous veils.

Stellate cystoid retinoschisis of the macula is present in all affected patients.[2,3]

Retinoschisis of the peripheral fundus includes two main types of lesions: (1) a mottled appearance of the retina and (2) large intraretinal translucent cysts. In most cases the mottled retinal appearance involves the superior quadrants, whereas the large intraretinal cysts involve the inferior quadrants. Large, bullous retinal cysts extending to the superior quadrants are usually observed only in boys under 4 years of age. It seems likely that the mottled appearance of the superior retina seen in older boys or adults results from spontaneous flattening of bullous retinoschisis seen in very young boys.[4] The inner layer of large intraretinal cysts usually shows large holes (Fig. 191). Most branches of the retinal vessels are situated in the inner layer of the retinoschisis, however branches of the retinal vessels may also be found in the outer layer. Tufts of new vessels can develop at the edges of the retinoschisis or at the edges of the inner layer holes. New vessels are associated with extensive capillary nonperfusion of the peripheral retina.[5] They may bleed or regress spontaneously.

Translucent mobile veils in the vitreous cavity are a constant clinical finding, which are mainly localized in the temporal half of the vitreous cavity.[4] In most cases they are free in the vitreous cavity. These translucent, intravitreal membranes are closely similar to those seen in Wagner's disease.

The natural course of X-linked retinoschisis is not yet fully understood. The disease may progress, remain stationary, or spontaneously regress.[4] Regression is characterized by flattening of the intraretinal cysts and formation of pigmented scars, which outline the boundaries of the schisis and the inner holes.

Two severe complications of X-chromosome-linked retinoschisis may occur: (1) vitreous hemorrhage and (2) retinal detachment.

Vitreous hemorrhage is the most frequent complication. It is probably caused by vitreous traction on the retinal vessels, which extend throughout the elevated inner layer of the schisis cavity. Hemorrhage in the schisis cavity[6] is uncommon.

Retinal detachment complicating juvenile retinoschisis is infrequent. There are wide variations in the incidence of retinal detachment complicating juvenile retinoschisis reported in the literature: 22%,[7] 13%,[4] 7.6%,[3] and 5.2%.[8] The author has followed more than 30 patients with juvenile retinoschisis for several years. Three of them developed vitreous hemorrhage; only one of them developed retinal detachment.

The most appropriate management of retinal de-

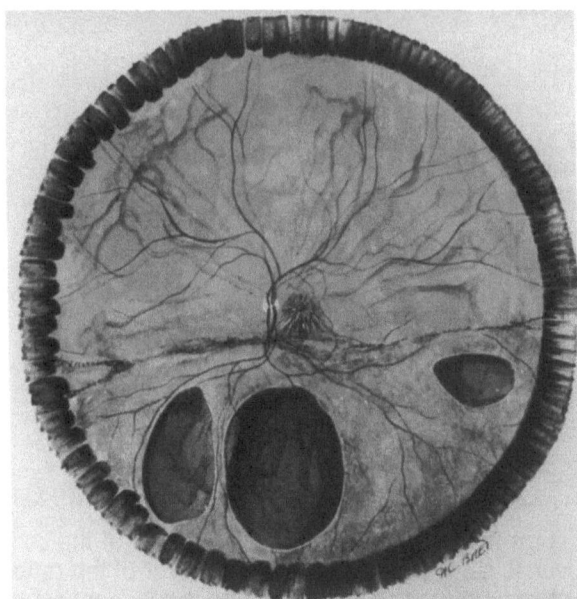

Figure 191. X-chromosome-linked retinoschisis in a 3-year-old boy. Bullous retinoschisis of the inferior retina is associated with three large holes in the inner layer of intraretinal cysts. Peripheral retinoschisis is associated with stellate appearance of the macula and pigmented lines at the superior border of the schisis (left eye. Right eye shows similar changes).

tachment complicating X-linked retinoschisis has not yet been clearly established. Restricted experience of retina surgeons in this specific field probably accounts for this fact. The prognosis for retinal reattachment after scleral buckling is poor: 25% anatomical success rate.[4] It is not known whether vitrectomy, which has been used in the treatment of vitreous hemorrhage in selected cases,[9] may improve the prognosis of retinal detachment. The retina may spontaneously reattach.[8] The value of prophylactic treatment with photocoagulation or cryotreatment, in an attempt to prevent retinal detachment remains to be established.

Retinal detachment is an uncommon complication of juvenile retinoschisis. Prophylactic photocoagulation may have adverse effects. In Brockhurst's series,[10] photocoagulation applied to the retinoschisis cavity caused breaks in the outer layer or both layers and subsequent retinal detachment. Photocoagulation applied posteriorly to the schisis cavity seems unnecessary, since the disease is self-limited to the inferior retina.[4] Photocoagulation of capillary nonperfusion areas of the peripheral retina in eyes with new-vessels has been suggested,[5] however, the new-vessels usually regress spontaneously.

Observation with periodic fundus examination probably is the least hazardous management of patients with X-linked juvenile retinoschisis.

SENILE RETINOSCHISIS

Acquired or senile retinoschisis is a common, asymptomatic, and benign fundus condition in adults.

The condition is frequent: it is present in 3.7% of the population and in 7% of individuals over 40 years of age.[11] It is significantly more frequent in hyperopic patients. The condition is revealed by routine fundus examination. It is asymptomatic and bilateral.

Clinical Findings and Differential Diagnosis

CLINICAL FINDINGS

Senile retinoschisis is asymptomatic and revealed by routine fundus examination. It is bilateral in 82% of individuals.[11] The area of maximal involvement is the inferior temporal quadrant in 74% of eyes.[12]

Histologically, two types of senile retinoschisis have been described: (1) flat[13] or typical,[14] and (2) bullous[13] or reticular.[14] Flat retinoschisis is confined to the retina anterior to the equator and exhibits no break in either layer. Bullous retinoschisis often extends posterior to the equator and frequently shows outer layer breaks.[13–14]

Clinically, flat retinoschisis and bullous retinoschisis can also be distinguished. However, the differences between the two relate to the height and posterior extent of the schisis rather than the basic clinical findings, which are similar in both cases.

Splitting of the peripheral retina, which characterizes degenerative retinoschisis, results in an increased retinal thickness. This is best recognized by slit lamp examination, which shows an increased distance beween the outer retinal layers and the internal limiting membrane. Retinoschisis is transparent and may escape detection during a rapid fundus examination. It is best recognized using retroillumination of the inner retinal layer adjacent to the slit illumination. The inner surface is convex toward the vitreous cavity. It is immobile with eye movement. The inner layer of the retinoschisis shows a beaten metal appearance, which is characteristic. Multiple, yellow-white, glistening dots are present in the inner layer in 70% of the eyes examined.[11] Anteriorly, the retinoschisis extends up to the ora serrata. The posterior extension varies. Extension posterior to the equator is seen in 43% of patients.[11] Posterior extension up to the inferior temporal vascular arcade is exceptional. The author has seen only one such case in a 70-year-old woman. The lesion has remained unchanged for 10 years. Retinal breaks in the outer layer are present in approximately

10% of eyes. They are usually irregular in shape, and roughly round or oval. In most cases they are located posteriorly to the equator. Characterstically, the edges of large outer layer breaks tend to roll inward. Inner layer breaks are uncommon.

DIFFERENTIAL DIAGNOSIS

The clinical characteristics of senile retinoschisis are typical and specific. Therefore, the lesion should easily be distinguished from other fundus lesions that are also associated with an increased thickness of the neurosensory retina, in particular, primary and secondary cystoid degeneration of the peripheral retina. Confusion between degenerative retinoschisis and secondary cystoid retinal degeneration associated with longstanding duration retinal detachment is a common error of beginners. A number of patients with longstanding retinal detachment associated with secondary cystoid degeneration are referred to the University Eye Clinics with the diagnosis of progressive degenerative retinoschisis. Advice is asked for an indication for photocoagulation treatment at the posterior edge of the pseudoretinoschisis, in an attempt to prevent further posterior extension. Other patients are referred with the diagnosis of degenera-

tive retinoschisis complicated by retinal detachment. Most patients referred to the author with the diagnosis of senile retinoschisis complicated by retinal detachment actually show longstanding subclinical retinal detachment complicated by secondary cystoid degeneration of the detached retina.

Longstanding retinal detachment associated with secondary cystoid degeneration of the detached retina may remain subclinical for an extended period of time. Retinal detachment can be either rhegmatogenous or tractional. Most longstanding rhegmatogenous retinal detachments associated with secondary cystoid degeneration of the detached retina are caused by oral dialysis (see p. 184) and round atrophic holes in lattice (see p. 175). In a few cases retinal detachment is caused by a tiny horseshoe tear in eyes with partial posterior vitreous detachment confined to the area of the detachment (Fig. 192). Localized longstanding traction retinal detachments associated with secondary cystoid degeneration of the detached retina are observed in a series of fundus diseases, such as proliferative diabetic retinopathy, Eales' disease, and cicatricial retinopathy of prematurity.

Longstanding traction retinal detachments associated with secondary cystoid degeneration of the detached retina are easily differentiated from senile

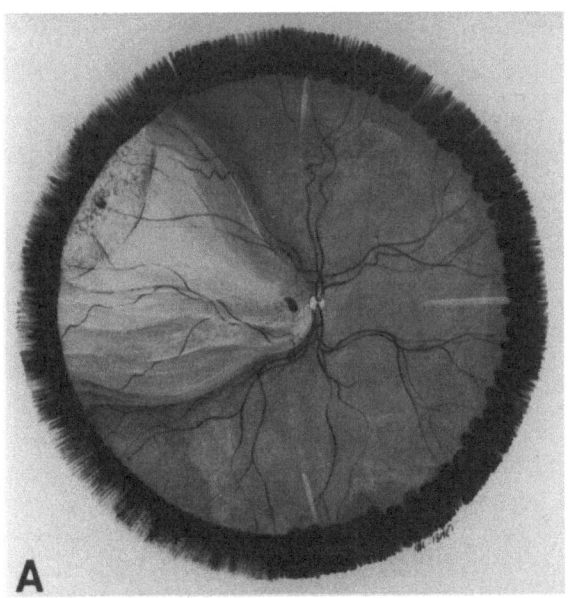 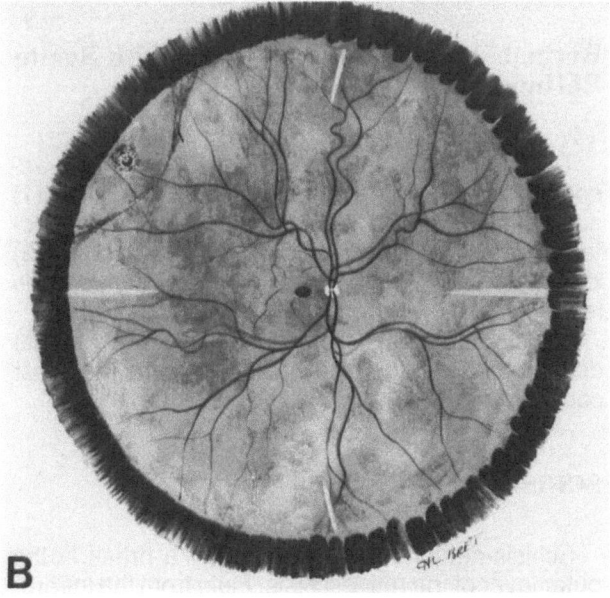

Figure 192. Two-step rhegmatogenous retinal detachment mimicking senile retinoschisis complicated by retinal detachment in a 61 year old patient. (A) Preoperative fundus appearance. Retinal detachment is associated with a tiny horse-shoe tear at 10 o'clock. It consists of two components: 1) a peripheral detachment with secondary cystoid degeneration of the detached retina outlined by a pigmented demarcation line and 2) a posterior detachment of recent onset with mobile retinal folds. (B) Postoperative fundus appearance. Total retinal reattachment was achieved by two cryoapplications on the tiny tear associated with intravitreal injection of 0.4 cc of pure SF6. The pseudo-retinoschisis has flattened with no sequelae but the pigmented demarcation line.

retinoschisis because of their specific clinical features and the associated lesions of the underlying fundus disease.

In contrast, longstanding rhegmatogenous retinal detachments may be misinterpreted as progressive retinoschisis or senile retinoschisis, complicated by retinal detachment because the retinal break, which is very small, and very peripheral in most cases, may be difficult to disclose (Fig. 192). Clinical findings associated with longstanding retinal detachments are helpful in differentiating the lesion from senile retinoschisis. These clinical findings include: (1) pigmented demarcation lines, (2) subretinal proliferation, (3) intraretinal macrocysts,, and (4) absolute scotoma. Equatorial retinal new-vessels in the detached retina may also be present (see p. 175), but the latter clinical finding is uncommon. When one or, most often, several of such clinical fndings are present, repeated fundus examination should be performed to identify the small full-thickness retinal break(s). Segmental scleral buckling and cryotreatment, strictly confined to the area of the tiny retinal break(s), will result in spontaneous absorption of subretinal fluid and total flattening of the pseudoretinoschisis within a few days (Fig. 192). After retinal reattachment no sequela of cystoid degeneration of the peripheral retina and intraretinal macrocyst is detectable by fundus examination.

Retinal Detachment Associated with Senile Retinoschisis

Three distinct types of retinal detachment associated with senile retinoschisis may be seen: (1) schisis-detachment, (2) rhegmatogenous retinal detachment related to the retinoschisis, and (3) rhegmatogenous retinal detachment unrelated to the retinoschisis.

Schisis-detachment and rhegmatogenous retinal detachment unrelated to the schisis are the most common.

SCHISIS-DETACHMENT

Schisis-detachment is caused by a break in the outer layer of the retinoschisis. Fluid from the intraretinal schisis cavity leaks toward the subretinal space through the outer layer break. This type of detachment has been documented histopathologically.[13,15] This detachment is self-limited and asymptomatic in most cases.[12,16] It is revealed by routine fundus examination. The fundus changes are subtle and may escape the observer. The outer layer of the

schisis cavity is detached from the pigment epithelium in the vicinity of an outer layer break. In a number of eyes, the outer layer break shows rolled edges. A pigmented demarcation line is helpful in identifying the presence of a schisis-detachment.[12] Outer layer breaks in senile retinoschisis are associated with a high incidence of schisis-detachment (58%).[12] Schisis-detachments are asymptomatic and relatively nonprogressive in most cases.[12] No treatment is required in most cases. Only schisis-detachment involving the posterior pole may require treatment when detachment of the outer retinal layer involves or threatens the macula. Photocoagulation treatment of the outer layer break with simultaneous scleral depression in combination with gas injection is the least traumatic surgical technique in such eyes. Pars plana vitrectomy may be required to create intravitreal space for injection of a gas bubble of therapeutic volume.

RETINAL DETACHMENT RELATED TO THE RETINOSCHISIS

Symptomatic retinal detachment related to the retinoschisis is caused by a combination of outer layer

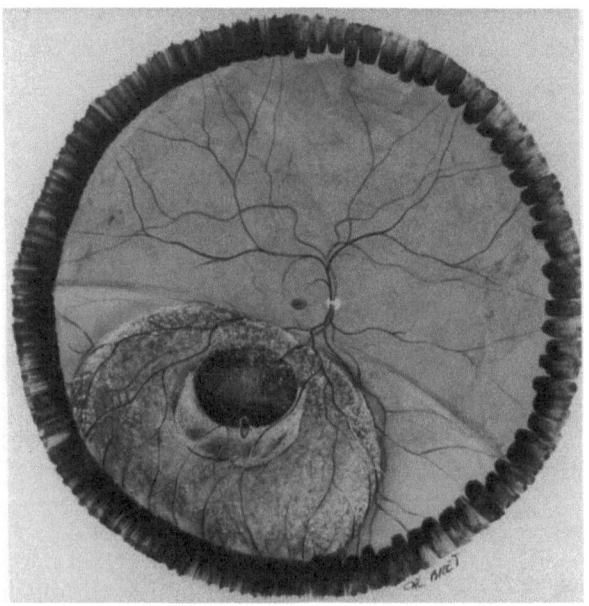

Figure 193. Acquired retinoschisis complicated by retinal detachment in a 45-year-old patient. Retinal detachment extends beyond the schisis cavity. It is associated with a large outer layer break and a small inner layer break. Characteristically the edge of the outer layer break is rolled toward the schisis cavity.

breaks and inner layer break(s). It is characterized by acute visual symptoms, mainly floaters and visual field defects. Fundus examination shows retinal detachment extending beyond the schisis cavity limits and communicating directly with an outer layer break[16] (Fig. 193). The inner layer break is usually small and tractional. Partial or complete posterior vitreous detachment is present. This type of detachment is most uncommon (0.05%).[16] Retinal reattachment, with persistence of the retinoschisis, can be achieved by segmental scleral buckling of the inner layer break(s).

RETINAL DETACHMENT UNRELATED TO THE RETINOSCHISIS

Patients with senile retinoschisis may develop rhegmatogenous retinal detachment caused by horseshoe tears unrelated to the retinoschisis. The horseshoe tears are situated in areas distant from the retinoschisis. They develop at the time of senile posterior vitreous detachment. The management and the prognosis of such retinal detachments are not modified by the association of the unrelated retinoschisis. This type of symptomatic retinal detachment is the most common in eyes with senile retinoschisis.

Prophylactic Treatment

The indications for prophylactic treatment by photocoagulation or cryotherapy in senile retinoschisis remain controversial. Prophylactic treatment does not prevent progression of retinoschisis and is associated with a relatively high incidence of complications, such as retinal detachment, maculopathy, vitreous hemorrhage, and proliferative vitreoretinopathy.[17–23] Retinal detachment caused by senile retinoschisis is infrequent (0.05%).[16] Therefore, the most appropriate management of senile retinoschisis is observation with periodic retinal examination. Fundus examination is carried out at 2-year-intervals when no break is present in the retinoschisis layers. It is carried out at 6 month intervals when outer layer breaks are present. Nontreatment of uncomplicated senile retinoschisis carries less risk of complications than does prophylactic treatment[12]

REFERENCES

1. Yanoff M, Rahn EK, Zimmerman LE: Histopathology of juvenile retinoschisis. Arch Ophthalmol 79:49–53, 1968
2. Deutman AF: Twenty vitreoretinal dystrophies. In, Krill AE (ed) Krill's hereditary retinal and choroidal diseases. Hagerstown: Harper and Row 1977, 11:1043–1062
3. Francois P, Turut P, Soltysik C, Hache JC: Le retinoschisis juvenile lié au sexe. Arch Ophtalmol (Paris) 36:113–126, 1976
4. Rousseau A: Congenital retinoschisis. In, Blankenship G, Daicker B, Gailloud B, Gloor B, et al: Currents concepts in diagnosis and treatment of vitreoretinal diseases. Dev Ophthalmol 2, Basel, Karger 43–52, 1981
5. Brancato R, Menchini U, Pece A: Retinoschisis maculaire idiopathique du sujet jeune associé À des néovaisseaux prérétiniens et papillaires. J Fr Ophtalmol 7:685–688, 1984
6. Conway BP, Welch RB: X-chromosome-linked juvenile retinoschisis with hemorrhagic retinal cyst. Am J Ophthalmol 83:853–855, 1977
7. Kraushar MF, Schepens CL, Kaplan JA, Freeman HM: Congenital retinoschisis. In, Bellows JG (ed) Contemporary ophthalmology honoring Sir Steward-Duke-Elder, Baltimore, Williams and Wilkins, 265–290, 1972
8. Verdaguer J: Juvenile retinal detachment Am J Ophthalmol 93: 145–156, 1982
9. Schulman J, Peyman GA, Jednock N, Larson B: Indications for vitrectomy in congenital retinoschisis Brit J Ophthalmol 69:482–486, 1985
10. Brockhurst RJ: Photocoagulation in congenital retinoschisis Arch Ophthalmol 84:158–165, 1970
11. Byer NE: Clinical study of senile retinoschisis Arch Ophthalmol 79:36–44, 1968
12. Byer NE: Long-term natural history study of senile retinoschisis with implications for management. Ophthalmology 93:1127–1136, 1986
13. Foos RY: Senile retinoschisis. Relationship to cystoid degeneration. Trans Am Acad Ophthalmol Otolaryngol 74:33–50, 1970
14. Straatsma BR, Foos RY: Typical and reticular degenerative retinoschisis. Am J Ophthalmol 75:551–575, 1973
15. Göttinger W: Retinoschisis und ablatio. Klin Monatsbl Augenheilkd 169:14–21, 1976
16. Gutman FA: Discussion. Byer N.E. Long term natural history study of senile retinoschisis with implications for management. Ophthalmology 93:1136–1137, 1986
17. Dorbie JG: Cryotherapy in the management of senile retinoschisis. Trans Am Acad Ophthalmol Otolaryngol 73:1047–1059, 1969
18. Shea M, Schepens CL, Von Pirquet SR: Retinoschisis. I—senile type: a clinical report of one hundred seven cases. Arch Ophthalmol 63:1–9, 1960
19. Okun E, Cibis PA: The role of photocoagulation in the management of retinoschisis. Arch Ophthalmol 72:309–314, 1964
20. Boniuk I, Okun E, Johnston GP, Arribas N: Xenon photocoagulation Vs cryotherapy in the prevention of retinal detachment. Mod Probl Ophthalmol 12:1281–1292, 1974
21. Constantinides G, Madelain F, Francois P: Résultats du traitement par photocoagulation du rétinoschisis bulleux. Bull Soc Ophtalmol Fr 76:817–818, 1976
22. Gerhard JP, Risse JF, Flament J: La photocoagulation dans le traitement du retinoschisis. Indications et techniques. Bull Soc Ophtalmol Fr 76:813–814, 1976
23. Forest A, Girard P, Bodard E, et al: Le traitement chirurgical du retinoschisis. J Fr Ophtalmol 2:109–114, 1979

23

Retinal Detachment Complicating Proliferative Retinopathies

Proliferative retinopathies can be complicated by two types of retinal detachment: (1) traction retinal detachment and (2) rhegmatogenous retinal detachment.

Proliferative retinopathies that may be complicated by retinal detachment include: (1) diabetic retinopathy, (2) tributary retinal vein occlusion, (3) Eale's disease, (4) sickle-cell hemoglobinopathy, (5) retinopathy of prematurity, (6) autosomal dominant exsudative vitreoretinopathy, and (7) retinal angiomatosis (Von Hippel's disease).

In France, proliferative diabetic retinopathy is the leading cause of retinal detachments caused by proliferative retinopathies. A few retinal detachments associated with tributary retinal vein occlusion are also observed. Retinal detachments complicating other proliferative retinopathies, including retinopathy of prematurity, are infrequent.

The basic principles of the treatment of such retinal detachments are similar, regardless of the etiology. They include (1) relief of vitreous traction and (2) specific treatment of the retinal break(s) when a rhegmatogenous component is associated with traction detachment. Development of closed vitreous surgery has brought about significant improvement in the treatment of these difficult detachments. Vitreous surgery in particular, has made hopeless cases, such as traction detachments involving the macula in advanced proliferative diabetic retinopathy, and late stages of retinopathy of prematurity, amenable to surgical management. The surgical difficulties encountered in the treatment of these detachments vary widely from one case to another, depending on the extent and severity of the vitreoretinal changes. The prognosis for permanent retinal reattachment and visual recovery also shows a wide range of variations depending on the etiology of the proliferative retinal disease, the stage of the disease at the time of surgical management, and the patient's age.

RETINAL DETACHMENTS COMPLICATING DIABETIC RETINOPATHY

Traction retinal detachment is one of the most severe complications of proliferative diabetic retinopathy and occurs at a late stage of the disease. It is caused by contraction of the posterior vitreous cortex, secondary to fibrovascular proliferation and it may be associated with a rhegmatogenous component.

Before the development of closed vitrectomy, a significant number of cases were hopeless and left untreated. Selected cases were managed by transvitreous membrane cutting and scleral buckling.[1-6] Retinal reattachment could initially be obtained by these techniques in a number of cases.[5,6] However, these methods did not remove the cause of traction retinal detachment and a significant number of cases failed to reattach. In addition retinal reattachment in eyes successfully operated on, was often of short duration owing to the continuing progression of the vitreoretinal disease.

Closed vitrectomy has made hopeless cases amenable to surgical management.[7-10] It has improved the initial and long-term anatomical results.[8,11-17] However, the percentage of severe postoperative complications resulting in loss of any light perception is still high. The visual results in successful cases are often poor, owing to the severity of underlying retinal disease.

The incidence of traction retinal detachment complicating proliferative diabetic retinopathy has been significantly decreased since the introduction of photocoagulation treatment of diabetic retinopathy by Meyer-Schwickerath[18] and the development of panretinal photocoagulation.[19–23] Due to early panretinal photocoagulation of proliferative diabetic retinopathy, the incidence of traction diabetic retinal detachment has become significantly low in the author's own experience.[24,25]

A large number of diabetic patients are treated in the author's clinic, however severe complications of proliferative diabetic retinopathy account for only about 6% of all vitrectomies performed there during the last years.[26] Seventy percent of diabetic patients who required vitrectomy have been referred from foreign countries.[15] However the large series of vitrectomies for complications of proliferative diabetic retinopathy reported in the recent literature[8,11,13,16,17] demonstrate that severe complications of this disease have not been totally eradicated by photocoagulation treatment.

Pathophysiology

Retinal detachment complicating proliferative diabetic retinopathy, either purely tractional, or tractional and rhegmatogenous, is caused by vitreous changes secondary to fibrovascular proliferation.

TRACTION RETINAL DETACHMENT

Traction retinal detachment is caused by contraction of the posterior vitreous cortex. Characteristically, the vitreous gel is partially detached from the retina. Areas of posterior vitreous detachment extend between sites of firm vitreoretinal adhesion.

Firm vitreoretinal adhesions are located at the sites of fibrovascular proliferation. Most islands of fibrovascular prolilferation and firm vitreoretinal adhesion are typically located in the close vicinity of the posterior pole, particularly along the temporal vascular arcades.

Contraction of the proliferative tissue on the posterior vitreous surface exerts traction on areas of firm vitreoretinal adhesions. In most cases the traction forces are oriented in two main directions: (1) an anterior-posterior direction, between the vitreous base and areas of fibrovascular proliferation on the posterior pole and (2) a tangential direction between areas of fibrovascular proliferation. In a number of cases the condensed posterior vitreous cortex is firmly adherent to the temporal vascular arcades and the optic disc.

RHEGMATOGENOUS-TRACTION RETINAL DETACHMENT

The traction forces that cause retinal detachment are basically similar to those of purely tractional detachment.

Retinal breaks are caused by strong vitreous traction and retinal atrophy. In most cases the breaks are located posteriorly, in atrophic retina, and in close vicinity of fibrovascular proliferative islands.

Clinical Findings

The complexity of retinal detachments complicating proliferative diabetic retinopathy requires detailed preoperative examination with the slit lamp and the three-mirror contact lens using bright illumination and high magnification. In a significant number of cases, however, detailed preoperative examination is uneasy, due to poor pupillary dilation, lens opacities or vitreous hemorrhage. The complexity of fundus lesions depends on four main parameters: (1) the extent of retinal detachment, (2) the presence, or absence, of retinal breaks, (3) the location, extent, and morphology of the fibrovascular proliferation, and (4) the extent and topography of partial vitreous detachment.

RETINAL DETACHMENT

Two types of retinal detachment can be observed: tractional and combined rhegmatogenous-traction retinal detachments. Rhegmatogenous-traction retinal detachment is less frequent than traction retinal detachment.

Traction Retinal Detachment. The clinical characteristics of traction retinal detachments are as follows:

The detachment is partial (Fig. 194). It is confined to the posterior pole or the midperiphery of the fundus in most cases. Advanced and severe cases may show an extensive detachment. Even in such cases, however, the detachment does not involve the preequatorial region. Limited detachments are shallow in most cases. The height of the detachment shows wide topographical variations. The maximum height of the detachment is located in the vicinity of retinal proliferation and vitreoretinal adhesions. The anterior surface of the detachment is concave, and the detachment is fixed. Progression of traction retinal detachment is most gradual. Progression occurs in approximately 40% of eyes.[27] Progression of extramacular traction detachment toward the macula is

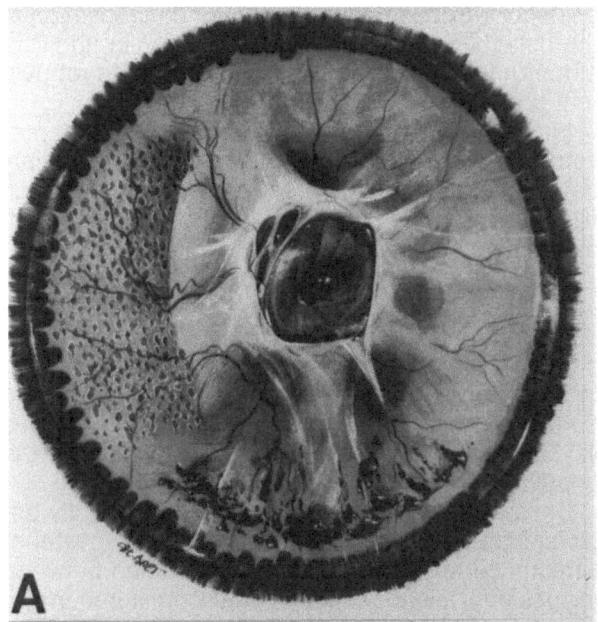 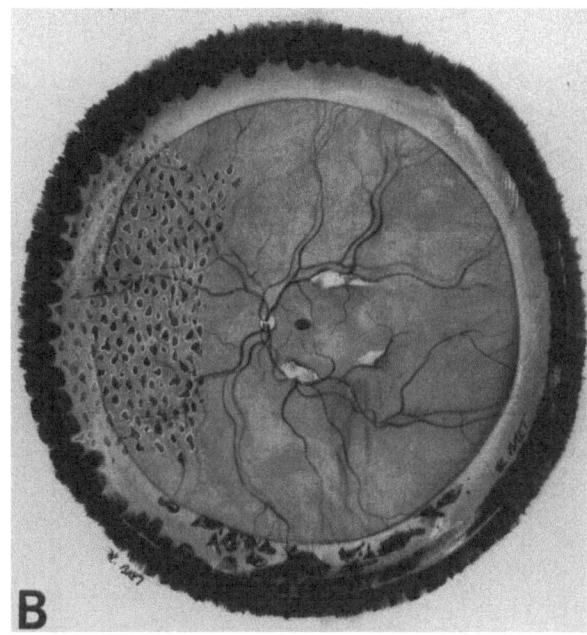

Figure 194. Traction retinal detachment complicating proliferative diabetic retinopathy in a 31-year-old patient. (A) Preoperative fundus appearance: Retinal detachment is confined to the posterior pole and the midperiphery of the fundus. It is associated with fibrous proliferation on the optic disc and along the temporal arcades. Photocoagulation scars are visible in the nasal quadrants. Traction detachment is associated with intravitreal blood in the inferior fundus. (B) Postoperative fundus appearance: retinal reattachment has been achieved by vitrectomy. Small islands of fibrous tissue remain on the temporal arcades.

observed in approximately 15% of eyes per year.[27,28] Traction retinal detachment may improve spontaneously in some cases.

Rhegmatogenous-Traction Retinal Detachment. When a retinal break develops, a rhegmatogenous retinal detachment converts the tent-like configuration of traction retinal detachment to a ballooning retinal detachment with a convex, undulating surface (Fig. 195). Progression of the detachment is often rapid, and subretinal fluid spreads to the peripheral fundus in most cases. Such clinical findings should lead to a meticulous search for retinal break(s).

In contrast with traction retinal detachment, rhegmatogenous-traction retinal detachment never improves spontaneously.

RETINAL BREAKS

Thorough examination of the fundus to disclose retinal break(s) should be repeated when the clinical characteristics of the detached retina are those of a detachment with a rhegmatogenous component.

Characteristically, retinal breaks are located posteriorly to the equator (Fig. 195). The posterior location of retinal breaks in diabetic retinal detachment is nearly a constant finding. However, careful examination of the periphery should not be omitted, since approximately 10% of breaks are located anteriorly to the equator.[5] In most cases the retinal breaks are located in atrophic retina adjacent to fibrovascular proliferation or along retinal blood vessels.

Retinal breaks are small; breaks as large as one disc diameter in size are uncommon. They are round or oval in shape. Most eyes have only one or two break(s). Breaks may be difficult to differentiate from intraretinal cysts, which are common in tractional retinal detachments of long duration. They may be hidden by fibrovascular proliferation or hemorrhage. In a few cases, a retinal break suspected on the configuration of the detachment that cannot be identified preoperatively may be found only intraoperatively.

FIBROVASCULAR PROLIFERATION

The degree, extent, and location of the fibrovascular proliferation associated with the retinal detachment show a wide range of variations. The amount

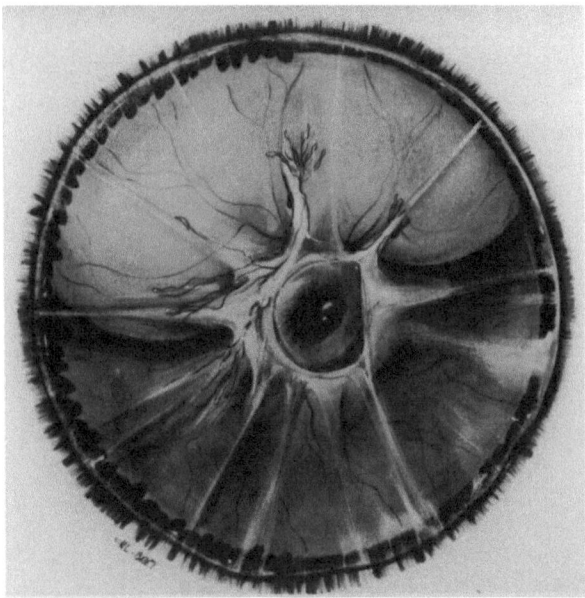

Figure 195. Rhegmatogenous-traction retinal detachment complicating proliferative diabetic retinopathy in a 56-year-old patient. Tent-like detachment of the posterior pole is associated with a bullous detachment of the superior retina. A small posterior break is present at twelve o'clock along fibrovascular tissue. Fundus changes are associated with rubeosis iridis (see Fig. 196).

of active new vessels in the fibrovascular tissue also shows important variations. Most traction retinal detachments associated with active new vessels are also associated with vitreous hemorrhage. Their surgical management is more difficult due to the potential for intraoperative bleeding. Surgical management is often easier and the postoperative outcome better in retinal detachments associated with proliferative tissue that is mainly fibrous, particularly in eyes previously treated by photocoagulation.

In most traction retinal detachments involving the macula, fibrovascular tissue extends from the optic disc in an arcuate direction along the superior and inferior temporal arcades. Fibrovascular tissue often extends also, although to a lesser degree, on the nasal side of the optic disc. Isolated islands of fibrovascular tissue may also be present in the midperiphery of the fundus.

VITREOUS BODY

Modifications of the vitreous body in diabetic traction retinal detachment were first described by Tolentino et al.,[29] and are still constant findings.

They include liquefaction of the vitreous gel, partial

posterior vitreous detachment, and condensation of the detached posterior vitreous cortex. In addition, hemorrhages of the vitreous cavity and the retrovitreal space may be present.

In eyes with dense vitreous hemorrhage that prevent fundus examination, the diagnosis of retinal detachment is made by preoperative A- and B-scan ultrasonography. Precise evaluation of the vitroretinal anatomy is made intraoperatively.

The degree and extent of vitreous gel liquefaction vary depending on the patient's age, as well as the duration and severity of proliferative diabetic retinopathy. The vitreous gel shows extensive liquefaction in most proliferative diabetic retinopathies of long duration. In contrast, it remains often highly viscous in young diabetic patients with florid proliferative retinopathy.

Characteristically, the vitreous gel is partially detached from the retina. The condensed posterior vitreous cortex has a funnel-configuration between the posterior islands of fibrovascular proliferation and the vitreous base. Posteriorly, the partially detached posterior vitreous cortex bridges between the islands of fibrovascular tissue. Localized vitreoretinal adhesions are present in areas of new vessels, along the major retinal vessels, in particular the temporal arcades, and in the proximity of the optic disc.

ASSOCIATED CLINICAL FINDINGS

Complete clinical evaluation of diabetic retinal detachment should include additional investigations, which can provide useful information with regard to management and prognosis.

When the media are sufficiently clear, panretinal fundus fluorescein angiography is performed. It provides useful information regarding the stage of the retinal new-vessels. Profuse dye leakage is indicative of florid neovascularization. In such cases photocoagulation treatment of the attached retina should be performed. When vitrectomy is required because the macula is detached, photocoagulation treatment of the attached retina is performed 2–3 weeks before surgery. This therapeutic approach decreases the risk of uncontrolled intraoperative bleeding and improves the postoperative outcome.[13,15–17]

In all cases clinical examination includes complete eye and systemic examination. Assessment of the visual function and the potential for postoperative visual recovery includes visual acuity measurement, light localization evaluation, and E.R.G. A nonrecordable E.R.G. is not an absolute contraindication for surgical management. It is a sign, however, of poor prognosis.[15] In such eyes, adequate evaluation of light perception and localization has a major value in the therapeutic decision. In addition, visually evoked or electrically-evoked potentials are performed. Surgery is contraindicated when light localization is inaccurate and the evoked potentials are nonrecordable.

Biomicroscopic examination of the anterior segment is first performed on the nondilated pupil to disclose iris neovascularization of the pupillary margin and the anterior chamber angle. The presence of iris new-vessels is not an absolute contraindication for treatment. However the prognosis is more guarded.[15–17] Incipient rubeosis iridis may be invisible in highly pigmented eyes. It will be disclosed by iris fluorescein angiography.

Biomicroscopy of the anterior segment is then performed on a dilated pupil to assess the lens status. Lens opacities will make vitreous surgery more difficult to perform and increase the likelihood of late postoperative cataract. Lens removal before vitrectomy is necessary when lens opacities prevent satisfactory visualization of the fundus. However aphakia is associated with a more guarded postoperative prognosis,[15,16,30–33] therefore, lens removal should be avoided whenever possible.

Iris fluorescein angiography makes it possible to disclose subtle iris new-vessels that may be invisible by biomicroscopic examination. The absence of iris dye leakage is a sign of good prognosis. In eyes with rubeosis iridis, the extent and degree of iris dye leakage are correlated with the prognosis (Fig. 196).[15,34]

Measurement of intraocular pressure is routinely performed. Surgery for retinal detachment management is contraindicated in eyes with neovascular glaucoma.

Choroidal thickness on the posterior pole is measured by A-scan ultrasonography. Increased choroidal thickness over 2 mm is a sign of poor prognosis.

Complete evaluation of diabetes mellitus and associated complications particularly obliterative arterial disease, renal, and cardiac failure are also important parameters to be taken into account in determining indications for surgical management of the vitreoretinal disease.

Indications for Surgical Management

A number of parameters should be taken into account for the indication of surgical management of diabetic retinal detachment. These parameters are related to the specific clinical characteristics of the detachment, the associated clinical findings (see above), and the condition of the other eye.

An indication for surgical management is considered in eyes with traction retinal detachment involving the macula and eyes with rhegmatogenous-traction retinal detachment.

Tractional retinal detachment that does not extend to the macula may remain stable or even improve without surgery.[27] Therefore, owing to the hazards involved by vitreous surgery in diabetic eyes, traction retinal detachments that do not extend to the macula are not an indication for surgery. The patients are followed at regular intervals. An indication for surgical management is considered when there is a documented progression to the macula.

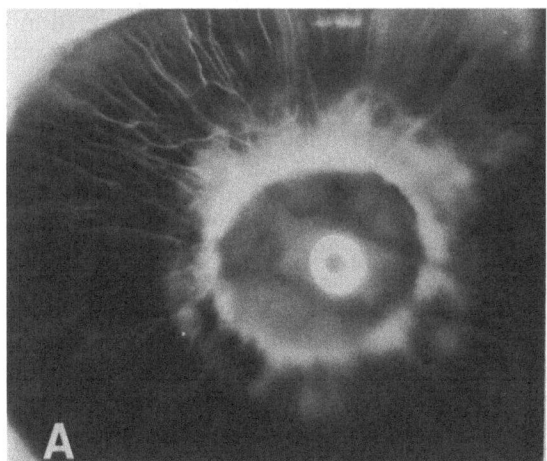 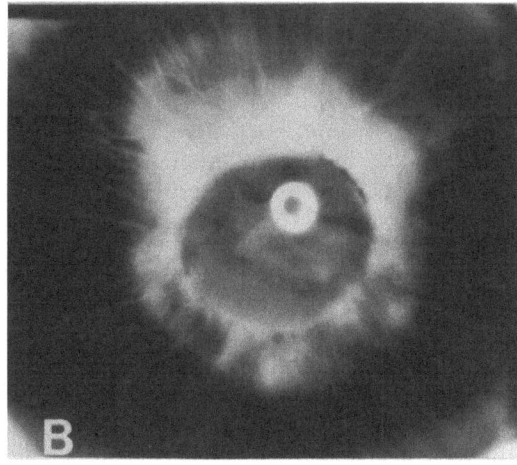

Figure 196. Iris fluorescein angiography in retinal detachment complicating proliferative diabetic retinopathy (Fundus of the same eye is shown in Figure 195). (A) Early phase shows early dye leakage on 360° of the pupil. (B) Late phase shows profuse dye leakage. In spite of the high likelihood of postoperative neovascular glaucoma, retinal reattachment was achieved by vitrectomy combined with extensive cryotreatment of the hypoxic retina and gas injection. Iris dye leakage partially regressed postoperatively.

Whenever possible ablation of the hypoxic attached retina by argon laser photocoagulation treatment is perfomed in eyes with traction detachment and florid new vessels.

Preoperative photocoagulation treatment improves the prognosis in eyes requiring surgical management.[15,16] In any case it decreases the risk of subsequent vitreous hemorrhage. Photocoagulation scars should remain distant from the detached retina and areas of vitreoretinal traction to avoid worsening of the retinal detachment.

In eyes that require surgery, at least a 2-week period is recommended between completion of the photocoagulation treatment and vitrectomy. Although the macula is detached, waiting that period of time before surgery will not worsen the prognosis for postoperative visual recovery. Postoperative visual improvement is modest in most eyes because of associated macular lesions due to diabetic retinopathy, rather than the duration of macular detachment.

Surgical Management

At present, the surgical techniques for management of diabetic retinal detachments include closed vitreous surgery in most cases and scleral buckling in selected cases. Other methods, such as argon laser photocoagulation and cryotreatment, are adjuncts to the former techniques in selected cases.

In the future, new laser therapic methods, such as the pulsed Neodymium-Yag laser[35,36] may be alternatives or adjuncts to surgery in selected cases.

VITREOUS SURGERY

Rationale for Vitreous Surgery. The objectives of vitreous surgery in the management of diabetic retinal detachment are twofold: (1) relief of anterior-posterior traction and (2) relief of tangential traction. In addition, opacities in the vitreous cavity, when present, can be removed by vitrectomy.

Relief of traction can be achieve by (1) a 360° cut of the funnel-like posterior vitreous cortex between the vitreous base and the islands of fibrovascular proliferation in the posterior fundus and (2) segmentation of the posterior vitreous cortex and sheets of epiretinal fibrovascular tissue to completely isolate the islands of fibrovascular proliferation and vitreoretinal attachment in the posterior fundus.

Total removal of the condensed posterior vitreous cortex and fibrovascular proliferation is unnecessary to achieve permanent retinal reattachment, provided all vitreoretinal tractions are relieved. After mere sec-

tion, the cut edges of the posterior vitreous cortex and fibrous sheets usually separate 1 mm or further, owing to traction relief. In most cases increasing separation occurs postoperatively. When vitreous traction is totally relieved the islands of fibrovascular proliferation spontaneously regress postoperatively.[15,37]

Surgical Technique. In most diabetic retinal detachments, vitreous surgery is difficult, owing to the complexity of the vitreoretinal anatomy and the frequent association of other complications of diabetes mellitus, such as vitreous hemorrhages and weakness of the corneal epithelium adhesion. The presence of florid new-vessels significantly increases the likelihood of intraoperative bleeding.

- Whenever possible the crystalline lens should not be removed, since better surgical results can be expected in phakic eyes.[15,16]
- When lens opacities prevent adequate visualization of the posterior segment lens removal and vitrectomy are done as a two step procedure. Lens removal is performed through a limbal approach 3–4 weeks before vitrectomy. Better surgical results can be expected with the two-step procedure compared to lens removal at the time of vitrectomy.[15]
- The anterior vitreous cortex should be left untouched, since it plays no determining role in retinal detachment. In addition, leaving the anterior vitreous may decrease postoperative iris neovascularization.[38]

Excision of the vitreous gel is begun in the center of the vitreous cavity. It is easy and rapid in eyes with advanced vitreous gel liquefaction. In contrast, great care should be taken in young patients with florid proliferative retinopathy. In such eyes, most of the vitreous gel may remain highly viscous. Low-suction force, which is just supraliminal, is used to avoid traction on the retina. In eyes with vitreous hemorrhage, intravitreal blood is removed as much as possible using the vitrectomy probe. Nonclotted blood in the preretinal space is removed either actively by using linear suction force, or passively by venting a flute needle to the atmosphere. Great care is taken not to aspirate the detached retina.

When opacities in the vitreous cavity or viscous vitreous have been removed, dissection of the posterior vitreous cortex and fibrous tissue is meticulously conducted step by step.

The first step is a 360° cut of the funnel-like posterior vitreous cortex between the vitreous base and the posterior islands of fibrovascular proliferation. A hole is made with the vitrectomy probe approximately halfway between the posterior border of the vitreous base and the most peripheral islands of fibrovascular proliferation. This hole is made in a quadrant of attached retina. Next the hole is enlarged. When the posterior vitreous cortex is opaque, it is removed as completely as possible with the vitrectomy probe in areas of attached retina. When the posterior vitreous cortex is not opaque, removal is unnecessary. A circular cut posterior to the vitreous base is made on 360°. Great care should be taken not to leave portion of the funnel uncut. Cutting should be conducted entirely from the initial opening of the posterior vitreous face toward it on 360° of the eye circumference, in one step. In areas of detached retina, sectioning of the posterior vitreous face with the vitrectomy probe may be hazardous. The atrophic, thin, and nearly avascular detached retina may be difficult to distinguish from the posterior vitreous face. It may tear under traction from the suction force. Therefore, automated right-angle scissors are used rather than the vitrectomy probe to cut the posterior vitreous face in areas of detached retina. The scissors are used in combination with the aspirating fiberoptic probe connected to linear aspiration (Fig. 197). Linear aspiration is used to gently lift one cut edge of the posterior vitreous face. This maneuver makes differentiation of the posterior vitreous face from the underlying thin detached retina easier. A gentle lifting of the posterior vitreous face increases space between the posterior vitreous face and the detached retina. Insertion and progression of the posterior scissor blade beneath the posterior vitreous face therefore is less hazardous.

When the 360° peripheral cut in the posterior vitreous face is completed, segmentation of the posterior vitreous cortex and fibrous tissue in the posterior fundus is begun. This is the most difficult and hazardous part of the procedure. Segmentation of the posterior vitreous face and fibrous tissue should be conducted meticulously to completely isolate all epicenters of fibrovascular proliferation, and so as not to create iatrogenic retinal breaks.[39] Bipolar diathermy is used to close prominent new-vessels before dissection. Hemostatic agents, such as intravitreal thrombin[40] may be useful adjuncts to prevent uncontrolled intraoperative bleeding in eyes with severe neovascularization.

Whenever possible, dissection of the posterior vitreous cortex and fibrous tissue is conducted from the posterior pole toward the periphery. It is begun in an area of the attached retina. In most eyes the posterior vitreous cortex, which is firmly attached to the temporal vascular arcades and the optic disc bridges the posterior pole. A hole is made in this bridge using the vitrectomy probe or a Khunt-Bregeat straight needle. Next, the posterior blade of automated right-angle scissors is inserted in the hole

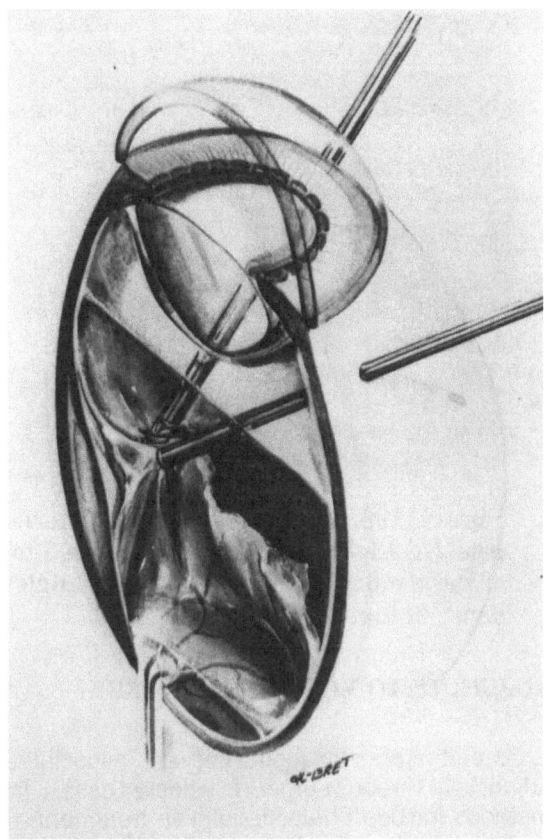

Figure 197. Section of the posterior vitreous face in areas of detached retina. Automatic scissors rather than the vitrectomy probe are used to cut the posterior vitreous face and relieve anterior posterior traction. The aspirating fiberoptic probe is used to gently lift the posterior vitreous face before section.

and the posterior vitreous cortex and fibrous tissue are cut along the inner side of the temporal arcades (Fig. 198). Next each island of fibrovascular proliferation is isolated using scissors. The linear aspiration-fiberoptic probe is useful to gently lift the posterior vitreous cortex before segmentation in areas of the detached retina. Dense fibrovascular proliferation around the optic disc and along the temporal arcades is present in most eyes. It is usually possible to create a cleavage plane at several points.[39] Cleavage is performed using the posterior blade of the right-angle scissors (Fig. 198). Several cuts are done to relieve traction from these tangential sheets of proliferative tissue. When dissection of the posterior vitreous face and fibrous tissue is completed, additional endodiathermy is applied to an oozing new vessel. The entire retina is then carefully examined to disclose any retinal break.

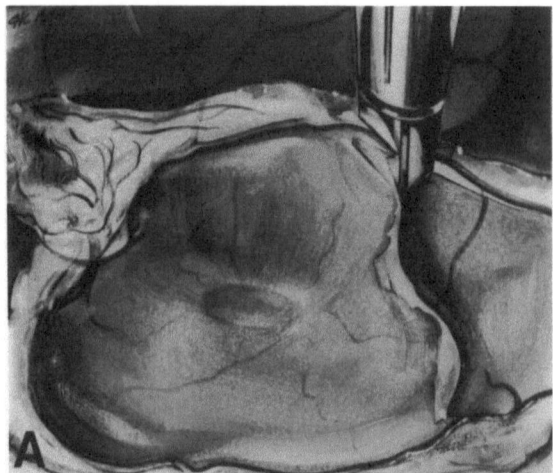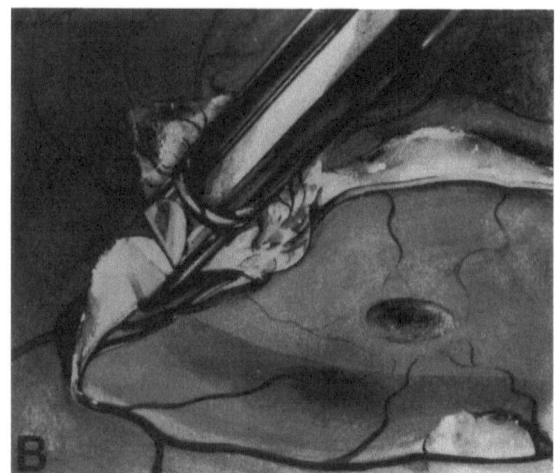

Figure 198. Dissection of the posterior vitreous face and fibrous tissue on the posterior pole. (A) Right angle scissors are used to cut the posterior vitreous face along the inner side of the temporal arcades. (B) Right angle scissors are used to create a clivage plane beneath dense fibrous tissue.

ADJUNCTS TO VITREOUS SURGERY

Other therapeutic modalities are associated as adjuncts to vitreous surgery in selected cases. These methods include photocoagulation treatment, cryotreatment, scleral buckling, and gas injection.

When the retinal detachment is purely tractional, and no iatrogenic break has been created, no surgical adjunct to vitrectomy is necessary, except for photocoagulation treatment in selected cases. Photocoagulation treatment is performed intraoperatively in eyes with florid new-vessels to decrease the potential for recurrent vitreous hemorrhage postoperatively. It is applied to the attached hypoxic retina using either endovitreal or transpupillary argon laser photocoagulation (see p. 41).

When the retinal detachment is associated with a preoperative rhegmatogenous component, the break is managed after completion of the vitrectomy.

When all vitreous tractions on the retina surrounding the break(s) have been relieved by vitrectomy, scleral buckling is unnecessary. Transscleral cryotreatment under biomicroscopic control of the fundus is applied to the retina surrounding the break(s). Gas is used to seal the break during the period of time necessary for the development of the induced retinochoroidal scar. Sulfur hexafluoride is used for the necessary short-duration retinal tamponade (see p. 119). Great care should be taken not to induce increased intraocular pressure (see p. 63), since diabetic eyes have severely compromised retinal blood circulation and would not tolerate even a moderate increase in intraocular pressure.

When the surgeon cannot make certain that all vitreous tractions on the retina surrounding the break(s) have been relieved by vitrectomy, scleral buckling of the retinal break(s) is necessary. Segmental scleral buckles are used. Rather large buckles are used since localization of the scleral projection of a posterior break may not be perfectly accurate in a vitrectomized eye. Special technique is used for the placement of the posterior scleral sutures (see p. 107). Gas injection is associated with scleral buckling in most cases.

When iatrogenic break(s) has (have) been created during segmentation of the posterior vitreous face and fibrous tissue, their treatment is performed after completion of the vitrectomy procedure. Posterior breaks are managed by cryotreatment and gas injection when all vitreoretinal tractions have been relieved by vitrectomy. Breaks that remain under vitreous traction should be supported by scleral buckles.

Complications

Vitreous surgery has made intractable diabetic retinal detachments amenable to surgical management. However, due to the complexity of such detachments and the fragility of diabetic eyes with advanced proliferative retinopathy, vitreous surgery is fraught with serious complications. Certain complications will result in loss of light perception. As a rule, eyes that are not functionally improved or stabilized by vitreous surgery are severely worsened; most failed eyes loose light perception. Severe postoperative complications that result in loss of light perception, are more likely to develop when serious intraoperative complications occur.

INTRAOPERATIVE COMPLICATIONS

Corneal clouding, lens opacification, iatrogenic retinal breaks, uncontrolled bleeding, and the inability to relieve all vitreoretinal tractions are the main complications of vitreous surgery for diabetic retinal detachment.

Corneal Clouding. Owing to the loose adhesion of the corneal epithelium to the basement membrane[39] corneal clouding is more likely to occur during vitrectomy in diabetic eyes. It is a most serious complication when it prevents adequate visualization of the fundus. It may be the cause of severe intraoperative complication or inability to complete the mechanical objectives of the procedure (For prevention of this complication see p. 52).

Lens Opacification. The lens of diabetic patients can develop subcapsular feather-like opacification during vitrectomy. This can decrease intraoperative visualization. However, intraoperative lens opacification that prevents proper completion of the vitrectomy procedure or requires lens removal is infrequent. Use of an enriched irrigating solution may lessen or prevent intraoperative lens opacification.[41] Whenever possible the lens should not be removed, since aphakia significantly increases the risk of postoperative neovascular glaucoma.[15,31,33,42]

Iatrogenic Retinal Breaks. Iatrogenic retinal breaks are a serious complication. They result from excessive traction or the surgeon's inability to differentiate the posterior vitreous face from the thin, hypoxic retina. The incidence of iatrogenic retinal breaks shows a wide range of variations depending on the series. It is approximately 10% in certain series,[8,15] approximately 20% in most series,[13,43,44] and higher in other series.[45]

The incidence of iatrogenic retinal breaks depends on three main parameters: (1) case selection, (2) surgical expertise, and (3) instruments and surgical technique. In the author's experience, the incidence of iatrogenic breaks has been significantly decreased by the use of linear aspiration separate from the cutting instrument. Iatrogenic retinal breaks are associated with a more severe prognosis.

Uncontrolled Bleeding. Intraoperative bleeding from retinal new-vessels is common during vitrectomy for diabetic retinal detachment. It can be minimized, however, by presetting the intraocular pressure between 25 mm and 30 mm of Hg and

by applying bipolar diathermy to the new-vessels before dissection of the posterior vitreous face and fibrous tissue. In most cases bleeding is limited and can be controlled by a temporary increase in intraocular pressure and endodiathermy. Uncontrolled bleeding that prevents proper completion of the procedure occurs in less than 2% of vitrectomies for diabetic retinal detachment. It is associated with a poor prognosis.

POSTOPERATIVE COMPLICATIONS

Any complication of vitrectomy (see p. 150) can develop. Certain complications, such as late lens opacification and fibrovascular ingrowth are more frequent in diabetic eyes. Postoperative complications that are more likely to occur include recurrent corneal epithelium erosion, vitreous hemorrhage, iris neovascularization, neovascular glaucoma, and phthisis bulbi. Several of these complications are frequently associated.

Prolonged and recurrent defect of the corneal epithelium in the early postoperative period is almost specific to diabetic eyes.[7,39] Decreased corneal sensitivity, intraoperative lensectomy, and removal of the corneal epithelium intraoperatively are predisposing factors.[46,47] It may result in permanent corneal dystrophy.[39]

Postoperative vitreous hemorrhage is more likely to occur in young patients with florid proliferative retinopathy, or in eyes that received no photocoagulation treatment. The incidence of this complication can be decreased by meticulous endodiathermy of new-vessels[11,48] and photocoagulation treatment of the hypoxic attached retina. Spontaneous clearing is more rapid in aphakic eyes compared to phakic eyes.[49] Reoperation should be considered in eyes with dense vitreous hemorrhage with no clinical evidence of spontaneous clearing after 4 weeks, especially in eyes that had no photocoagulation treatment when the hemorrhage occurred or when iris new-vessels develop.[50] Removal of vitreous blood should be associated with revision of the vitreoretinal anatomy, endodiathermy of active new-vessels, and photocoagulation or cryotreatment of the hypoxic retina.

Rubeosis iridis is more likely to occur or worsen postoperatively in eyes with florid proliferative retinopathy, eyes that had no previous photocoagulation treatment, and when retinal reattachment was not achieved.[39] It is significantly more frequent in aphakic eyes,[15,30,31,42] and can result in intractable neovascular glaucoma. Neovascular glaucoma develops in 11%[15] to 23%[8] of eyes. Phthisis bulbi develops in approximately 7% of eyes.[8,15] Successful eyes can develop late open-angle glaucoma. This late complication is more frequent in aphakic eyes.[14]

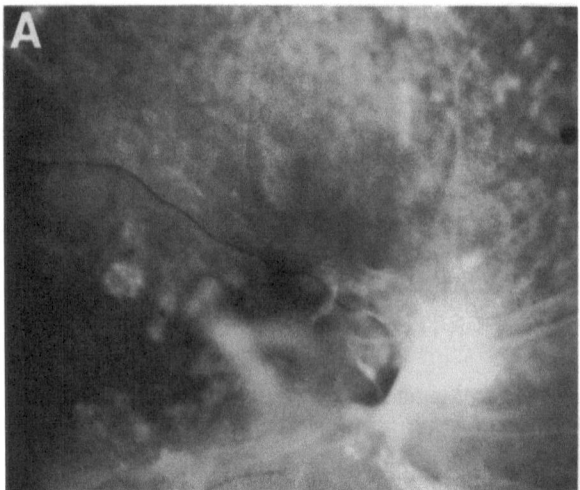 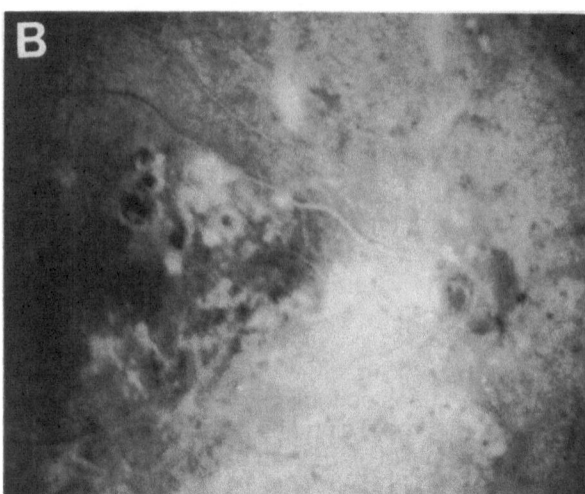

Figure 199. Traction retinal detachment of the posterior pole complicating proliferative diabetic retinopathy, managed by vitrectomy. (A) Fundus photograph before vitrectomy. (B) Postoperative fluorescein angiography. Macular changes due to diabetic retinopathy and prolonged detachment of the retina account for poor postoperative visual recovery in spite of macular reattachment. Central vision is counting finger.

Results

Total retinal reattachment, or at least reattachment of the macula, can be achieved in 45%–65% of eyes, depending on the series.[8,11,12,15–17,51] The anatomical success rate is apparently no better than that achieved in other series of eyes managed by scleral buckling.[5,6] Comparison of the results achieved by the two therapeutic approaches has little value, owing to different case selection. A number of cases included in the vitrectomy series would have been intractable by scleral buckling. The anatomical and visual results achieved by vitreous surgery are stable on a long-term basis in approxiately 80% to 90% of eyes that were successful at 6 months postoperatively.[13,14] However visual improvement is modest in most eyes. Macular lesions caused by diabetic retinopathy, mainly capillary loss and cystoid macular edema, limit the visual recovery after reattachment of the macula. Most patients recover only ambulatory vision (Figs. 199 and 200). Preoperative

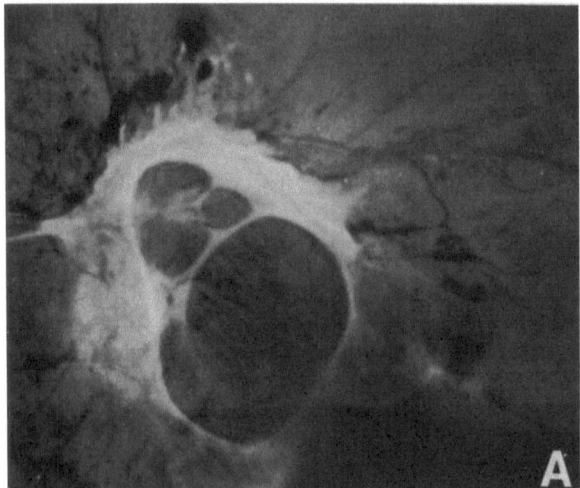 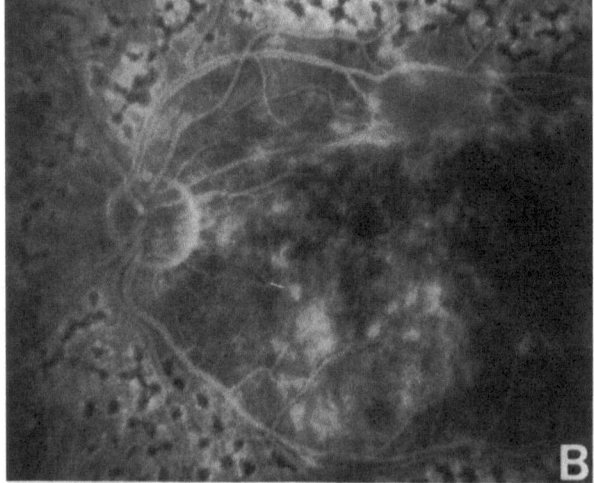

Figure 200. Traction retinal detachment of the posterior pole complicating proliferative diabetic retinopathy, managed by vitrectomy. (A) Fundus photograph before vitrectomy. (B) Fluorescein angiography after vitrectomy and panretinal photocoagulation. Due to cystoid macular edema central vision is reduced to 20/400.

factors associated with a better visual prognosis are as follows:[16] (1) preoperative visual acuity of 5/200 or better, (2) absence of iris new-vessels, (3) absence or only mild vitreous hemorrhage, (4) a clear crystalline lens, (5) previous panretinal photocoagulation of at least one-fourth of the retina, and (6) absence of severe neovascularization. Preoperative factors associated with a guarded prognosis include: (1) association of vitreous hemorrhage,[13,16] (2) florid retinal neovascularization,[16,44] (3) absence of preoperative photocoagulation,[13,15] and (4) iris neovascularization.[15,16] Intraoperative factors associated with a more severe prognosis include: (1) lens removal and (2) iatrogenic retinal breaks. The prognosis is more severe in eyes with rhegmatogenous traction retinal detachment compared to eyes with purely tractional retinal detachment.[17,42]

RETINAL DETACHMENT COMPLICATING OTHER PROLIFERATIVE RETINOPATHIES

Retinal Detachment after Tributary Retinal Vein Occlusion

Retinal detachment is an infrequent complication of tributary retinal vein occlusion. It has been observed in only the ischemic type complicated by retinal neovascularization. Purely tractional retinal detachment is uncommon. Most cases that the author has observed and that are reported in the literature[52–56] are combined, rhegmatogenous-traction detachments.

In most cases the retinal breaks are located very posteriorly. They are situated in atrophic nonperfused retina and in close vicinity of retinal new-vessels. The retinal breaks are round atrophic holes or operculated tears.[56] Their size usually ranges from 0.5 to one disc diameter. They may be difficult to disclose in the thin atrophic retina.

Peripheral retinal tears are much less common. They are horseshoe tears,[52] which develop at the time of acute posterior vitreous detachment and may be unrelated to retinal vein occlusion.

Most retinal detachments associated with peripheral tears are successfully managed by segmental scleral buckling.

Vitreous surgery is indicated in: (1) traction retinal detachment extending to the macula, (2) traction-rhegmatogenous retinal detachment with retinal breaks situated very posteriorly Fig. 201, and (3) retinal detachment associated with vitreous hemorrhage precluding adequate visualization of the fundus and identification of the retinal breaks. In

such cases the retinal breaks are managed by cryo-treatment or photocoagulation treatment and gas injection.

The surgical results are good in terms of retinal reattachment, however, the results in terms of central vision recovery are often poor, due to the macular sequelae of retinal vein occlusion.

Retinal Detachment Complicating Eale's Disease

Both traction retinal detachment and combined rhegmatogenous-traction retinal detachment can develop at a late stage of Eale's disease.

Surgical management is basically similar to that of retinal detachment associated with diabetic retinopathy. In the few cases that the author has managed, retinal reattachment has been achieved. However the long-term visual prognosis has been rather poor owing to the severity and relentless progression of the retinal disease in spite of photocoagulation treatment.

Retinal Detachment Complicating Sickle-Cell Hemoglobinopathy

Both traction retinal detachment and rhegmatogenous traction retinal detachment can develop in patients with sickle-cell hemoglobinopathy. Management of such cases requires special care because these patients are most vulnerable to surgical trauma. In particular, anterior segment ischemia can develop as a complication of scleral buckling,[57] or vitreous surgery.[58]

Retinal Detachment Complicating Retinopathy of Prematurity

Retinal detachment can develop either at the active stage of retinopathy of prematurity, or years later at the cicatricial stage.

In active retinopathy of prematurity, the occurrence of retinal detachment characterizes Stage 4.[59] Retinal detachment can be exudative and tractional. Traction retinal detachment is caused by vitreoretinal changes secondary to proliferation and contraction of tissue originating in the shunt area.[60] Scleral buckling, in combination with cryotreatment, can be effective in reattaching the retina in selected patients with retinopathy of prematurity grade IV.[61–65] However, recurrent detachment can occur from continuing vitreoretinal traction.[61–65] In addi-

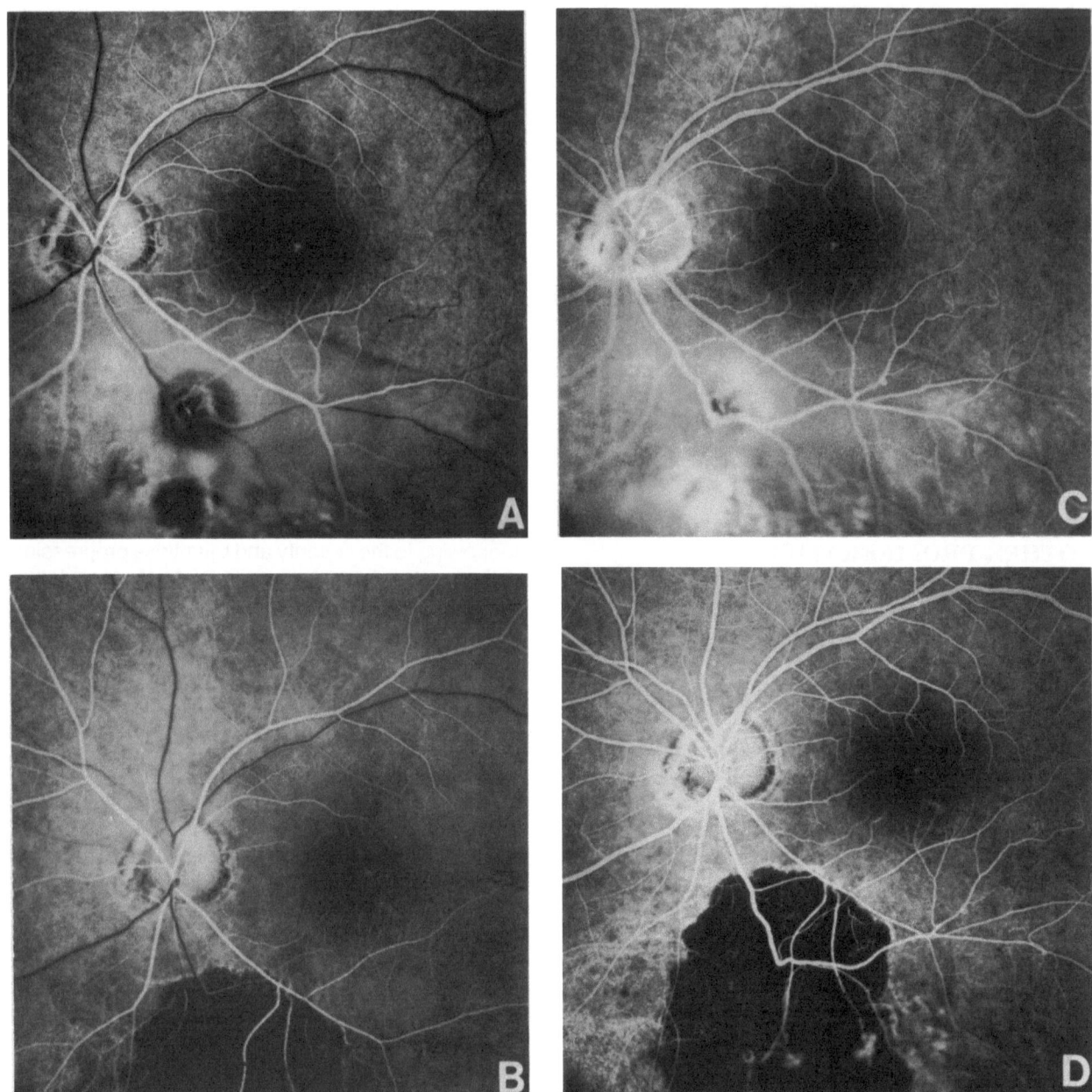

Figure 201. Preoperative and postoperative fluorescein angiography of retinal detachment complicating tributary vein occlusion associated with a posterior retinal break. (A) Preoperative early phase. The retinal break is on the inner side of the inferior temporal vein. (B) Early phase of fluorescein angiography after vitrectomy combined with argon laser photocoagulation and intravitreal injection of pure SF6. The retina is reattached. (C) Preoperative late phase. (D) Late phase of postoperative fluorescein angiography. The dark area corresponds to photocoagulation scars that cover the retinal break area and the hypoxic peripheral retina.

tion, scleral buckling in infants who have active retinopathy of prematurity with tractional and serous detachment remains controversial, because some cases will reattach spontaneously. Vitrectomy in active retinopathy stage IV and V was first attempted in 1977. [66–67] Since then, an improved understand-

ing of the surgical anatomy and pathogenesis has led to improved results. At present, retinal reattachment can be achieved in 22% of eyes with open-sky vitrectomy[68] and approximately 45% of eyes with closed vitrectomy.[69–71] The visual results are, however, rather disappointing.[70] Fixing and follow-

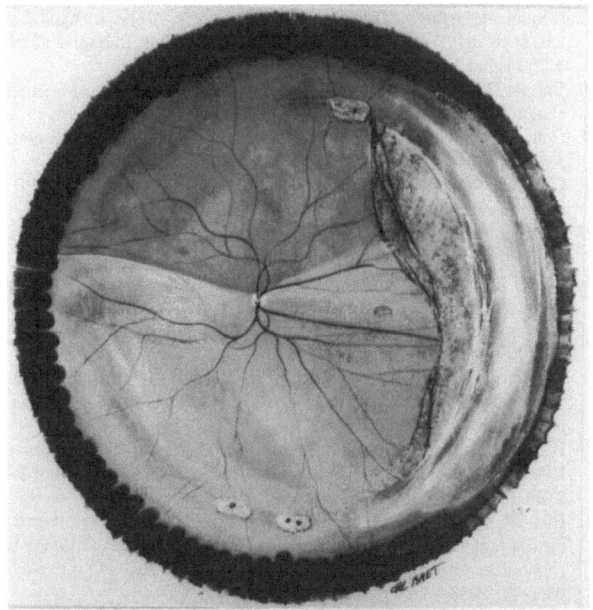

Figure 202. Retinal detachment complicating cicatricial retinopathy of prematurity in an 11-year-old boy. Retinal detachment consists of two components: (1) traction detachment of long duration of the retina adjacent to cicatricial fibrous tissue in the temporal quadrants and (2) rhegmatogenous retinal detachment of recent onset in the lower quadrants. Traction detachment is associated with cystoid degeneration of the retina and pigmented demarcation lines. Rhegmatogenous retinal detachment is related to small atrophic holes in islands of lattice degeneration.

ing visual function is achieved in only about 40% of the successful eyes.[69–70] Assessment of vision is difficult in these children. Longer follow-up is required to determine whether these children will develop and maintain useful vision.

Rhegmatogenous retinal detachment can develop as a late complication in eyes with cicatricial retinopathy of prematurity (Fig. 202).[72–75] Most cases have been observed in children. However rhegmatogenous retinal detachment can also develop in adults with cicatricial retinopathy of prematurity. A higher incidence of lattice degeneration is observed in patients with cicatricial retinopathy of prematurity Stage II and III as compared to the general population (lattice incidence 15% versus 7%). Patients who develop late rhegmatogenous retinal detachment show characteristic ocular changes of cicatricial retinopathy of prematurity. These changes include myopia, chorioretinal scarring, dense vitreous membranes temporally, dragging of the blood retinal vessels, and macular ectopia. In most cases, the retinal breaks are situated in the temporal quadrants with

a prevalence in the lower temporal quadrant (Fig. 202).[72] Round holes can be observed.[72] However small horseshoe tractional tears are more frequent. The tears are usually small. They may be difficult to disclose in areas of cicatricial fibrovascular proliferation. Progression of the detachment is generally slow.[73] In children the detachment is usually disclosed only when the macula is detached. In spite of advanced vitreous gell syneresis and marked vitreoretinal traction, most cases can be reattached merely by scleral buckling.[72–73] Patients with cicatricial retinopathy of prematurity should be examined at regular intervals for life.

Retinal Detachment Complicating Autosomal Dominant Exsudative Vitreoretinopathy

Traction retinal detachment associated with fundus changes similar to those of retinopathy of prematurity can develop in patients with autosomal dominant exsudative vitreoretinopathy.[76–78] However, only few patients affected by the fundus disease progress to retinal detachment.[78] Progression and complications of the disease are observed only in patients under 20 years of age.[78] Retinal reattachment was achieved by scleral buckling alone in one patient.[78] More severe cases require vitrectomy.[66]

Retinal Detachment Complicating Retinal Angiomatosis

Most retinal detachments complicating retinal angiomatosis are exsudative retinal detachments. They are caused by large and multiple capillary angiomas. Subretinal fluid absorbs when the angioma can be destroyed by cryotreatment[79,80] or penetrating diathermy.[81]

Occasionally, a rhegmatogenous retinal detachment may develop in eyes with angiomatosis retinae.[82] The retinal break is caused by vitreoretinal traction at the site of fibrovascular proliferation on the angioma. Characteristically, the break is situated at the posterior border of a large retinal angioma, between the afferent and efferent vessels.[82] The retinal break can be sealed with segmental scleral buckling. The prognosis for retinal reattachment is good.[82]

Total retinal detachments observed at the end-stage of Von Hippel's disease are mainly exsudative retinal detachments, although a tractional component is often associated. Due to the severity of the underlying fundus disease, no treatment can restore any vision to these eyes.

REFERENCES

1. Okun E, Fung WE: Therapy of diabetic retinal detachment, in Symposium on Retina and Retina Surgery: Transactions of the New Orleans Academy of Ophthalmology. St. Louis, C.V. Mosby Co, 1969, 319–327
2. Tasman W: Retinal detachment secondary to proliferative diabetic retinopathy. Arch Ophthalmol 87:286–289, 1972
3. Boniuk I, Okun E, Johnston GP: Scleral buckling in diabetic retinal detachment. Mod Probl Ophthalmol 10:341–349, 1972
4. Wetzig PC: Surgical treatment of advanced cases of proliferative diabetic retinopathy. Mod Probl Ophthalmol 10: 350–353, 1972
5. Gragoudas ES, McMeel JW: Treatment of rhegmatogenous retinal detachment secondary to proliferative diabetic retinopathy. Am J Ophthalmol 81:810–819, 1976
6. Miller SA, Shafrr F, Bresnick GH, Davis MD, Myers FL: Scleral buckling procedure for retinal detachments secondary to proliferative diabetic retinopathy. Am J Ophthalmol 89:103–112, 1980
7. Mandelcorn MS, Blankenship G, Machemer R: Pars plana vitrectomy for the management of severe diabetic retinopathy. Am J Ophthalmol 81:561–570, 1976
8. Tolentino FI, Freeman HM, Tolentino FL: Closed vitrectomy in the management of diabetic traction retinal detachment. Ophthalmology 87:1078–1089, 1980
9. Machemer R: Vitrectomy in diabetic retinopathy: removal of pre-retinal proliferation. Ophthalmology (Rochester) 79: op 394, 1975
10. Michels RG: Vitrectomy for complications of diabetic retinopathy. Arch Ophthalmol 96:237–246, 1978
11. Aaberg TM: Pars plana vitrectomy for diabetic traction retinal detachment. Ophthalmology 88:639–642, 1981
12. Peyman GA, Huamonte FU, Goldberg MF, et al: Four hundred consecutive pars plana vitrectomies with the vitrophage. Arch Ophthalmol 96:45–50, 1978
13. Rice TA, Michels RG, Rice EF: Vitrectomy for diabetic traction retinal detachment involving the macula. Am J Ophthalmol 95: 22–33, 1983
14. Blankenship GW, Machemer R: Long-term diabetic vitrectomy results: report of ten years' follow-up. Ophthalmology 92:503–506, 1985
15. Bonnet M, Grange JD: Photocoagulation et vitrectomie dans les rétinopathies prolifératives neo-vasculaires. Bull Soc Ophtalmol Fr 11:1399–1406, 1986
16. Thompson JT, De Bustros S, Michels RG, Rice TA: Results and prognostic factors in vitrectomy for diabetic traction retinal detachment of the macula. Arch Ophthalmol 105:497–502, 1987
17. Thompson JT, De Bustros S, Michels R, Rice TA: Results and prognostic factors in vitrectomy for diabetic traction. Rhegmatogenous retinal detachment. Arch Ophthalmol 105:503–507, 1987
18. Meyer-Schwickerath G: Lichtcoagulation. Eine Methode zur Behandlung und Verhütung der Netzhautablösung. Von Graefe Arch Ophthalmol 156:2–34, 1954
19. Meyer-Schwickerath G, Wessing A: Treatment of diabetic retinopathy with photocoagulation. Fluorescein studies. 21 st concilium ophthalmologicum, Mexico 1970, Part 1: 959–967. (Exerpta Medica, Amsterdam 1971)
20. James WA, L'Esperance F: Treatment of diabetic optic nerve neovascularization by extensive retinal photocoagulation. Am J Ophthalmol 78:939–947, 1974
21. Little H, Zweng C, Jack R, Vassiliadis A: Techniques of argon laser photocoagulation of diabetic disk new-vessels. Am J Ophthalmol 82:675–683, 1976
22. L'Esperance FA, James WA: Diabetic retinopathy: clinical evaluation and management St Louis, C.V. Mosby Co, 1981
23. Diabetic Retinopathy Research Group: Photocoagulation treatment of proliferative diabetic retinopathy: The second report of diabetic retinopathy study finding. Ophthalmology (Rochester) 85:82–705, 1978
24. Bonnet M, Grange JD, Pingault CL: Note technique sur la photocoagulation pan:rétinienne Bull Soc ophtalmol Fr 76:239–240, 1976
25. Bonnet M, Grange JD, Pingault CL: Panretinal photocoagulation and optic disc neovascularization. Mod Probl Ophthalmol 20:389–395 Basel, Karger, 1979
26. Bonnet M: Indications de la vitrectomie dans le décollement rétinien rhegmatogène. Ophtalmologie 1:95–100, 1987
27. Cohen HB, McMeel JW, Franks EP: Diabetic traction detachment. Arch Ophthalmol 97:1268–1272, 1979
28. Charles S, Flinn CE: The natural history of diabetic extramacular traction retinal detachment. Arch Ophthalmol 99:66–68, 1981
29. Tolentino FI, Lee PF, Schepens CL: Biomicroscopic study of vitreous cavity in diabetic retinopathy. Arch Ophthalmol 75:238–246, 1966
30. Irvine AR, Shorb S: Removal of the lens at vitrectomy. Its advantages and disadvantages in McPherson A (ed) New and controversial aspects of vitreoretinal surgery. St. Louis, C.V. Mosby 295–300, 1977
31. Blankenship G, Cortez R, Machemer R: The lens and pars plana vitrectomy for diabetic retinopathy complications. Arch Ophthalmol 97:1263–1267, 1979
32. Blankenship GW: The lens influence on diabetic vitrectomy results. Report of a prospectiive randomized study. Arch Ophthalmol 98: 2196–2198, 1980
33. Rice TA, Michels RG, Maguire MG, Rice EF: The effect of lensectomy on the incidence of iris neovascularization and neovascular glaucoma after vitrectomy for diabetic retinopathy. Am J Ophthalmol 95:1–11, 1983
34. Machemer R: Iris angiography study before and after vitrectomy. Vail Vitrectomy Seminar, 1983
35. Brown GC, Benson WE: Treatment of diabetic traction retinal detachment with the pulsed neodymium-yag laser. Am J Ophthalmol 99:258–262, 1985
36. Frankhauser F, Kwasniewska S, Van der Zypen E: Vitreolysis with the Q-switched laser. Arch Ophthalmol 103:1166–1171, 1985
37. Federman JL, Boyer D, Breit P: An objective analysis of proliferative diabetic retinopathy before and after pars plana vitrectomy. Ophthalmology 86:278–282, 1979
38. Charles S: Vitreous surgery. Baltimore, Williams and Wilkins, 65, 1981
39. Michels RG: Vitreous surgery. St. Louis, C.V. Mosby Co 166–167, 173–174, 213–229, 1981
40. Thompson JT, Glaser BM, Michels RG, et al: The use of intravitreal thrombin to control hemorrhage during vitrectomy. Ophthalmology 93:279–282, 1986
41. Haimann MH, Abrams GW: Prevention of lens opacification during diabetic vitrectomy. Ophthalmology 91:116–121, 1984
42. Blankenship GW: Posterior retinal holes secondary to diabetic retinopathy. Arch Ophthalmol 101:885–887, 1983
43. Hutton WL, Bernstein I, Fuller D: Diabetic traction retinal detachment. Factors influencing final visual acuity. Ophthalmology 87: 1071–1077, 1980
44. Machemer R, Blankenship G: Vitrectomy for proliferative diabetic retinopathy associated with vitreous hemorrhage. Ophthalmology 88:643–646, 1981
45. Blankenship G: Pars plana vitrectomy for diabetic retinopathy. A report of eight years' experience. Mod Probl Ophthalmol 20:376–385, 1979
46. Brightbill FS, Myers FL, Bresnick GH: Postvitrectomy keratopathy. Am J Ophthalmol 85:651–655, 1978
47. Foulks GN, Thoft RA, Perry HD, et al: Factors related to corneal epithelial complications after closed vitrectomy in diabetics. Arch ophthalmol 97:1076–1078, 1979
48. Machemer R, Aaberg TM: Vitrectomy. 2nd ed. Orlando FL, Grune & Stratton, 82, 1979
49. Novak MA, Rice TA, Michels RG, Auer C: Vitreous hemorrhage after vitrectomy for diabetic retinopathy. Ophthalmology 91:1485–1489, 1984
50. Blankenship GW: Management of vitreous cavity hemorrhage following pars plana vitrectomy for diabetic retinopathy. Ophthalmology 93:39–44, 1986
51. Miller SA, Butler JB, Myers FL, Bresnick GH: Pars plana vitrectomy. Treatment for tractional macula detachment secondary to

proliferative diabetic retinopathy. Arch Ophthalmol 98:659–664, 1980

52. Zauberman H: Retinopathy of retinal detachment after major vascular occlusions. Br J Ophthalmol 52:117–121, 1968
53. Joondeph HC, Goldberg MF: Rhegmatogenous retinal detachment after tributary retinal vein occlusion. Am J Ophthalmol 80:253–257, 1975
54. Constantinides G, Francois P, Madelain F: Déchirures rétiniennes au décours des thromboses veineuses. Ann Oculist (Paris) 204:1249–1250, 1971
55. Gutman FA, Zegarra H: Retinal detachment secondary to retinal branch vein occlusion. Trans Am Acad Ophthalmol Otolaryngol 81:491–496, 1976
56. Regenbogen L, Godel V, Feiler-Ofri V, et al: Retinal breaks secondary to vascular accidents. Am J Ophthalmol 84:187–196, 1977
57. Ryan S, Goldberg MF: Anterior segment ischemia following scleral buckling in sickle-cell hemoglobinopathy. Am J Ophthalmol 72:35–49, 1971
58. Michels RG: Vitreous Surgery. Philadelphia, C.V. Mosby Co, 231, 1981
59. Committee for the classification of retinopathy of prematurity: The international classification of retinopathy of prematurity (ROP). Arch Ophthalmol 102:1130–1134, 1984
60. Machemer R: Description and pathogenesis of later stages of retinopathy of prematurity. Ophthalmology 92:1000–1004, 1985
61. Topilow HW, Ackerman AL, Wang FM: The treatment of advanced retinopathy of prematurity by cryotherapy and scleral buckling surgery. Ophthalmology 92:379–387, 1985
62. Tasman W: Management of retinopathy of prematurity. Ophthalmology 92:995–999, 1985
63. Mc Pherson AR, Hittner HM: Scleral buckling in 2½ to 11 month-old premature infants with retinal detachment associated with acute retrolental fibroplasia. Ophthalmology 86:819–835, 1979
64. Mc Pherson AR, Hittner HM, Lemos R: Retinal detachment in young premature infants with acute retrolental fibroplasia. Thirty two new cases: Ophthalmology 89:1160–1169, 1982
65. Mc Pherson AR, Hittner HM, Kretzer FL: Treatment of acute retinopathy of prematurity by scleral buckling. in Mc Pherson AR, Hittner HM, Kretzer FL (Eds) Retinopathy of prematurity. Current concepts and controversies. Philadelphia, B.C. Decker, Inc, 1986, 179–192
66. Treister G, Machemer R: Results of vitrectomy for rare hemorrhagic and proliferative diseases. Am J Ophthalmol 84:394–412, 1977
67. Hirose T, Schepens CL: Complications in open-sky vitrectomy In Freeman HM, Hirose T, Schepens CL (eds): Vitreous surgery and advances in fundus diagnosis and treatment. New York, Appleton-century-crafts, 1977, 479

68. Mc Pherson AR, Hittner HM, Moura RA, Kretzer TL: Treatment of retrolental fibroplasia with open-sky vitrectomy. in Mc Pherson AR, Hittner HM, Kretzer FL (Eds): Retinopathy of prematurity. Current concepts and controversies. Philadelphia, B.C. Decker, Inc. 193–208, 1986
69. Trese MT: Visual results and prognostic factors for vision following surgery for stage V retinopathy of prematurity. Ophthalmology 93: 574–579, 1986
70. Chong LP, Machemer R, De Juan E: Vitrectomy for advanced stages of retinopathy of prematurity. Am J Ophthalmol 102:710–716, 1986
71. Charles ST: Vitrectomy with ciliary entry for retrolental fibroplasia, in Mc Pherson AR, Hittner HM, Kretzer FL (eds): Retinopathy of prematurity. Current concepts and controversies. Philadelphia, BC Decker, inc. 225–234, 1986
72. Tasman W, Annesley W: Retinal detachment in the retinopathy of prematurity. Arch Ophthalmol 75:608–614, 1966
73. Faris BM, Brockhurst RJ: Retrolental fibroplasia in the cicatricial stage. The complication of rhegmatogenous retinal detachment. Arch Ophthalmol 82:60–65, 1969
74. Harris GS: Retinopathy of prematurity and retinal detachment. Can J Ophthalmol 11:21–25, 1976
75. Starzycka M, Ciechanowska A, Gergovich A: Retinal detachment in retrolental fibroplasia. Ophthalmologica 181:261–265, 1980
76. Criswick VG, Schepens CL: Familial exsudative vitreoretinopathy. Am J Ophthalmol 68:578–594, 1969
77. Grow J, Oliver CL: Familial exsudative vitreoretinopathy. Arch Ophthalmol 86:150–155, 1971
78. Ober RR, Bird AC, Hamilton AM, Sehmi K: Autosomal dominant exsudative vitreoretinopathy. Brit J Ophthalmol 64:112–120, 1980
78. Annesley WH, Leonard BC: Fifteen year review of treated cases of retinal angiomatosis. Trans Am Acad Ophthalmol Otolaryngol 83:446–453, 1977
80. Bonnet M, Garmier G: Les Angiomes capillaires rétiniens de la maladie de Von Hippel. J Fr Ophtalmol 7:545–555, 1984
81. Cardoso R, Brockhurst RJ: Perforating diathermycoagulation for retinal angiomas. Arch ophthalmol 94:1702–1719, 1976
82. Nicholson DH, Anderson LS, Blodi C: Rhegmatogenous retinal detachment in angiomatosis retinae. Am J Ophthalmol 101:187–189, 1986

24

Retinal Detachment after Penetrating Injury of the Eye

ETIOLOGY

Incidence

According to statistics, which were published before the development of vitrectomy techniques in the management of penetrating injury of the eye, retinal detachment occurs in approximately 30%[1,2] to more than 50% of eyes[3,4] with penetrating injury of the posterior segment. At present, early vitrectomy enables the salvaging of some severely injured eyes that would otherwise be lost.[5-6] In addition, early vitrectomy may be helpful in preventing late retinal detachment in eyes with less severe initial damage from injury.[8] However, it is not yet known whether this new surgical approach to selected eye injuries decreases the overall incidence of retinal detachment. Some studies have shown that the incidence of retinal detachment after removal of intraocular foreign bodies is significantly decreased in eyes managed with vitrectomy techniques compared to eyes treated without vitrectomy.[4] However, the results of other studies[9,10] are much less optimistic. Evaluation of vitrectomy as a prophylactic measure of retinal detachment after penetrating eye injury is difficult because of the marked heterogeneity of trauma cases.

Age and Sex Distribution

Age and sex distribution shows a significant prevalence of males and young individuals. Males account for 77%[11] to 91%[12] of all patients. The mean patient age is approximately 25 years.[13] The age and sex distribution reflects the frequent participation of young males in hazardous activities.

Penetrating Eye Injuries

Retinal detachment may develop after any penetrating eye injury involving the vitreous gel. Most cases are observed in eyes with scleral wounds. However a few cases occur in eyes with purely corneal wounds. In the latter group, the vitreous gel is invariably incarcerated in the corneal wound.

Scleral wounds of the ciliary region, and in particular penetrating wounds of the limbus, are those that involve the highest risk of secondary retinal detachment. In a series of retinal detachments after penetrating eye injuries[11] the penetrating wound was purely corneal in 9% of patients. It was scleral and anterior to the ora serrata in 77% of patients. The wound involved the sclera posterior to the ora serrata in only 14% of eyes. In the same series of patients, 14% of the eyes had a double perforation and 20% had a removed or retained intraocular foreign body.

Latent Interval

The time interval between the eye injury and the diagnosis of the retinal detachment shows a wide range of variations. Retinal detachment may develop and be recognized a few days to several years after the trauma. A relationship between the severity of the penetrating eye injury and the duration of the latent interval is most likely. Severely injured eyes are more likely to develop early retinal detachments, whereas months or years may elapse before the retinal detachment is recognized in eyes with small penetrating wounds. In a retinal referral center, where trauma cases are not primarily repaired, only 10% of the retinal detachments after penetrating eye injury were diagnosed within a month of the trauma, and 57% within 6 months.[11] In the same series, retinal detachment was recognized more than a year after the trauma in 28% of patients. Latent intervals over 10 years have been observed.[12,13] It should be emphasized that a latent interval of several years does not rule out the etiologic significance of the injury.

PATHOPHYSIOLOGY

The pathophysiology of retinal detachments after penetrating eye injury is helpful in understanding the clinical characteristics of such detachments and establishing a rationale for surgical management.

Histopathologic examinations of eyes enucleated after penetrating eye injuries as well as experimental models[14–18] have demonstrated that most retinal detachments after penetrating injury of the eye are secondary to intraocular proliferation of fibrous tissue through the penetrating wound. The retinal detachment is primarily a traction retinal detachment in most cases. A rhegmatogenous component is associated to the traction detachment in approximately 65% of the eyes.[11,12]

Traction Retinal Detachment

The sequence of events that result in traction retinal detachment are as follows[14,15]: a fibrous, or fibrovascular tissue proliferates along the scaffold of vitreous gel incarcerated in the wound. Cell proliferation is induced by the inflammatory response to the penetrating injury. It is enhanced by intravitreal blood and poor wound apposition. Intraocular cell proliferation participates to the formation of transvitreal bands and fan-shaped membranes, a cyclitic membrane on the anterior vitreous face, and periretinal membranes.

Then, the fibrous ingrowth contracts and pulls onto the retina. Traction retinal detachment develops. In most cases traction retinal detachment begins in the peripheral retina and ciliary epithelium. At the end stage, the retina is totally detached and dragged towards the penetrating wound.

Rhegmatogenous Component

Traction retinal detachment is associated with retinal breaks in approximately 65% of the eyes.[11] Retinal breaks may develop at the time of the penetrating injury. This is the case for retinal lacerations by a foreign body or penetrating object. Most often, how-

ever, retinal breaks develop later on. Most retinal breaks are induced by secondary changes of the vitreous gel.

Gradual shrinkage of the vitreous gel and intravitreal membranes may result in retinal dialysis at the ora serrata. The dialysis is located opposite to the scleral wound in most cases. It will gradually enlarge as the vitreous gel shrinkage increases. Ultimately, the dialysis may involve nearly 360° of the eye circumference, and the retina remains adherent to the eye wall only at the perforation site and around the optic disc.

Vitreous liquefaction and the resultant posterior vitreous detachment may result in horseshoe retinal tears and operculated retinal tears. The retinal tears develop at the site of localized vitreoretinal adhesions. They are located in the equatorial region or the posterior edge of the vitreous base in most cases. Paravascular linear retinal tears, located more posteriorly, are much less common.

CLINICAL FINDINGS

Retinal detachments after penetrating eye injury show a wide variety of clinical characteristics, which depend on the wide variety of penetrating eye injuries. In spite of the disparity of clinical cases, ocular findings may be categorized into four distinct groups: the status of the vitreous body, the status of the retina, the retinal breaks, and the associated lesions. Careful preoperative analysis of all findings is most important because it will be the basis for the therapeutic protocol to be applied in any given clinical case.

Status of the Vitreous Body

Status of the vitreous body depends mainly on the severity of the penetrating injury and the time interval between the injury and the diagnosis of the retinal detachment.

In early retinal detachments that develop within a month after the eye injury the vitreous body most often is opaque due to vitreous hemorrhage. Vitreous hemorrahge may be so dense that the retina is not visible. Opaque media, particularly trauma cataract, may also prevent fundus examination. The diagnosis of retinal detachment is made by ultrasonography. There is an indication for immediate vitrectomy. The protocol to reattach the retina will be established after intraoperative examination of the retina. When opaque media or intraoperative bleeding prevent satisfactory examination of the retina, it is sometimes advantageous to inject gas and postpone surgical management of the retinal detachment until 2–3 weeks later.

In retinal detachments that develop several weeks, months, or years after the injury, the clarity of the vitreous body and media is usually sufficient, although not perfect, to allow detailed examination of the vitreous body and retina. The status of the anterior vitreous face, vitreous gel, posterior vitreous face, and vitreous base should be carefully evaluated by slit lamp examination.

ANTERIOR VITREOUS FACE

In phakic eyes, the anterior vitreous gel may appear normal. In particular, some eyes show no modification of the normal clarity, orientation, and mobility of the anterior vitreous fibrils. This finding indicates that removal of the clear lens will be unnecessary to complete the retinal reattachment operation. In contrast, other eyes exhibit a cyclitic membrane on the anterior vitreous face and fine strands that fan out, in a frontal plane into the anterior vitreous gel from the incarceration site. The clear lens should be removed for satisfactory completion of the retinal reattachment procedure in such eyes.

In aphakic eyes there is a cyclitic membrane on the anterior vitreous face in most cases. Special care should be taken to identify fibrous or fibrovascular ingrowth connected to the corneal wound and vitreous strands incarcerated into the corneal wound. All tractions from such abnormal tissue should be relieved during vitrectomy.

VITREOUS BODY

All eyes with retinal detachments secondary to penetrating eye injury show modifications of the vitreous gel. These modifications may be subtle and missed by the observer during rapid examination, or so marked that they prevent complete examination of the entire retina. They show two main clinical aspects. The first aspect is that of multiple strands that fan out from the scleral wound (Fig. 203). The strands may be fine and almost translucent, or dense with a gray-white color. They may be localized in the vicinity of the incarceration site or extend to the opposite side of the vitreous cavity. The second clinical aspect is that of a single vitreous strand that crosses the vitreous cavity in the path of an intraocular foreign body or an object that made a double perforation. The vitreous strand may be a dense opaque vitreous cord (Fig. 204).

Remnants of vitreous hemorrhage are often present in the lower part of the vitreous cavity.

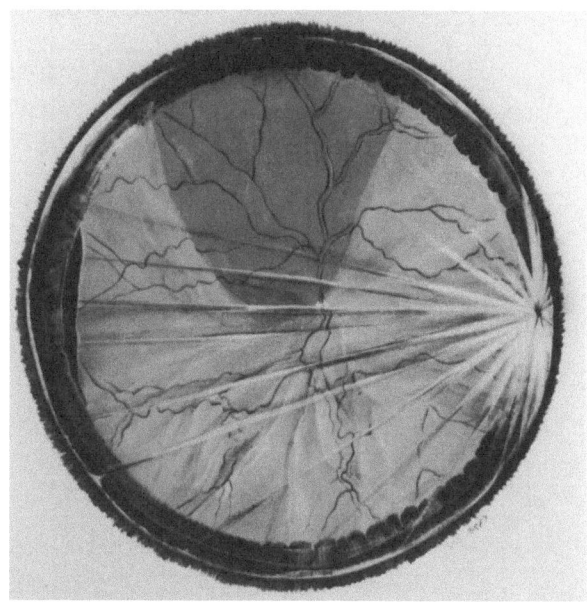

Figure 203. Retinal detachment after penetrating injury of the ciliary region in a 12-year-old boy (right eye). White strands of fibrous ingrowth fan out from the penetrating wound into the vitreous gel. Retinal dialysis related to static vitreous traction has developed in the temporal quadrants. The nonpigmented ciliary epithelium is detached from eight o'clock to ten o'clock (Courtesy of BONNET M. Opthalmologica 194:164–168, 1987).

POSTERIOR VITREOUS FACE

Whenever possible the situation of the posterior vitreous face should be determined by preoperative slit lamp examination. The posterior vitreous face may not be detached, particularly in recent onset retinal detachments that develop early after the injury. This clinical finding has a guarded prognosis. In most eyes it will be impossible to detach and remove the posterior vitreous face during vitrectomy. Vitrectomized eyes with the posterior vitreous face remaining adherent to the retina are more prone to develop severe proliferative vitreoretinopathy and recurrent retinal detachment postoperatively.

VITREOUS BASE

In penetrating wounds of the ciliary region, ingrowth of the fibrous or fibrovascular tissue from the wound usually extends into the vitreous base as well as the vitreous cavity. Dense fibrous condensation of the vitreous base will require radial cuts during surgery to relieve the anterior ring traction.

In most eyes, significant condensation of the vitre-

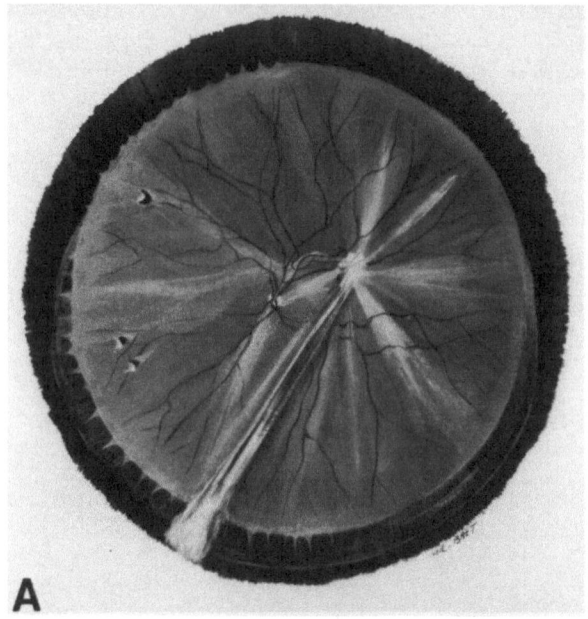 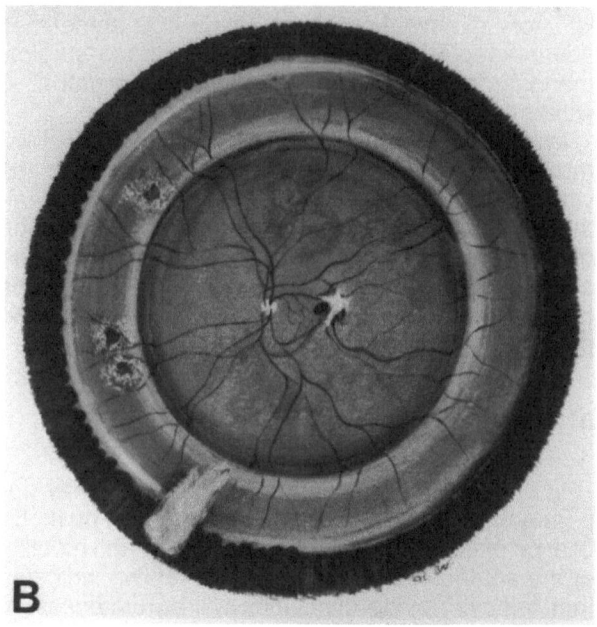

A   B

Figure 204. Retinal detachment after penetrating injury by a magnetic foreign body in a 28-year-old man. (A) Fundus appearance at initial examination. Retinal detachment developed weeks after removal of the intraocular foreign body. Direct retinal damage from the foreign body has resulted in a fibrous scar on the posterior pole. Dense vitreous strands are stretched from the fibrous scar on the posterior pole to the pars plana incision at 7 o'clock. They are related to removal rather than penetration of the foreign body. Three small horseshoe tears at the posterior border of the vitreous base in the nasal quadrants are associated with traction retinal detachment (Courtesy of BONNET M. Ophthalmologica 194:164–168, 1987). (B) Postoperative fundus appearance. Permanent retinal reattachment was achieved by a single operation. The surgical procedure consisted of vitrectomy, cryotreatment limited to the retinal tears, a 360° scleral buckling procedure and retinal tamponade with SF6. Remnants of fibrous scar on the posterior pole and fibrous ingrowth from the pars plana incision for foreign body removal are still visible.

ous base is associated with detachment of the ciliary epithelium and a circumferential retinal fold at the posterior edge of the vitreous base. Retinal dialyses at the ora serrata or small horseshoe tears at the posterior border of the vitreous base are often present in such eyes (Fig. 203). The fibrous ingrowth may also extend anteriorly to a limbal wound and drag the retinal anteriorly onto the ciliary region.

Retinal Detachment

The clinical characteristics of the retinal detachment are most helpful in establishing the surgical protocol and for predicting the surgical prognosis.

The orientation of the retinal folds indicates the main direction of the vitreous traction forces and the area where the most care should be taken during vitrectomy to relieve all vitreoretinal tractions.

Extension of the retinal detachment far beyond the limits of localized vitreous strands often indicate

that traction retinal detachment is associated with a rhegmatogenous component (Fig. 204). Therefore, thorough biomicroscopic examination of the retina should be performed to identify the retinal breaks.

Detachment of the ciliary epithelium and circumferential retinal folds parallel to the ora serrata indicate major vitreous base contraction that will require specific treatment. The limits of the ciliary epithelium detachment, as well as the location of the retina dragged anteriorly onto the pars plana should be precisely recorded on the preoperative fundus chart to avoid these areas for the pars plana incisions.

The height of the retinal detachment may provide indirect information on the presence and extent of posterior vitreous detachment. A shallow detachment, with a smooth surface, generally indicates the absence of posterior vitreous detachment. In contrast, most bullous retinal detachments are associated with posterior vitreous detachment.

Cystoid degeneration of the detached retina, that may be associated with large retinal cysts, is indicative of a longlasting retinal detachment of very gradual progression (Fig. 207). Similarly, subretinal membranes and cords are associated with longlasting and very gradual detachments (Fig. 207). The prognosis for retinal reattachment is excellent in most eyes, when there are no associated preretinal membranes.

In contrast preretinal proliferation with full thickness fixed retinal folds indicates a more guarded surgical prognosis. All grades of proliferative vitreoretinopathy may be observed in retinal detachments after penetrating injury. Epiretinal membrane dissection will be required in such eyes.

Retinal Breaks

Traction retinal detachment is associated with a rhegmatogenous component in approximately 65% of eyes.[11] Retinal breaks show several distinct aspects. They include: (1) retinal lacerations, (2) retinal dialysis at the ora serrata (Fig. 203) (3) horseshoe (Fig. 204) and operculated retinal tears, and (4) linear paravascular retinal breaks (Fig. 210)

RETINAL LACERATIONS

According to Cox and Freeman,[12] retinal lacerations by a penetrating object or a foreign body are present in approximately 20% of eyes. In the authors own experience, retinal lacerations are rarely responsible for a rhegmatogenous retinal detachment. In most cases, spontaneous healing of the retinal wound at the perforation site, as well as the posterior retinal wound in eyes with a double perforation, has occurred when retinal detachment develops. In most eyes the retinal laceration plays a role in the development of the traction retinal detachment rather than the associated rhegmatogenous retinal detachment.

RETINAL DIALYSIS

Retinal dialysis are present in approximately 12%[11] to 15%[12] of eyes. They may be due to severe blunt trauma associated with the penetrating injury.[12] In such circumstances the dialysis develops at the time of the injury. Its clinical characteristics are those of any dialysis after blunt injury. The dialysis is most often located in the upper nasal quadrant and associated with an avulsed vitreous base (see p. 188)

Retinal dialysis may also be due to gradual vitreoretinal traction resulting from fibrous ingrowth and vitreous contraction. In such instances, the dialysis develops long after the penetrating eye injury. It is invariably associated with dense gray-white condensation of the vitreous base and fan-shaped vitreous bands (Fig. 203). In most eyes the dialysis is opposite to the perforation site. In a few eyes there are two dialyses located on each side of the fibrous ingrowth. These dialyses slowly extend laterally with time. In extreme cases the dialysis involves the entire circumference of the eye except for the area of fibrous ingrowth. Small dialyses may be difficult to identify because they are hidden by fibrous proliferation onto the vitreous base. In addition, the retina is often dragged anteriorly and the dialysis may appear to be located on the pars plana. The ora serrata bays dragged anteriorly on both sides of the dialysis make it possible to identify the nature of the lesion. Scleral depression is a requisite for identification and accurate clinical analysis of the dialysis.

HORSESHOE AND OPERCULATED RETINAL TEARS

Small horse-shoe and/or operculated retinal tears are present in 27%[12] to more than 50%[11] of eyes. They develop at the site of vitreoretinal adhesions at the time of the injury[12] or later on.[11] The latter are related to posterior vitreous detachment secondary to vitreous gel degeneration and gradual contraction of the vitreous base. In most eyes the retinal tears are very small, often multiple, located in the equatorial region or at the posterior edge of the vitreous base (Fig. 204), and may be hidden by the opaque peripheral vitreous.

Associated Lesions

A wide range of lesions secondary to the penetrating eye injury may be associated with the retinal detachment. They include lesions of the anterior segment and retained intraocular foreign bodies. Sequelae of previous surgery may be present. Some eyes show signs of severely compromised trophicity.

A retained intraocular foreign body may be hidden by fibrous tissue. It should be removed during the operation for retinal reattachment when it is chemically active.

Modifications of the anterior segment include corneal scars, vitreous incarceration and fibrous or fibrovascular ingrowth from the corneal wound, posterior synechiae, cyclitic membranes, and lens opacification. The lesions may prevent precise preoperative evaluation of the posterior segment. In such eyes surgical management may require combined anterior and posterior surgical approaches. Signs of severely compromised eye trophicity are contraindications for surgery in patients with useful vision of the fellow eye. They include: (1) significant reduction of the axial length of the posterior segment of the eye, (2) increased choroidal thickness over 3 mm, and (3) poor or no light perception.

SURGICAL MANAGEMENT

The basic surgical procedure includes five steps: (1) pars plana vitrectomy, (2) cryotreatment of the fibrous ingrowth remnants after vitrectomy, (3) treatment of the retinal breaks, (4) scleral buckling of the vitreous base, and (5) retinal tamponade with gas.

Additional surgical steps, such as reconstruction of the anterior segment anatomy and removal of a retained intraocular foreign body are required in some eyes.

Preoperative formulation of a plan of treatment is frequently complicated by opacification of the media and vitreous hemorrhage. Therefore, the surgical protocol should be based upon intraoperative clinical findings.

Vitreous Surgery

Relief of tractions on the detached retina is the main objective of vitreous surgery. This requires removal of the vitreous gel and the fibrous ingrowth in all eyes. In specific circumstances, surgery through the pars plana may include additional steps: (1) removal of a clear or opaque lens, (2) reconstruction of the anterior segment anatomy, (3) radial cuts in the vitreous base, (4) epiretinal membrane dissection, (5) retinotomies, and (6) removal of a retained intraocular foreign body.

QUADRANTIC LOCATION OF THE PARS PLANA INCISIONS

The quadrantic location of the pars plana incisions is determined according to three parameters: (1) the location of the performation site, (2) the presence and extent of ciliary epithelium detachment, and (3) the extent of retina that is dragged anteriorly onto the pars plana, towards the perforation site. The pars plana incision sites should be distant from these areas. In particular, the pars plana incisions must never involve the perforating wound. In the most severe cases the ciliary epithelium may be detached on 360° of the eye circumference, and the retina may also be dragged anteriorly on nearly 360° of the eye circumference. In such eyes the author uses

an infusion cannula 2 mm longer than the usual cannula. A longer infusion cannula eliminates the risk of fluid infusion into the subretinal space. When the anatomical conditions make it unavoidable to make the pars plana incision for the vitreous probe in an area where the retina is dragged anteriorly, a pilot-tube is used to minimize retinal laceration during entry and removal of the working instruments. Even so, a break is made in the retina dragged onto the pars plana. It will require specific treatment when the vitrectomy procedure is completed. Whenever possible, the pars plana incision for the vitreous probe should be opposite to the perforation site.

REMOVAL OF THE LENS

Removal of an associated traumatic cataract is performed as the first step of the surgical procedure. In most patients, it is performed through the pars plana. Removal of a clear lens may also be required in eyes with a dense cyclitic membrane on the anterior vitreous face or condensed strands in the anterior vitreous gel. In such eyes removal of the lens is necessary to allow complete relief of vitreous traction in a frontal plane. Removal of the clear lens can be performed with the pars plana approach in most eyes since most patients with retinal detachment after penetrating injury are young. In patients over age 40, lens removal is performed through the limbus.

RECONSTRUCTION OF THE ANTERIOR SEGMENT ANATOMY

Reconstruction of the anterior segment anatomy is required in eyes with severe lesions. This should be done as the first step of the surgical procedure. In most eyes reconstruction of the anterior segment anatomy can be done through the pars plana approach. However, severely injured eyes may require combined anterior segment microsurgery via the limbus. Posterior iris synechiae are cut with a spatula. Iris synechiae to the corneal wound should be cut with scissors because they are strong in most cases and often associated with fibrovascular ingrowth from the corneal wound. Endodiathermy is applied to the fibrovascular tissue before and after section. Special care should be taken to completely cut any vitreous incarceration in a corneal or limbal wound. The vitreous strands or sheets incarcerated into the wound are generally condensed. Manual vitreous microscissors are the most appropriate instrument to be used in most cases. The above surgical maneuvers can be performed through the pars plana approach in most eyes.

In contrast, the anterior approach is more appropriate for the management of heavy fibrovascular ingrowth from a limbal wound. In most eyes the fibrovascular ingrowth is very thick and extends in a frontal plane through the anterior segment. The corneal incision should involve 90°. Two cuts are made with vannas scissors at both extremities of the fibrovascular sheet; the fibrovascular sheet is then removed in one piece from the eye. A continuous suture with 10–0 nylon monofilament is placed to tightly close the corneal wound. The anterior approach for removal of thick fibrovascular ingrowth in the pupillary plane is more rapid and less traumatizing as compared to the pars plana approach.

REMOVAL OF THE VITREOUS GEL AND POSTERIOR FIBROVASCULAR INGROWTH

Removal of the cyclitic membrane on the anterior vitreous face is started at the center of the pupil and continued up to the vitreous base. Removal of the vitreous gel and posterior fibrovascular ingrowth is carried out from the front of the fibrovascular ingrowth towards the perforation site (Fig. 205). The intraocular pressure is temporarily increased to prevent or stop bleeding from the new vessels. When removal of the fibrovascular ingrowth up to its root in the perforating site is completed, endodiathermy is applied to the cut ends of the new vessels. Then the intraocular pressure is lowered to 25 mm of mercury and vitreous gel removal is completed. Thick vitreous cords on the path of a foreign body or penetrating object are cut with automated microscissors (Fig. 206). Usually, a large gap develops between the cut ends as a result of the relieved elasticity of the fibrous cord (Fig. 207).

Removal of the posterior vitreous face is easy in eyes with posterior vitreous detachment. It is completed up to the posterior edge of the vitreous base. In contrast, removal of the posterior vitreous face may be hazardous in eyes with no posterior vitreous detachment.

In eyes with dense fibrous ingrowth on the vitreous base, radial cuts of the fibrous tissue are made with the microscissors. The goal of radial cuts is to relieve ring contraction of the vitreous base.

Preretinal membranes are segmented and full thickness retinal folds are open with the technique described on p. 245.)

In severe cases, with the retina dragged anteriorly towards a perforation site located in the ciliary or limbal region, the retina may appear too short to settle on the pigment epithelium. Scleral shortening with a wide scleral fold, or a relaxing retinotomy should be considered.

Removal or segmentation of subretinal sheets and cords is unnecessary in all eyes without preretinal membranes. In eyes with associated preretinal membranes the value of the surgical approach of subretinal proliferation remains to be fully demonstrated.

REMOVAL OF A RETAINED INTRAOCULAR FOREIGN BODY

Removal of a retained intraocular foreign body is performed after completion of the vitrectomy. The surgical technique depends on the shape, size, and location of the foreign body. Foreign bodies less than 5 mm at the smallest diameter are removed through a pars plana incision. The pars plana incision used for the vitreous probe is enlarged according to the foreign body size. Large foreign bodies are removed through a corneal incision.

An intravitreal foreign body is mobilized and held with the suction fiber optic probe before any attempt to grasp it with forceps. It is then grasped with the most appropriate forceps and suction pressure of the fiber optic probe is relieved. The forceps to be used should be chosen according to the size and shape of the foreign body.

Retained foreign bodies incarcerated into the retina are encapsulated. The fibrous capsule should be extensively incised before any attempt to grasp the foreign body with forceps (Fig. 208). The capsule incision is carried out using a sharp 20-gauge needle or kuhnt's knife. A cruciate incision completely frees the foreign body. Photocoagulation or cryotreatment of the retina around the capsule incision is unnecessary in most cases (Fig. 209).

Cryotreatment of Fibrous Ingrowth Remnants

The root of the fibrous ingrowth cannot be removed by vitrectomy in eyes with perforating sites located in the ciliary region. Remnants of the fibrous tissue in the vitreous base may result in further cell proliferation onto the vitreous base or the retina. This may play a role in surgical failures and recurrent retinal detachments.[11,13] Therefore, an adjunct to vitrectomy is required to destroy the root of the fibrovascular ingrowth and prevent further intraocular cell proliferation.[13] Cryotreatment with the multiple thaw-freeze cycle technique is an effective method for destruction of selected intraocular cell proliferations.[19–21] This method is used for fibrous ingrowth remnants after vitrectomy. Cryoapplications are carried out with simultaneous observation of the inner surface of the scleral wound. No corneal contact lens is used. Scleral depression with the

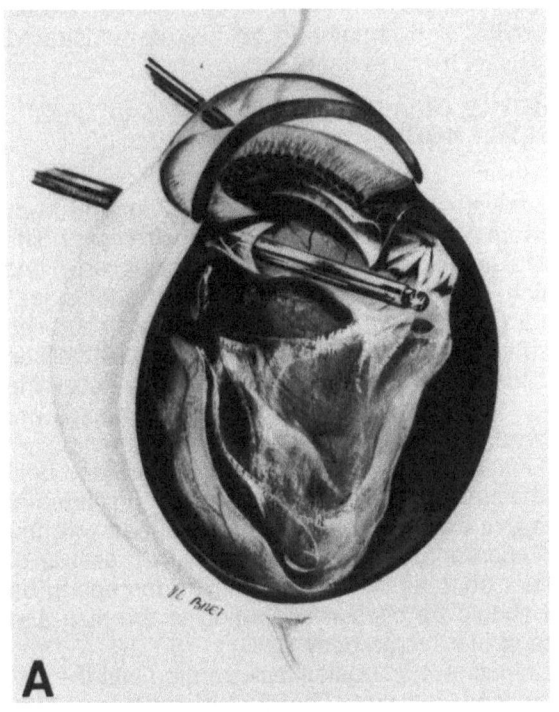

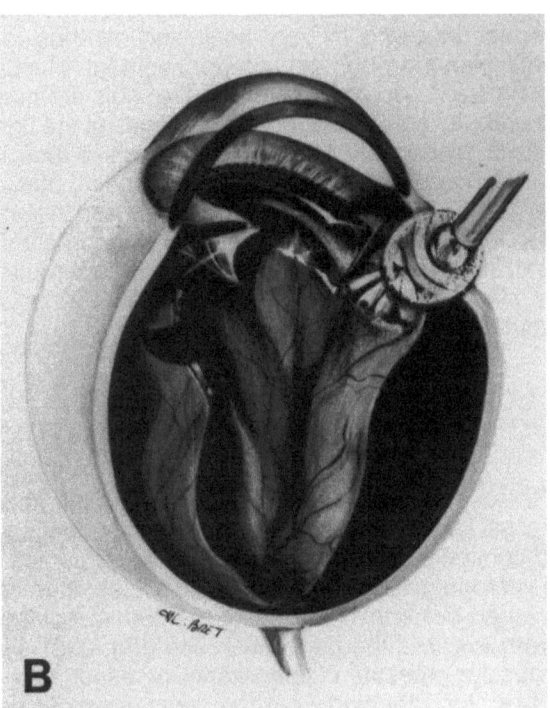

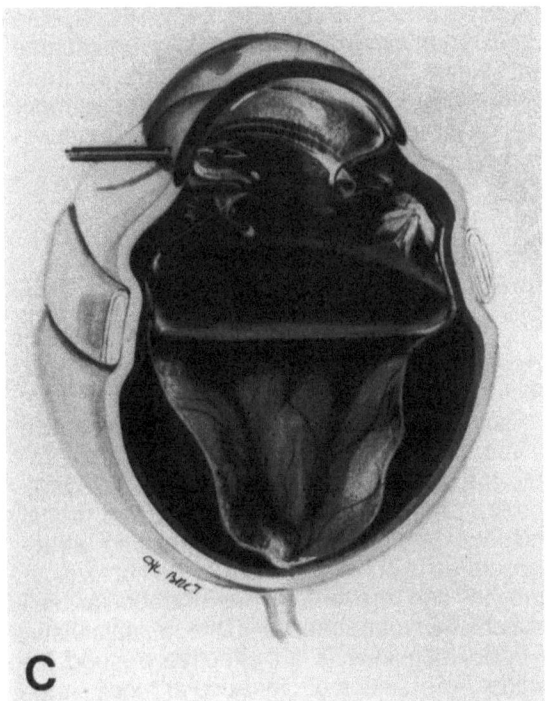

Figure 205. Surgical management of retinal detachment after penetrating eye injury (Preoperative fundus appearance of same case is shown in Figure 203). (A) Lensectomy through the pars plana has been completed. Vitreous gel and fibrous ingrowth are being removed up to the vitreous base. (B) Cryotreatment is carried out on the root of fibrous ingrowth remnants at the perforation site. (C) After cryotreatment of the temporal dialysis and scleral buckling, 1.5 cc of pure SF6 are being injected through the limbus.

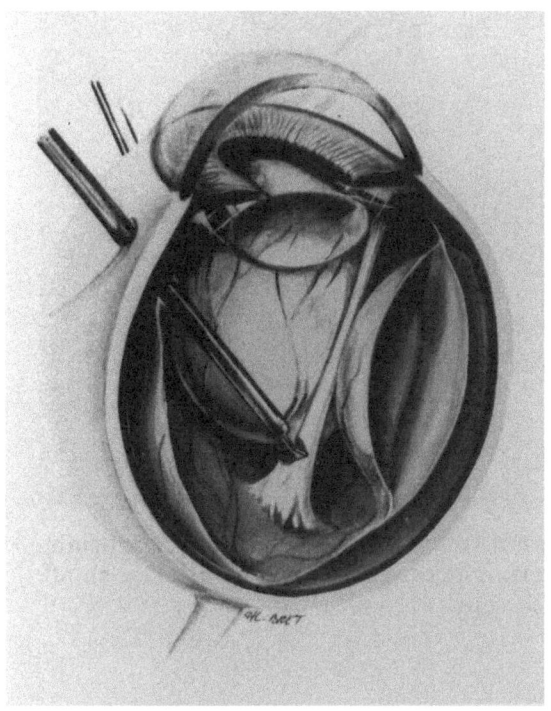

Figure 206. Surgical management of traction retinal detachment after penetrating injury. A thick vitreous cord on the path of a penetrating object is being cut with automatic microscissors. (Preoperative and postoperative fundus appearance of same case shown in Figure 207).

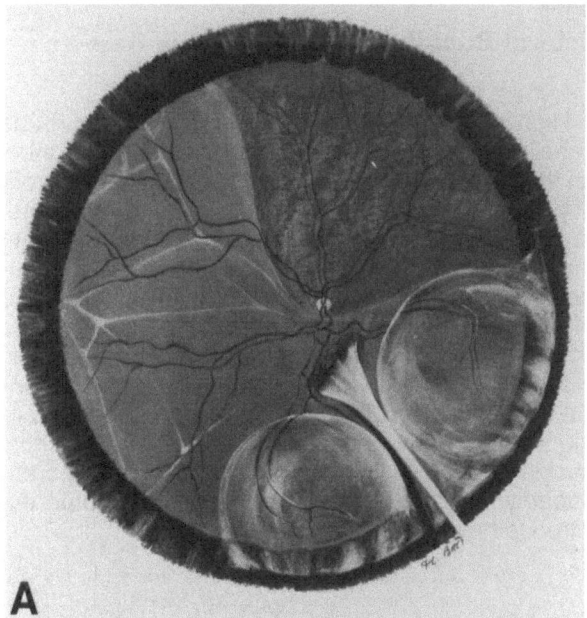

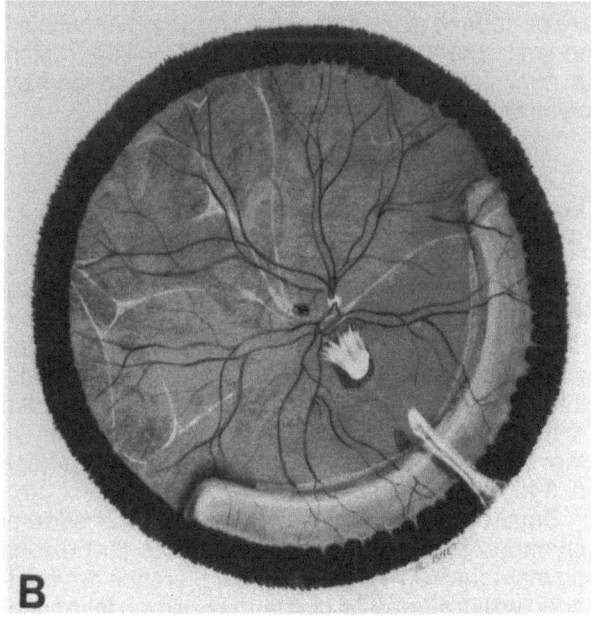

A

B

Figure 207. Longstanding traction retinal detachment after penetrating injury by an arrow. (A) Preoperative fundus appearance. Retinal detachment was recognized 3 years after trauma. It is associated with white strands of subretinal proliferation, two intraretinal macrocysts, and detachment of the pars plana epithelium in the inferior nasal quadrant. A thick white cord has developed in the vitreous gel on the path of the penetrating arrow. (B) Postoperative fundus appearance. Permanent retinal reattachment was achieved by vitrectomy combined with segmental scleral buckling of the vitreous base in the area of detached ciliary epithelium. A large gap has developed between the cut ends of the vitreous cord. Intraretinal cysts have spontaneously flattened.

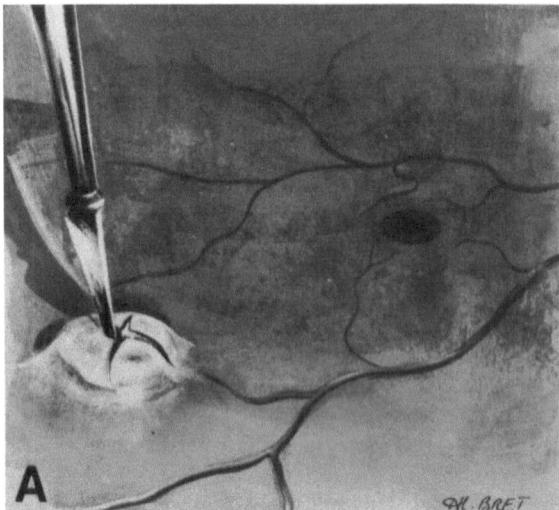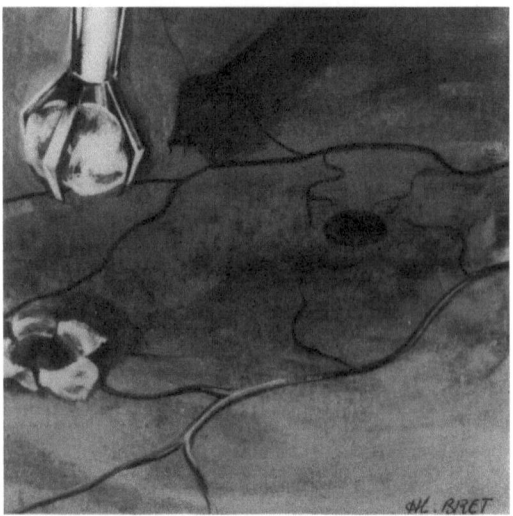

Figure 208. Removal of a retained foreign body incarcerated in the retina. (A) A cruciate incision is performed in the fibrous capsule using a straight discision needle. (B) The small foreign body is removed through the pars plana using forceps.

cryoprobe tip is sufficient to put the fibrous ingrowth root into direct view. Cryoapplication is continued until freezing of the inner surface of the scleral wound is obtained (Fig. 205). Two or three cryoapplications are performed at the same site. The treatment should be limited to the scleral wound in the ciliary region to minimize the inflammatory reaction induced by cryotreatment.

Treatment of the Retinal Breaks

Thorough examination of the peripheral retina using the three-mirror contact lens and scleral depression should be performed after completion of the vitrectomy procedure. Retinal breaks that were invisible at preoperative examination because of opaque media and iatrogenic retinal breaks, particularly at the entry site of the vitrectomy instruments, (see p. 149) must be identified.

Small retinal breaks are managed with transscleral cryoapplications. Large retinal dialyses that extend on more than 90° of the eye circumference are managed with transscleral diathermy or argon laser photocoagulation to avoid excessive cryotreatment that may stimulate further cell proliferation (see p. 234). Argon laser photocoagulation is carried out 3–4 days postoperatively when the gas bubble has reached maximal expansion (see p. 81).

Broad and high scleral buckling should be performed. Segmental radial buckles are used for retinal breaks located in the equatorial region. Retinal breaks located more anteriorly are supported by the

circumferential buckle used to counteract ring contraction of the vitreous base.

Scleral Buckling of the Vitreous Base

High and broad scleral buckling of the vitreous base is necessary in all eyes with fibrous proliferation on the vitreous base and with proliferative vitreoretinopathy with ring contraction of the vitreous base. In areas where the retina is dragged anteriorly onto the pars plana, the anterior bites of the scleral mattress sutures should be placed 1 mm anteriorly to the muscle ring. The circumferential extent of the scleral buckle is determined according to the specific vitreoretinal anatomy of the eye. A 180° circumferential buckle is used in eyes with limited changes of the vitreous base (Fig. 210). A 360° circumferential buckle is used in eyes with proliferative vitreoretinopathy and/or extensive fibrous ingrowth onto the vitreous base (Fig. 204).

Gas Injection

Intravitreal gas injection is the last step of the procedure (Fig. 205). Pure SF6 is used in eyes with no preretinal proliferation. Pure C3F8 is used in eyes with preretinal proliferation. The volume of pure gas to be injected is determined according to 3 parameters; (1) the size and location of the retinal breaks, (2) the biometry of the eye, and (3) the amount of

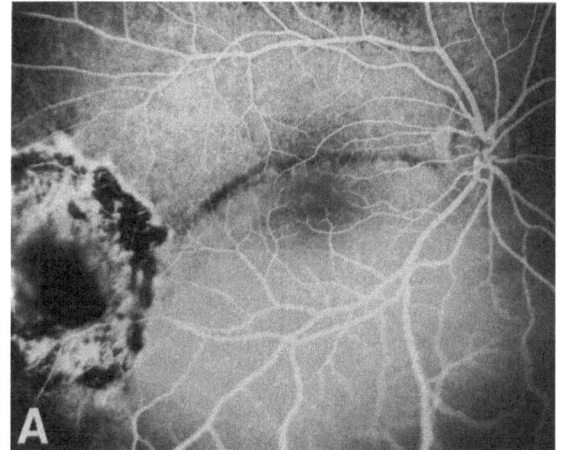

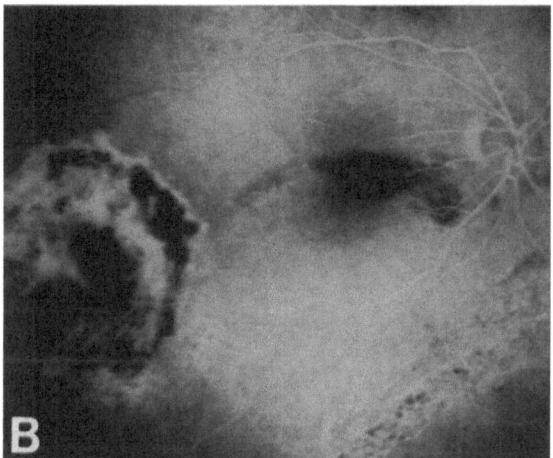

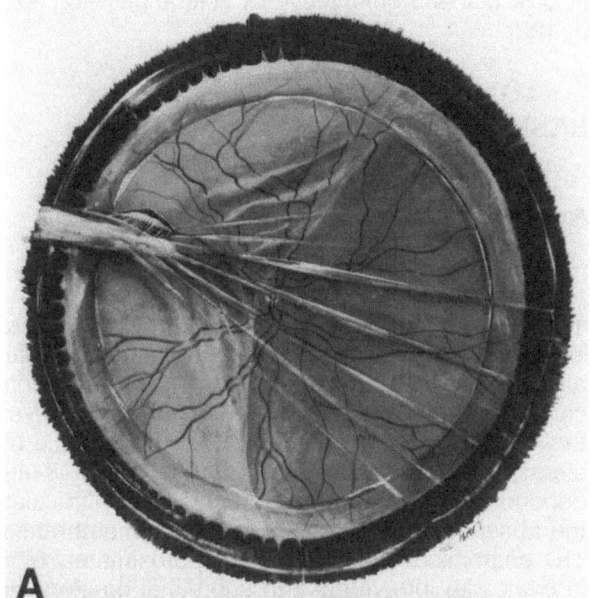

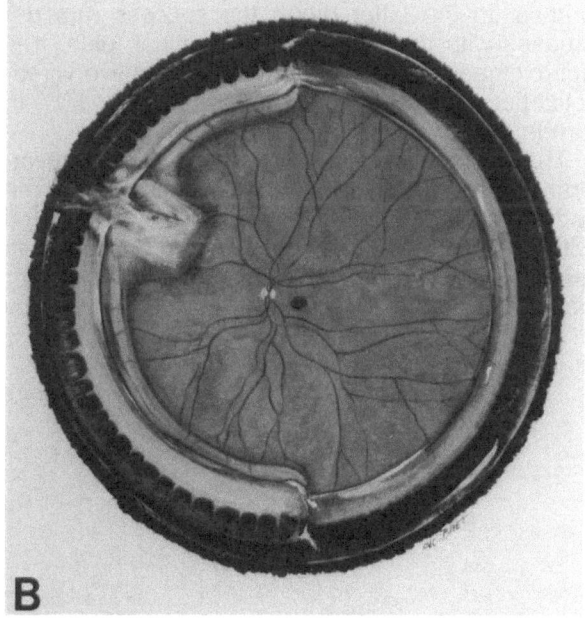

Figure 209. Retinal detachment associated with an intraocular foreign body encapsulated in the paramacular region. (A) Preoperative fluorescein angiography. Retinal detachment involves the macula. Scars around the encapsulated foreign body are related to photocoagulation treatment performed elsewhere. (B) Postoperative fluorescein angiography. The foreign body was removed through the pars plana. The vitrectomy procedure was combined with scleral buckling of a small horseshoe tear in the superior nasal quadrant. Subretinal fluid has absorbed. Demarcation lines remain visible.

Figure 210. Retinal detachment after penetrating injury of the ciliary region. (A) Fundus appearance at initial examination: Traction retinal detachment related to fibrous ingrowth is associated with rhegmatogenous detachment. The tractional tear developed at the superior border of fibrous scar along a retinal vessel. (B) Postoperative fundus appearance. Permanent retinal reattachment was achieved by a single operation: vitrectomy, radial buckling of the tear, and segmental circumferential scleral buckling of the vitreous base. Central vision is 20/20.

fluid displaced from the eye by scleral buckling (see p. 122).

RESULTS

Anatomical Results

Since the advent of vitreoretinal microsurgery, many eyes have been saved that previously were lost. Total and permanent retinal reattachment, with at least a 6-month follow-up after gas absorption, can be achieved in approximately 80% of the eyes that are judged operable[11] (Fig. 211). It should be stressed, however, that the anatomical success rate depends mostly on case selection, and in particular, the absence or presence of preretinal membranes. The anatomical success rate is approximately 87% in eyes with intravitreal and subretinal proliferation compared to only 73% in eyes with preretinal membranes. In the latter group the success rate decreases with the extent of fixed retinal folds. It is approximately 84% in eyes with proliferative vitreoretinopathy, Grade C as compared to only 50% in Grade D.[11]

The success rate in eyes with preretinal membranes and fixed folds is rather higher than in eyes with severe proliferative vitreoretinopathy associated with primary rhegmatogenous retinal detachments (see p. 252). The fact that retinal detachments after penetrating injury develop in eyes that were healthy before trauma may account for the difference between the two groups.

It should also be stressed that in our series,[11] permanent retinal reattachment could be achieved with a single successful operation in only 64% of eyes. Two or even three operations were necessary in the remaining eyes. Recurrent proliferative vitreoretinopathy or increasing contraction of the vitreous base were the cause of all recurrent detachments after the first operation. Some of those eyes developed sequential retinal breaks in the vitreous base area. Repeated surgery is fully justified in young patients and all patients with no useful vision of the fellow eye.

Visual Results

Visual results depend on three parameters: (1) the duration of macular detachment, (2) the extent and severity of preretinal membranes, and (3) the associated lesions due to the penetrating injury. In our series,[11] postoperative visual acuity of 20/40 or better was achieved in 50% of eyes successfully operated on.

REFERENCES

1. Percival SP: Late complications from posterior segment intraocular foreign bodies with particular reference to retinal detachment. Br J Ophthalmol 56:462–468, 1972

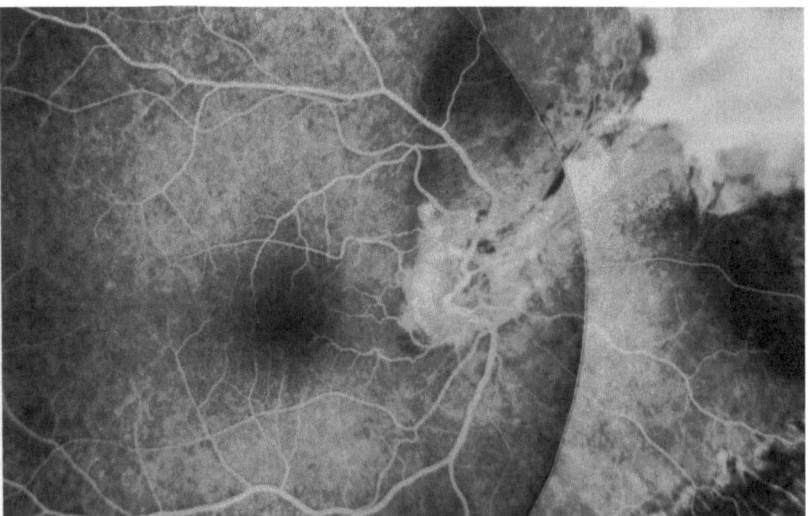

Figure 211. Postoperative fluorescein angiography of a retinal detachment after double perforation by a blunt bullet. Remnants of fibrous ingrowth are visible on the nasal side. The macula is normal. (Courtesy of BONNET MJ, Fr Ophtalmol 7:801–806, 1984).

2. Hutton WL: Retinal detachments associated with intraocular foreign bodies. Mechanisms of detachment and role of vitreous surgery. Mod Probl Ophthalmol 20:260–263, 1979

3. Hutton WL, Snyder WB, Vaiser A: Vitrectomy in the treatment of perforating injuries of the eye. Am J Ophthalmol 81:733–739, 1976

4. Barthelemy F, Girard P, Bonnissent JF, Kohen D: Décollement de la rétine après extraction d'un corps étranger intra-oculaire. Influence de la vitrectomie. J Fr ophtalmol 6:823–827, 1983

5. De Juan E, Sternberg P, Michels RG: Penetrating ocular injuries. Ophthalmology 90:1318–1322, 1983

6. Coleman DJ: Early vitrectomy in the management of the severely traumatized eye. Am J Ophthalmol 93:543–551, 1982

7. Heiman K, Neubauer H, Paulmann H, Tavakolian U: Pars plana vitrectomy after intraocular foreign bodies. Mod Probl Ophthalmol 20:247–255, 1979

8. Ryan SJ, Allen AW: Pars plana vitrectomy in ocular trauma. Am J Ophthalmol 88:483–491, 1979

9. Slusher MM, Sarin LK, Federman JL: Management of intra retinal foreign bodies. Ophthalmology 89:369–373, 1982

10. De Juan E, Sternberg P, Michels R: Evaluation of vitrectomy in penetrating ocular trauma. Archives Ophthalmol. 102:1160–1163, 1984

11. Bonnet M: Treatment of retinal detachment after penetrating injury: heavy cryotreatment of the fibrous ingrowth as an adjunct to vitreoretinal microsurgery. Ophthalmologica (Basel) 194:164–168, 1987

12. Cox MS, Freeman HM: Retinal detachment due to ocular penetration. 1 - clinical characteristics and surgical results. Arch Ophthalmol 96:1354–1361; 1978

13. Bonnet M: Microchirurgie des décollements de la rétine après traumatisme perforant: J Fr Ophtalmol 7:801–806, 1984

14. Cleary PE, Ryan SJ: Methods of production and natural history of experimental posterior penetrating eye injury in the rhesus monkey. Amer J Ophthalmol 88:212–220, 1979

15. Cleary PE, Ryan SJ: Histology of wound, vitreous and retina in experimental posterior penetrating eye injury in the rhesus monkey. Amer J Ophthalmol 88:221–231, 1979

16. Cleary PE, Minckler DS, Ryan S: Ultrastructure of traction retinal detachment in rhesus monkey eyes after a posterior penetrating ocular injury. Am J Ophthalmol 90:829–845, 1980

17. Topping TM, Abrams GW, Machemer R: Experimental double-perforation injury of the posterior segment in rabbit eyes. The natural history of intraocular proliferation. Arch Ophthalmol 97:735–742, 1979

18. Ryan SJ: Experimental posterior penetrating eye injury in the rhesus monkey. British J Ophthalmol 64:801–808, 1980

19. Lincoff H, McLean JM, Long R: The cryosurgical treatment of intraocular tumors. Am J Ophthalmol 63:389–399, 1967

20. Amoils SP, Smith R: Cryotherapy of angiomatosis retinae. Arch Opthalmol 81:689–691, 1969

21. Moreau PG, Haut J: Cryo ophtalmologie, Paris, Masson, 1971, 246–247

25

Retinal Detachment Following Inflammatory Diseases

Traction and rhegmatogenous retinal detachment can occur as a complication of various, acute or chronic, intraocular inflammatory diseases. Traction and rhegmatogenous retinal detachment has been observed in chorioretinitis,[1,2] particularly in toxoplasmosis,[1–6] pars planitis,[1,2,7,8] toxocariasis,[1] ophthalmomyasis interna posterior,[9] acute retinal necrosis syndrome,[10–12] cytomegalovirus retinitis in the immunedeficiency syndrome,[13–16] and endophthalmitis.

COMMON CLINICAL FEATURES

All traction and rhegmatogenous retinal detachments associated with inflammatory diseases show common clinical features:

1. They are infrequent and account for approximately 1% of all rhegmatogenous or traction detachments.
2. Most cases occur in young patients.
3. Rhegmatogenous retinal detachment that occurs at the acute stage of the inflammatory disease should be distinguished from exsudative retinal detachment.
4. In many cases adequate examination of the fundus and identification of all retinal tears is difficult, owing to vitreous haze, vitreous membranes, poor pupillary dilation, and sometimes complicated cataract. When the retinal tear cannot be disclosed it may be difficult to determine whether the detachment is purely exudative or rhegmatogenous. Shifting subretinal fluid is indicative of exsudative rather than rhegmatogenous detachment.

5. In most cases the retinal breaks are related to vitreous traction. Horseshoe tears are the most common.[1] Round or oval holes are less common and are situated in areas of firm vitreo-retinal adhesion. Giant tears are uncommon.
6. Rhegmatogenous retinal detachments that develop at the acute stage of the inflammatory disease are more severe compared to detachments developing at the cicatricial stage. Increased severity is related to a difficulty in identifying the retinal breaks and an increased incidence of proliferative vitreoretinopathy.

SPECIFIC CLINICAL FEATURES

Rhegmatogenous or traction retinal detachment following inflammatory diseases shows clinical variations that depend on clinical characteristics of the associated inflammatory disease.

Chorioretinitis

The incidence of retinal detachment associated with chorioretinitis, particularly toxoplasmic retinochoroiditis, is low. Friedman and Knox[5] reported a 4.7% incidence of retinal detachment in a series of 63 patients with toxoplasmic retinochoroiditis. Case selection probably accounts for this high incidence. Except for Havener's case of bilateral exsudative detachment, all cases reported in the literature were rhegmatogenous.[4–6,17]

Retinal detachment or retinal breaks can occur in eyes with either active or cicatricial retinochoroiditis. Rhegmatogenous retinal detachment following prophylactic photocoagulation of retinochoroidal scars has been reported.[17]

Two types of retinal breaks have been observed: (1) peripheral horseshoe tears distant from foci of retinochoroiditis (Fig. 212) and (2) breaks at the edge of atrophic retinochoroidal scars.[6] Both types are related to vitreous traction and are associated with partial posterior vitreous detachment, vitreous strands, and condensations of the partially detached posterior vitreous face. Breaks at the edge of atrophic retinochoroidal scars are related to dense vitreous strands. In most cases the retinal breaks are located in the superior quadrants.[6] They are difficult to disclose in eyes with active retinochoroiditis, owing to vitreous haziness. Prognosis for retinal reattachment following scleral buckling procedures is good in eyes with peripheral retinal breaks and inactive or mild retinochoroiditis.[1,6] In contrast, prognosis for retinal reattachment is more guarded in eyes with severe active intraocular inflammation and clinical evidence of proliferative vitreoretinopathy. Vitrectomy combined with scleral buckling is required in such eyes. It is associated with systemic antiin-

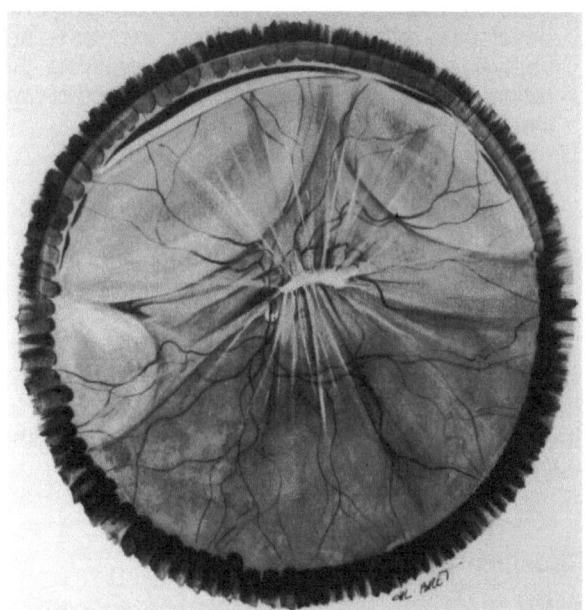

Figure 212. Traction-rhegmatogenous retinal detachment complicating chorioretinitis in a 20-year-old patient. Retinal detachment developed as a late complication of chorioretinitis in the region of the superior temporal arcade. It is associated with a large superior tear at the posterior border of the vitreous base and multiple vitreous strands. The eye is emmetropic. Permanent retinal reattachment was achieved by scleral buckling combined with vitrectomy.

flammatory treatment, which is given preoperatively and postoperatively.

Pars Planitis

The incidence of rhegmatogenous retinal detachment complicating pars planitis has been reported to be 5%,[18] 9%,[19] and 22%.[7] Patient selection likely accounts for the differences between the series. The incidence of rhegmatogenous retinal detachment and the severity of the inflammatory process are positively correlated.[7] The severity of retinal detachment and the severity of pars planitis are also positively correlated. Brockhurst described four types of rhegmatogenous retinal detachment according to the severity of the peripheral uveitis, which can be benign, mild, severe, and relentless.[7] With regard to the prognosis, two distinct groups of retinal detachment should be distinguished: (1) retinal detachment associated with quiescent and mild pars planitis, and (2) retinal detachment associated with severe active pars planitis.

RETINAL DETACHMENT COMPLICATING QUIESCENT OR MILD PARS PLANITIS

Rhegmatogenous retinal detachment develops years after clinical remission of a benign pars planitis, or multiple exacerbations and remissions of a chronic and mild disease (Fig. 213). In both cases the vitreous base is coated by a thick fibrous proliferation that is located, or more pronounced in the lower quadrants. New vessels may be present in the fibrous tissue. Exudates are absent or slight.

In most cases the retinal detachment progresses slowly, over months. It is often disclosed by routine examination. The detachment involves one or two quadrants. The detached retina shows cystoid degeneration that is more marked in the peripheral fundus. Cystoid degeneration is secondary to the long duration of the detachment. It may show the aspect of a secondary bullous retinoschisis.[20] Demarcation lines are frequent.[7] The retinal breaks are usually horseshoe tears situated at the posterior border of the vitreous base; they are small and may be hidden by the fibrous peripheral tissue and difficult to disclose. In most cases these retinal breaks are located in the inferior and superior temporal quadrants.[8] Retinal holes are less frequent than horseshoe tears.[8]

The prognosis for retinal reattachment with segmental scleral buckling is excellent. A nearly 100% anatomical success rate can be expected.[7,8] The scleral buckle should be high, broad, and permanent to counteract further potential contraction of the fi-

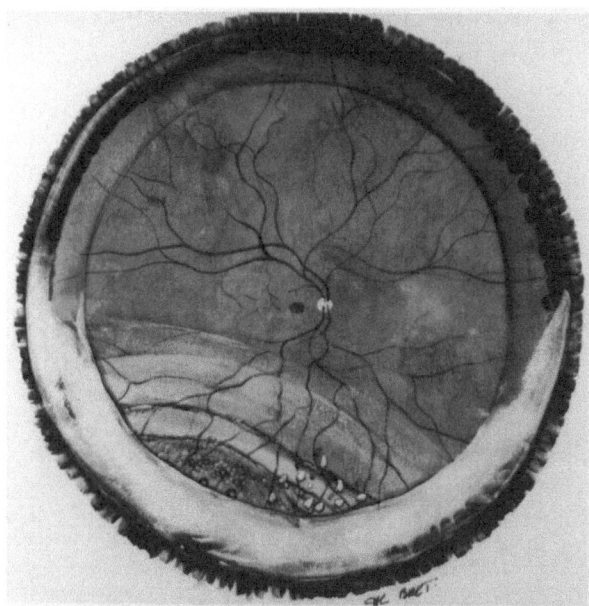

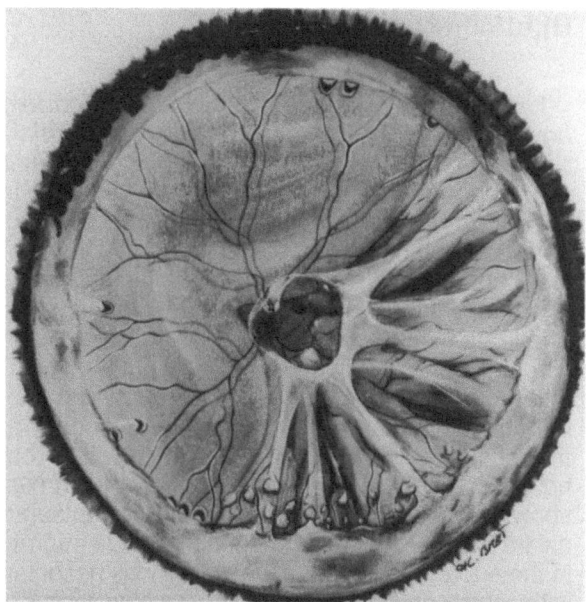

Figure 213. Retinal detachment complicating mild pars planitis in a 9-year-old boy. The inferior vitreous base is coated by thick fibrous proliferation. Intraocular inflammation is slight. Retinal detachment is associated with cystoid degeneration of the detached retina in the equatorial region and demarcation lines. Two tiny tears are present at the posterior border of the condensed vitreous base at 7 o'clock. The macula is attached and retinal detachment was disclosed by routine examination. Permanent retinal reattachment was achieved by scleral buckling.

Figure 214. Retinal detachment complicating severe pars planitis in a 29-year-old patient. Retinal detachment developed 5 months after clinical recognition of the pars planitis. It is associated with extensive yellowish exudates on the vitreous base, condensation of the posterior vitreous face, incomplete posterior vitreous detachment, multiple horseshoe tears, and clinical evidence of proliferative vitreoretinopathy. Retinal reattachment was achieved by vitrectomy combined with a 360° scleral buckling procedure. However, recurrent proliferative vitreoretinopathy and intractable detachment developed 2 months postoperatively.

brous peripheral ring. Recurrences are uncommon. The visual results are limited by the common association of other complications of pars planitis, such as cataract and macular degeneration secondary to cystoid macular edema.

RETINAL DETACHMENT COMPLICATING SEVERE ACTIVE PARS PLANITIS

Rhegmatogenous retinal detachment develops a few months after clinical recognition of the inflammatory disease, and the onset of the detachment is acute. In most cases the detachment becomes total in a few days (Fig. 214). The eye shows clinical evidence of severe inflammation with vitreous haze and yellowish exsudates on the vitreous base. The peripheral exsudates are more pronounced in the lower fundus. However, they often involve the superior fundus as well. Examination under scleral depression may disclose dilated new-vessels on the

anterior part of the vitreous base. Inflammatory sheathing of the peripheral retinal vessels is common. The retinal detachment is due to horseshoe tears that are often multiple and located in more than two quadrants.[8] Identification of all retinal tears is difficult due to vitreous gel haze and exsudation in the peripheral fundus. The retinal detachment is often associated with early proliferative vitreoretinopathy. Surgical management should be associated with systemic administration of corticosteroids to be given preoperatively and postoperatively. A 360° high and broad scleral buckle is required in most of these eyes. Early vitrectomy is indicated in eyes with preretinal membranes and fixed folds. Initial retinal reattachment can be achieved in approximately 70% of eyes.[8] However, recurrent detachment due to proliferative vitreoretinopathy and relentless contraction of the peripheral fibrovascular ring is common. Most eyes eventually develop secondary cataract, glaucoma, or phthisis bulbi.

Ophthalmomyasis

Larvae of various flies, particularly *Hypoderma bovis, Hypoderma lineatum, Cochliomyia hominivorax, Dermatobia hominis, Gastrophilus intestinalis, Oedemagena Tarandi* (Reindeer warble fly),[21] and *Curetebra sp* (rodent botfly)[22] can penetrate the eye and lead to anterior or posterior uveitis. Rhegmatogenous retinal detachment can develop as a complication of ophthalmomyasis interna posterior.[9,23,24] The larva migrates from the subretinal space to the vitreous cavity making a hole in the retina.[9,21] The author has seen two cases, both in young boys. In both cases the larva was in the vitreous cavity and the retinal detachment was associated with a round hole in the equatorial region (Fig. 215). Both cases showed lens subluxation and criss-crossing subretinal tracks, which are characteristic of larva migration in the subretinal space.[25] One case was associated with severe posterior uveitis. The larva was removed by vitrectomy and the retina was permanently reattached by segmental scleral buckling of the retinal hole. In the other case, the eye was quiet and the

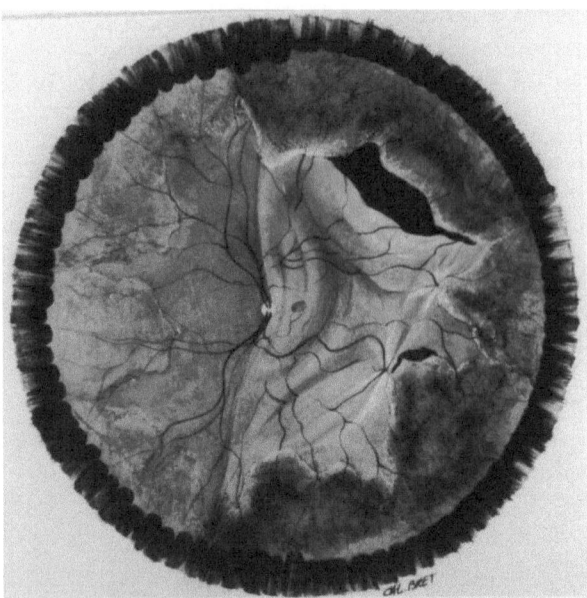

Figure 216. Retinal detachment complicating acute retinal necrosis syndrome in a 40-year old patient with acquired immune deficiency syndrome (AIDS). Retinal detachment is associated with large tears at the junction of necrotic and normal retina, and two star-shaped folds.

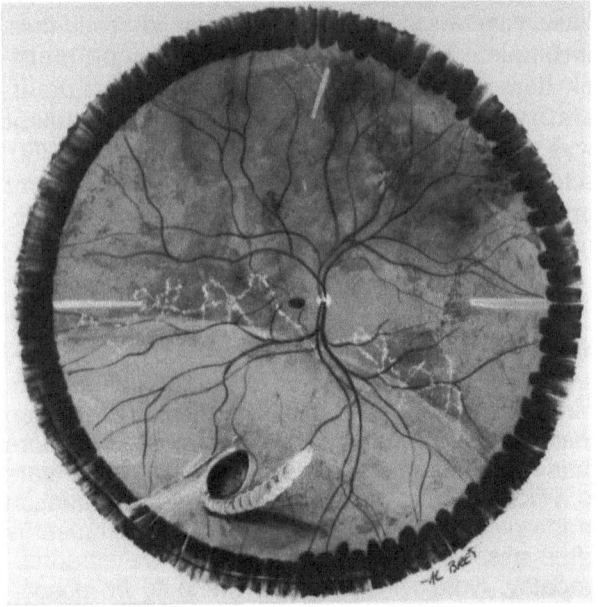

Figure 215. Retinal detachment complicating ophtalmomyasis interna posterior in a 5-year-old boy. Retinal detachment is associated with a hole made by the larva in the inferior temporal quadrant. Criss-crossing subretinal tracks made by the larva are visible on the posterior pole. The larva in the vitreous gel is dead. Permanent retinal reattachment was achieved by scleral buckling of the retinal hole combined with vitrectomy to remove the larva.

dead larva in the vitreous cavity was well tolerated. No attempt was made to remove the dead larva in this case. The retina was permanently reattached by segmental scleral buckling of the retinal hole.

Acute Retinal Necrosis Syndrome

The acute retinal necrosis syndrome is characterized by necrotizing confluent peripheral retinitis, retinal arteritis, papillatis, and vitritis occurring in otherwise healthy patients of any age,[11,12,26] or in patients with acquired immune deficiency syndrome.[16] It can be caused by a number of virus including cytomegalovirus.[13-15] Rhegmatogenous retinal detachment is a common complication. It has been observed in approximately 75% of eyes.[11,12] In most cases, retinal detachment develops within 3 months after the onset of symptoms, after resolution of the retinitis. The retinal detachment is associated with large holes within the area of previously necrotic retina as well as breaks located at the junction of involved and uninvolved retina (Fig. 216).[12] It is associated with clinical evidence of vitreous traction. Proliferative vitreoretinopathy is common.[12] The cumulative success rate achieved by scleral buckling alone is approximately 22%.[12] This success rate can be improved to 70% by combination of vitreous surgery and scleral buckling.[12] Approximately one-third of eyes are inoperable, however, because of associated lesions such as neovascular glaucoma. Visual function in eyes successfully reattached remains poor due to macular pucker.[12] Prophylactic treatment with argon laser photocoagulation to produce chorioretinal adhesion posterior to the retinal necrosis areas has been considered as an attempt to prevent development of retinal detachment.[27] It should be performed within a month to 6 weeks after the onset of symptoms, however, vitreous opacification may delay or preclude prophylactic treatment.

Endophthalmitis

The overall risk of rhegmatogenous retinal detachment following endophthalmitis successfully managed by vitrectomy and antibiotic injections is approximately 15%.[28–29] Several mechanisms may contribute to the development of such detachments: (1) Penetrating trauma or surgical trauma complicated by endophthalmitis, (2) vitreoretinal changes secondary to intraocular inflammation, or (3) vitreoretinal lesions caused by intraocular antibiotic injections or vitrectomy. Retinal detachment is more frequent in eyes managed by intraocular antibiotic injection and vitrectomy (21%) as compared with eyes managed by antibiotic injection alone (9%).[29] The increased incidence of retinal detachment in eyes managed by vitrectomy may be related to increased severity of endophthalmitis in eyes managed by vitrectomy[28,29] or surgical complications. Endophthalmitis is likely to increase the risk of retinal detachment following vitrectomy.[28,29]

Retinal detachment may develop either intraoperatively or months after endophthalmitis. A retinal detachment that develops during vitrectomy has a more severe prognosis.[29,30] A retinal detachment that develops months after resolution of endophthalmitis can be associated with retinal breaks at foci of cicatricial retinitis.[29,31]

REFERENCES

1. Hagler WS, Jarrett WH, Chang M: Rhegmatogenous retinal detachment following chorioretinal inflammatory disease. Am J Ophthalmol 86, 3:373–379, 1978
2. Schepens CL: Retinal detachment and allied diseases. Philadelphia, W.B. Saunders Co 1983, 53, 261, 677
3. Havener WH, Harris WR: Retinal detachment in toxoplasmosis. Am J Ophthalmol 54:451–452, 1962
4. Dobbie JG: Cryotherapy in the management of toxoplasma retinochoroiditis. Trans Am Acad Ophthalmol Otolaryngol 72:364–373, 1968
5. Friedmann CT, Knox DL: Variations in recurrent active toxoplasmosis retinochoroiditis. Arch Ophthalmol 81:481–493, 1969
6. Lucier AC: Retinal detachment associated with ocular toxoplasmosis. Trans Am Acad Ophthalmol Otolaryngol 78:882–889 1974
7. Brockhurst RJ, Schepens CL: Uveitis, IV Peripheral uveitis: the complication of retinal detachment. Arch ophthalmol 80:747–753, 1968
8. Bonnet M, Aracil P: Pars planitis et décollement de la rétine. Bull Soc Ophtalmol Fr 86:479–483, 1986
9. Ducournau D, Bonnet M: Les ophtalmomyases internes postérieures: Bull Soc Ophtalmol Fr 82; 12:1527–1530, 1982
10. Willerson DJ, Aaberg TM, Reeser FH: Necrotizing vaso-occlusive retinitis. Am J Ophthalmol 84:209–219, 1977
11. Fisher JP, Lewis ML, Blumenkranz M, et al: The acute retinal necrosis syndrome. Part 1: clinical manifestations. Ophthalmology 89:1309–1316, 1982
12. Clarkson JG, Blumenkranz M, Culbertson WW et al: Retinal detachment following the acute retinal necrosis syndrome. Ophthalmology 91:1665–1668, 1984
13. Broughton WL, Cupples HP, Parver LM: Bilateral retinal detachment following cytomegalovirus retinitis. Arch Ophthalmol 96:618–619, 1978
14. Aaberg TM, Cesarz T, Rytal M: Correlation of virology and clinical course of cytomegalovirus retinitis. Am J Ophthalmol 74:407–415, 1972
15. Chumbley L, Robertson D, Smith T, et al: Adult cytomegalovirus inclusion retino-uveitis. Am J Ophthalmol 80:807–816, 1975
16. Freeman WR, Lerner CW, Mines JA, et al: A prospective study of the ophthalmologic findings in the acquired immune deficiency syndrome. Am J Ophthalmol 97:133–142, 1984
17. O'Connor GR: Discussion on techniques employed in selected uveitis surveys. In Aronson SB, Gamble CN, Goodner EK, et al (Eds): Clinical methods in uveitis. St. Louis, C.V. Mosby, 93, 1968
18. Smith RE, Godfrey WA, Kimura SJ: Complications of chronic cyclitis. Am J Ophthalmol 82:277–282 1976
19. Moron-Morel F: La pars planitis: analyse de 46 observations et résultat du traitement chirurgical sur 19 yeux. Thèse doctorat université Lyon, 1984
20. Brockhurst RJ: Retinoschisis. Complication of peripheral uveitis Arch Ophthalmol 99:1998–1999, 1981
21. Syrdalen P, Stenkula S: Ophthalmomyasis interna posterior. Graefe's Arch Clin Exp Ophthalmol 225:103–106, 1987
22. Custis PH, Pakalnis VA, Klintworth GK, et al: Posterior internal ophthalmomyasis. Ophthalmology 90:1583–1590, 1983
23. De Boe MP: Diphterous larva passing from the optic nerve into the vitreous chamber. Arch Ophthalmol 10:824–825, 1933
24. Purtscher A: Entfemung einer lebenden Larve von Hypoderma bovis aus dem Glaskörper. Z Aughenheilkd 57:601–605, 1925
25. Gass JD, Lewis RA: Subretinal tracks in ophthalmomyasis Trans Am Acad Ophthalmol Otolaryngol 81:483–490, 1976
26. Martenet C: "Nécrose" rétinienne périphérique et décollement rétinien total d'origine vasculaire. In François (Ed) Fifth congress of the European Society of Ophthalmology, Hamburg 1976, Stuttgart Enke 1978, 180–182
27. Han DP, Lewis H, Williams GA, et al: Laser photocoagulation in the acute retinal necrosis syndrome. Arch Ophthalmol 105:1051–1054, 1987
28. Olson JC, Flynn HW, Forster RK, Culberston WW: Results in the treatment of postoperative endophthalmitis. Ophthalmology 90:692–697, 1983
29. Nelsen PT, Marcus DA, Bovino JA: Retinal detachment following endophthalmitis. Ophthalmology 92:1112–1117, 1985
30. Brinton GS, Topping TM, Hyndiuk RA:, et al: Posttraumatic endophthalmitis. Arch Ophthalmol 102:547–550, 1984
31. Landers JH, Chappell CW: Bilateral metastatic endophthalmitis. Retina 1:175–178, 1981

Index

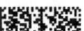